PRIMARY CARE SECRETS

PRIMARY CARE SECRETS

JEANETTE MLADENOVIC, M.D.
Professor of Medicine and
    Vice-Chair for Educational Affairs
University of Colorado School of Medicine
Chief, Department of Medicine
Denver General Hospital
Denver, Colorado

HANLEY & BELFUS, INC./ Philadelphia
MOSBY/ St. Louis • Baltimore • Boston • Chicago
    London • Philadelphia • Sydney • Toronto

Publisher: HANLEY & BELFUS, INC.
210 S. 13th Street
Philadelphia, PA 19107
(215) 546-7293
FAX (215) 790-9330

North American and worldwide sales and distribution:

MOSBY
11830 Westline Industrial Drive
St. Louis, MO 63146

In Canada: Times Mirror Professional Publishing, Ltd.
130 Flaska Drive
Markham, Ontario L6G 1B8
Canada

Library of Congress Cataloging-in-Publication Data

Primary care secrets / |edited by| Jeanette Mladenovic.
    p.   cm.
    Includes bibliographical references and index.
    ISBN 1-56053-105-3
    1. Internal medicine—Miscellanea.   2. Primary care (Medicine)—Miscellanea.   I. Mladenovic,
Jeanette, 1949–   .
    |DNLM: 1. Primary Health Care—examination questions.   2. Internal Medicine—examination
questions.   W 18 P9515 1994|
    RC48.P736   1994
    616'.0076—dc20
    DNLM/DLC
    for Library of Congress   94-31931
        CIP

PRIMARY CARE SECRETS   ISBN 1-56053-105-3

Last digit is the print number: 9 8 7 6 5 4 3 2

DEDICATION

To my total support system,

Steve

and

Ben, Jessica, Amy, Jeffrey

CONTENTS

IV. DISORDERS OF THE EYES, EARS, NOSE, AND THROAT

V. ENDOCRINE AND METABOLIC DISORDERS

VI. PROBLEMS OF THE GASTROINTESTINAL TRACT

VII. GENDER-SPECIFIC CARE

VIII. COMMON DISORDERS OF THE RENAL AND URINARY SYSTEM

CONTRIBUTORS

Irene Aguilar, M.D.
Assistant Professor, Department of Medicine, Division of Internal Medicine, University of Colorado School of Medicine; Attending Physician, Primary Care Physician, Community Health Services, Denver General Hospital, Denver, Colorado

Stephen F. Albert, D.P.M.
Assistant Clinical Professor and Chief, Podiatric Section, Department of Surgery, University of Colorado School of Medicine; Chief, Podiatric Section, Surgery Service, Veterans Affairs Medical Center, Denver, Colorado

Catherine M. Amlie-Lefond, M.D.
Neurology Fellow, University of Colorado School of Medicine, Denver, Colorado

C. Alan Anderson, M.D.
Department of Neurology, University of Colorado School of Medicine, Denver, Colorado

Joseph C. Anderson, M.D.
Clinical Instructor of Medicine, State University of New York at Stony Brook Health Sciences Center School of Medicine, Stony Brook, New York

Roberta K. Beach, M.D., M.P.H.
Associate Professor of Pediatrics, University of Colorado School of Medicine; Assistant Director of Community Health, Denver Department of Health and Hospitals, Denver, Colorado

Leonard Berry, Jr., M.D.
Fellow, Department of Medicine, Division of Gastroenterology, University of Colorado School of Medicine, Denver, Colorado

Daniel H. Bessesen, M.D.
Assistant Professor of Medicine, University of Colorado School of Medicine, Denver, Colorado

Bahri Bilir, M.D.
Assistant Professor, Department of Medicine, Division of Gastroenterology, University of Colorado School of Medicine, Denver, Colorado

Nuray Bilir, M.D., M.S.
Instructor, Department of Medicine, Division of Gastroenterology, University of Colorado School of Medicine, Denver, Colorado

Jon M. Braverman, M.D.
Assistant Professor, Department of Ophthalmology, University of Colorado School of Medicine; Director, Division of Ophthalmology, Denver General Hospital, Denver, Colorado

Elizabeth C. Brew, M.D.
Resident, Department of Surgery, University of Colorado School of Medicine, Denver, Colorado

John F. Bridges, M.D.
Assistant Clinical Professor of Psychiatry, University of Colorado School of Medicine; Medical Director, Alcohol, Drug and Psychiatric Emergency Services, Denver General Hospital, Denver, Colorado

Christina Hope Brown Bryan, M.D.
Assistant Clinical Professor, Department of Medicine, University of Colorado School of Medicine, Denver, Colorado

Edmund Casper, M.D.
Associate Professor of Psychiatry, University of Colorado School of Medicine; Director, Alcohol, Drug and Psychiatric Service, Denver General Hospital, Denver, Colorado

Arlene Chapman, M.D.
Assistant Professor of Medicine, University of Colorado School of Medicine, Denver, Colorado

David H. Collier, M.D.
Associate Professor of Medicine, University of Colorado School of Medicine; Chief of Rheumatology, Denver General Hospital, Denver, Colorado

Alan B. Cooper, M.D.
Fellow in Nephrology, Department of Medicine, University of Colorado School of Medicine, Denver, Colorado

Thomas V. Davis, D.O.
Fellow, Department of Medicine, Division of Gastroenterology, University of Colorado School of Medicine, Denver, Colorado

Mary Ann DeGroote, M.D.
Fellow in Infectious Diseases, Department of Medicine, University of Colorado School of Medicine, Denver, Colorado

Jeffrey A. DesJardin, M.D.
Chief Resident, Department of Medicine, University of Colorado School of Medicine, Denver, Colorado

Susan J. Diem, M.D., M.P.H.
Duke University School of Medicine, Durham, North Carolina

Robert H. Eckel, M.D.
Professor of Medicine and of Biochemistry, Biophysics and Genetics, University of Colorado School of Medicine, Denver, Colorado; Adjunct Professor of Food Science and Human Nutrition, Colorado State University, Fort Collins, Colorado

Raymond O. Estacio, M.D.
Instructor, Department of Medicine, University of Colorado School of Medicine, Denver, Colorado

Richard C. Fisher, M.D., M.S.
Associate Professor, Department of Orthopaedics, University of Colorado School of Medicine; Director of Orthopaedics, Denver General Hospital, Denver, Colorado

John E. Fitzgerald, M.D.
Fellow, Pulmonary and Critical Care Medicine, University of Colorado School of Medicine, Denver, Colorado

Mark E. Fogarty, M.D.
Instructor, Department of Medicine, University of Colorado School of Medicine, Denver, Colorado

Paul A. Foley, M.D.
Department of Neurology, University of Colorado School of Medicine, Denver, Colorado

Carlos E. Girod, M.D.
Instructor, Department of Medicine, University of Colorado School of Medicine, Denver, Colorado

Loren E. Golitz, M.D.
Professor of Dermatology and Pathology, University of Colorado School of Medicine; Chief of Dermatology, Clinical Director, Ambulatory Care Center, Denver General Hospital, Denver, Colorado

Michael E. Hanley, M.D.
Assistant Professor of Medicine, University of Colorado School of Medicine; Staff Physician, Denver General Hospital, Denver, Colorado

Donald B. Hansen, B.S.(Pharm), Pharm.D.
Pharmacy Clinical Coordinator, Denver General Hospital, Denver, Colorado

Fred D. Hofeldt, M.D.
Professor of Medicine, University of Colorado School of Medicine, Denver, Colorado

Richard L. Hughes, M.D.
Assistant Professor of Neurology, University of Colorado School of Medicine, Denver, Colorado

Evelyn Hutt, M.D.
Assistant Professor of Medicine, University of Colorado School of Medicine, Denver, Colorado

Lori Jensen, M.D.
Fellow, Department of Medicine, Division of Medical Oncology, University of Colorado School of Medicine, Denver, Colorado

Joyce Seiko Kobayashi, M.D.
Associate Professor of Psychiatry, University of Colorado School of Medicine, Denver, Colorado

Randall Lee, M.D.
Assistant Professor, Department of Medicine, Division of Gastroenterology, University of Colorado School of Medicine, Denver, Colorado

David W. Lehman, M.D., Ph.D.
Assistant Professor of Medicine, University of Colorado School of Medicine; Clinical Director, HIV Early Intervention Services, Denver Department of Health and Hospitals, Community Health Services, Denver, Colorado

Michael L. Lepore, M.D., FACS
Professor, Vice Chairman, and Program Director, Department of Otolaryngology–Head and Neck Surgery, University of Colorado School of Medicine; Chief, Division of Otolaryngology, Denver Department of Health and Hospitals; Chief, Division of Otolaryngology, Rose Medical Center, Denver, Colorado

Allan Liebgott, M.D.
Associate Clinical Professor of Medicine, University of Colorado School of Medicine; Medical Director of Managed Care, Denver General Hospital, Denver, Colorado

Stuart L. Linas, M.D.
Professor of Medicine, and Head, Section of Hypertension, Division of Renal Diseases and Hypertension, University of Colorado School of Medicine, Denver, Colorado

Richard P. Lofgren, M.D., M.P.H.
Associate Professor of Medicine, and Chief, Division of General Internal Medicine, Medical College of Wisconsin, Milwaukee, Wisconsin

Thomas D. MacKenzie, M.D.
Assistant Professor, Department of Medicine, Division of Internal Medicine, University of Colorado School of Medicine, Denver, Colorado

Eric T. McFarling, M.D.
Instructor of Medicine, University of Colorado School of Medicine, Denver, Colorado

Philip S. Mehler, M.D.
Associate Professor of Medicine, and Head, Division of General Internal Medicine, University of Colorado School of Medicine; Attending Physician, Denver General Hospital, Denver, Colorado

Lawrence A. Meredith, M.D.
Instructor and Fellow in Behavioral Neurology, University of Colorado School of Medicine, Denver, Colorado

Jeanette Mladenovic, M.D.
Professor of Medicine and Vice-Chair for Educational Affairs, University of Colorado School of Medicine; Chief, Department of Medicine, Denver General Hospital, Denver, Colorado

Louis A. Morris, M.D.
Clinical Instructor, Department of Medicine, Division of Gastroenterology, University of Colorado School of Medicine, Denver, Colorado

Kristin L. Nichol, M.D. M.P.H.
Associate Professor of Medicine, University of Minnesota Medical School; Chief, Section of General Internal Medicine, VA Medical Center, Minneapolis, Minnesota

Kathleen M. Ogle, M.D.
Director, Medical Oncology, Park-Nicollet Medical Center, St. Louis Park, Minnesota

David L. Olson, M.D.
Assistant Professor of Medicine, University of Colorado School of Medicine; Clinical Director, Adult Medicine, Eastside Health Center, Denver, Colorado

Marcelle Owens, M.D.
Fellow, Department of Medicine, Division of Gastroenterology, University of Colorado School of Medicine, Denver, Colorado

Norman Peterson, M.D.
Professor of Surgery (Urology), University of Colorado School of Medicine; Associate Director of Surgery, and Chief, Division of Urology, Denver Department of Health and Hospitals, Denver, Colorado

Jeffrey Pickard, M.D.
Associate Professor of Medicine, University of Colorado School of Medicine, Denver, Colorado

Kamasamudram Ravilochan, M.D.
Instructor, Department of Neurology, University of Colorado School of Medicine, Denver, Colorado

Douglas J. Redosh, M.D.
Clinical Instructor, Department of Neurology, University of Colorado School of Medicine, Denver, Colorado

Randall R. Reves, M.D.
Associate Professor, Department of Medicine, Division of Infectious Diseases, University of Colorado School of Medicine; Co-Director, Infectious Diseases/AIDS Clinic, Denver Department of Health and Hospitals, Denver, Colorado

Julie Rifkin, M.D.
Assistant Professor, Department of Medicine, Division of Internal Medicine, University of Colorado School of Medicine; Primary Care Internist, Denver General Hospital, Denver, Colorado

Hanna Bloomfield Rubins, M.D., M.P.H.
Assistant Professor, Department of Medicine, University of Minnesota Medical School, Minneapolis, Minnesota

Roshan Shrestha, M.D.
Fellow, Department of Medicine, Division of Gastroenterology, University of Colorado School of Medicine, Denver, Colorado

Jeffrey M. Sippel, M.D.
Instructor, Department of Medicine, Division of Internal Medicine, University of Colorado School of Medicine, Denver, Colorado

Jonathan Slater, M.D.
Fellow in Nephrology, Department of Medicine, University of Colorado School of Medicine, Denver, Colorado

Lawrence Smith, M.D.
Associate Professor of Medicine, Mt. Sinai School of Medicine; Attending Physician, Mt. Sinai Hospital, New York, New York

Andrew Steele, M.D., M.P.H.
Assistant Professor of Medicine, University of Colorado School of Medicine, Denver, Colorado

Stephen E. Steinberg, M.D.
Professor of Medicine, Division of Gastroenterology, University of Colorado School of Medicine, Denver, Colorado

Eugene J. Sullivan, M.D.
Fellow, Department of Medicine, Division of Pulmonary and Critical Care Medicine, University of Colorado School of Medicine, Denver, Colorado

John Towbin, M.D.
Department of Neurology, University of Colorado School of Medicine, Denver, Colorado

Thomas E. Trouillot, M.D.
Fellow, Department of Medicine, Division of Gastroenterology, University of Colorado School of Medicine, Denver, Colorado

Valerie K. Ulstad, M.D.
Assistant Professor, Department of Medicine, Division of Cardiology, University of Minnesota Medical School, Minneapolis, Minnesota; Director, Coronary Care Unit, Saint Paul–Ramsey Medical Center, St. Paul, Minnesota

Thomas R. Vendegna, M.D.
Fellow, Department of Medicine, Division of Pulmonary and Critical Care Medicine, University of Colorado School of Medicine, Denver, Colorado

Rafael Villalobos, M.D.
Department of Neurology, University of Colorado School of Medicine, Denver, Colorado

Danny C. Williams, M.D., M.S.
Assistant Professor of Medicine, Division of Rheumatology, University of Colorado School
of Medicine, Denver, Colorado

Timothy J. Wilt, M.D., M.P.H.
Assistant Professor, Department of Medicine, Minneapolis VA Medical Center, Minneapolis,
Minnesota

PREFACE

Primary Care Secrets is aimed at those medical students, residents, retraining physicians, and other health care providers who must develop and maintain a practical and scholarly breadth of knowledge to deliver the necessary daily care to their patients. As the first professional contact for both preventive and therapeutic needs, primary care providers are often faced with problems much different from those intensive experiences that led to educational opportunities on the classic inpatient service. For this reason, the abbreviated topics selected from this overwhelmingly broad subject matter were organized (where possible) according to problems commonly facing the health care professional in the outpatient setting. Answers to the questions posed are not meant to be proscriptive in nature, but rather to address approaches, rationales, and often cost-effectiveness. The contributors include medical and surgical specialists and subspecialists, in addition to generalists. They have frequently provided opinions about which patients should be referred for the next level of care or admitted to the hospital. While the subject matter does not specifically address the primary care of newborns and children, issues unique to the pediatric patient are discussed in several, especially nonmedical, chapters.

Primary Care Secrets is another text in the popular and unique Secrets Series® originated by the late Dr. Charles Abernathy, who cleverly acknowledged the time-honored Socratic educational approach in written format. Dr. Abernathy was a practicing academic surgeon whose energy and passion for life and medicine were infectious and apparent to all who were fortunate enough to cross his path. His intense commitment to the art of medicine, the fun of learning, and the fundamentals of teaching are embodied in his own chapters and Secrets. These should serve as his reminder to us that the practice of medicine is based upon "secrets" divulged within a relationship between physician and patient, and interpreted in the light of sound clinical evidence.

I would like to express my appreciation to all the contributors for their time and efforts, and to Vicky Kalasountas for her exceptional organizational skills in preparation of manuscripts and coordination of this project.

Jeanette Mladenovic, M.D.

I. Health Maintenance

1. PRINCIPLES OF PREVENTIVE MAINTENANCE AND TEST SELECTION

Richard P. Lofgren, M.D., M.P.H.

1. Why buy a test?
There are three reasons to obtain a laboratory or diagnostic test.

1. **Screening or case finding.** The purpose is to detect a condition before symptoms occur in the hope of altering the natural history of the disease.

2. **Diagnosis of disease.** The purpose is to refine the diagnostic hypothesis either to "rule in" a disease if the likelihood of disease is high or to "rule out" a disease if the likelihood is low.

3. **Patient management.** Tests can aid patient management by (a) monitoring the status of diseases, (b) identifying complications, (c) providing prognostic information, and (d) ensuring therapeutic levels.

2. What is the most important characteristic of a test used to monitor the status of a patient?
The reproducibility of the test.

3. How is an "abnormal" test result defined?
Differentiating normal from abnormal is often more difficult than it seems. A test may be abnormal based on three different definitions:

1. **Normal distribution.** For most analytic tests, normal limits are determined by measurements done in a large number of subjects and are arbitrarily defined as the range encompassed by 2 standard deviations from the mean. With a normal curve distribution, 95% of observations are within 2 standard deviations from the mean.

2. **Biologically normal.** The results of tests that are statistically normal may not be biologically normal. The classic example is cholesterol. There is a three-fold increase in the risk of cardiovascular disease with a high-normal cholesterol versus a low-normal cholesterol level.

3. **Abnormal as treatable.** Abnormal not only refers to a value that increases the risk of bad outcome, but also to a result that, if treated, results in improved outcome. Initially hypertension was defined as a diastolic blood pressure above 105 mmHg, since studies had shown that treatment at that level was beneficial. With further studies the definition of "normal" has steadily decreased and may vary for different populations such as diabetic versus nondiabetic patients.

4. What are the limitations inherent in using the normal distribution as a definition of normal?
There are several limitations:

- **Chance phenomenon.** By definition, 5% of subjects will have results that lie at the extremes and will be labeled abnormal. With any given test, a normal individual has a 1 in 20 chance of having an "abnormal" result. The likelihood of having an abnormal

1

result increases in proportion to the number of independent tests performed. Sixty-four percent of normal individuals will have at least one abnormal result on a chemistry panel of 20 tests. Therefore, it is distinctly abnormal for a normal person to have a normal screening "chem 20" panel.

- **Physiologic variable.** Some physiologic variables, such as the alkaline phosphatase, have a skewed distribution.
- **Reference group.** Often the normal range is determined in young healthy volunteers (such as medical students). For many tests the distribution will vary by age, gender, or other important parameters.

5. What are the sensitivity and specificity of a test?

Although the terms are often defined mathematically, it is helpful to remember what they mean in simple language.

Sensitivity is the probability that a test will be positive if the disease is present.

Specificity is the probability that a test will be negative if the disease is absent.

The terms can also be defined using a 2 × 2 table:

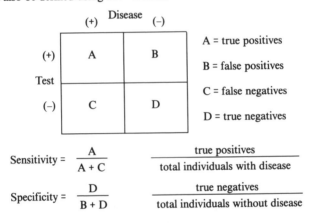

$$\text{Sensitivity} = \frac{A}{A + C} \qquad \frac{\text{true positives}}{\text{total individuals with disease}}$$

$$\text{Specificity} = \frac{D}{B + D} \qquad \frac{\text{true negatives}}{\text{total individuals without disease}}$$

6. If a test to detect a disease whose prevalence is 1/1000 has a 95% sensitivity and 95% specificity, what is the chance that a person found to have a positive result actually has the disease?

The answer is < 2%. There is a 95% chance that the test will detect the one individual out of 1000 with the disease. However, with a 95% specificity or a 5% false-positive rate, 50 normal individuals will have an abnormal result. Therefore, only 1 of the 51 individuals with a "positive" result will actually have the disease.

This question was asked of 20 students, 20 residents, and 20 attending physicians, and only 18% gave the correct answer. The most common answer given was "95%," a gross overestimation of the likelihood of disease! Appropriately interpreting test results is not intuitively obvious. In order to interpret test results properly, it is essential the clinician make a "guesstimate" of the likelihood (or prevalence) of disease prior to obtaining the test. The most common mistake made in interpreting test results is failing to consider the probability of disease before the results are known. Once the results are in hand, clinicians tend to be swayed by the findings and inflate the accuracy of the test.

7. What is predictive value?

Sensitivity and specificity are characteristics of a test. They tell you the likelihood a test will be positive or negative if you already know if the disease is present or absent. Knowledge of test characteristics does not, per se, permit the accurate interpretation of the test result. In practice, the clinician needs to know the likelihood that the disease is absent or present when the result is positive or negative. This is the **predictive value** of a test. It is determined by the sensitivity and specificity of the test and the prevalence of the disease in the population. **Positive predictive value** is the probability that the disease is present given a positive test result. **Negative predictive value** is the probability that the disease is absent given a negative test result.

In order to accurately interpret the test results (i.e., the positive and negative predictive value), one has to know (or make an a priori educated guess) about the prevalence of the disease before obtaining the test. The predictive value can be calculated using Bayes' theorem or a 2 × 2 table if prevalence is known.

$$\text{Positive predictive value} = \frac{A}{A + B} \qquad \frac{\text{true positives}}{\text{total individuals with positive result}}$$

$$= \frac{(Se)(P)}{(Se)(P) + (1 - Sp)(1 - P)} \qquad \begin{aligned} Se &= \text{sensitivity} \\ Sp &= \text{specificity} \\ P &= \text{prevalence of disease} \end{aligned}$$

$$\text{Negative predictive value} = \frac{D}{C + D} \qquad \frac{\text{true negatives}}{\text{total individuals with negative result}}$$

$$= \frac{(1 - P)(Sp)}{(1 - P)(Sp) + (P)(1 - Se)}$$

8. When ruling out a disease, what kind of test is needed?

When ruling out a disease, the clinician suspects that the probability of disease is low (i.e., "it is possible but I doubt it"). In these situations, you must select a test that is almost always positive when the disease is present (a sensitive test). If such a test is negative, then the clinician can be confident that the likelihood of disease is remote. However, sensitive tests are not as specific and are subject to many false-positive results. If the pretest likelihood of disease is low and the test is positive, then it is likely a false-positive result. When the probability of disease is low, negative result using a sensitive test yields a very high negative predictive value.

Conversely, when ruling in disease, the clinician strongly suspects the disease is present. In these situations, the clinician wants a test that is rarely positive in people without the disease (a specific test). A positive result confirms the diagnosis, whereas a negative result is likely a false negative. When the probability of disease is high, a positive result using a specific test yields a very high positive predictive value.

In summary, there are two important rules to remember when interpreting laboratory results. When "ruling out" a disease, you should select a very sensitive test and you want the result to be negative. If it is positive, it is most likely a false-positive result and is not helpful (try to ignore the result). When "ruling in" disease, you should select a very specific test. If the result is positive, the diagnosis is confirmed. However, if the result is negative it is likely a false-negative result and not useful. Armed with these two simple rules, the clinician can correctly interpret test results without necessarily calculating the exact predictive value. Clinicians must resist being unduly influenced if the "unexpected" result is obtained.

9. How can you increase the sensitivity and specificity of your diagnostic strategy?

Often there is no single test that is sufficiently sensitive to rule out a disease (or sufficiently specific to rule in a disease). The clinician can improve the sensitivity or specificity of the diagnostic approach by using multiple tests. Using several tests in combination, or in parallel, will significantly increase the sensitivity (while decreasing the specificity) and thus the negative predictive value of the diagnostic strategy. If all of the tests used in combination are negative, then it is unlikely the disease is present. Conversely, using multiple tests in sequence, or series, significantly increases the specificity (while decreasing the sensitivity). If you do test A and if positive, do test B and if positive test C, then the clinician can be fairly certain the disease is present if all three tests are positive (a strong positive predictive value).

10. When should you screen for a disease?

There are important factors to consider before screening for a disease.

1. **Common disease.** The disease must be relatively common for a screening program to be cost effective. If the disease is rare, a significant number of normal individuals will have a false-positive result and the predictive value will be poor. Individuals with a false-positive result may be subject to further expensive and perhaps invasive procedures.

2. **Cause significant morbidity.** The disease must result in significant suffering. For example, tinea pedis may be common but does not cause sufficient problems to warrant a screening program.

3. **An effective screening test must exist.** A screening program needs to have a test with reasonable test characteristics (sensitivity and specificity) and be practical, convenient, and inexpensive with few side effects. Because the majority of individuals will not have the disease, the screening process has to be acceptable to the patient. Although the complications of a cerebral aneurysm may be preventable, a screening program using cerebral angiograms is not practical or acceptable. However, screening for hypertension is simple and effective.

4. **Therapy must alter the natural history of disease.** Treatment early in the asymptomatic period should be superior to therapy started once symptoms develop. Data strongly suggest that removal of adenomatous colonic polyps decreases the incidence of colon cancer. Similarly, therapy of stage I breast cancer is superior to treatment of stage III disease. On the other hand, it is not clear that early treatment of asymptomatic hyperglycemia improves patient outcomes. Since early therapy is not clearly beneficial, screening for this important disease is questionable.

11. What is the difference between primary, secondary, and tertiary preventive care?

Primary prevention is an intervention designed to prevent a pathologic condition or disease from occurring. Examples include immunizations to prevent specific infectious diseases or wearing a seat belt to prevent bodily injury during an accident.

Secondary prevention is an intervention designed to prevent future morbidity and/or mortality by treating a condition during the asymptomatic period. Often early intervention is relatively simple and more effective therapy. Screening and treating malignancies such as cervical cancer, colon cancer, and breast cancer are examples of secondary prevention.

Tertiary prevention is an intervention designed to prevent complications in patients with an established disease. For example, treating an elevated cholesterol to prevent the progression of atherosclerosis in a patient with coronary artery disease is a tertiary preventive measure. Primary care physicians often spend considerable time delivering tertiary preventive services.

The distinction between the various types of preventive care can be blurred. For example, the treatment of hypertension could be primary intervention to prevent heart disease or tertiary intervention to prevent the progression of renal disease in a diabetic patient.

12. What is the purpose of the periodic health examination?

The value of the periodic health examination (PHE) is multifaceted and includes:

1. **Preventing disease** (primary prevention), such as providing immunization
2. **Identifying risk factors** for common chronic disease such as hyperlipidemia and obesity
3. **Case finding** (secondary prevention) to detect asymptomatic disease, such as screening for cervical or colorectal cancer, hypertension, and glaucoma
4. **Counseling and educating patients to promote health behavior such as diet, exercise, and smoking cessation**
5. **Updating the patient's clinical data**, including any new medical conditions, such as surgeries or allergies
6. **Enhancing patient/physician communication.** It is important that the patient knows and trusts the physician and becomes an active partner in his or her own health. Periodic examinations can help nurture this relationship.

The PHE is a time-honored but often maligned practice. Few preventive medicine procedures have been demonstrated to reduce mortality and morbidity by randomized trials. Discussions about the value of the PHE often fail to recognize the importance of points 5 and 6.

13. How well do physicians do in providing preventive service?
Unfortunately, not well. Studies from a variety of clinical settings report compliance rates from 75–99% for blood pressure determination, 40–80% for breast examination, 20–80% for Pap smears, 20–65% for hemoccult tests, 10–54% for mammograms, 8–20% for pneumococcal vaccines, and 5–40% for yearly influenza vaccines. Physicians fail to recognize more than 50% of patients with alcoholism and substance abuse. Physicians are knowledgeable, generally recognize the importance of preventive services, and typically overrate their own success. Providing preventive services often is not the top priority during an office visit.

14. How can physicians improve their success in providing preventive care?
To effectively implement a preventive medicine program into a busy practice setting, physicians need to develop a specific plan. Important elements include:
  1. **Use of PHE.** Performance of the PHE improves provision of preventive measures. However, attendance rates are lower for purely preventive visits. It is often necessary to incorporate the services into regular office visits.
  2. **Guidelines.** There are a number of competing and conflicting guidelines. The practice should adopt a set of guidelines that is acceptable and post it throughout the clinic setting.
  3. **Flow sheet.** The use of a preventive medicine flow sheet in a prominent part of the medical records may help.
  4. **Reminders.** A number of different strategies have been used to remind busy physicians to perform preventive service. In large clinics, automatic computer reminders, customized to individual patients, are effective.
  5. **Allied health personnel.** Involving nursing and other professionals in the practice to initiate and implement preventive services can be effective.

15. Why and how do the recommended guidelines for preventive services vary?
Many professional organizations and societies, advisory panels, and federal organizations have issued guidelines. The content and frequency of the recommended preventive services are controversial and may vary significantly among published guidelines. In general, guidelines from specific professional societies, such as the American Cancer Society or the American Diabetes Association, are the most aggressive in recommending specific screening procedures.

On the other hand, the Canadian and U.S. Task Forces are more conservative in their recommendations. These task forces use explicit rules of evidence and criteria to generate recommendations. Recommendations to perform or not to perform a preventive service are based on the quality of the evidence that its performance would be beneficial. The strongest recommendations are reserved for interventions proved to be effective in well-designed studies. Measures are described as "clinically prudent" only if there is compelling *indirect* evidence. Many procedures receive no recommendations because the evidence of efficacy is lacking.

16. What is the difference between efficacy and effectiveness of preventive service?
Efficacy refers to the ability of an intervention to produce the desired outcome under optimal circumstances. Effectiveness is the performance of an intervention in a practice setting (i.e., does it still work in the heterogeneous environment of clinical practice?). Clinical studies usually involve highly motivated, select patients with equally motivated health professionals. Oftentimes preventive services are not nearly as effective when applied in "real world" conditions. Unfortunately, the effectiveness of an intervention is rarely studied.

BIBLIOGRAPHY

1. Canadian Task Force on the Periodic Health Examination: Periodic health examination, 2: 1989 update. Can Med Assoc J 141:1136–1140, 1989.
2. Fletcher RH, Fletcher SW, Wagner EH: Clinical Epidemiology: The Essentials. Baltimore, Williams & Wilkins, 1982, pp 18–74.
3. Hayward RS, Steinberg EP, Ford DE, et al: Preventive care guidelines—1991. Ann Intern Med 114:758–783, 1991.
4. Holbrook JH: Periodic health examination for adults. In Stults BM, Dere W (eds): Practical Care of the Ambulatory Patient. Philadelphia, W.B. Saunders, 1989, pp 415–422.
5. Kern DE: Preventive medicine in ambulatory practice. In Barker LR, Burton JR, Zieve PD (eds): Principles of Ambulatory Medicine. Baltimore, Williams & Wilkins, 1991, pp 13–25.
6. US Preventive Services Task Force: Guide to Clinical Preventive Services. Baltimore, Williams & Wilkins, 1989.
7. Woolf SH: Analytic principles in assessing the effectiveness of clinical preventive services. In Goldbloom RB, Lawrence RS (eds): Preventing Disease Beyond the Rhetoric. New York, Springer-Verlag, 1990, pp 5–11.

2. EARLY CANCER DETECTION

Timothy J. Wilt, M.D., M.P.H.

1. List and describe the major biases that can result in invalid conclusions about the effectiveness of cancer screening methods.

- **Lead time** is the length of time between detection of cancer with a screening test and the time at which the disease, by the presence of signs and symptoms, would otherwise have been detected in the absence of screening. Lead time bias occurs when survival appears to be lengthened because screening simply advances the time of diagnosis, lengthening the period to time between diagnosis and death without altering the natural history of the disease.
- **Length bias** can also overestimate the benefits of cancer screening. This occurs because less aggressive tumors (slower growing) with relatively good prognosis are detected by screening programs more frequently than aggressive tumors due to their longer detectable preclinical phase. Therefore, aggressive tumors are underrepresented in screening programs, resulting in apparently improved survival of malignancies detected by screening.
- **Overdiagnosis bias** results when screening detects lesions that may not be clinically significant. Very early "cancers" detected during screening might never have caused symptomatic disease if they had been left undetected. Screening programs may overreport the number of malignancies that would have caused problems if not found by early detection.
- **Selection bias** occurs because individuals who participate in screening programs are often different from the general population. They may participate because they are at higher risk for disease, are more likely to comply with screening and treatment programs, and frequently have other health care practices that result in improved health outcome independent of the screening program.

2. Why is the positive predictive value (PPV) for cancer screening programs generally lower than the PPV for detecting cancer?

Because the goal of cancer screening programs is to detect curable cancers, the PPV then becomes lower than that calculated to detect all cancers, which include cancer precursors and curable and incurable tumors. For example, the hemoccult test that is recommended for colorectal cancer detection has a PPV of 5–10% for detecting colorectal cancer and 30% for adenomatous polyps in asymptomatic average-risk individuals over age 50. However, not all adenomatous polyps become cancerous. Therefore, some polyps discovered by screening may not have required detection and removal. Furthermore, not all cancers detected by this method are localized cancer and thus may not be curable.

3. Current evidence supports the practice of screening chest roentgenograms and/or sputum cytology to reduce lung cancer mortality. True or false?

False. Chest roentgenograms and sputum cytology have been proposed as tests for early detection of lung cancer. If the tumor is detected while it is still localized, surgical resection has generally been considered the only possibility for cure. However, several randomized controlled trials, a nonrandomized controlled trial, and two case-controlled studies have failed to demonstrate a reduction in lung cancer mortality from frequent screening with chest roentgenograms and sputum cytology. The United States Preventive Services Task Force (USPSTF) therefore concluded that there is good evidence to recommend against the use of either of these procedures to screen for lung cancer even in high-risk smokers.

4. What is the best method of preventing lung cancer?

Lung cancer is the leading cause of cancer-related mortality in both men and women. In 1991 there were an estimated 161,000 new cases of lung cancer and 143,000 lung-cancer-related deaths. The 5-year survival of individuals with lung cancer is less than 15%. Up to 80% of lung cancers are related to cigarette smoking, and therefore should be preventable. Decreased use of tobacco is the best method of preventing lung cancer. Specific screening for this disease is not recommended.

5. Does screening for colon cancer with annual fecal occult-blood tests reduce colon cancer mortality?

Colorectal cancer is one of the most common malignancies, with approximately 150,000 new cases and 61,000 deaths annually. A randomized controlled trial demonstrated that annual fecal occult-blood testing with rehydration of samples resulted in a 33% reduction in mortality from colorectal cancer compared with a control group. This reduction in mortality was accompanied by a shift to detection at an earlier stage of cancer and improved survival in those in whom cancer developed as compared with the control group. People who are offered testing every other year did not show a significant reduction in mortality, although they also had a shift to the detection of cancers at earlier stages.

6. Which patients should be screened by flexible sigmoidoscopy for colon cancer?

Some evidence suggests that in addition to fecal occult-blood testing, screening with a 65-cm flexible sigmoidoscope should be performed every 3–5 years (and possibly as infrequently as every 10 years) for average-risk men and women between 50 and 75 years of age.

Men and women at high risk should be referred for screening by colonoscopy. High-risk patients to be considered include those with a family history of colon cancer in first-degree relatives, and those with a family history of cancer syndromes, polyposis syndromes, past polyps, colon cancer, or inflammatory bowel disease.

7. Should all men be screened routinely for prostate cancer?

While several orag nizations recommend annual digital rectal examination and prostate specific antigen (PSA) testing, the efficacy of these or other tests in reducing prostate-specific mortality or total mortality has not yet been demonstrated.

Prostate cancer is currently the most frequently diagnosed cancer and second leading cause of cancer-related mortality in men. The biggest risk factor is age. The median age at diagnosis is 72 years. The average annual incidence rates in 1986–90 were 23/100,0000 for men under age 65 and 884/100,0000 for men $\geq$ 65. In 1993 it was estimated that approximately

200,000 men would be diagnosed with prostate cancer, and that 40,000 men would succumb to the disease. From 1989 to 1990, the incidence of prostate cancer rose 16%. This increased incidence is most likely because more men are receiving tests and procedures that detect asymptomatic cancers. Despite the increased number of patients with localized prostate cancer that is diagnosed and treated, death rates from prostate cancer have increased. This finding has led to speculation that early detection and treament programs may not be effective in reducing morbidity and mortality related to prostate cancer.

Before early detection strategies can be rationally recommended, treatment efficacy must first be demonstrated. Results from a small clinical trial, surgical, radiation, and expectant management case series, a structured literature review, and decision analysis modeling all suggest that therapy reserved for palliative relief of symptomatic disease progression (expectant management) may provide similar survival rates to that of early intervention. Men with large or poorly differentiated prostate cancer that metastasizes early are at high risk for death from prostate cancer. However, in these individuals, even when the cancer is judged to be localized to the prostate gland, early intervention with surgery or radiation is unlikely to prevent disease persistence or recurrence. Early intervention with radical prostatectomy or radiation may not be effective. Several randomized clinical trials are currently under way to address the issue of the effectiveness of early detection and treatment of prostate cancer.

8. What is the purpose of the Pap smear?

The Papanicolaou smear, developed by Dr. George Papanicolaou in the 1930s, is the recommended screening test for cervical cancer. Although the incidence and mortality of cervical cancer are relatively low compared with lung, breast, and colon cancer, the natural history of this disease (long preinvasive stage) and the availability of the Pap smear make screening practical. Since the widespread use of Pap smears, the mortality from cervical cancer has decreased from 23/100,000 in the 1960s to approximately 14/100,000 currently.

9. How often should Pap smears be performed? What should be done if the results are "atypical"?

Pap smears should be performed at intervals of 1–3 years beginning at the age of sexual intercourse and continuing until age 65 if multiple smears have been normal. The frequency of examination depends on the presence of risk factors, which include early onset of sexual intercourse, multiple sexual partners, low socioeconomic status, or history of genital warts.

Unlike many objective laboratory tests, the Pap smear depends entirely on human evaluation. The cytologic appearance of cells obtained from the tip of an instrument placed in the endocervical canal and/or from a sample of the vaginal pool cells is evaluated for evidence of atypical or malignant cells. Preparation of the slide is important, as it may affect the cytopathologic appearance of the specimen. The laboratory should be provided with clinical data such as age, obstetric and gynecologic history, and a description of clinical findings. The principal goal of cervical smears is not to diagnose overt clinical cancer but to detect occult small carcinomas and precancerous abnormalities that may lead to invasive cancer. Therefore clinicians should conduct further evaluation with colposcopy rather than repeat a Pap smear in women with "atypical" or "precancerous lesions."

10. Should CA-125 be used to screen patients for ovarian cancer?

CA-125 should not be used as a screening test to detect ovarian cancer in average-risk or low-risk women. The annual incidence and mortality of ovarian cancer are low (14 and 8.5/100,000, respectively), with the greatest risk factor being increasing age. While CA-125 is a tumor-specific marker for ovarian cancer, the sensitivity of the test is only 50% for early stage I-II neoplasms. The combined specificity of transvaginal ultrasound (TVS) and CA-125 for detecting ovarian cancer is estimated to be 99.95%, although the sensitivity is only 45%. Thus it is estimated that the benefit of screening in terms of life expectancy is probably small owing to the low prevalence of the disease, and therefore may not yet be justified.

The sensitivity and specificity of TVS in detecting an ovarian mass are approximately 90 and 98%, respectively. When a mass is detected, CA-125 should be used to screen for ovarian carcinoma. Average-risk patients (those at risk in the general population and those at risk due to increasing age), however, should not be confused with patients at extremely high risk due to a family history of sibling or maternal ovarian cancer. High-risk patients should be carefully screened for ovarian cancer regularly and referred to a specialist in this area for consideration of surgical prevention or entry into study protocols.

11. What type of early detection and treatment recommendations would you make to an individual concerned about skin cancer?

The most serious of the dermatologic malignancies is malignant melanoma, which produces 3% of all fatal cancers. Basal and squamous cell carcinomas grow slowly, rarely metastasize, and do not produce sufficient morbidity to warrant screening. Patients should be encouraged to report any lesion noted to bleed, ulcerate, or develop a horn.

A case-control study of risk for melanoma identified five significant risk factors: fair skin, six or more moles > 0.5 cm in diameter, previously diagnosed basal or squamous carcinoma of the skin, a parental history of skin cancer, and poor tolerance of sunlight. Persons with dysplastic moles, a family history of melanoma, or excessive sun exposure are also at increased risk for melanoma. Individuals should be encouraged to use sun screens with a sun protective factor (SPF) of at least 15. Wide-brimmed hats are helpful. Fair-skinned individuals should be advised to minimize exposure from 11:00 a.m. to 2:30 p.m. when about 70% of the harmful ultraviolet radiation occurs. One third of newly diagnosed melanomas occur on non–sun-exposed areas that may not be routinely seen. Therefore, a complete skin examination at least once is important. Individuals with multiple large moles or dysplastic moles should probably receive at least annual skin evaluation. In black, Hispanic, and Asian patients, attention to palmar, plantar, and subungual areas is important because of a greater incidence of acral lentiginous melanomas in these populations.

12. Who is at risk for breast cancer?

Breast cancer is the most frequent cancer and second leading cause of cancer-related deaths in women. Approximately 1 in 8 women will develop breast cancer. Important risk factors include a family history of premenopausal breast cancer, previous breast cancer, a history of benign breast disease, and increasing age. Other factors that may be associated with breast cancer include first pregnancy after age 30, menarche before age 12, menopause after age 50, obesity, and high socioeconomic status. Breast implants as a risk factor for breast cancer have not been demonstrated but probably makes early detection of small malignancies more difficult. Recent reports have failed to find an association between dietary fat and development of breast cancer. A clinical trial is currently in progress to determine whether low-dose tamoxifen decreases the incidence of breast cancer in high-risk women.

13. Should all women be taught self breast examination (SBE) to detect breast masses?

Not necessarily. Women who are trained to perform SBE detect approximately 50% of lumps ranging in size from 0.25 to 3.0 cm in diameter. However, SBE also increases the false detection rate. No study has yet demonstrated the additional benefit of including SBE with clinical breast examination (CBE) and mammography. The USPSTF states that there is insufficient evidence to recommend for or against SBE. SBE should probably be recommended on an individual basis that incorporates the woman's desire to be trained in SBE.

14. How should women be screened for breast cancer?

Annual mammography and clinical breast examination (CBE) by a health care provider are recommended for all women beginning at age 50. In this group, this combination of tests has been shown to be effective in detecting early breast cancer and reducing breast cancer mortality. In women less than age 50 who are at high risk for breast cancer (particularly from a history of maternal or sibling breast cancer), annual mammography has been shown to be beneficial in reducing breast cancer mortality and is recommended. CBE alone is probably not sufficiently sensitive to be used as a primary screening modality in this group but is complementary to mammography.

The effectiveness of mammography and CBE has not been demonstrated in women of average risk under the age of 50. Two recent trials investigating the benefits of annual screening with mammography and CBE showed no effect on the rate of breast cancer deaths in the average-risk woman under age 50.

Given these findings, a reasonable approach for women of average risk and less than 50 years of age might include a single mammography at age less than 50, and an annual CBE beginning at age 40. An annual CBE is recommended by the USPSTF for women at average risk over the age of 40 (see Breast Mass chapter).

15. Is fecal occult-blood testing a good screening test for upper gastrointestinal (GI) bleeding?
No. Fecal occult-blood testing is not performed as a screening test for upper GI bleeding, and upper GI evaluation is generally not warranted in asymptomatic patients presenting with positive fecal occult-blood specimens. Guaiac is the reagent used in fecal occult-blood cards to detect hemoglobin via an oxidation reaction. Fecal occult-blood tests detect unoxidized heme and require that the patient be losing approxiately 20 ml/day. A normal individual loses between 0.5 and 2.0 ml/day. Because hemoglobin is altered as it passes through the GI tract, it loses its pseudoperoxidase activity and its ability to oxidize guaiac. Therefore, upper GI bleeding is less likely to produce a positive result than lower GI tract bleeding.

16. What can you do to decrease the false-positive results of fecal occult-blood testing?
In general, it is recommended that screening for colon cancer be performed on spontaneously passed stool specimens and not from stool obtained during a digital rectal examination. Anal trauma during rectal exam may increase the false-positive results.

Ideally, you should restrict high doses of aspirin and nonsteroidal anti-inflammatory agents, iron, vitamin C, and foods high in peroxidase (beets) for 3 days before obtaining fecal occult-blood tests. In randomized trials, patients were placed on high-residue, meat-free diets during testing to reduce the number of false-positive tests. While these recommendations may not be totally practical or meet with complete compliance, they should be taken into account by the physician as he or she requests guaiac testing, but should not negate a positive test without further evaluation.

17. In performing fecal occult screening for colon cancer, your patient is noted to have only 1 out of 3 cards positive. You notice that he is on an aspirin a day for cardiac disease. What is the best approach in this patient?
In screening for colorectal cancer, any fecal occult positive test should be followed up with a full evaluation of the colon. This approach was taken in the randomized clinical trial described above that demonstrated a 33% reduction in colorectal cancer mortality. Colon cancer and its precursor (adenomatous polyps) frequently bleed intermittently or in small amounts. Furthermore, the hemoccult procedure samples only a portion of the stool specimen. Evaluating only when 3/3 tests are positive could result in missing clinically important lesions. Adenomas smaller than 2 cm probably do not bleed enough to be detected. The PPV for occult blood tests is about 10% for carcinoma and 30% for adenomas. Some evidence suggests that aspirin may not produce false-positive results in clinical practice.

While digital rectal examination may be useful in evaluating anal and rectal pathology, it evaluates only a small portion of the colon and should not be substituted for a complete colonic evaluation. Colonoscopy is the gold standard and allows for evaluation of the colon, biopsy of suspicious lesions, and removal of many polyps. It does, however, require a trained examiner. When a trained examiner is not available, the combination of flexible sigmoidoscopy and air contrast barium enema is acceptable. Colonoscopy should be performed if a lesion looks suspicious or visualization is inadequate.

BIBLIOGRAPHY

1. Fleming C, Wasson JH, Albertsen PC, et al. for the Prostate Patient Outcomes Research Team: A decision analysis of alternative treatment strategies for clinically localized prostate cancer. JAMA 269:2650–2659, 1993.
2. Friedman GD: Primer of Epidemiology, 3rd ed. New York, McGraw-Hill, 1987.
3. Mandel JS, Bond JH, Church TR, et al: Reducing mortality from colorectal cancer by screening for fecal occult blood. N Engl J Med 328:1365–1371, 1993.
4. Oboler SK, LaForce FM: The periodic physical examination in asymptomatic adults. Ann Intern Med 110:214–226, 1989.
5. Richert-Boe KE, Humphrey LL: Screening for cancers of the lung and colon. Arch Intern Med 152:2398–2404, 1992.
6. Richert-Boe KE, Humphrey LL: Screening for cancers of the cervix and breast. Arch Intern Med 152:2405–2411, 1992.
7. Schapira MM, Matchar DB, Young MJ: The effectiveness of ovarian cancer screening. A decision analysis model. Ann Intern Med 118:838–843, 1993.
8. United States Preventive Services Task Force. Fisher M (ed): Guide to Clinical Preventive Services. Baltimore, Williams & Wilkins, 1989.
9. Whitmore WF: Localised prostatic cancer: management and detection issues. Lancet 343:1263–1267, 1994.

3. CARDIOVASCULAR DISEASE PREVENTION

Hanna Bloomfield Rubins, M.D., M.P.H.

Cardiovascular disease is the leading cause of death for both women and men in the United States, claiming nearly 1 million lives a year. It is estimated that 70 million Americans have one or more manifestations of cardiovascular disease, including high blood pressure, stroke, and coronary heart disease. Coronary heart disease (CHD) alone affects close to 12 million Americans and every year half a million people suffer an acute stroke. This chapter focuses on the actions that primary care physicians can take to reduce the risk of cardiovascular disease (specifically CHD, cerebrovascular disease, and peripheral vascular disease) in their patients. Treatment of hypertension and certain other cardiovascular risk factors (e.g., obesity and dyslipidemia) is covered in detail in other chapters.

1. Is there a simple way to assess a patient's overall risk for atherosclerotic cardiovascular disease?

The major risk factors for atherosclerotic cardiovascular disease are listed below.

Major Risk Factors for Atherosclerotic Cardiovascular Disease

Fixed	Modifiable
Advanced age	Cigarette smoking
Male gender or postmenopausal female	Dyslipidemia (high LDL-C and/or low HDL-C)
Family history of premature coronary heart disease	Hypertension
	Sedentary lifestyle
	Diabetes
	Obesity

Multivariate risk functions that use a patient's risk factor profile to quantitate cardiac risk are available in either handbook or pocket calculator form. However, it is generally sufficient to assess a patient's risk status less quantitatively. High-risk patients are those with two or more major risk factors or with a very strong family history of premature CHD (even without other evident risk factors). Patients with one risk factor are considered to be at moderate risk and patients without any are at low risk. Although some risk factors appear to be more important than others for specific manifestations of atherosclerotic disease (e.g., hypertension is a strong determinant of stroke, whereas dyslipidemia is not), this is of little practical importance because the goal is to prevent all cardiovascular disease.

A thorough assessment of all risk factors should be made at the initial visit and shared with the patient. A plan of action for any identified modifiable risk factors should be initiated and close follow-up provided.

2. Should asymptomatic patients be screened for occult cardiovascular disease?
Screening for modifiable risk factors (e.g., hypertension, dyslipidemia, smoking) is strongly recommended, but screening asymptomatic people to detect occult atherosclerotic disease with modalities such as resting electrocardiography, exercise electrocardiography, noninvasive carotid and peripheral vascular evaluation, is not. These tests have poor predictive value in asymptomatic populations and, furthermore, the benefit of treating any uncovered disease in asymptomatic patients is not established. There are, however, certain asymptomatic individuals in whom cardiac screening might be appropriate, including persons at very high risk for CHD (e.g., men over age 40 with several cardiac risk factors); persons in whom a catastrophic cardiac event would endanger public safety (e.g., airline pilots); and persons at moderate or high risk for CHD who wish to initiate a vigorous exercise program.

3. What can the physician do during a routine office visit to help patients quit smoking?
The National Cancer Institute recommends that physicians use the four As approach: Ask, Advise, Assist, and Arrange.
- **Ask** about smoking at every visit. This should include an assessment of the person's current motivation to quit smoking.
- **Advise** all smokers to stop with a clear, unequivocal statement. Personalize the message, if possible, with reference to the patient's particular social or health concerns.
- **Assist** the patient in stopping. This includes setting a "quit date," providing self-help materials, and possibly prescribing nicotine replacement therapy for highly addicted patients. Patients who are currently unmotivated to stop smoking should be given motivational literature and the issue should be raised again at the next visit.
- **Arrange** follow-up visits. Patients should be reminded of the "quit date" by letter and contacted soon after the "quit date" to provide support and help prevent relapse. (These tasks can be delegated to office staff.)

4. What useful diet advice can be given in 5 minutes or less?
The American Heart Association Step I diet, outlined in the table below, is recommended for all individuals over the age of 2.

Recommended Diet for the General Population

1. Achieve ideal body weight
2. Limit fat intake to 30% of calories
Saturated fatty acids: 8–10%
Polyunsaturated fatty acids: 10%
Monounsaturated fatty acids: 10–15%
3. Limit cholesterol to 300 mg/day
4. Derive 50–60% of calories from carbohydrates

The following recommendations are intended to translate this formal dietary plan into easily "digestible" nuggets for patients. It is helpful to acknowledge to the patient that lifetime habits are hard to change while introducing just two or three of these suggestions at any one visit.

- For packaged foods, choose those with fewer than 3 grams of fat (and no more than 1 gm of saturated fat) per 100-calorie serving. Don't be fooled by foods advertised as "cholesterol free" or "low cholesterol," since these may contain a lot of saturated fat.
- Use only low or nonfat dairy products.
- Use only lean beef.
- Avoid processed meats (bologna, salami, hot dogs, sausages) and organ meats.
- Increase your intake of fruits, vegetables, legumes (beans, peas), grains, and fish.
- Eat no more than 4 egg yolks/week.
- Use spray or liquid fats for cooking (good choices: canola oil, olive oil).

It is extremely helpful to suggest specific alternatives for foods your patients likes (pretzels rather than potato chips; nonfat frozen yogurt rather than ice cream; turkey breast rather than bologna; mustard instead of mayonnaise; jam instead of butter, etc.). The emphasis should be on substitution, not denial.

5. What advice should a physician give about alcohol?
Light to moderate alcohol consumption (<3 drinks a day) has been linked with decreased risk of myocardial infarction and CHD death. This association may be at least partially explained by alcohol's propensity to raise high-density lipoprotein-cholesterol (HDL-C). The relation between moderate alcohol intake and ischemic stroke is not clear; some data suggest that alcohol may increase the risk of both ischemic and hemorrhagic stroke. It is generally agreed that physicians should not actively recommend that nondrinkers start drinking alcohol. However, patients who drink 3 or fewer alcoholic beverages a day and have no associated social or medical problems may be reassured that this level of drinking is acceptable and may even be cardioprotective.

6. What are the benefits of exercise?
Numerous observational studies indicate that physical activity is associated with a reduced risk of CHD and total mortality, independent of its beneficial effect on other risk factors such as serum lipids, obesity, diabetes, and hypertension. Physical activity also protects against osteoporosis and promotes mental well-being. It used to be thought that only vigorous exercise would produce the desired health benefits; it is now believed that even a modest exercise program can have substantial positive effects.

7. When is it safe to start an exercise program?
The safety of starting an exercise program in an individual patient can be assessed with the Physical Activity Readiness questionnaire:

*Physical Activity Readiness Questions**

1. Have you ever been told you have heart trouble?
2. Do you frequently get pain in your chest?
3. Do you often feel faint or have severe dizzy spells?
4. Have you ever been told you have high blood pressure?
5. Have you ever been told you have problems with bones or joints (such as arthritis) that might be made worse by exercise?
6. Is there any other physical problem you have that might prevent you from exercising?
7. Are you older than 65 years and not used to regular, vigorous exercise?

*Adapted from Harris et al, JAMA 261:3590–3598, 1989.[7]

A patient answering "no" to all these questions can safely undertake an exercise program without further testing or medical supervision. Patients answering "yes" to any of these questions should be further evaluated. Exercise electrocardiography should be considered for older patients and patients with cardiac disease or risk factors who wish to undertake a vigorous exercise program. Screening exercise electrocardiography for young, asymptomatic patients with no cardiac risk factors is not recommended.

8. What should an "exercise prescription" include?

Prescriptions for exercise should specify **intensity, duration,** and **frequency.** Recommended intensity of exercise is in the range of 50–85% of maximal oxygen uptake (VO_2 max), which corresponds to 65–90% of the maximal heart rate. (The maximal heart rate is approximately equal to 220 minus the person's age). Patients should be told their target heart rate (e.g., for a sedentary 60-year-old, this might be 104: ([220 – 60] × .65) and shown how to take their pulse. For duration and frequency, 15–45 minutes of exercise 3–5 times a week are generally recommended. Patients should be told to work towards their exercise goal gradually. Brisk walking is in many ways the ideal exercise. It is easy, convenient, free, and has minimal risk of adverse effects (such as sudden death or musculoskeletal injury).

9. How often should a patient's cholesterol level be checked?

Adults without CHD. Current national guidelines suggest that adults (over 20 years of age) without CHD should have a total cholesterol and an HDL-C measured once. If the cholesterol is less than 200 mg/dl and the HDL-C is greater than 35 mg/dl, the measurements should be repeated every 5 years. The approach for those with either cholesterol greater than 200 mg/dl or HDL-C less than 35 mg/dl on initial screening is outlined in the figure.

Adults with CHD. In adults with known CHD a full lipoprotein analysis (fasting total cholesterol, HDL-C, low-density lipoprotein cholesterol [LDL-C], triglycerides) should be done initially. Those with an LDL-cholesterol less than 100 mg/dl should have a full lipoprotein analysis repeated annually. Patients with an initial LDL-C greater than 100 mg/dl will require diet and/or drug intervention, which will then determine the frequency of repeat testing.

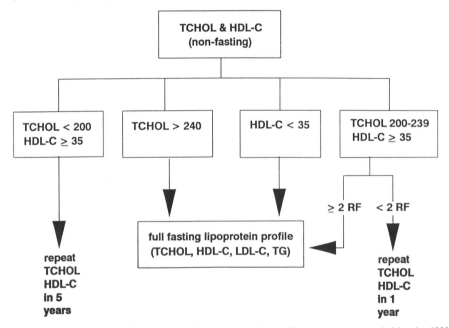

Algorithm for lipid screening in patients without coronary heart disease as recommended by the 1993 National Cholesterol Education Program Adult Treatment Panel. TCHOL: total cholesterol; HDL-C: high-density lipoprotein cholesterol; RF: risk factors; LDL-C: low-density lipoprotein cholesterol; TG: triglycerides.

10. What should be done about low levels of HDL-C or high levels of triglycerides?

Although both low levels of HDL-C and high levels of triglycerides have been linked epidemiologically to increased risk of CHD, there are no clinical trial data on which to base firm treatment recommendations. Patients with HDL-C less than 35 mg/dl should be advised to achieve ideal body weight, discontinue smoking, and exercise regularly. Drug therapy is not recommended.

Patients with triglycerides greater than 200 mg/dl should be advised to achieve ideal body weight, limit alcohol intake, and control diabetes (if present). Drug therapy is not recommended for the prevention of CHD. Patients with persistent elevations of fasting triglycerides above 750–1000 mg/dl should be considered for drug therapy (niacin or gemfibrozil) to reduce the risk of acute pancreatitis.

For patients with high levels of LDL-C requiring drug treatment (see chapter 30), the level of HDL-C and triglycerides should be considered in choosing the most appropriate regimen.

11. Is hormone replacement therapy indicated for postmenopausal women to prevent CHD?
In the absence of definitive data from randomized, controlled clinical trials, the decision to initiate hormone replacement therapy must be individualized. The physician should discuss the "pros" and "cons" with each patient to help her make an informed decision based on her medical history and personal values. The following information may be useful for this discussion.

CHD. Observational data strongly suggest that unopposed estrogen reduces a woman's risk of CHD by about 35%; however, no randomized clinical trial data are yet available to confirm this observation. Adding progestin may attenuate this benefit.

Hip and vertebral fractures. Limited evidence suggests that unopposed estrogen reduces risk for hip and vertebral fractures by 25% and 50%, respectively. Adding progestin probably does not attenuate this benefit.

Endometrial cancer. The risk of endometrial cancer is increased about eight-fold with prolonged use of unopposed estrogens. Addition of progestins eliminates this increased risk.

Breast cancer. The evidence linking hormone replacement therapy and breast cancer is inconsistent. One estimate is that long term (over 10 years), use of unopposed estrogen increases breast cancer risk by 25% (i.e., from a 10.2% to a 13% lifetime risk in an average-risk 50-year-old woman). Addition of progestins may increase this risk further.

Side effects. These include vaginal bleeding, headaches, bloating, breast tenderness, and need for endometrial monitoring (e.g., endometrial biopsy) for unopposed estrogen use. Adding progestin may cause other symptoms such as weight gain, irritability, and depression, but will obviate the need for endometrial monitoring.

Recent guidelines recommend:

1. Unopposed estrogens for women who have had a hysterectomy and are not at increased risk for breast cancer

2. Unopposed estrogens or combination therapy for women at high risk or with already established CHD

3. No hormone replacement therapy in women at high risk for breast cancer

4. Individualized decisions for all other women.

12. Which patients should be on aspirin and what is the best dose?
Recent American Heart Association guidelines recommend aspirin therapy in the following situations (assuming no contraindications exist):

1. For all patients with known CHD (dose 75–325 mg/day)

2. For men over age 40 years without CHD but with one or more risk factors for cardiovascular disease (dose 75–325 mg/day).

3. For all patients with a history of noncardiogenic stroke or transient ischemic attack (dose may need to be as high as 975–1500 mg/day, although a recent study indicated lower doses are equally effective).

13. Are vitamins indicated for the prevention of CHD?
This is an area of great interest and insufficient data. Many vitamins (such as vitamins C, E, and beta-carotene) have antioxidant properties. Oxidation of LDL-C is now thought to be a key factor in the initiation of the atherosclerotic lesion. Some observational studies report that

people with higher intake of these vitamins have lower rates of CHD than those with lower intake. There are no randomized controlled clinical trials to confirm these findings nor are the observational data as strong and consistent as for some other associations (e.g., postmenopausal hormone replacement). Some physicians recommend a single multivitamin tablet a day together with a diet rich in fruits and vegetables (e.g., citrus fruits, carrots, spinach) for patients who express an interest. Patients should understand that the possible dangers of high-dose vitamins available over-the-counter are not known.

14. What are the most important things a physician can do to prevent stroke?
The most important risk factors for stroke are age, hypertension, atrial fibrillation, and history of transient ischemic attack. Other cardiac risk factors such as smoking, dyslipidemia, and diabetes may also play a role. In order to prevent stroke the following are recommended:

- **Control of both systolic and diastolic hypertension** (see chapter 12).
- **Anticoagulation of patients with atrial fibrillation.** Several well-designed, randomized controlled clinical trials have now established that low-intensity anticoagulation (international normalized ratio: 2–3) with warfarin reduces the risk of stroke in patients with atrial fibrillation by 50–80%. It is unclear whether aspirin therapy is equally efficacious; results of ongoing trials are expected to answer this question within a few years.
- **Antiplatelet treatment in patients with a history of transient ischemic attack,** either with aspirin (see question 12) or with ticlopidine for patients who cannot tolerate aspirin.

15. What is the role of carotid endarterectomy for stroke prevention?
One large, well-designed, randomized controlled clinical trial has shown that carotid endarterectomy reduces stroke and total mortality in patients who have had a recent (within 4 months) transient ischemic attack or nondisabling stroke and who have high-grade (70–99%) ipsilateral carotid stenosis. This procedure should be recommended to eligible patients if the surgical mortality rate locally is comparable to the rate seen in the study (<3% major stroke; <1% mortality). Carotid endarterectomy is not currently recommended for patients with asymptomatic carotid bruit or for symptomatic patients with only moderate-grade carotid occlusion (30–69%).

16. Is aggressive risk factor treatment appropriate in elderly patients?
Elderly patients are at very high risk for CHD, stroke, and peripheral vascular disease. Treating hypertension with medication and anticoagulating elderly patients in atrial fibrillation to prevent stroke have both been proved beneficial in clinical trials that enrolled the elderly. Smoking cessation, a reasonable exercise regimen, and weight control should be encouraged in patients of all ages.

Most of the controversy revolves around drug treatment of dyslipidemia in the elderly. Elderly patients were not included in the clinical trials demonstrating that treatment of hypercholesterolemia resulted in decreased CHD morbidity and mortality. Furthermore, in several epidemiologic studies serum cholesterol levels were not as strongly associated with CHD risk in the elderly as in middle-aged people. However, because the elderly are at such high baseline risk for CHD and stroke, dyslipidemia in this population leads to a high number of cardiovascular events. Therefore, although decisions must be individualized, drug treatment of dyslipidemia should be considered in otherwise healthy elderly people.

17. Do the usual risk factors matter after a patient has had a myocardial infarction?
In the past, the importance of risk factor reduction in patients following a myocardial infarction was not emphasized, partly because prognosis was felt to be overwhelmingly determined by degree of myocardial damage sustained. It has been recently recognized that many modifiable risk factors, including cigarette smoking, dyslipidemia, physical inactivity, obesity, and hypertension, remain important predictors of recurrent cardiac events. Treating these risk factors in patients with established heart disease ("secondary prevention") may have

a more substantial impact on CHD incidence than treating people without known disease ("primary prevention"), since the absolute risk of myocardial infarction and CHD death is so much higher in the group with known disease. Clinical trials demonstrating beneficial effects of secondary prevention have been reported for hypercholesterolemia, hypertension, and exercise programs.

CONTROVERSY

18. Does lowering serum cholesterol increase the risk of all-cause mortality?
In several large observational studies the relationship between serum cholesterol and all-cause mortality is "J-shaped," i.e., those with the lowest and the highest levels of serum cholesterol have higher mortality than those in the middle range. The higher mortality in those with the lowest serum cholesterol was initially thought to reflect the fact that people with terminal disease (such as cancer) tend to develop low levels of cholesterol as a result of their disease. In other words, the terminal disease causes the low cholesterol and not vice versa. In order to explore this possibility, recent analyses have excluded early deaths; the J-shaped relationship has nevertheless persisted. Furthermore, in some clinical trials, the lowering of cholesterol resulted in decreased CHD mortality but increased mortality from other causes in the intervention group. It is unclear whether these findings are spurious or whether they are true findings that reflect either the side effects of specific drugs or the actual effect of cholesterol-lowering on all-cause mortality.

BIBLIOGRAPHY

1. Albers GW, Atwood JE, Hirsh J, et al: Stroke prevention in non-valvular atrial fibrillation. Ann Intern Med 115:727–736, 1991.
2. American College of Physicians: Guidelines for counselling postmenopausal women about preventive hormone therapy. Ann Intern Med 117:1038–1041, 1992.
3. Denke MA, Grundy SM: Hypercholesterolemia in elderly persons: Resolving the treatment dilemma. Ann Intern Med 112:780–792, 1990.
4. Expert Panel on Detection, Evaluation, and Treatment of High Blood Cholesterol in Adults: Summary of the second report of the National Cholesterol Education Program (NCEP) Expert Panel on detection, evaluation, and treatment of high blood cholesterol in adults (Adult Treatment Panel II). JAMA 269:3015–3023. 1993.
5. Fuster V, Dyken ML, Vokonas PS, Hennekens C: Aspirin as a therapeutic agent in cardiovascular disease. Circulation 87:659–675, 1993.
6. Glynn TJ, Manley MW: How to help your patients stop smoking. National Cancer Institute. NIH Publication No. 90-3064, 1990.
7. Harris SS, Caspersen CJ, DeFriese GH, Estes EH: Physical activity counselling for healthy adults as a primary preventive intervention in the clinical setting: Report for the U.S. Preventive Services Task Force. JAMA 261:3590–3598, 1989.
8. North American Symptomatic Carotid Endarterectomy Trials Collaborators: Beneficial effect of carotid endarterectomy in symptomatic patients with high-grade stenosis. N Engl J Med 325:445–453, 1991.
9. Siegel D, Grady D, Browner WS, Hulley SB: Risk factor modification after myocardial infarction. Ann Intern Med 109:213–218, 1988.
10. U.S. Preventive Services Task Force. Guide to Clinical Preventive Services. Baltimore, Williams & Wilkins, 1989.

4. IMMUNIZATIONS AND SCREENING FOR INFECTIOUS DISEASES

Kristin L. Nichol, M.D., M.P.H.

1. Which vaccines are recommended for children?

Current recommendations are for children to receive the following vaccines:

Diphtheria/tetanus/pertussis (DTaP)	5 doses
Polio	4 doses
Measles/mumps/rubella (MMR)	2 doses
Hemophilus influenzae B (HIB—conjugate vaccine)	3 to 4 doses
Hepatitis B	3 doses

These vaccines are administered at various intervals from birth to age 12 years, with 80% of injections scheduled to be given during the first 15–18 months of life. Several of these recommendations are new or have been modified within the last few years. These include the recommendations for universal childhood immunization against hepatitis B (1991), for the use of the conjugate form of HIB vaccine (1991), for the two-dose measles schedule (1989), and for the use of the acellular form of pertussis vaccine for the fourth and fifth doses of DTaP (1992).

2. Which vaccinations are recommended for adults?

Vaccinations for adults, in contrast to those for children, are largely recommended for persons only in specific risk groups.

Vaccines Most Often Administered to Adults

VACCINE	DOSE/TARGET GROUP
Influenza vaccine	Yearly: elderly, high-risk
Pneumococcal vaccine	Once: elderly, high-risk
Tetanus/diphtheria	Booster every 10 years after primary series has been completed
Hepatitis B	3 doses: high-risk
MMR	2 doses or other evidence of immunity (prior physician diagnosis of measles, laboratory evidence of immunity, or birth before 1957): high-risk

Persons aged 65 and older and other persons with chronic medical conditions (especially chronic heart and lung disease) are at particularly increased risk for complications from influenza and pneumococcal disease and should be offered these vaccines. Tetanus/diphtheria boosters are recommended routinely for all adults who have previously completed their primary series of three doses. Hepatitis B vaccine is recommended for persons with high-risk lifestyles (e.g., intravenous drug users, bisexual or homosexual persons, persons with other sexually transmitted diseases), for persons with high-risk occupations (e.g., health care providers), or for persons who live or work in high-risk environments (e.g., prison inmates). MMR is recommended for health care providers and for persons attending colleges and other educational institutions after high school who have not previously received two doses of the vaccine and who lack evidence of adequate immunity (prior physician diagnosis of measles, laboratory evidence of immunity, born before 1957).

In addition to routine immunizations, persons travelling outside of the country should also be assessed for need for any other vaccines. These special immunization requirements are geographically defined and may include immunizations for yellow fever, cholera, typh hepatitis B, and others. Local and state health departments and the Centers foɪ ᴅisease Control and Prevention may be consulted for up-to-date information on recommendations for immunizations for international travellers.

3. Why do the morbidity and mortality associated with vaccine-preventable diseases persist? The past several decades have seen dramatic decreases in the numbers of reported cases of vaccine-preventable diseases in this country. Nevertheless, vaccine-preventable diseases continue to be major causes of illness and death each year in all age groups (see tables below). Recent outbreaks of measles, congenital rubella syndrome, pertussis, and mumps underscore the continuing importance of these diseases among children. In addition, influenza and pneumonia continue to rank as the sixth leading cause of death in the United States, killing up to 60 times more persons (85% or more of whom are elderly) than all other vaccine-preventable diseases in all age groups combined.

Occurrences of Vaccine-preventable Diseases by Age Group, 1991*

VACCINE-PREVENTABLE DISEASE	TOTAL REPORTED CASES (1991)	CASES BY AGE GROUP		
		<20	20–59	60+
Diphtheria	5	2	2	—
Pertussis	2719	2289	249	15
Tetanus	57	4	22	30
Measles	9643	7713	1874	6
Mumps	4264	2754	548	25
Rubella	1401	798	305	1
Polio	6	3	2	1
H. influenzae B	2764	1734	398	493
Hepatitis B	18,003	1884	14,491	1060

*Data adapted from Centers for Disease Control: Summary of Notifiable Diseases, United States, 1991. MMR 40(53):1991.

Deaths Due to Vaccine-preventable Diseases, 1985–1989*

DISEASE	TOTAL CASES	TOTAL DEATHS
Influenza	—	50,000–200,000[†]
Pneumococcal	—	200,000[†]
Diphtheria	11	1
Pertussis	18,214	27
Tetanus	301	87
Measles	34,348	43
Mumps	34,198	7
Rubella	2108	10
Polio	35	4
Hepatitis B	125,230	2974

*Data from Centers for Disease Control: Summary of Notifiable Diseases, United States, 1991. MMWR 40(53):1991.
[†]80–90% of these occurred among persons age 65 and older.

The major reason that vaccine-preventable diseases continue to take a significant toll among children and adults is that vaccination rates often fall far short of national goals. Among children, for example, only 52–71% have been vaccinated against measles by their second birthday, with series-complete immunization levels ranging from 10–42%. The lowest vaccination rates may be seen in certain difficult-to-reach groups, including the urban poor and racial and ethnic minorities. Among adults, only 15% of targeted persons have received pneumococcal vaccine; only about 30–40% have received influenza vaccine; and up to 66% of adults may lack adequate immunity to tetanus.

4. How can vaccination rates be improved?

Even though many opportunities have been missed to ensure adequate immunity to vaccine-preventable diseases among targeted persons in this country, many opportunities also exist for improving levels of immunity by increasing vaccination rates. Strategies to improve vaccination rates should address known contributors to successful vaccination efforts:

Patient Issues
- Physician's recommendation
- Access to provider
- Cost
- Awareness of disease severity, vaccine efficacy, and vaccine safety

Provider Issues
- Up-to-date knowledge about vaccines (recommendations, efficacy, side effects)
- Reimbursement
- Effective organizational structures in practice settings to ensure that vaccine is offered and administered (including patient identification, tracking, and recall systems)

Public Policy Issues
- Public and provider education
- Reimbursement
- Vaccine purchase and distribution
- Regulations requiring evidence of immunity in specific situations (e.g., school enrollment, college matriculation requirements, etc.)

5. What is the most important predictor of patient immunization compliance?

Studies have shown that a physician's recommendation for immunization is among the most potent predictors of patient behavior regarding immunization. For providers, strategies aimed at improving organizational structures within their practice setting seem to be most effective in improving vaccination rates.

6. What are special considerations with regard to vaccinations and the immunocompromised host?

Persons who are immunocompromised may be at increased risk for vaccine-preventable diseases. This risk is determined by the nature and severity of the underlying process. These persons may also be at increased risk for adverse reactions to live-virus vaccines because viral replication after administration of live virus vaccines can be enhanced in severely immunocompromised persons. Killed or inactivated vaccines, however, do not represent a danger to immunocompromised persons and therefore generally should be administered as recommended for otherwise healthy persons.

Most Common Vaccines: Live versus Killed or Inactivated

LIVE (ATTENUATED) VACCINES*	KILLED/INACTIVATED VACCINES[†]
Measles[‡]	Diphtheria
Mumps[‡]	Pertussis
Rubella[‡]	Tetanus (toxoid)
Oral polio vaccine	Hepatitis B
	Influenza
	Pneumococcal
	H. influenzae B
	Enhanced inactivated polio vaccine

*These vaccines may be contraindicated for certain immunocompromised persons.
[†]These vaccines are generally considered to be safe for administration to immunocompromised persons.
[‡]Including MMR.

The specific conditions that result in an impaired immune response and that are of special importance with reference to vaccines include:

A. Persons who are severely immunocompromised as a result of non-HIV diseases (e.g., congenital immunodeficiency, leukemia, lymphoma, generalized malignancy, therapy with alkylating agents, antimetabolites, radiation, or large amounts of corticosteroids)

B. Persons with HIV infection

C. Persons with conditions that cause limited immune deficits (e.g., asplenia, renal failure) that may require the use of special vaccines or higher doses but that do not contraindicate use of any particular vaccine, including live-virus vaccines.

Live-virus vaccines are contraindicated for persons in group A. In addition, oral polio vaccine should not be given to any household contact or nursing personnel in close contact with a severely immunocompromised person because of shedding of vaccine virus by the vaccine recipient. For persons in group B, oral polio vaccine should also be avoided; if there is need for administration of polio vaccine, then the enhanced inactivated form of the vaccine should be used (eIPV). MMR vaccine for persons in group B should be considered and administered when indicated. Limited studies of MMR in both asymptomatic and symptomatic HIV-infected persons have not documented serious or unusual adverse events after administration of this vaccine. For persons in group C, live-virus vaccines may be administered according to the usual schedules.

Persons with certain medical conditions that impair immune responses may be at increased risk for specific diseases. For these people, bacterial polysaccharide (especially pneumococcal vaccine) and influenza vaccines are often recommended. Some of the conditions include renal failure, asplenia, and diabetes.

7. What general precautions should be exercised in the use of vaccines in pregnant or potentially pregnant women?

Several general precautions exist for the use of vaccines during pregnancy. Because of potential risk to the developing fetus, live-virus vaccines (particularly MMR) usually should be avoided altogether both for pregnant women and for women who are likely to become pregnant within 3 months. In addition, while there is no convincing evidence of increased risk to the fetus from immunizing pregnant women with inactivated virus or bacteria vaccines or toxoids, it is nevertheless a reasonable precaution to delay, if possible, until the second or third trimester, the administration of any vaccine or toxoid that must be given during pregnancy. This would minimize any possible or theoretical risk of teratogenicity for the fetus. Tetanus/diphtheria toxoid and influenza vaccine, for example, may be administered to pregnant women in this fashion if otherwise indicated. All considerations regarding the use of vaccines during pregnancy should weigh the benefits to the mother and/or fetus against the possible risks; current immunization recommendations should be consulted before administering vaccines in this setting.

8. Which vaccines are recommended for health care providers?

Health care providers, including medical students, residents, and practicing physicians, are at increased risk for contracting and transmitting vaccine-preventable diseases such as influenza, measles, mumps, rubella, and hepatitis B. Accordingly, health care professionals should have adequate immunity against these diseases. Often this means that they should receive annual influenza immunization, two doses of MMR (unless they were born before 1957 or have other evidence of immunity as described above), and hepatitis B vaccine. In addition, it is prudent for health care professionals to receive tetanus/diphtheria boosters every 10 years.

9. Should you worry about adverse events caused by immunization?

Modern vaccines are remarkably safe and effective. Although adverse events have been reported following the administration of all vaccines, the most frequent events are usually minor, local reactions. Hypersensitivity reactions are uncommon following immunization and are almost always caused by hypersensitivity to one or more vaccine components: (1) animal protein (e.g., residual egg protein from egg-grown virus vaccines such as measles, mumps, and influenza vaccines); (2) antibiotics (e.g., trace neomycin found in MMR); (3) preservatives (e.g., thimerosal found in influenza vaccine); and (4) stabilizers. Other severe, systemic effects are rare, and often a cause-and-effect relationship between symptom and vaccine may be difficult or impossible to establish.

Even though serious side effects are uncommon, health care providers may encounter patients who have temporally-associated events serious enough to require medical attention. Since 1988, health care providers and vaccine manufacturers have been required by law to report certain of these adverse events following immunization with MMR or its component vaccines, DTP or its component vaccines, and polio vaccines. These events—and adverse events following administration of any vaccine—should be reported to the Vaccine Adverse Event Reporting System (VAERS) of the U.S. Department of Health and Human Services.

10. Identify common contraindications to administration of vaccines.
Contraindications include certain disease states (e.g., live-virus vaccines are contraindicated for severely immunocompromised persons); other medical conditions (e.g., live-virus vaccines are generally contraindicated during pregnancy); and known hypersensitivity to previous doses of vaccine or to vaccine components (e.g., persons with a history of anaphylactic reactions to eggs or egg products should not receive egg-grown virus vaccines such as mumps, measles, and influenza vaccines). In addition, severe reactions to previous doses may preclude subsequent doses of certain immunizations (e.g., encephalopathy occurring within 7 days of DTP vaccination).

Certain conditions are commonly **misunderstood** to be contraindications of administration of vaccines. Physicians and other health care providers should maintain up-to-date knowledge on vaccine components and the indications and contraindications for vaccine administration to ensure appropriate immunization activities in their practices. Sources for this information include current vaccine package inserts and vaccination recommendations from expert groups such as the Advisory Committee on Immunization Practices (ACIP) of the Public Health Service.

Situations that Do Not *Represent Contraindications to Vaccination*

- Reaction to a previous dose of DTP or other vaccine that involved only a mild to moderate local reaction or fever less than 40.5°C
- Mild acute upper respiratory or gastrointestinal illness with a fever less than 38°C
- Current antimicrobial therapy or the convalescent phase of illnesses
- Prematurity in an infant
- Pregnancy of a household contact
- Recent exposure to an infectious disease
- Breastfeeding
- Personal history of nonspecific allergies
- Family history of allergies or seizures

11. Describe some of the new developments in vaccine research.
Vaccine research is currently focusing on a number of areas including:
- The development of new vaccines (e.g., for AIDS, hepatitis A)
- Improvement of existing vaccines to enhance their immunogenicity (e.g., research on adjuvant vaccines to enhance the antigenic response to pneumococcal vaccine and the recent release of the conjugate form of the HIB vaccine)
- Improvement of existing vaccines to decrease associated side effects (e.g., the recent release of acellular pertussis vaccine, which is used for the fourth and fifth doses of routine childhood DTP vaccination)
- New ways to combine multiple antigens into a single vaccine to decrease the numbers of injections required for the adequate immunization of children (e.g., the recent licensing of the combination DTP and HIB conjugate vaccine)
- ACIP is considering recommendations for the routine vaccination of children and other persons against varicella (chickenpox).

12. Who should be screened for HIV infection?

HIV infection, including acquired immunodeficiency syndrome (AIDS), is now the sixth leading cause of years of potential life lost in the United States, and the number of persons diagnosed with AIDS increases each year. It is estimated that 1–1.5 million persons are infected with HIV in the United States, and that 0.3–6.0% of persons receiving care in acute-care hospitals are HIV positive. Persons at increased risk for HIV and for whom screening may be indicated include persons receiving treatment for sexually transmitted diseases, homosexual/ bisexual men, intravenous drug users, persons with a history of multiple sexual partners or prostitution, residence or birth in an area with high prevalence of HIV infection, persons undergoing treatment for tuberculosis or drug abuse, and a history of a blood transfusion between 1978 and 1985. Some authorities also recommend offering HIV tests to pregnant women, particularly in areas of high HIV seroprevalence.

13. What considerations must be taken into account when ordering an HIV test?

Screening is usually performed initially with an enzyme-linked immunosorbent assay (ELISA), which detects antibodies to HIV. Even though this test reportedly has a sensitivity and specificity of about 99%, because of the implications of false-positive results, the ELISA test should be repeated before being reported as positive. Positive ELISA results should then be confirmed by the Western blot test before a diagnosis of HIV infection is made (if the true prevalence of HIV positivity in a population were 0.5%, even with 99% sensitivity and specificity, the positive predictive value of a single ELISA would be only 33%). In addition, because it may take 6–12 weeks after an exposure for a person to develop detectable antibodies to HIV, persons with a history of a recent, significant exposure and an initial negative ELISA test should be considered for re-testing. All screening should be accompanied by appropriate counseling and informed consent; persons with positive tests should receive additional information, counseling, and follow-up as appropriate, and should be informed of the need to notify sexual partners, persons with whom intravenous needles have been shared, and others at risk of exposure. All seropositive cases should be reported to local public health officials according to state guidelines.

14. Which populations are at high risk for tuberculosis?

In contrast to the steady decline in incidence of tuberculosis (TB) from 1953 through 1984, over the past 9 years there has been a 20% increase in cases of tuberculosis, with more than 28,000 excess cases being reported from 1985 through 1990 alone. Adverse social and economic factors, the HIV epidemic, and immigration of persons with TB infection are contributing factors. Screening programs should focus on high-risk populations, including:

- Persons with HIV infection
- Household members and close contacts of persons with known or suspected TB, including health care workers with significant exposures or increased risk of exposure
- Persons with medical risk factors known to increase the risk of disease, including diabetes mellitus, conditions requiring prolonged high-dose corticosteroid therapy, gastrectomy, and chronic renal failure
- Foreign-born persons from countries with high TB prevalence, including migrant and seasonal farm workers
- Medically underserved low-income populations, including high-risk racial and ethnic minorities
- Alcoholics and intravenous drug users
- Residents of long-term care facilities, correctional institutions, mental institutions, nursing homes/facilities, and homeless shelters

15. What are the screening methods for TB?

The tuberculin skin test is the standard method for demonstrating tuberculous infection. The most commonly used formulation of tuberculin is purified protein derivative (PPD), and the usual dose administered is 5 tuberculin unit (TU) dose (.1 mm of PPD). The tuberculin may be administered intracutaneously (Mantoux test) or with the multiple-puncture technique and should be read at 48 and 72 hours after injection. The tuberculin skin tests are interpreted according to the amount of induration at the injection site. Persons are considered to have positive reactions with the Mantoux test in the following situations:

Induration ≥5 mm
- Persons with HIV infection
- Close contacts of infectious cases
- Persons with chest radiographs with fibrotic lesions

Induration ≥10 mm
- All other persons with risk factors for TB

Induration ≥15 mm
- All other persons

For persons who received the multiple-puncture test, any vesicular reaction is considered positive. All papular reactions from the multiple-puncture test should be followed by a Mantoux test for further diagnostic evaluation.

Persons with positive skin reactions should be evaluated further to assess whether they have active disease. This evaluation usually includes a clinical examination, chest radiographs, and sputum smear examination. Based on this further evaluation, decisions are then made about the need for antimicrobial prophylaxis or treatment. All cases of active TB should be reported to the local public health official according to state guidelines.

16. Which sexually transmitted diseases (STDs) require screening?

STDs that Require Screening

DISEASE	POPULATIONS TO BE SCREENED
HIV	See above (question 12).
Hepatitis B	Pregnant women at first prenatal visit. Test may be repeated in the third trimester for high-risk persons (intravenous drug users, persons exposed to hepatitis B).
Syphilis	Prostitutes, persons who engage in sex with multiple partners in areas in which syphilis is prevalent, persons undergoing treatment for STDs, sexual contacts of persons with syphilis, and pregnant women at first prenatal visit and additional testing at 28 weeks or later for women at increased risk for acquiring syphilis during pregnancy. Depending on local prevalence rates, other high-risk populations may also benefit from screening such as jail or prison inmates.
Gonorrhea	Prostitutes, persons with multiple sexual partners, sexual contacts of persons with gonorrhea, persons with history of repeated episodes of gonorrhea, persons undergoing treatment for other STDs, and pregnant women at first prenatal visit with repeat testing later in pregnancy if the woman is at increased risk for acquiring gonorrhea during the pregnancy.
Chlamydia	Persons who attend clinics for STDs, persons who attend other high-risk health care facilities (e.g., adolescent and family planning clinics), or persons who have other risk factors (age <20, multiple sexual partners, have sexual partner with more multiple sexual contacts). Pregnant women with other risk factors should be screened at the first prenatal visit.

To ensure adequate partner notification, all newly identified cases of STDs should be reported to the local public health officials according to state guidelines.

17. Which tests should be used in screening for syphilis?

Tests used for screening for syphilis include treponemal tests (which detect antibodies against *Treponema pallidum* or its components) and nontreponemal tests (which detect antibodies directed against lipoidal antigens). The main nontreponemal tests are the Venereal Disease

Research Laboratory (VDRL) and rapid plasma reagin (RPR) tests. The main treponemal tests are the fluorescent treponemal antibody absorption test (FTA-ABS) and microhemagglutination test (e.g., MHA-TP). The VDRL or RPR tests usually become reactive at some time during primary syphilis, remain at a peak in the first year of infection, and then fall slowly thereafter. After adequate treatment, the patient usually becomes seronegative after 6–12 months, depending on the duration of infection. The FTA-ABS and MHA-TP tests usually become reactive during primary syphilis and remain reactive for the patient's lifetime, regardless of treatment. For asymptomatic persons, screening is usually done with the VDRL or RPR tests, with confirmation of positive tests by a treponemal test.

18. For which infectious diseases should pregnant women be screened?
Screening during pregnancy should take into account the particular risk profile of the patient. Routine screening for hepatitis B, syphilis, and gonorrhea is recommended because of the potential risk to the newborn. Pregnant women with risk factors for HIV infection should receive an HIV test. Some authorities recommend offering HIV tests to all pregnant women, particularly in areas with high HIV seroprevalence. Screening for other STDs such as chlamydia should be undertaken if the woman has other risk factors for the disease. In addition to being screened for STDs, pregnant women should also routinely be screened for rubella. If the woman is seronegative, then the vaccine should be administered after delivery but before discharge from the hospital (such women should be counselled to avoid conception for 3 months following vaccination).

BIBLIOGRAPHY

1. American College of Physicians Task Force on Adult Immunization and Infectious Diseases Society of America: Guide for Adult Immunizations, 2nd ed. Philadelphia, American College of Physicians, 1990.
2. Beneson AS (ed): Control of Communicable Diseases in Man. Washington: American Public Health Association, 1990.
3. Centers for Disease Control and Prevention: Public health burden of vaccine-preventable diseases among adults: Standards for adult immunization practice. MMWR 39:725–729, 1990.
4. Centers for Disease Control and Prevention: Standards for pediatric immunization practices. MMWR 42(RR-5), 1993.
5. Centers for Disease Control and Prevention: General recommendations on immunization. MMWR 43(RR-1), 1994.
6. Immunization Practices Advisory Committee: Update on adult immunization. MMWR 40(RR-12), 1991.
7. Peter G: Childhood immunizations. N Engl J Med 327:1794–1800, 1992.
8. U.S. Preventive Services Task Force: Guide to Clinical Preventive Services. Baltimore, Williams & Wilkins, 1989.
9. Williams WW, Hickson MA, Kane MA, et al: Immunization policies and vaccine coverage among adults: The risk for missed opportunities. Ann Intern Med 108:616–625, 1988.

ADDITIONAL REFERENCES ON SPECIFIC TOPICS

10. Advisory Committee for the Elimination of Tuberculosis: Screening for tuberculosis and tuberculous infection in high-risk populations. MMWR 39(RR-8), 1990.
11. Advisory Committee on Immunization Practices (ACIP): Pertussis vaccination: Acellular pertussis vaccine for the fourth and fifth doses of the DTP series: Update to supplementary ACIP statement. MMWR 41(RR-15), 1992.
12. Advisory Committee on Immunization Practices: Use of vaccines and immune globulins for persons with altered immunocompetence. MMWR 42(RR-4), 1993.
13. Advisory Council for the Elimination of Tuberculosis: Prevention and control of tuberculosis in US communities with at-risk minority populations and prevention and control of tuberculosis among homeless persons. MMWR 41(RR-5), 1992.
14. Advisory Council for the Elimination of Tuberculosis: Prevention and control of tuberculosis in migrant farm workers. MMWR 41(RR-10), 1992.
15. American Thoracic Society: Diagnostic standards and classification of tuberculosis, 1990. Am Rev Respir Dis 1990 142:725–735, 1990.

16. Centers for Disease Control and Prevention: Recommendations for HIV testing and services for inpatients and outpatients in acute-care hospital settings. MMWR 42(RR-2):1–6, 1993.
17. Centers for Disease Control and Prevention: Recommendations for the prevention and management of *Chlamydia trachomatis* infections. MMWR 42(RR-12), 1993.
18. Centers for Disease Control and Prevention, 1993: Sexually transmitted diseases treatment guidelines. MMWR 42(RR-14), 1993.
19. Centers for Disease Control: Vaccine adverse event reporting system—United States. MMWR 39:730–733, 1990.
20. Hart G: Syphilis tests in diagnostic and therapeutic decision making. Ann Intern Med 104:368–376, 1986.
21. Immunization Practices Advisory Committee: *Haemophilus b* conjugate vaccines for prevention of *Haemophilus influenzae* type b disease among infants and children two months of age and older. MMWR 40(RR-1), 1991.
22. Immunization Practices Advisory Committee: Hepatitis B virus: A comprehensive strategy for eliminating transmission in the United States through universal childhood vaccination. MMWR 40(RR-13), 1991.
23. Immunization Practices Advisory Committee: Measles prevention. MMWR 38(S-9), 1989.
24. Immunization Practices Advisory Committee: Pertussis vaccination: Acellular pertussis vaccine for reinforcing and booster use—Supplementary ACIP statement. MMWR 41(RR-1), 1992.
25. Immunization Practices Advisory Committee. Rubella prevention. MMWR 39(RR-15), 1990.

5. ETHNIC DIVERSITY AND DISEASE

Irene Aguilar, M.D.

1. What is an ethnic group?

An ethnic group is an aggregate of people who share a real or presumed common origin, a mutual historical past, and cultural symbols or social norms that shape the thought and behavior of individual members. Examples of symbols and norms include values (family dynamics), beliefs (religion), customs (food preferences, holidays), behaviors (sex roles), and language or distinctive dialects. Ethnic groups usually have a shared sense of identity within the larger social system.

2. What is the difference between "behavioral" and "ideological" ethnicity?

With behavioral ethnicity, values, beliefs, behavioral norms, and languages are learned during growth and development. Here ethnicity permeates all interactions. In the United States this is seen primarily in first- and second-generation residents and by ethnic minorities with a history of exclusion from the mainstream (e.g., blacks, Hispanics, and Native Americans). Ideological ethnicity is based mainly on customs that are not central to a person's daily functioning but are symbols of a cultural heritage. This involves voluntary identification, such as observance of holiday customs and celebrations among third- or fourth-generation white ethnic immigrants (e.g., Germans).

3. How commonly might ethnic minority groups be encountered in primary care settings?

The 1990 Census demonstrates significant changes in the population of the United States. The white majority is shrinking and aging; many of the minority ethnic populations are young and growing. In California there is expected to be a "minority majority" by 2005.

	% Total Population	% Population below Poverty
Black	12.1	31
Hispanic	9	21.5
Asian and Pacific	2.9	12.2
Native Americans	0.8	19–45
Whites	80.3	10

The black population increased by 13.2% from 1980 to 1990. There is no breakdown by country of origin. Black Americans have been in the U.S. since as early as 1619.

The Hispanic population, which includes Spanish-origin people of any race (black or white), increased by 53% from 1980 to 1990. The greatest numbers of the Hispanic population are of Mexican-American descent—62.6%. Puerto Rican—11.1%, Cuban—4.9%, and Central and South American—13.7% make up most of the remainder.

Asian and Pacific Islander populations increased by 108% from 1980–1990. Of these, 24% are Chinese, 21% Filipino, 10% Japanese, 10% Asian Indians, 10% Korean, 7% Vietnamese, 3.4% Hawaiian, 1.2% Samoan, and 1% Gaumians.

The Native-American, Eskimo, and Aleut populations in the United States increased by 37.7% from 1980 to 1990. The majority (96%) are American Indians, 3% are Eskimos, and 1% are Aleuts. The percentage of people who fell below the poverty level in 1990 varied from a high of 44.8% for reservation Indians to a "low" of 19.5% for Aleuts.

By contrast, the white population of the United States (and this includes Hispanics who may be of any race) constitutes 80.3% of the total population. This represents a population increase of 6% from 1980, but an overall 3% decrease of the total population. Ten percent of white persons were below the poverty level in 1990.

4. Why is it difficult to study health patterns or clinical research in ethnic groups?

Although technically different, ethnicity and social class are closely interrelated in the United States, making it difficult to interpret clinical research on health patterns of ethnic groups.

5. Why is it important to recognize ethnic diversity in the care of patients?

1. **Ethnic groups may vary in rates of morbidity and mortality for specific diseases.** These differences may result from: biases in vital statistics; nonbehavioral factors, such as genetic predisposition; shared risk factors (largely due to class membership) such as poverty, poor nutrition, or exposure to different pathogenic agents; or from ethnically patterned pathogenic cultural standards or behaviors. Specific diseases may have different prognoses solely dependent on ethnic status.

2. **Ethnicity influences concepts of disease and illness, which in turn influence other aspects of health behavior, i.e., how symptoms are perceived, evaluated, and acted upon (or not acted upon).** Problems in patient interactions or compliance may be ameliorated by an understanding of traditional beliefs. Fundamental differences often exist between the health beliefs of health care providers and patients. Understanding the patient's behavior and beliefs may allow physicians to comfortably ask patients their interpretation of symptoms and potential remedies. These recognitions allow the health care provider to meet the patient's needs more effectively.

3. **Ethnicity affects utilization of mainstream medical services.** This may be evident by the location of mainstream care (i.e., emergency room, hospital, clinic). Ethnic residential segregation may result in patient populations in hospitals, clinics, or private practices composed preponderantly of specific local ethnic groups. Use of alternative providers of health care before, during, or after accessing mainstream care may occur. Providers should be familiar with formal and informal sources of help that exist outside the traditional medical community.

4. **Ethnicity often dictates styles of interaction.** Attitudes toward authority figures, gender roles, and ways of expressing emotion and asking for help are carried into health-care situations. For example, Southeast Asians expect health professionals to be experts and consequently tend not to contribute much information and do not question or oppose authority figures openly so as not to offend or embarass them.

By knowing and respecting ethnically determined factors, physicians can tailor interventions to meet the patient's needs.

6. A 62-year-old Native-American man with constipation has seen a medicine man and was prescribed medicinal herbs for his symptoms, but his wife insisted he see you. Should you change his treatment?

Recognition of the health beliefs and practices of local ethnic groups permits the physician to gain patient trust and avoid creating a feeling of alienation in the patient. Every effort should be made to combine folk treatment with standard Western treatment, as long as the two are not antagonistic and as long as the patient will come to no harm with the prescribed folk therapy. If the regimen is harmful, you might suggest that because this treatment has not seemed to work, something else might be tried.

7. A 28-year-old Mexican-American woman comes to see you for the sixth time in 3 months, complaining of restlessness, insomnia, anorexia, anergia, and anhedonia. After a comprehensive evaluation, you treat her for depression, with little apparent improvement in her symptoms. To which specialist should you refer her?

She should be referred to a traditional Mexican-American healer, a *curandero*. *Curanderos* believe in both natural and supernatural illness and often refer patients to traditional physicians if they feel they are unable to diagnose and treat a natural illness. *Curanderos* deal with problems of a social, psychological and/or spiritual nature as well as physical ailments.

The most likely diagnosis here is susto. *Susto* involves "soul loss" and is a folk illness believed to arise from fright. The "soul" is believed to have left the body to wander freely as a result of a dream or a particularly traumatic event. The symptoms of the disease, listed above, may also include hallucinations and various painful sensations. The *curandero* coaxes the soul back into the person's body through prayer, barridas (sweeping over the body), and herb teas.

Other common Mexican-American folk illnesses are:

Empacho: an illness caused by a ball of food sticking to the wall of the stomach. Symptoms include stomachache, cramps, anorexia, diarrhea, and vomiting. Massaging the stomach, pinching the spine, and drinking a purgative tea are commonly prescribed by the *curandero*.

Mal ojo (evil eye): an illness to which all children are susceptible. It results from an admiring or covetous look from a person with a "strong" eye. Symptoms are vomiting, fever, crying, and restlessness. The evil eye may be prevented if the person with the strong eye touches the child as he admires him, or by the wearing of protective amulets. The illness is treated by a *curandero* using a barrida and prayer.

Envidia (envy) is considered to be a cause of illness and bad luck. If one's success provokes the envy of friends and neighbors, misfortune can befall him and his family.

8. An elderly Cambodian woman comes to see you for diarrhea. On physical examination you notice cigarette burns on her abdomen. She is not a smoker. Should you report her family to adult protective services?

No. Cigarette burns are a traditional method of folk healing seen in Asian populations. Moxibustion and/or dermabrasive practices are one of the Chinese folk remedies widely practiced among Vietnamese, Khmer, Hmong, and Mien peoples. The dermal methods are seen as ways to relieve headaches, muscle pains, sinusitis, colds, sore throat, coughs, difficulty breathing, diarrhea, or fever. **Burning**, touching a cigarette or piece of burning cotton to the skin, usually the abdomen, is done to compensate for "heat" lost through diarrhea. **Cupping** involves placing a heated cup on the skin; as it cools, it contracts and draws the skin and excess energy or "wind" or toxicity into the cup. This procedure leaves circular ecchymoses on the skin. **Pinching** produces bruises or welts at the site of treatment. **Rubbing** of skin with a spoon or coin is done to bring the toxic "wind" to the body surface and also produces bruises or welts.

Other traditional practices used by Asians include acupuncture, massage, and herbal concoctions and poultices. These practices rarely represent a threat to the person and almost always nurture their sense of being cared for and their ability to actively alleviate bothersome symptoms.

These remedies relate to Chinese theories of health as a state of balance among the different components of the body and of the body with its environment. Therapeutic diets require consideration of the "hot" or "cold" natures of foods, cooking methods, and the person's ailment. The various parts of the human body correspond to the dualistic principles of "yin" and "yang" and must be kept in harmony.

9. How do you recognize cutaneous color-related signs in dark-skinned persons?

Very few signs cannot be recognized in dark-skinned persons with proper technique. Lighting (nonglare daylight), positioning (examine part of body at heart level), environmental temperature, and the person's emotional state all contribute to an accurate exam in any patient. Color changes are best observed where pigmentation from melanin, melanoid, and carotene is least: the sclera, conjunctiva, nail beds, lips, buccal mucosa, tongue, palms, and soles (unless heavily calloused). Blacks commonly have brown freckle-like pigmentation of the gums, buccal cavity, border of the tongue, and even the nail beds.

Jaundice is best seen in sclera. However, many darkly pigmented patients have heavy deposits of subconjunctival fat which may mimic jaundice. Therefore, if inspection of the portion revealed naturally by the lid slit reveals icterus, then inspection to the edges of the cornea and of the posterior portion of the hard palate should be undertaken.

Pallor is best diagnosed by the absence of underlying red tones, so the brown skin appears more yellowish brown and black skin appears ashen gray. The conjunctivae are also an excellent place to assess pallor.

Petechiae are more easily seen on the abdomen, buttocks, and volar surface of the forearm. In very dark brown skin, they may be more difficult to see except in mucous membranes.

Cyanosis is the most difficult to diagnose. The mucous membranes show bluish discoloration. Applying light pressure to create pallor and observing for the return of color, and following the exam serially over time are helpful approaches.

10. A 24-year-old Laotian woman comes to see you for a physical examination before getting pregnant. How does her ethnic background influence your search for possible disease or prevention considerations?

Knowledge of an ethnic group's genetic disorders and disease prevalences can strongly influence evaluation. The following six potential diagnoses should be considered in light of her desire to become pregnant.

1. **Hemoglobinopathies.** Microcytosis in persons of Southeast Asian origin is most commonly related to alpha- and beta-thalassemia and hemoglobin E carrier states. A study of Southeast Asians in California found that 8% of persons from Viet Nam and 3% of those from Cambodia and Laos have the beta-thalassemia trait; 36% of refugees from Cambodia and 28% of those from Laos were carriers of the hemoglobin E trait. Correct diagnosis is necessary in order to provide genetic counseling and avoid inappropriate treatment of carriers with iron (risking iron overload) for microcytic anemia.

2. **G6PD deficiency**

3. **Lactose intolerance**

4. **Hepatitis B carrier state.** The carrier state for hepatitis B was as high as 8.6% in one study of this population.

5. **Parasitic infestation.** As many as 35% of Southeast Asian refugees will have positive stool for parasites.

6. **Tuberculosis.** Up to 52% have a positive PPD. The age-specific incidence of tuberculosis is 14–70 times higher than that for the U.S. population as a whole. Drug resistance is common.

11. Which chronic illness disproportionately affects Hispanics? Why?

The prevalence of diabetes is 1.7 to 2.4 times higher in Hispanics at all age groups than in non-Hispanic whites. Among 65- to 74-year-olds, diabetes is present in 33% of Hispanics (compared to 17% of non-Hispanic whites and 25% of non-Hispanic blacks). The age-adjusted death rate from diabetes is twice as high in Hispanics as in non-Hispanic whites.

The excess prevalence is believed to be related to multiple factors, including the high incidence of obesity, hyperinsulinemia, family history, and the high frequency of Native-American genes in Hispanics.

Despite the excess prevalence, macrovascular complications are not increased in Hispanics. However, microvascular complications of retinopathy, nephropathy, and neuropathy have been found to be increased in Mexican-Americans.

12. How has AIDS affected ethnic minorities?
Many ethnic minority populations are disproportionately affected by AIDS compared with the proportion of the U.S. population they represent. In 1991 blacks represented 33.3% of AIDS cases but only 12.1% of the U.S. population, whereas Hispanics represented 14.7% of AIDS cases but only 9.0% of the total population.

This disparity is even greater among women and children. Hispanic and black women of childbearing age represented 74.4% of all reported AIDS cases in women through 1989. Hispanic and black children accounted for 75.1% of all childhood AIDS cases through 1989. Intravenous drug use represents the primary route of HIV transmission in these populations.

In 1990 HIV disease became the leading cause of death for black men between the ages of 35 and 44, and the second leading cause of death for black men and women between the ages of 25 and 35, and remains so currently.

13. What is the major health problem of Native Americans?
Alcohol abuse is the major cause of morbidity and mortality in the Native-American community. Alcohol abuse contributes to death and illnesses from accidents, suicide, homicide, diabetes, congenital anomalies in infants, pneumonia, heart disease, and cancer. Alcoholism has been implicated in 50% of adult crime on Indian reservations. There is a high rate of unintentional injuries as well as chronic liver disease and cirrhosis-related deaths in Native Americans. The incidence of fetal alcohol syndrome is 4 per 1000 live births in Native Americans and Alaska Natives compared to 0.8 per 1000 live births in black Americans.

14. What factors contribute to alcoholism in American Indians?
A multifactorial etiology of alcohol abuse includes genetic, physiologic, and social factors. Native Americans may be genetically predisposed to crave ever-increasing doses of alcohol during a rapid loss of control of their senses. There are differences in alcohol absorption and metabolism between Native Americans and whites. Passive aggressiveness and emotional repression as well as socioeconomic conditions and failure to develop social sanctions against drunkenness contribute to alcoholism. Self-esteem of Native Americans is often very low, perhaps related to inadequate formal education, poverty, and a traditional value system that has been ignored by the dominant society.

CONTROVERSY

15. Are American blacks at increased risk for cardiovascular morbidity and mortality?
Many recent articles have addressed racial disparity in morbidity and mortality from heart disease. Two studies from the southeastern United States suggest that black men may be relatively protected from coronary disease. A more recent study in Chicago suggests that blacks are at increased risk for sudden death and have lower survival rates than whites.

Excess morbidity and mortality may more importantly be related to unequal access to treatment. Three major reasons should be acknowledged:

1. **Lack of a primary care physician.** Black patients are more likely to use the emergency room as a source of primary care and hence be seen for noncardiac chest pain or cardiac chest pain without adequate treatment. Likewise, they are more often seen for severe, uncontrolled hypertension in emergency rooms. Hypertension remains uncontrolled due to poor follow-up, lack of health insurance, and poor compliance with medication due to cost, dosing frequency, or lack of knowledge about the severity of illness.

2. **The patient may lack knowledge of signs and symptoms of cardiovascular disease.** Blacks are less likely to go to an emergency room within 6 hours of an acute myocardial infarction, resulting in poor outcome of therapy.

3. **Black patients are less likely to be aggressively evaluated and treated for cardiovascular disease.** Blacks are less likely than whites to undergo a wide range of major medical procedures, including cardiac catheterization. This difference has not been explained by variable

disease severity, type of hospital, or socioeconomic status. The black/white disparity in the use of procedures is greatest when decision making is less clearly dictated by the clinical situation. Additionally, white patients may be more likely to request procedures, whereas black patients may refuse recommended treatment. This reluctance may reflect poor communication about treatment options between physicians and black patients. Physicians must make an effort to explain and offer choices in a nonbiased, ethnically accessible way.

BIBLIOGRAPHY

1. Ayanian JZ: Heart disease in black and white. N Engl J Med 329:656, 1993.
2. Becker LB, et al: Racial differences in the incidence of cardiac arrest and subsequent survival. N Engl J Med 329:600, 1993.
3. Buchwald D, Carolis PV, Gany F, et al: Five vignettes of cross-cultural care. Patient Care 28:120–123, 1994.
4. Chesney AP, et al: Mexican American folk medicine: Implications for the family physician. J Fam Pract 11(4):567, 1980.
5. Gayle JA, et al: Surveillance for AIDS and HIV infection among Black and Hispanic children and women of childbearing age, 1981–1989. MMWR 39(ss-30), 1990.
6. Harwood A (ed): Ethnicity and Medical Care. Cambridge, MA, Harvard University Press, 1981.
7. Henderson G, Primeaux M (eds): Transcultural Health Care. Menlo Park, CA, Addison-Wesley, 1981.
8. Johnson PA, et al: Effect of race on the presentation and management of patients with acute chest pain. Ann Intern Med 118:593, 1993.
9. Lamarine R: The dilemma of native American health. Health Educ 20:15, 1989.
10. Lamarine R: Alcohol abuse among native Americans. J Commun Health 13:143, 1988.
11. Lin-Fu JS: Population characteristics and health care needs of Asian Pacific Americans. Public Health Rep 103:18, 1988.
12. Muecke MA: Caring for Southeast Asian refugee patients in the USA. Am J Public Health 73:431, 1983.
13. Roach LB: Color changes in dark skin. In Henderson G, Primeaux M (eds): Transcultural Health Care. Menlo Park, CA, Addison-Wesley, 1981.
14. Shea S, et al: Predisposing factors for severe, uncontrolled hypertension in an inner city minority population. N Eng J Med 327:776, 1992.
15. Smith DK: HIV disease as a cause of death for African Americans in 1987 and 1990. J Natl Med Assoc 84:481, 1992.
16. Spector RE: Cultural Diversity of Health and Illness. Norwalk, Appleton & Lange, 1991.
17. Stern MP, Haffner MP: Type II diabetes and its complications in Mexican Americans. Diabetes Metab Rev 6(1):29, 1990.
18. Trotter RT II, Chavira JA: Curanderismo: An ethnic theoretical perspective of Mexican-American folk medicine. Med Anthropol Fall 1980, p 423.
19. U.S. Congress, Office of Technology Assessment. Indian Health Care, OTA-H-290. Washington, DC, U.S. Government Printing Office, 1986.
20. Whittle J, et al: Racial differences in the use of invasive procedures in the Department of Veterans Affairs medical system. N Engl J Med 329:621, 1993.
21. 1990 Census of Population and Housing. Summary tape file 1c (computer file). Washington, DC, Bureau of the Census, Data Users Services Division, 1992.

II. Behavioral Medicine

6. DEPRESSION

Edmund Casper, M.D., and Allan Liebgott, M.D.

1. How frequently does the primary care provider encounter patients with clinically relevant depression?

The prevalence of depressive disorders in primary care practice may be greater than 20% and even higher in patients with chronic medical illnesses. Among adolescents, the prevalence is approximately 5%. Thus, the primary care provider must recognize depressive disorders, be comfortable providing the first level of care, and recognize danger signs and symptoms that require referral to a psychiatrist.

2. Describe the spectrum of depression.

Depression ranges from normal signs of bereavement to major depression accompanied by frank psychoses. Major depression is usually an episodic illness, often beginning in adolescence, with remissions and exacerbations throughout life. A chronic form of less severe depression without acute major episodes is termed dysthymia. Patients with depression may have a bipolar manic-depressive disorder.

3. What is the epidemiology of depression?

Depression occurs more frequently in women than men. The incidence decreases with age in women but increases with age in men and is higher among single individuals. Depression is inversely related to social class but shows no racial, urban, or rural predilection. Major depressive episodes frequently follow a stressful life event in predisposed individuals.

4. How can the primary care provider recognize depression?

1. By recognition of classic symptoms: depressed mood accompanied by changes in sleep patterns, weight, and/or energy level and feelings of hopelessness, loss of self worth, and/or disinterest in usual activities.

2. By the responses to screening questionnaires on routine physician visits. Routine questionnaires for new patients should include items related to depression or a standard depression screening test (such as the Center for Epidemiologic Studies Depression Scale).

3. By carefully pursuing concomitant depression in patients who abuse alcohol or drugs. Up to one-third of substance abusers have concurrent mood disorders.

4. By suspecting depression in patients who somaticize. Patients who are depressed may present with physical symptoms that cannot be supported by the severity or diagnosis of a physical disorder. Such vague symptoms as dizziness, headache, palpitations, or other complaints that result in multiple physician visits should suggest depression.

5. By being alert to medical conditions with a high rate of accompanying depression (see question 8).

5. What criteria lead to a diagnosis of a major depressive episode?

The diagnosis requires the 2-week presence of depressed mood and/or disinterest, accompanied by four of the following:

Weight changes	Feelings of worthlessness or guilt
Sleep disturbances	Poor concentration
Daily fatigue	Thoughts of death
Observed psychomotor agitation or retardation	

The depression should not be due to loss of a loved one or other organic causes. The patient should not carry a diagnosis of schizophrenia or other psychotic disorders. Although severe depression may be accompanied by psychotic symptoms (e.g., delusional thinking—hallucinations), such symptoms should not be seen in the absence of depression.

6. Describe manifestations of depression in the child or adolescent.
Children and adolescents may have symptoms similar to adults, including substance abuse and hypochondriasis. Depression also should be suspected with mood irritability, difficulty in family relationships or with the law, or fall in school grades.

7. How does one distinguish between normal depressive reaction to loss of a loved one and a major depressive episode?
Definitive distinction between bereavement and major depression may be difficult, because grieving may result in all of the symptoms of a major depression. However, prolonged symptoms that lead to a significant threat to health should be treated similarly to a major depressive episode.

8. Which medical diseases are associated with a high incidence of depression?

	Approximate Prevalence (%)
1. Stroke	50
2. Chronic fatigue syndrome	50
3. Diabetes mellitus	30
4. Malignancies (especially of the pancreas or lung)	25
5. Myocardial infarction	25
6. Rheumatoid arthritis	20

Reference: Katon W, Sullivan MD: Depression and chronic medical illness. J Clin Psychiatry 51 (Suppl 6):3–11, 1990.

9. Which drugs are particularly likely to induce depression?
Drugs that may frequently precipitate depression include the phenothiazines, steroids, propranolol, cimetidine, levodopa, indomethacin, and withdrawal from CNS stimulants.

10. Which persons are at highest risk for suicide?
1. Persons who have developed a specific plan for suicide
2. Persons who are socially isolated
3. Elderly men
4. Substance abusers
5. Persons with terminal malignancies

11. How does the patient's personal or family history aid in the diagnosis of depression?
A history of mood disorder in a first-degree relative or a major previous depression predisposes the patient to depression.

12. How should patients with major depression be treated?
Patients with a major depressive episode should be treated pharmacologically. Although many drugs are available, the primary care physician should restrict therapy to widely accepted agents. Although tricyclic antidepressants are the traditional drug of choice, the physician also should consider agents that have resulted in improvement in previous episodes. Therapy should be continued for 6–12 months; the highest risk of recurrence occurs within 2 months of tapering off medication.

Drug therapy for patients with less severe depression or dysthymia has been less effective. Behavior therapy and/or self-help groups may be as effective as antidepressants in patients with mild-to-moderate depression.

13. Does therapy for depression differ in patients with comorbid medical illness and other patients with major depression?

Aggressive therapy of the underlying illness and return to function may ameliorate depression caused by illness. However, specific therapy for depression may be needed to allow complete return to health.

14. What response is anticipated with treatment?

Approximately 65% of patients with depression respond to therapy with one or more agents. However, the chance of recurrence is high; the majority of patients experience a recurrent episode and one-fourth follow a chronic course with debilitating symptoms.

15. Describe the mortality and morbidity associated with major depression.

Up to 15% of patients with recurrent major depressive disorders die of suicide, and over three-quarters of completed suicides occur in patients with major mood disorders. In medical patients major depression or dysthymia causes greater disability than hypertension, diabetes, arthritis, and chronic lung disease. In addition, untreated patients with chronic depression often function poorly.

16. Which patients with major depression should be referred to a psychiatrist?

1. Patients who are suicidal
2. Patients who have a past history of mania or who become manic on antidepressive therapy
3. Patients with accompanying psychosis
4. Patients who show no response to treatment after 4 weeks

17. What are the side effects of tricyclic antidepressant drugs (TCAs)?

As a class, TCAs cause sedation, postural hypotension, and anticholinergic effects (dry mouth, urinary retention, tachycardia, constipation). Newer drugs (such as nortriptyline or desipramine) have fewer side effects than older drugs (amitriptyline, imipramine, doxepin) and may be less expensive than second-generation antidepressants. Before beginning therapy patients should undergo a physical exam, and have normal values on hemogram, liver function tests, and electrocardiogram. Side effects may be minimized by initiating therapy with lower doses and slowly reaching therapeutic doses by 7–10 days. Elderly patients should be treated with 30–50% of recommended doses. Full therapeutic efficacy is not reached for up to 28 days.

18. When are TCAs contraindicated or likely to prove problematic?

Contraindicated:

1. In patients with cardiac conduction defects, TCAs have a quinidinelike effect and may induce arrhythmias; thus, alternative drugs should be used.
2. In patients with narrow-angle glaucoma, because of the anticholinergic effects of TCAs.

Problematic:

1. In patients with preexisting conditions that may be exacerbated by TCAs. Prostatism and mild congestive heart failure may worsen because of the anticholinergic effects (urinary retention and tachycardia, respectively).
2. In patients taking phenothiazines, cimetidine, and other anticholinergics (e.g., antihistamines), TCAs should be used cautiously and at lower doses. Patients also should be instructed to refrain from alcohol.

19. What is the advantage of newer second-generation antidepressants?

Newer agents include drugs that are tricyclic derivatives or inhibit uptake of serotonin and have fewer anticholinergic side effects, including less effect on the cardiac conduction system.

Examples include fluoxetine, bupropion, sertraline, and paroxetine. Several of the newer agents have demonstrated an efficacy similar to that of TCAs . Despite their promise, their cost requires careful consideration.

BIBLIOGRAPHY

1. Frank E, Prien RF, Jarrett RB, et al: Conceptualization and rationale for consensus definitions of terms in major depressive disorder. Arch Gen Psychiatry 48:851, 1991.
2. Judd LL, Britton KT, Braff DL: Mental disorders. In Isselbacher KJ, et al (eds): Harrison's Principles of Internal Medicine, 13th ed. New York, McGraw-Hill, 1994, pp 2400–2420.
3. Katon W, Sullivan MD: Depression and chronic medical illness. J Clin Psychiatry 51(Suppl 6):3–11, 1990.
4. McGreery JF, Franco K: Depression in the elderly: The role of the primary care physician in management. J Gen Intern Med 3:498–507, 1988.
5. Michaels R, Marzuk PM: Progress in psychiatry. N Engl J Med 329:552, 628, 1993.
6. Stewart Al: Functional status and well-being of patients with chronic conditions. Results from the medical outcomes study. JAMA 262:907, 1989.

7. SLEEP DISORDERS

Eric McFarling, M.D.

1. Describe the stages of normal sleep.

By monitoring sleep in a laboratory, using electroencephalography (EEG), electrooculography (EOG), electromyography (EMG), and other recording methods, normal sleep patterns have been described. Sleep is divided into rapid eye movement (REM) sleep and non-REM sleep. REM sleep is characterized by eye movement bursts, a high-frequency EEG with low voltage, and atonia of skeletal muscles. In addition, REM is the stage of sleep during which most dreams occur.

Non-REM sleep is divided into four stages based on EEG patterns, and accounts for the majority of time spent sleeping. Stages 1 and 2 (light sleep) are identified by a low-amplitude, high-frequency EEG tracing, and stages 3 and 4 (deep sleep) by high-amplitude, slow (delta wave) pattern. Initial sleep is non-REM sleep.

A period consisting of stages 1 through 4 and REM sleep is a sleep cycle, and a night's sleep commonly consists of 3–5 cycles. As waketime nears, deep sleep is less prevalent, and a greater proportion of sleep is spent in REM.

2. How common are problems with sleep patterns in an otherwise healthy population?

Surveys show that approximately 1 in 3 individuals had problematic insomnia at some time over the past year. Prevalence is higher among women, the elderly, and those of high socioeconomic status.

Approximately 1 in 20 adults complain of problems with excessive daytime sleepiness, which may include falling asleep at inappropriate times (e.g., during conversation, during work, or while driving).

3. What questions should be asked when taking a sleep history?

Primary care physicians often fail to ask patients about sleep problems, even though they are common and often readily treatable. A sleep history results in diagnosis of the majority of sleep disorders. Useful adjuncts to the sleep history include talking to a sleep partner and having the patient keep a 1- or 2-week sleep log. These specific questions supplement the medical and psychiatric history.

Sleep History Questions

Do you fall asleep during the day, or do others notice that you are excessively sleepy?
Do you have problems getting enough sleep?
When did the symptoms begin?
What is your daily schedule, including work, meals, exercise and naps?
What is your bedtime routine?
What medications are you taking?
Do you know of unusual movements, abnormalities in breathing, or snoring during sleep?
What treatments have been tried in the past? Which were effective?

4. How does the time course of insomnia help with classification?

Insomnia is classified as recent onset (i.e., less than 3 weeks) or chronic. Insomnia of recent onset is usually transient and may develop in patients with previously normal sleep due to a stressful life change. Examples are hospitalization, bereavement, academic exams, and disturbance of circadian rhythms because of air travel across time zones or shift changes at work. Chronic insomina of months' or years' duration has a poorer prognosis and a high association with psychiatric or medical disorders.

5. Which medical disorders commonly interfere with sleep?

Many medical disorders cause symptoms that interfere with sleep (i.e., nocturia, pain, or dyspnea). Examples of medical conditions that specifically disrupt sleep include the following:

Respiratory disease, including asthma, emphysema, and cystic fibrosis
Congestive heart failure
Gastroesophageal reflux
End-stage renal disease
Endocrine disease
  Hypo- or hyperthyroidism
  Addison's or Cushing's syndrome
  Diabetes mellitus (due to
    nocturnal hypoglycemia)

Rheumatoid arthritis (pain)
CNS neoplasms
Headaches, especially cluster headaches
Seizure disorders
Parkinson's disease
Fibromyalgia (associated with
  nonrestorative sleep)
Alzheimer's disease

Therapy directed specifically at the medical problem may relieve the insomnia.

6. What is "sleep hygiene"?

Sleep hygiene is a set of behaviors used to promote sleep and improve sleep quality. The following are recommended measures:

The bedroom should be dark, quiet, and comfortable in temperature.
Reading, watching TV, or working in the bedroom should be avoided. Only sleep and sexual relations should occur there.
Caffeine (present in coffee, tea, chocolate, some soft drinks, and some analgesic preparations) should be restricted for at least 8 hours before bedtime. Nicotine should also be minimized.
Patients should attempt to keep a regular sleep-wake schedule with consistent bed and wake times regardless of the amount of sleep achieved. Naps should be avoided.
Regular exercise, finished at least 3–4 hours before bedtime, appears to promote sleep.
Heavy meals at dinner should be avoided. A light snack before bedtime may aid sleep.
Alcohol may hasten sleep onset, but its metabolites may cause sleep interruption later in the night, and its use should be avoided.
If sleep is not achieved 10–20 minutes after bedtime, the patient should leave the bedroom and do a quiet activity such as reading. When sleepiness recurs, the patient returns to bed. If sleep is again not achieved, the cycle is repeated.
Illuminated bedroom clocks (the insomniac's nemesis) should be removed.

The goal of sleep hygiene is to associate the bedroom with falling asleep quickly, minimizing frustration and anxiety.

7. What medications are used as hypnotics (sleep promoters)?

Commonly used prescription hypnotics are benzodiazepines and sedating antidepressants. Barbiturates have a high incidence of tolerance, addiction, and death (if overdosed) and should not be used as hypnotics. Chloral hydrate (a "Mickey Finn," when mixed with alcohol) may be safer than barbiturates but can cause gastritis. Nonprescription medications sold as hypnotics include antihistamines, scopolamine (an anticholinergic), and salicylates. Tryptophan, in high doses, was used as a "natural" hypnotic before it was associated with the eosinophilia-myalgia syndrome.

8. When are hypnotic medications indicated?

Sleep medications may be useful in the management of short-term insomnia. They should be used on an intermittent and temporary basis, usually no more than 3–4 weeks. It is important to prescribe them in the context of a secure doctor-patient relationship and in combination with nonpharmacologic measures.

9. Which hypnotics are most appropriate?

The benzodiazepines are most commonly used and have a reasonable safety record. Benzodiazepines currently marketed as hypnotics are triazolam (Halcion), temazepam (Restoril), and flurazepam (Dalmane). They vary chiefly in rates of absorption and elimination, with triazolam having the shortest half-life, flurazepam the longest, and temazepam, an intermediate duration.

Antihistamines are not as potent as benzodiazepines and may have anticholinergic side effects, such as urinary retention. Low-dose sedating antidepressants (e.g., amitriptyline or trazodone) have advantages in that they are nonaddictive and safe in sleep apnea, but data on safety and efficacy for chronic insomnia are unavailable.

Agitation and insomnia in hospitalized elderly patients ("sundowning") may be paradoxically worsened by benzodiazepines; low-dose haloperidol is a more effective treatment.

10. What precautions must be observed when using benzodiazepines for insomnia?

Most importantly, the insomnia should be fully investigated before prescribing sleep medications. Many medical and psychiatric disorders can present as insomnia and can be masked or worsened with benzodiazepines. They may depress respiratory drive and can worsen sleep apnea and emphysema. Rebound insomina (worsening of sleeplessness after discontinuation of hypnotics) can occur after only one dose. It should also be kept in mind that any benzodiazepine can be addictive. Short-acting drugs (e.g., triazolam) may reduce sleep latency, but unwanted effects include early-morning awakening, anterograde amnesia, and increased daytime anxiety. Long-acting benzodiazepines (e.g., temazepam) may prevent early-morning awakening, but can result in daytime sleepiness. Flurazepam has a long-acting metabolite tht may cause daytime sedation after multiple doses, especially in the elderly. Drug interactions (e.g., alcohol, phenobarbital) may be dangerous. Tolerance to benzodiazepines is the rule, and no study shows a difference between hypnotics and placebo after 3–4 weeks of therapy.

11. My patient complains of falling asleep during the day. What diagnoses should be considered?

For patients with excessive daytime somnolence, sleep apnea, narcolepsy, and idiopathic hypersomnolence (sleepiness of unknown cause, but not meeting criteria for narcolepsy) should be considered. Medical disorders such as thyroid disease, anemia, hydrocephalus, and medications (e.g., clonidine, antihistamines, neuroleptics, and tricyclic antidepressants) can cause sleepiness. Schizophrenia and depression may present with somnolence. Patients with transient hypersomnia have excessive daytime sleepiness and loss of energy, usually due to a stressful event, and recover in less than 3 weeks. Also, some patients are simply getting insufficient amounts of sleep to participate in their daily schedules.

12. Describe classic narcolepsy.

Narcolepsy is characterized by the sudden onset of daytime sleep with abnormally prompt entry into REM sleep. Classic narcolepsy includes the following:

Cataplexy—the sudden, temporary loss of skeletal muscle tone, often following excitement or fear

Sleep paralysis—a transitory but frightening inability to move or speak occurring at transitions between wakefulness and sleep

Hypnagogic hallucinations—dream-like visual or auditory hallucinations at the transitions of wakefulness and sleep

Abnormal nocturnal sleep—with frequent awakenings

The diagnosis is confirmed in the sleep lab by repetitively measuring the time from attempting sleep to sleep onset (multiple sleep latency testing, or MSLT). Sleep latency is usually less than 5 minutes in narcolepsy, and greater than 10 minutes in normals. The majority of narcoleptics also are found to have direct entry from wakefulness into REM sleep.

Current therapy includes stimulants to prevent daytime sleepiness, tricyclics such as imipramine or protriptyline to control cataplexy and scheduled daytime naps.

13. What is sleep apnea?

Sleep apnea is the repetitive cessation of airflow through the nose or mouth for at least 10 seconds during sleep. Apneas may occur hundreds of times per night and result in partial arousal from sleep. Sleep apnea may result from obstruction of the upper airway (obstructive sleep apnea), a failure of respiratory drive (central sleep apnea), or a combination of the two.

14. When should sleep apnea be suspected?

Sleep apnea should be considered in any patients with excessive daytime sleepiness and a history of snoring. Suspicion is heightened in males, the elderly, the obese, and probably alcoholics. Other clues include long pauses without audible respiration (reported by bed partner), frequent arousals, and early-morning headaches. Patients with obstructive sleep apneas may have large necks and a narrow upper airway on physical exam.

15. How is sleep apnea syndrome diagnosed?

Sleep apnea is diagnosed in a sleep laboratory. Polysomnographic monitoring for sleep apnea includes nasal and oral thermistors to measure airflow, chest and abdominal strain gauges to measure respiratory effort, ear oximetry to follow arterial oxygen saturation, EKG to detect heart rhythm abnormalities, and monitoring to determine sleep stage. Simple ear oximetry is used by some centers for screening, but a normal study does not rule out significant sleep apnea.

Patients having more than five apneas per hour are abnormal. Hypopneas (a decrease in ventilation severe enough to cause a fall in arterial oxygen saturation without complete cessation of ventilation) are also quantitated.

Results of polysomnography must be interpreted in the context of signs and symptoms before the diagnosis of sleep apnea syndrome can be considered certain.

16. What consequences result from sleep apnea?

Complications of sleep apnea are believed to result from cessation of ventilation with acute oxygen desaturation and carbon dioxide retention. The immediate consequence is sleep disruption from intermittent nocturnal asphyxiation. Resulting daytime sleepiness may impair the ability to stay awake while working or driving. Short-term consequences may also include personality changes, intellectural deterioration, memory impairment, and impotence.

Systemic blood pressure rises during apneas and sustained daytime hypertension, often refractory to medicines, is commonly found. Some studies have shown that treatment of sleep apnea can lower systemic blood pressure.

Effects on cardiac rhythm during sleep are commonly noted, and probably contribute to the overall decrease in survival found in patients with sleep apnea. Sleeping EKG may show bradycardia, sinus pauses, atrioventricular block and ventricular premature beats.

Chronic sleep apnea, usually in concert with primary pulmonary disease or severe obesity, may result in pulmonary hypertension and right-sided heart failure.

17. How is obstructive sleep apnea treated?

Conservative measures include weight loss (when modest weight loss can be effective), abstinence from alcohol and other sedatives, oxygen therapy to prevent severe desaturation, and training patients to sleep on their side rather than supine.

Drugs result in mild, if any, improvement in obstructive sleep apnea. The tricyclic antidepressant protriptyline appears to be the most effective. It appears to reduce REM sleep, during which the upper airway muscles are most relaxed.

Mechanical measures are indicated for more severe cases. Nasal continuous positive airway pressure (CPAP) used during sleep appears to "splint" the upper airway and prevents soft-tissue collapse during inspiration. CPAP is delivered through a close-fitting nasal mask used at home. Though successful when used, patients often find the device uncomfortable, and long-term compliance is variable. Removal of parts of the soft palate, uvulopalatopharyngoplasty (UPPP), results in improvement in approximately half of those treated, but it is currently difficult to predict who will benefit. Experience with prostheses designed to hold the pharynx open during sleep has been limited. Tracheostomy remains the definitive therapy for severe obstructive sleep apnea refractory to other therapies.

18. My patient complains that his legs jerk and keep him awake. How can I help him?

Periodic leg movements of sleep are stereotypical leg jerks that occur after sleep onset that may cause frequent awakenings in the patient. They occur more commonly with age, and are rare before age 40. They may be worsened by tricyclic antidepressants. Short-acting benzodiazepines do not reduce twitching but suppress arousal from sleep.

Restless leg syndrome is a waketime disorder consisting of unpleasant "crawling" muscular sensations in the legs that cause an almost irresistible urge to move the legs. This condition makes sleep onset difficult. Small doses of the antiparkinsonian drug Sinemet (carbidopa/L-dopa, 25/100) may enable sleep onset.

Hypnic jerks are sudden movements usually involving all extremities and occur in the transition of wakefulness to sleep. They are commonly experienced in normal people and seldom impair sleep.

19. Who should have a sleep study?

Most patients with excessive daytime sleepiness should be studied in a sleep lab (polysomnography). This may include MSLT (usually done the day following polysomnography) during which the time from wakefulness to sleep during several daytime naps is measured. Insomnia has not routinely been an indication for polysomnography.

BIBLIOGRAPHY

1. Aldrich MS: Narcolepsy. N Engl J Med 323:389, 1990.
2. Brownell LG, West P, Sweatman P, et al: Protriptyline in obstructive sleep apnea. N Engl J Med 307:1037, 1982.
3. Fletcher EC, DeBehnke RD, Lovoi MS, Gorin AB: Undiagnosed sleep apnea in patients with essential hypertension. Ann Intern Med 103:190, 1985.
4. Gillin JC, Byerly WF: The diagnosis and management of insomnia. N Engl J Med 322:239, 1990.
5. Hauri JH, Esther MS: Insomnia. Mayo Clin Proc 65:869, 1990.
6. Hoffstein V, Szalai JP: Predictive value of clinical features in diagnosing obstructive sleep apnea. Sleep 16:118, 1993.
7. Krueger BR: Restless legs syndrome and periodic movements of sleep. Mayo Clin Proc 65:999, 1990.

8. Kryger MH, Roth T, Dement WC: Principles and Practice of Sleep Medicine. Philadelphia, W.B. Saunders, 1989.
9. Nakra BRS, Groosberg GT, Peck B: Insomnia in the Elderly. Am Fam Physician 43:477, 1991.
10. Reite ML, Nagel KE, Ruddy JR: The Evaluation and Management of Sleep Disorders. Washington, D.C., American Psychiatric Press, Inc., 1990.
11. Shapiro CM, Devins GM, Hussain MRG: ABC of sleep disorders: Sleep problems in patients with medical illness. BMJ 306:1532, 1993.
12. Swift CG, Shapiro CM: ABC of sleep disorders: Sleep and sleep problems in elderly people. BMJ 306:1468, 1993.
13. Wiggins RV, Schmidt-Nowara WW: Treatment of the obstructive sleep apnea syndrome. West J Med 147:561, 1987.
14. Young T, Palta M, Dempsey J, et al: The occurrence of sleep-disordered breathing among middle-aged adults. N Engl J Med 328:1230, 1993.

8. ALCOHOL AND SUBSTANCE ABUSE

Philip S. Mehler, M.D.

1. What are the societal implications of alcoholism?

Alcohol abuse and its sequelae present some of the most serious social and medical problems in the United States. The toll on human life is staggering; approximately 70,000 Americans died in 1990 as a result of alcohol abuse. After heart disease and cancer, alcoholism is America's third largest health problem. Moreover, the alcohol trauma syndrome is an enormous problem; 41% of patients experiencing trauma have measurable blood alcohol levels on initial evaluation in the emergency department. Alcohol is also involved in about 25% of suicides. The annual cost to society is estimated to be $136 billion/year.

2. Given the magnitude of alcohol abuse and the paramount importance of early detection, what types of screening instruments are available?

Two types of screening instruments are available: (1) self-report questionnaires and structured interviews and (2) clinical laboratory tests that detect pathophysiologic changes associated with excessive alcohol usage.

The **CAGE** questionnaire, a mnemonic for attempts to cut down on drinking, annoyance with criticism about drinking, guilt about drinking, and using alcohol as an eye-opener, is a self-report screening instrument that appears to be suited to a busy medical practice in which time for patient interviews is limited. Two "yes" answers correctly identify 75% of alcoholics. The specificity of the test is 95%. The sensitivity of the CAGE questionnaire is dramatically enhanced by an open-ended introduction. Another questionnaire, the Michigan Alcoholism Screening Test (MAST), is a formal 25-item test that requires 25 minutes to complete. A shortened 10-item MAST (B-MAST) has been constructed with items from the original test that are highly discriminating for alcoholism. A cut-off score of "6" is suggestive for the B-Mast.

CAGE Questionnaire

Have you ever felt you ought to	Cut down on your drinking?
Have people	Annoyed you by criticizing your drinking?
Have you ever felt bad or	Guilty about your drinking?
Have you ever had a drink first thing in the morning to steady your nerves or get rid of a hangover?	Eye-opener

Brief MAST

Points
- (2) *1. Do you feel you are a normal drinker?
- (2) *2. Do friends or relatives think you are a normal drinker?
- (5) 3. Have you ever attended a meeting of Alcoholics Anonymous?
- (2) 4. Have you ever lost friends or girlfriends/boyfriends because of drinking?
- (2) 5. Have you ever gotten into trouble at work because of drinking?
- (2) 6. Have you ever neglected your obligations, your family, or your work for two or more days in a row because you were drinking?
- (2) 7. Have you ever had delirium tremens (DTs), severe shaking, heard voices, seen things that weren't there after heavy drinking?
- (5) 8. Have you ever gone to anyone for help about your drinking?
- (5) 9. Have you ever been in a hospital because of drinking?
- (2) 10. Have you ever been arrested for drunk driving or driving after drinking?

---

* Negative responses are alcoholic responses.
Scoring: ≤ 3 points, nonalcoholic; 4 points, suggestive of alcoholism; 5 indicates alcoholism

Clinical laboratory tests frequently are used to corroborate results of questionnaires. Several tests provide objective evidence of problem drinking, especially in patients who deny an alcohol problem. Increased levels of serum gamma-glutamyl transferase (GGT) is a relatively sensitive index of alcohol use. Although serum GGT is the most widely used laboratory screening test for alcoholism, it lacks diagnostic specificity. Results are more specific in conjunction with an elevated mean corpuscular volume (MCV), which increases with excessive alcohol intake. The ratio of the liver enzyme aspartate aminotransferase (AST) to alanine aminotransferase (ALT), if greater than 1, may be a useful marker of alcoholic liver disease.

3. What major organ systems are affected by alcohol abuse?
Alcohol affects almost every organ system in the body.

Cardiovascular system
   Cardiomyopathy
   Atrial and ventricular dysrhythmias
Endocrine system
   Testicular atrophy
   Femininization
   Amenorrhea and premature menopause
   Pseudo-Cushing's syndrome
Gastrointestinal system
   Hepatitis and cirrhosis
   Esophagitis and gastritis
   Peptic ulcer disease
   Esophageal carcinoma
   Malabsorption with diarrhea
   Pancreatitis

Hematologic system
   Anemia due to folate deficiency
      or sideroblastosis
   Thrombocytopenia
   Diminished neutrophil migration
Nervous system
   Cognitive impairment
   Dementia
   Korsakoff's psychosis
   Wernicke's encephalopathy
   Peripheral neuropathy

4. Are gender differences observed in alcohol-related liver disease?
Yes. Although the cirrhosis-induced death rate is higher for men than for women, women are more susceptible to alcohol-related liver damage and develop liver disease with shorter durations of alcohol abuse.

5. What are the consequences to the fetus of alcohol use during pregnancy?
Alcohol is a teratogen. Although a critical dosage or exposure level has not been determined, observations of human infants and experimental animals make clear that a mother who drinks heavily during pregnancy may severely damage her fetus. The distinct pattern of birth defects, which has been labeled the fetal alcohol syndrome, includes growth retardation, a characteristic

constellation of craniofacial anomalies, central nervous system dysfunction, and malformations of major organ systems.

6. Describe the manifestations of alcohol withdrawal syndrome.

Alcohol withdrawal may have several different and occasionally overlapping manifestations. Minor withdrawal begins 6–12 hours after a significant decrease or cessation of drinking in heavy drinkers. Withdrawal syndrome may occur with significant blood levels of alcohol. This stage, which lasts 3–5 days, is characterized by tremors, sweating, anxiety, diarrhea, nausea, and insomnia; patients may not require pharmacologic therapy. Approximately 12–24 hours after the last drink, alcohol-dependent patients may develop marked tremulousness, hyperactivity, tachycardia, and visual hallucinations. Withdrawal seizures, usually single episodes of grand mal that last < 15 minutes, also occur 12–48 hours after abstinence. However, if the seizures are multiple, focal, or accompanied by a fever, further neurologic evaluation is imperative.

The risk for delirium tremens (DTs), which is a medical emergency, occurs 72–120 hours after cessation of drinking. Essential for the diagnosis is the presence of acute delirium with confusion and disorientation, fever, and tachycardia. Patients experiencing DTs are agitated, belligerent, profusely diaphoretic, tremulous, and hypertensive. This syndrome may last for 3–4 days and requires aggressive management.

7. Outline the principles of management in patients with alcohol withdrawal syndromes.

Although outpatient treatment of minor alcohol withdrawal has its place, patients with hyperactivity of the sympathetic nervous system, concurrent medical problems, lack of a social support system, and previous history of complications during withdrawal episodes require inpatient treatment. Delirium tremens require management in the intensive care unit. Although patients experiencing mild withdrawal symptoms can be managed without adjunctive pharmacologic therapy, current guidelines recommend treatment for most patients experiencing alcohol withdrawal.

The proper management of alcohol withdrawal is aimed at alleviating patient suffering and preventing minor symptoms from progressing to major symptoms. Normalization of vital signs and moderate sedation are two desired endpoints of treatment. Sedation is accomplished by substituting another sedative hypnotic agent for alcohol, such as a benzodiazepine, in a gradually tapering dose. In patients with significant liver disease, lorazepam (Ativan) or oxazepam (Serax) should be used, because they are not extensively oxidized by the liver. Intravenous use of benzodiazepines until mild sedation occurs prevents the physiologic storm that may be seen with delirium tremens. Haloperidol (Haldol) may also be used to control agitation and belligerence, but only after benzodiazepines have been given, because haloperidol lowers the seizure threshold. In all stages of alcohol withdrawal, compulsive attention to fluid and electrolyte status is required. Beta blockers such as atenolol (Tenormin) also have been successfully used to reduce the adrenergic signs of withdrawal. A daily dose of 50 mg during the withdrawal period shortens hospital stays and reduces the total dose of benzodiazepine required for treatment. In addition to beta blockers, alpha$_2$-receptor agonists, such as clonidine (Catapres), also have been used to treat alcohol withdrawal because of their sedative as well as blood pressure- and pulse-lowering properties. The usual dosage is 0.2 mg twice a day.

8. What new pharmacotherapies are available to deter alcoholism?

Recent research has focused on agents that decrease the desire for alcohol. In randomized, placebo-controlled studies, inhibitors of serotonin reuptake, such as fluoxetine (Prozac), reduce alcohol intake. The mechanism of action is not known but may be related to alleviation of depression. Similar data are available for the narcotic antagonist, naltrexone. Disulfiram functions as an alcohol-deterrent agent by blocking aldehyde dehydrogenase; thus, the concentration of acetaldehyde, the first metabolic byproduct of alcohol oxidation, is increased. As a result, ingestion of alcohol in patients taking disulfiram results in flushing, tachycardia, palpitations, dyspnea, and headache. Although uncomfortable, most of these reactions are self-limiting without significant risk to the patient.

9. Which patients may benefit from disulfiram?
The ideal patient for disulfiram therapy is a daily rather than a binge drinker who is committed to treatment but prone to relapse. The main contraindications to its use are heart disease, history of seizures, cirrhosis, diabetes, pregnancy, and significantly elevated levels of transaminase.

10. Which classes of drugs are characterized by potentially dangerous withdrawal syndromes?
Drugs of abuse are generally divided into the following categories: sedatives, stimulants, opiates, psychedelic agents, and phencyclidine (PCP). Withdrawal is defined as the predictable development of physical and psychologic signs and symptoms in response to the abrupt discontinuation of a drug in dependent individuals. The only class of drugs connected with dangerous withdrawal syndromes is the central nervous system depressants, which include alcohol, benzodiazepines, barbiturates, chloral hydrate, and meprobamate.

11. Characterize the opiate withdrawal syndrome.
Mild withdrawal is characterized by yawning and dilated pupils. In more severe cases, vomiting, diarrhea, piloerection, rhinorrhea, and lacrimation are seen. Symptoms include anxiety, insomnia, abdominal cramping, irritability, and leg spasms. Withdrawal usually begins 6–12 hours after the last use of narcotics. Most of the withdrawal syndrome is effectively mitigated through the use of two medications: (1) clonidine, in doses of 0.8–1.2 mg/day with ancillary medications for pain and sleep, or (2) methadone, a longer-acting opioid that, in doses of 20–30 mg/day, is substituted for the opioid of abuse, whether it is heroin, meperidine, or codeine. Recently, buprenorphine hydrochloride has been shown to reduce heroin intake sharply in abusers. Because it is a mixed agonist-antagonist, it has a low potential for abuse and overdose.

12. Does discontinuance of hallucinogens result in withdrawal?
No. Hallucinogens and phencyclidine (PCP) do not produce withdrawal symptoms, although drug craving is present.

13. Describe characteristic syndromes associated with particular drugs of abuse.

Cocaine	Severe depression
Panic attacks	Lysergic acid diethylamide (LSD)
Flashbacks ("bad trips")	Hallucinogens
Psychoses	PCP, cocaine, amphetamines
Chronic organic brain syndrome	Alcohol, solvents, PCP

14. What are the physiologic effects of cocaine?
Cocaine is obtained by adding hydrochloric acid to coca leaves. The water-soluble crystal that forms may be absorbed through the nasal mucosa or injected intravenously. "Crack" is a highly purified form of the cocaine free base that makes a popping sound when heated. The physiologic response to cocaine is primarily related to excessive catecholamine discharge: hypertension, tachycardia, hyperthermia, agitation, and seizures.

15. Why must chest pain related to cocaine be seriously evaluated?
Cocaine is one of the most dangerous illicit drugs in use today because of its association with acute myocardial infarction in young people with normal coronary arteries. The cause of myocardial infarction is multifactorial but includes vasoconstriction of large epicardial coronary arteries and thrombosis, most commonly involving the left anterior descending artery. Recent evidence indicates that cocaine changes endothelium vasodilator capacity, exerts a potent myocardial depressant effect on myocytes, and may directly constrict vascular muscle, independently of alpha adrenergic stimulation.

Although chest pain is frequently encountered after cocaine use, the actual incidence of acute myocardial infarction is low, especially when the initial electrocardiogram is normal or a variant of normal. Most patients can be safely managed in a nonintensive care setting, and some may not even require hospital admission.

16. Which drug is contraindicated in cocaine-related chest pain?
If the chest pain is believed to indicate myocardial ischemia, beta blockers are contraindicated, because they result in unopposed coronary vasoconstriction mediated by alpha adrenergic agents. Nitroglycerin and calcium-channel blockers are the mainstay of therapy. Heparin, aspirin, and thrombolytic agents also have a role because of experimental evidence of cocaine-enhanced platelet aggregation and thrombosis.

17. Bidirectional nystagmus should suggest abuse of which recreational drug?
PCP is the only drug of abuse that produces bidirectional nystagmus; it has dopaminergic, anticholinergic, and adrenergic activities. Intoxicated patients present with hypertension, tachycardia, bidirectional nystagmus, hyperthermia, hallucinations, and marked agitation. The combination of a comalike state with open eyes, diminished pain perception, intermittent periods of excitation, and severe muscle rigidity indicates a PCP reaction. Patients are at risk for hypertensive crisis, rhabdomyolysis, seizures, and bizarre, often violent behavior. PCP is abused because of the sense of invisibility and power that it produces. It is most often smoked but also may be taken intravenously or orally. Management of acute PCP intoxication may be extremely challenging. The patient should be placed in a quiet environment; in most instances, this suffices. Patients who are severely agitated, however, should be sedated adequately with benzodiazepines, cooled rapidly if indicated, and hydrated. Drugs such as haloperidol are effective for treatment of terrifying hallucinations.

18. What drug of abuse imposes the largest health and economic burden on society?
The surprising answer is nicotine, one of the major preventable nemeses of public health. The 1989 Surgeon General's report estimated that 1 in 6 deaths in the United States was caused by cigarettes. Almost 400,000 deaths were directly attributable to smoking. Only recently have efforts been made to portray tobacco smoking as an addictive disease. Nicotine is a psychoactive drug associated with definite dependence, tolerance, and withdrawal syndrome. The withdrawal process is characterized by dysphoria, craving, irritability, and nervousness. Tobacco addiction is a complex process involving nicotinic cholinergic receptors in the brain. Because of the complexity of the addiction, many smokers are not able to quit by themselves. The pharmacotherapy of tobacco addiction involves maintaining a fairly constant level of nicotine in the body through nicotine-substitution therapy. Thus symptoms of abstinence are relieved. Nicotine chewing gum and transdermal delivery systems are available to achieve this end. However, without some form of concomitant behavioral support from a physician or other caregiver, substitution therapy is frequently unsuccessful. Reports about the effects of clonidine on decreasing cigarette usage are encouraging.

19. Although the margin of safety with benzodiazepines is reassuring compared with other central nervous system sedatives, which addiction issues should the health care provider consider?
Benzodiazepines produce significant physical and psychological dependence as well as a potentially dangerous withdrawal syndrome after prolonged use. In 1990, 60 million benzodiazepine prescriptions were dispensed. The effects are additive with other central nervous system depressants, such as alcohol and barbiturates. Certain medications, such as cimetidine and disulfiram, and certain conditions, such as older age and hepatic impairment, impede the metabolism of benzodiazepines. Medications such as phenytoin and carbamazepine enhance the metabolism of benzodiazepines.

20. Characterize benzodiazepine withdrawal and its therapy.
Benzodiazepines are divided into short-acting agents, such as temazepam (Restoril) and triazolam (Halcion); intermediate-acting agents, such as alprazolam (Xanax), lorazepam (Ativan), and oxazepam (Serax); and long-acting agents, such as clorazepate (Tranxene), diazepam (Valium), and clonazepam (Klonopin). Dependence may develop rapidly, often within a few weeks. In general, the shorter the half-life, the more intense the withdrawal syndrome. Signs

and symptoms of withdrawal occur within 24 hours of cessation with a short-acting benzo-diazepine and by the fifth day with longer-acting drugs. Benzodiazepine withdrawal produces a highly excitable state that is contrary to the usual sedative effects and may include palpitations, diarrhea, polyuria, tremor, and seizures. Detoxification is predicated on the premise that benzodiazepines have mutual cross-tolerance. Conversion for equivalent doses are easily calculated. In general, a long-acting benzodiazepine is preferable for suppressing withdrawal symptoms. A schedule of 7–10 days of gradual tapering is set up if the abused benzodiazepine is a short-acting one; a schedule of 10–14 days is used for longer-acting drugs.

Sedative Hypnotic Drugs Dose Conversions

DRUG	DOSE (mg)	DRUG	DOSE (mg)
Barbiturates		Benzodiazepines	
Pentobarbital	100	Alprazolam	1
Secobarbital	100	Chlordiazepoxide	25
Butalbital	100	Clonazepam	4
Amobarbital	100	Clorazepate	15
Phenobarbital	30	Diazepam	10
Nonbarbiturates		Flurazepam	15
Nonbenzodiazepines		Lorazepam	2
Ethchlorvynol	300	Oxazepam	10
Glutethimide	250	Quazepam	15
Methyprylon	200	Temazepam	15
Methaqualone	300	Triazolam	0.25
Meprobamate	400		
Carisoprodol	700		
Chloral hydrate	500		

21. How accurate is urine drug testing?

Because of a determined effort to reduce drug abuse, drug testing has become more common. Most urine drug panels screen for marijuana, cocaine, opiates, PCP, and amphetamines. The cost of such tests is $50–100. Positive results are confirmed by gas chromatography–mass spectrometry (GC-MS). Almost one-third of positive results on initial screening tests are found to be false. For example, sympathomimetic agents in over-the-counter decongestants test positive for amphetamines; confirmatory testing, however, is negative for the D-isomer of abused amphetamines.

Errors in handling or analysis also may result in false-negative results. In general, marijuana is detected for 1–3 days after occasional use and for up to 3–4 weeks in a heavy smoker because of accumulation in fatty tissues. The major metabolite of cocaine, benzoyl ecgonine, may be detected for 2–3 days after use. A positive test for PCP usually indicates drug use within the previous week.

Another caveat with drug testing is that poppy seeds used on baked goods contain sufficient amounts of morphine to produce a positive urine test. The result is not a false-positive, because the drug is actually present. Therefore, decision making in drug testing requires the expertise of a medical review officer (MRO) with specific training in addiction medicine. MROs help to protect the rights of a patient while contributing to the effort to reduce drug abuse.

CONTROVERSY

22. What is the role of anticonvulsants in preventing alcohol withdrawal seizures?

A seizure may herald the onset of a major withdrawal syndrome, and one-third of patients with alcohol withdrawal seizures may later develop delirium tremens. Nonetheless, the routine use of phenytoin to prevent seizures in patients withdrawing from alcohol is controversial. Three studies have focused on this issue: two do not support the use of phenytoin, whereas one does.

The efficacy of phenytoin in combination with a benzodiazepine thus remains uncertain. Current practice is to give phenytoin only to withdrawing patients with a documented history of nonalcohol-related seizures or a history of withdrawal seizures.

BIBLIOGRAPHY

1. Alldredge BK, Simon RP: Placebo-controlled trial of IV diphenylhydantoin for short-term treatment of alcohol withdrawal seizures. Am J Med 87:645–648, 1989.
2. Everett WD, Linden N: Drug testing in the workplace. Postgrad Med 91:164–170, 1992.
3. Ewing JA: Detecting alcoholism: The CAGE questionnaire. JAMA 252:1905–1907, 1984.
4. Has AA, Tavassoli M: Laboratory markers of alcohol intake and abuse. Am J Med Sci 303:415–428, 1992.
5. Henry JA, Jeffrey KJ, Dawling S: Toxicity and death from methamphetamine. Lancet 340:384–387, 1992.
6. Lee EW, D'Alonzo GE: Nicotine addiction and its pharmacologic treatment. Arch Intern Med 153:34–48, 1993.
7. Ling W, Wesson DR: Drugs of abuse—opiates. West J Med 152:565–572, 1991.
8. Miller NS, Gold MS: Benzodiazepines, tolerance, dependence, abuse, and addiction. J Psychol 122:1–11, 1990.
9. Mynor RL, Scott BD, Brown DP, Winford MD: Cocaine-induced myocardial infarction and patients with normal coronary arteries. Ann Intern Med 115:797–806, 1991.
10. Pokorny AD, Miller BA, Kaplan HB: The brief MAST. Am J Psychol 129:118–121, 1972.
11. Schwartz RH: Phencyclidine (PCP) overview. Substance Abuse 2:10–19, 1987.
12. Turnek RC, Lichftein PR, Peden JG, Waivers LE: Alcohol withdrawal syndrome: A review of pathophysiology and treatment. J Gen Intern Med 4:432–444, 1989.
13. Warner E: Cocaine abuse. Ann Intern Med 119:226–235, 1993.
14. Zitten RZ, Allen JP: Pharmacotherapies for alcoholism. Alcohol Clin Exp Res 15:623–633, 1991.

9. ANXIETY

Joyce Seiko Kobayashi, M.D.

1. Why does the primary care physician need to know more about the evaluation and management of anxiety in the medical setting?

Anxiety frequently is accompanied by specific physical symptoms and thus may trigger a major diagnostic work-up that the astute practitioner can avoid if the proper diagnosis is made early in the evaluation. Early diagnosis of anxiety spares unnecessary expense and protects the patient from unnecessary distress.

On the other hand, because a primary medical disorder may cause anxiety, the physician should avoid premature diagnosis of presenting symptoms as a strictly emotional disorder. The physician also may be able to help the patient to adjust to an anxiety-producing medical disorder more effectively than a consultant because of a longer-term relationship.

Furthermore, patients who express their anxiety through somatic symptoms often prefer to talk with their primary care physician and feel abandoned (which usually increases their anxiety) if referred to a psychiatrist. If the physician believes that a referral is necessary because of the severity of symptoms, acuity of presentation, or comorbid disorders, the patient should be assured that the physician will work closely with the psychiatrist.

2. What are the three most common errors that a primary care practitioner can make with a patient who presents with significant anxiety?

1. The primary care physician may be too quick to consider anxiety a psychiatric problem and either refer the patient to a mental health professional prematurely or rush to prescribe

benzodiazepines. Routine treatment of anxiety with benzodiazepines is no more appropriate than routine treatment of fever with penicillin. Anxiety is often treated as the diagnosis rather than a signal to pursue the source of the anxiety or to attempt to understand its meaning. If the anxiety is a symptom of medical illness or part of the patient's adjustment to medical illness, the physician may be in the best position to treat either, and should talk with the patient more specifically about his or her feelings.

2. The primary care physician may assume that he or she knows what the patient "must" be anxious about. A classic example is assuming that the patient about to undergo a course of chemotherapy is most concerned about the medically serious side effects rather than, for example, about losing hair or some other side effect that may feel more immediately threatening.

3. The primary care physician may rush to reassure the patient that "there is really nothing to worry about." Such statements in fact may increase the anxiety of the patient, who may feel that the physician is not taking his or her concerns seriously. Instead, the physician should reassure the patient of continued support and close monitoring of the cause of anxiety.

3. What are the primary causes of anxiety in the medical setting?

1. Anxiety as a normal alerting response to the perceived threat of medical illness and treatment interventions
2. Anxiety as a symptomatic manifestation of medical illness
3. Anxiety as a symptom of intoxication or withdrawal syndromes
4. Anxiety disorders or other psychiatric disorders

4. List the medical disorders that may present with anxiety as a primary symptom.

Endocrine disorders: hyperthyroidism, pheochromocytoma, hypoglycemia, hypo/hypercalcemia

Cardiac disorders: hypoxia, angina, arrhythmias, congestive heart failure, mitral valve prolapse

Pulmonary disorders: hypoxia, chronic obstructive pulmonary disease, pneumonia, hyperventilation, pulmonary embolism

Neurologic disorders: partial complex seizures, encephalitis, postconcussion syndrome, sleep disorders

Metabolic disorders: vitamin B12 deficiency, porphyria

Stimulant toxicity: caffeine, sympathomimetic medications or drugs

Withdrawal syndromes: alcohol, benzodiazepines, barbiturates, opiates, or delirium of any etiology. The reader also is referred to chapter 10 on Psychoses.

5. What physical symptoms frequently associated with anxiety disorder may be confused with medical illness?

General physical symptoms that often accompany anxiety may or may not be of sufficient severity to meet criteria for a specific disorder. Such symptoms may be classified in three categories:

1. **Motor tension:** trembling, twitching, feeling shaky, muscle tension or aches, restlessness, easy fatigability
2. **Autonomic hyperactivity:** shortness of breath or smothering sensations, palpitations or tachycardia, sweating or clammy hands, dry mouth, dizziness or lightheadedness, nausea, diarrhea or other abdominal distress, hot flashes or chills, frequent urination, trouble swallowing or "lump in throat"
3. **Vigilance or scanning:** feeling keyed-up or on edge, exaggerated startle response, difficulty concentrating or "mind going blank," trouble falling or staying asleep, irritability

Symptoms associated with panic attacks commonly precipitate major medical work-ups.

6. What aspects of medical illness and treatment are common sources of anxiety?

Many aspects of medical illness and treatment may cause anxiety depending on the patient's history, capacity to cope, support network, and the specific tasks of adjustment associated with a particular disease or its treatment. It is essential to start by asking general, open-ended questions about reactions to diagnosis, experiences with the proposed or related therapies, and major current concerns. Some patients may feel that the illness is a punishment; others may use it as an organizing focus for unmet dependency needs. The physician should attempt to understand the meaning of illness to each patient.

A number of predictable, deeper concerns are common and the physician should listen for them in the patient's discussions. Examples include fears of pain, abandonment, dependency, disfigurement, or social unacceptability; loss of control or function; and death. Asking about such deeper concerns too directly or prematurely, however, may increase the patient's anxiety; clinical judgment must be exercised. Reassuring the patient that he or she will not be abandoned, for example, does not require specific acknowledgement of this fear.

The physician also should assess whether the level of anxiety is adaptive or signals the patient's need for further treatment and whether it is pathologic and out of proportion to the situation. Reassurance focused on the medical aspects of the illness in patients with pathologic anxiety does not address their underlying concerns; psychiatric consultation may be considered, with reassurance that the physician will continue to be involved.

Finally, patients also may feel anxious about the doctor-patient relationship or unable to trust the efficacy of medical treatment or the health care system in general because of prior experiences, sociocultural barriers, or personal histories of abuse or neglect. Such patients often feel less anxious as the physician gains their trust through consistent caring and compassionate interaction.

7. Which psychiatric disorders present with anxiety as a major symptom?

Several categories of psychiatric disorders may present with anxiety, including adjustment disorders, posttraumatic stress disorders, and substance-induced anxiety disorder. Less common underlying disorders include the phobias, obsessive-compulsive disorder, and generalized anxiety disorder. In addition, patients with somatoform, conversion, and certain personality disorders often seek help in the primary care setting with similar presentations. Finally, comorbid disorders are quite common. Generalized anxiety disorder, for example, does not commonly occur in isolation (current and lifetime prevalence: 1.2%–6.6%) but has a lifetime comorbidity rate of 90%. One of the most common and treatable comorbid diagnoses that should always be kept in mind when anxiety is a presenting symptom is major depressive disorder. The reader is referred to the fourth edition of the Diagnostic and Statistical Manual of the American Psychiatric Association (DSM-IV) for a more specific listing of the diagnostic criteria of the above disorders.

8. What is a panic attack? What other disorders may be associated with panic attacks?

Patients with panic attacks often seek help first from their primary care physician. The essential element of a panic attack is a discrete period of intense fear or discomfort, in which four (or more) of the following symptoms develop abruptly and reach a peak within 10 minutes:

Palpitations	Feeling dizzy or faint
Sweating	Derealization (feelings of unreality)
Trembling	or depersonalization (being detached
Sensation of shortness of breath	from oneself)
or smothering	Fear of losing control or sanity
Feeling of choking	Fear of dying
Chest pain or discomfort	Paresthesias
Nausea or abdominal distress	Chills or hot flushes

Because such patients often feel as if they are going to have a heart attack or stroke or fear that they are dying, they are seen frequently in emergency departments. Some patients fear catastrophic outcomes from minor physical symptoms or medication side effects and may be mislabeled as histrionic or hypochondriacal, when direct reassurance and continuity of care may lessen their fears over time. They may receive multiple major medical work-ups (often at multiple sites) when an initial exclusionary work-up, thorough review of past records and careful history, may suffice. Accurate diagnosis and stabilization and continuity of care with a primary care physician and psychiatrist may prevent further mismanagement of panic disorder.

The diagnosis of panic attacks should promote a review of symptoms that may be related to frequently comorbid disorders, such as major depressive disorder (50–65%); social phobia (15–30%); specific phobia (10–20%); generalized anxiety disorder (25%); and obsessive-compulsive disorder (8–10%). Agoraphobia (fear of places or situations, such as crowded areas, where one may suffer embarrassment or be unable to escape if a panic attack occurs) is commonly associated with panic attacks (more than one-half of clinical populations) and may severely restrict activities as well as impair functioning. Chronic relapse over years is common, although one-third of patients may recover completely with appropriate treatment. Panic disorders occur 2–3 times more frequently in women than men, and first-degree relatives have a 4–7-fold higher risk of developing panic disorder.

9. What clues help the primary care physician to recognize other common psychiatric disorders that present with anxiety?

1. **Major depressive disorder** is one of the most common and readily treatable disorders that may present with clinically significant anxiety, with or without panic attacks. Depressive disorders are easily overlooked when anxiety and/or anhedonia (loss of pleasure) is more prominent than sadness.

2. **Adjustment disorder** with anxiety may be an acute or chronic condition and is characterized by the development of emotional or behavioral symptoms in response to an identifiable stressor(s) occurring within 3 months of the onset of symptoms. The degree of distress exceeds what normally would be expected, or social or occupational functioning is significantly impaired.

3. A **substance-induced anxiety disorder** is diagnosed when the anxiety is judged to be due to the direct physiologic effects of an illicit drug, medication, or toxin.

4. **Posttraumatic or acute stress disorders** are diagnosed by characteristic symptoms in response to an extreme traumatic stressor.

5. **Phobias** are common in the general population but rarely reach the level of clinical significance. Lifetime prevalence of diagnosable specific phobias is around 10%. However, specific phobias (categorized as animal, natural environment, blood-injection injury, situational, and other types) may have significant effect on health care behavior (e.g., fears of blood, needles, and choking [medications]) and should be consciously assessed for clinical severity with an in-depth history. Patients with such disorders are aware that their fears are out of proportion to the situation but may not say so unless asked.

6. **Obsessive-compulsive disorders** are important to note (lifetime prevalence of 2–5%), because they are more common than is realized, there are effective pharmacologic treatments available, they are often disabling, and fears of contamination may bring a patient to the primary care physician.

DSM-IV provides a more specific listing of the diagnostic criteria of the above disorders.

10. What is the DSM-IV?
DSM-IV, published in 1994, is the fourth edition of the American Psychiatric Association's Diagnostic and Statistical Manual of Mental Disorders. This manual was the product of 13 work groups whose comprehensive literature reviews were critiqued by 50–100 advisers representing a diversity of clinical and research expertise; two methods conferences; 40 data reanalyses; and 12 field trials of the revised diagnostic criteria, involving 70 sites and more than 6000 subjects. The APA acknowledges the limitations of any categorical approach, given the heterogeneity of human behavior, but the DSM-IV has begun to incorporate different cultural perspectives and represents a major step in standardizing clinical diagnosis, communication, and research about mental disorders.

11. Which medications, substances, and toxic agents may cause anxiety as a symptom in either intoxication or withdrawal?

Although the term "intoxication and withdrawal syndromes" appropriately brings to mind street drugs and alcohol, excess caffeine ingestion and nicotine withdrawal are two of the most commonly overlooked causes or contributors to anxiety. Caffeine is frequently underestimated as a toxic agent, and a careful history of all sources of caffeine (coffee, sodas, chocolate) should be included in the evaluation of the anxious patient. Symptoms may occur with 200 mg of caffeine daily (less than 2 cups of coffee), and individuals vary in susceptibility. Minor withdrawal from nicotine is usually self-medicated with more cigarettes, but patients who gradually increase tobacco consumption may not be conscious of withdrawal effects.

Withdrawal from benzodiazepines, barbiturates and other sedative/hypnotics, opiates, and alcohol commonly cause anxiety with or without tremulousness. Despite awareness of these pharmacologic effects, the physician may prescribe anxiolytics to a person who presents in great distress, without considering the possibility of a minor withdrawal syndrome.

Cocaine, phencyclidine, amphetamine, methamphetamine, and other stimulants, such as over-the-counter alpha-adrenergic medications (e.g., phenylpropanolamine, ephedrine, phenylephrine, and pseudoephedrine) may cause varying degrees of anxiety, irritability, agitation, and restlessness.

Among the major offending agents in causing anxiety, however, are commonly prescribed medications. The akathisia of neuroleptics is frequently accompanied by a subjective feeling of restlessness and anxiety that may be profoundly disturbing to the sensitive patient. Antidepressants, such as fluoxetine or imipramine; xanthines, such as theophylline and other bronchodilators (epinephrine, isoproterenol, metapropterenol, albuterol, isoetharine); and calcium channel blockers (verapamil, nifedipine, diltiazem) may cause anxiety at therapeutic doses.

Other medications that have been reported to cause anxiety as a side effect include antihistamines, baclofen, cycloserine, indomethacin, oxymetazoline, and quinacrine.

12. For what reasons may the primary care physician be hesitant to discuss an issue that causes anxiety in a particular patient?

1. The busy physician is sometimes concerned that such discussions will take too much valuable time. More often, however, they save time over the long term, because some patients escalate their presenting symptoms (somatic, interpersonal, emotional) to ensure that they will be heard.

2. The conscientious physician may feel "responsible" for solving the problem. Few patients, however, expect the physician to find a solution; they are nevertheless profoundly grateful that someone is willing to listen. Often the more "hopeless" the circumstances, the smaller the number of people who will listen; therefore, the patient is even more appreciative (and comforted) if the physician takes a few minutes to do so.

13. What clinical approaches to anxious patients may be useful?

The maxim, "Don't just do something, stand there," is important. Therefore, after ruling out medical etiologies, medication toxicity, and intoxication/withdrawal syndromes and reviewing psychiatric history, the following guidelines may be considered for approaching the anxious patient:

1. **Listen**, using a calm, responsive, but nondirect approach; do not rush to "solve" or "fix" the problem;

2. **Explore** the meaning of the illness, treatment, or situation for the patient;

3. **Target** the conscious reasons for the anxiety (such as fears of abandonment, dependency, and pain) by direct reassurance, while continuing to listen for other concerns;

4. **Understand** that it may be difficult for the patient to identify the immediate cause of anxiety, but that the physician's willingness to listen may be directly calming;

5. **Assess** whether the anxiety is out of proportion to the situation, and consider psychiatric consultation;

6. **Support** through continued discussions, marshalling the natural support network of friends and family or other support groups, trying to address concerns once they are identified, and considering pharmacologic approaches when indicated.

14. Should barbiturates be used to treat anxiety?

No. Barbiturates are no longer indicated for anxiety or associated insomnia. However, a small dose of barbiturates or benzodiazepines to promote sleep in patients suffering acute grief, on an as needed basis for a few days, is often helpful.

15. What conservative pharmacologic approaches may be safely used for anxiety?

When medical etiologies and intoxication/withdrawal syndromes have been ruled out, medication may be considered for a short time, along with supportive psychosocial and adjunctive approaches, such as meditation and relaxation exercises. Benzodiazepines are highly effective agents, and patients should not be denied their benefits in bona fide circumstances. They are also problematic because of their significant potential for tolerance and dependence. Thus, they should be used only after extensive patient education.

Lorazepam (Ativan), 0.5–1.0 mg; clorazepate (Tranxene), 7.5–15 mg; and diazepam (Valium), 2–5 mg—all up to 3 times/day as needed for anxiety, may be considered when the severity of the anxiety or circumstances warrants. Lorazepam has the advantage of a short half-life. Alprazolam (Xanax), 0.5 mg, has a relatively short half-life, and patients occasionally experience minor withdrawal anxiety before the next scheduled dose. Alprazolam may be more difficult for the patient to discontinue, although studies have shown that discontinuance is facilitated by sufficient patient education about withdrawal effects. It may be considered specifically for panic attacks. If the panic attacks are in the context of depressive symptoms, however, imipramine (Tofranil) in the range of 150 mg should be tried first. Clonazepam (Klonopin) 0.5 mg is more useful for severe insomnia and agitation because of its relative potency and long half-life.

Buspirone (Buspar), 5–20 mg 3 times/day, is a non-benzodiazepine anxiolytic and may be tried before the benzodiazepines because of its lack of sedation and low abuse potential. However, the patient must follow a regular dosage pattern (3 times/day) for a full month before noticing significant results; frequently there is a lag of at least several weeks before full efficacy is reached. Buspirone is not useful on an as needed basis and should not be used with inhibitors of monoamine oxidase because of the possibility of hypertensive crises.

Antidepressants may be useful if depression is a component of the anxiety or a concomitant disorder. Anxiety associated with a major depressive disorder often remits without anxiolytics when the depression is treated. Low-dose neuroleptics (such as trifluoperazine/Stelazine, 1 mg; loxapine/Loxitane, 5 mg; or liquid perphenazine/Trilafon, 2–4 mg) may be helpful for the patient with organic or extreme, disorganizing anxiety. Beta-blockers, such as propranolol/Inderal (5–20 mg 3 times/day or a single dose before a performance, for example) may be useful when somatic symptoms predominate.

Once medications have been used, exploration of issues to identify sources of anxiety, should continue, and nonpharmacologic approaches, such as meditation, self-relaxation exercise, support groups, or counseling should be encouraged.

BIBLIOGRAPHY

1. Diagnostic and Statistical Manual of Mental Disorders, 4th ed. Washington, DC, American Psychiatric Press, 1994.
2. Dubovsky S, Thomas M: Psychotic depression: Advances in conceptualization and treatment. Hosp Commun Psychiatry 43:1189–1218, 1992.
3. Fennig S, Bromet E, Jandorf L: Gender differences in clinical characteristics of first-admission psychotic depression. Am J Psychiatry 150:1734–1736, 1993.
4. Goldberg TE, Gold JM, Greenberg R, et al: Contrasts between patients with affective disorders and patients with schizophrenia on a neuropsychological test battery. Am J Psychiatry 150:1355–1362, 1993.

5. Hales RE, Yudofsky SC (eds): Textbook of Neuropsychiatry, 2nd ed. Washington, DC, American Psychiatric Press, 1992.
6. Kessler RC, McGonagle KA, Zhao S, et al: Lifetime and 12-month prevalence of DSM-III-R psychiatric disorders in the United States. Arch Gen Psychiatry 51:8–19, 1994.
7. Lipowski ZJ: Delirium. Springfield, IL, Charles C Thomas, 1980.
8. Popkin MK, Tucker GJ: Secondary and drug-induced mood, anxiety, psychotic, catatonic, and personality disorders: A reveiw of the literature. J Neuropsychiatry Clin Neurosci 4:369–385, 1992.
9. Severino S, Yonkers KA: A literature review of psychotic symptoms associated with the premenstruum. Psychosomatics 34:299–314, 1993.
10. Stoudemire A, Fogel BS (eds): Principles of Medical Psychiatry. New York, Grune & Stratton Inc., 1987.
11. Tsuang D, Coryell W: An 8-year follow-up of patients with DSM-III-R psychotic depression, schizoaffective disorder and schizophrenia. Am J Psychiatry 150:1182–1188, 1993.

10. PSYCHOSES

Joyce Seiko Kobayashi, M.D.

1. What are the common symptoms of a psychosis?
Psychotic symptoms generally reflect thinking that is out of touch with reality. Psychotic symptoms are often divided into "deficit" symptoms, which are discussed in relationship to schizophrenia (see question 9), and "positive" psychotic symptoms, which include the following:

Auditory or visual hallucinations

Delusions (paranoid, grandiose, romantic, mistaken identities)

Ideas of reference (e.g., a radio or television carrying a special message for an individual)

Thought insertion

Thought broadcasting

Thought control

Loosening of associations and disorganized thought process

2. How should a primary care provider identify and assess positive psychotic symptoms?
Patients often refer to positive symptoms in colloquial terms, and frank psychotic symptoms may go unrecognized if patients are not specifically asked about them. Questions should be simple and nonthreatening:

- Do you find that your thoughts sometimes feel like they are racing or come so fast that they feel out of control?
- Have you ever felt like you have special powers, such as being able to read other peoples' minds, or that your life has a special purpose?
- Do you ever feel that other people can control your thoughts or read your mind?
- Do you ever feel that others are trying to hurt you or make life difficult for you?
- Do you ever hear voices or see things that are not there?
- Do you ever feel that the television or radio is talking directly to you or that they have special messages intended just for you?

3. What are the most common diagnoses of patients who present with psychotic symptoms in the primary care setting?

Delirium or dementia	Mood disorders
Intoxication or withdrawal syndromes	Schizophrenia

4. Define delirium.
Delirium is an acute change of mental status with disturbance of attention and cognition. It has an organic cause and is characterized by abrupt onset (hours or days) and fluctuating

course. It may be associated with rambling, incoherent or muttering speech, perceptual disturbances, disruption of sleep-wake cycle, increased or decreased psychomotor activity, disorientation, or memory impairment.

5. Why should delirium be the first diagnosis considered in a patient with psychotic symptoms?

1. It is often iatrogenic (related to medications or to fluid and electrolyte disturbance).

2. It is the initial presentation of many serious and treatable medical disorders.

3. It is very common, particularly in high-risk populations. An elderly patient may be unaware of any symptoms from a urinary tract infection but present with delirium. A demented patient or a patient with an extensive history of alcohol abuse may become acutely delirious after taking a narcotic or anticholinergic medication. In one study, up to 85% of terminally ill patients with cancer manifested delirium.

6. How useful are the terms toxic psychosis, ICU psychosis, organic psychosis, and organic mental syndrome?

Delirium should replace these earlier terms, which reflect the presumed etiologies of the delirium. Many medications, substances, and other toxins may cause delirium. Theories about the causes of delirium in the intensive care unit (ICU) include sensory deprivation and sensory overload with sleep deprivation as well as the other medical etiologies of delirium to which such patients are susceptible. Psychoses caused by identifiable biologic factors were historically termed "organic" to differentiate them from the "functional" psychoses such as schizophrenia. This distinction is no longer useful. Although the term organic may be helpful as a descriptive term referring to the range of etiologies that are possible in a delirium (physiologic, metabolic, and structural), the general terms "organic mental syndrome" and "organic brain syndrome" should be discarded for a specific diagnosis of delirium or dementia.

7. What are the most common medications that may cause toxic psychosis or delirium in the medically ill patient?

Although any centrally active medication has the potential for toxicity in some patients or at high levels, the most common offenders should be kept in mind:

Narcotics	Anticonvulsants
Benzodiazepines	Antihypertensives
Anticholinergics (or drugs with	Cimetidine
anticholinergic side effects, such	Propranolol
as amitriptyline, thioridizine,	Digoxin
antihistamines)	Theophylline
Antidepressants	Antibiotics such as cephalosporins,
Barbiturates	aminoglycosides, and metronidazole
Steroids	(less common)

8. Which conditions predispose a patient to the development of delirium?

Head injury, mental retardation, dementia, or other neurologic disorders may predispose a patient to delirium of any etiology. Other patients at high risk for psychotic symptoms associated with delirium include

1. Patients over 65 years old with no prior psychiatric history

2. Patients with a history of significant substance abuse

3. Patients who have advanced medical illness or organ failure or are easily susceptible to infection

4. Patients who may be transiently vulnerable to psychotic symptoms because of other specific medical circumstances, (e.g., postpartum delirium)

A good history is necessary to determine exposure to medications, substances, or toxins; both intoxication and withdrawal syndromes should be considered. It is also important to determine the premorbid level of function, psychiatric history, and timing of onset in relation to acute events, such as trauma or hypoxia. Common additional etiologies that should be assessed include infection, metabolic or fluid and electrolyte disturbances, vitamin deficiencies, endocrinopathies, cerebrovascular events (strokes, hemorrhage), and other pathology of the central nervous system such as tumors, seizures, abscesses, cerebritis, and hydrocephalus.

Finally, the physician should consider a summation effect, in which factors such as sleep deprivation, dehydration, anemia, or stress may precipitate delirium in conjunction with other conditions, such as a low-grade infection in an elderly patient.

9. How is delirium differentiated from schizophrenia?

Helpful Clues

	DELIRIUM	SCHIZOPHRENIA
Age of onset	> Fifth decade	< Fifth decade
Speech	May be dysarthric	Usually clear articulation
Hallucinations	Visual > auditory	Auditory > visual
Disorientation	Frequent	Uncommon
Memory	Often abnormal	May be normal
Diurnal variation	May be worse at night (sundowning)	No change
Misinterpretation	Unfamiliar as familiar	Familiar as unfamiliar

The positive psychotic symptoms observed in schizophrenia usually occur in the context of a deteriorating level of function and are frequently associated with a more extensive course of deficit symptoms, such as marked social isolation or withdrawal, peculiar or bizarre behavior, marked impairment in personal hygiene, blunted or inappropriate affect, poverty of speech or speech content, or marked lack of initiative. Formal diagnosis generally requires at least 1 week of positive psychotic symptoms within a 6-month period of asymptomatic behavior.

10. When are psychotic symptoms seen in a patient with dementia?

The diagnosis of dementia requires a primary disturbance in memory and new learning as well as secondary disturbances in higher cortical functions such as abstract reasoning, judgment, language, or personality. Patients are generally diagnosed with dementia before they experience frank psychotic symptoms. However, a surprisingly high percentage of patients with moderate-to-severe dementia of all etiologies may experience psychotic symptoms at some point in their illness, most commonly auditory or visual hallucinations or paranoid delusions.

Patients who are very forgetful or feel vulnerable because of becoming more disorganized may begin to believe that someone is taking their (misplaced) possessions or intends to harm them. Others who have difficulty hearing or who have little social contact may begin to talk to themselves or imagine visits from dead relatives. Diminished cognitive capacity may result in diminished ability to distinguish the real from the imaginary.

The possibility of superimposed delirium must always be considered in a demented patient with psychotic symptoms, particularly if the symptoms have an acute onset. In addition, many disorders that were historically described as secondary dementias because the cognitive symptoms are due to a treatable or identifiable disease may present with mild cognitive dysfunction and prominent psychotic symptoms. Examples include porphyria, Huntington's chorea, endocrinopathies, nutritional deficiencies, temporal lobe epilepsy, and heavy metal toxicity.

Treatment of the delirium or secondary dementias obviously requires treatment of the underlying disorders, but psychotic symptoms of any etiology are often ameliorated by very low doses of neuroleptics.

11. In which medical conditions may a mood disturbance be a prominent manifestation of delirium?

Steroid toxicity, hypo- and hypercalcemia, thyroid disease, and tertiary syphilis may result in prominent mood disturbances, although any delirious patient may intermittently manifest emotional lability.

12. What disorders in addition to schizophrenia or delirium may present with psychotic symptoms?

1. **Mood disorders** such as major depressive disorder or bipolar (manic-depressive) disorder may or may not be associated with psychotic symptoms during an episode of depression or mania. Psychotic symptoms usually are congruent with the mood, such as delusions of guilt and punishment in depression or grandiose delusions in mania. Episodes frequently recur at variable intervals, but functioning generally returns to normal between episodes.

2. If psychotic symptoms also occur in the absence of a mood disorder (mood-incongruent positive psychotic symptoms), the diagnosis is usually a **schizoaffective disorder.**

3. The symptoms of a **brief reactive psychosis** are indistinguishable from psychotic symptoms that may occur in schizophrenia, but they appear in relationship to one or more markedly stressful events, and resolve within a short period of time (usually within hours to a few weeks). Reactive psychosis is usually accompanied by significant emotional turmoil and is not associated with the gradual deterioration of function that often precedes a schizophrenic psychosis. A brief reactive psychosis may be observed in a patient who has been sexually assaulted, for example.

Formal diagnostic criteria for these and less common psychotic disorders may be found in the revised third edition of the Diagnostic and Statistical Manual of the American Psychiatric Association (DSM-1V).

13. What behavioral, environmental, and pharmacologic approaches are useful in treating the psychotic patient with delirium?

Interventions that help to orient the patient, structure activities, and make the environment feel more familiar are helpful. Strategies include introducing anyone who enters the patients' room and reminding the patient of the date and purpose of the visit; maintaining a regular daily schedule without abrupt changes in location; keeping a diary, appointment book, or calendar visible in the patient's room; having a night light, clock, and familiar objects nearby; asking friends or relatives to accompany or visit the patient frequently; keeping information and discussions simple, with frequent repetition; and writing down specific instructions about medications or activities.

The most useful pharmacologic treatment for the delirious patient, besides treating the underlying disorder, is a trial of low-dose neuroleptic medication. High-potency antipsychotic medication in divided doses, such as haloperidol (0.5–4 mg/day) or trifluoperazine (1–4 mg/day), may have a remarkable effect on agitation and behavioral confusion, without significant orthostatic hypotension. Lower-potency medications, such as trifluoperazine (2–8 mg/day), thiothixene (2–10 mg/day), or loxapine (5–10 mg/day) may be substituted in the presence of extrapyramidal side effects rather than treating the side effects with anticholinergic agents or using thioridazine.

Benzodiazepines may be useful in the acute management of significant physical agitation but risk further confusion. Anticonvulsants at low doses and methylphenidate at titrated doses may be useful in chronic delirious states, such as cognitive dysfunction related to the human immunodeficiency virus (HIV).

14. What are the common side effects of antipsychotic medication in medically ill patients?

The most common side effects of antipsychotic medication derive from short- and long-term effects on the extrapyramidal system, including dystonia (stiffness), akathisia (restlessness), and tardive dyskinesia. Patients may complain of dry mouth, sialorrhea, or other anticholinergic side effects; orthostatic hypotension; diminished range of affect; or cognitive dysfunction. Less commonly, phenothiazines have been associated with hepatic dysfunction, agranulocytosis, gynecomastia and/or lactation, and pigmentary retinopathy. High-potency neuroleptics have been associated in rare cases with neuroleptic malignant syndrome.

BIBLIOGRAPHY

1. Barsky AJ, Cleary PD, Sarnie MK, et al: The course of transient hypochondriasis. Am J Psychiatry 150:484–488, 1993.
2. Brawman-Mintzer O, Lydiard RB, Emmanuel N, et al: Psychiatric comorbidity in patients with generalized anxiety disorder. Am J Psychiatry 150:1216–1218, 1993.
3. Chignon JM, Lepine JP, Ades J: Panic disorder in cardiac outpatients. Am J Psychiatry 150:780–785, 1993.
4. Clark DA, Beck AT, Beck JS: Symptom differences in major depression, dysthymia, panic disorder, and generalized anxiety disorder. Am J Psychiatry 150:205–209, 1994.
5. Coryell W, Endicott J, Winokur G: Anxiety syndromes as epiphenomena of primary major depression: Outcome and familial psychopathology. Am J Psychiatry 149:100–107, 1992.
6. Diagnostic and Statistical Manual of Mental Disorders, 4th ed. Washington, DC, American Psychiatric Press, 1994.
7. Fricchione GL, Howanitz E, Jandorf L, et al: Psychological adjustment of end-stage renal disease and the implications of denial. Psychosomatics 33:85–93, 1992.
8. Hales RE, Yudofsky SC (eds): Textbook of Neuropsychiatry, 2nd ed. Washington, DC, American Psychiatric Press, 1992.
9. Kessler RC, McGonagle KA, Zhao S, et al: Lifetime and 12-month prevalence of DSM-III-R psychiatric disorders in the United States. Arch Gen Psychiatry 51:8–19, 1994.
10. Kirmayer LJ, Robbins JM: Somatization and the recognition of depression and anxiety in primary care. Am J Psychiatry 150:734–741, 1993.
11. Lydiard RB, Brady K, Ballenger JC, et al: Anxiety and mood disorders in hospitalized alcoholic individuals. Am J Addict 1:325–331, 1992.
12. Massion AO, Warshaw MG, Keller MB: Quality of life and psychiatric morbidity in panic disorder and generalized anxiety disorder. Am J Psychiatry 150:600–607, 1993.
13. Pardis CM, Friedman S, Lazar RM, et al: Anxiety disorders in a neuromuscular clinic. Am J Psychiatry 150:1102–1104, 1993.
14. Popkin MK, Tucker GJ: Secondary and drug-induced mood, anxiety, psychotic, catatonic, and personality disorders: A review of the literature. J Neuropsychiatry Clin Neurosci 4:369–385, 1992.
15. Smith SL, Colenda CC, Espeland MA: Factors determining the level of anxiety state in geriatric primary care patients in a community dwelling. Psychosomatics 35:50–58, 1994.
16. Stoudemire A, Fogel BS (eds): Principles of Medical Psychiatry. New York, Grune & Stratton Inc., 1987.
17. Wald TG, Kathol RG, Noyes R, et al: Rapid relief of anxiety in cancer patients with both alprazolam and placebo. Psychosomatics 34:324–338, 1993.

11. THE DIFFICULT PERSONALITY

John F. Bridges, M.D.

1. What is personality?

Although it is a common and intuitive concept, personality is a difficult term to define with specificity and completeness. Personality encompasses both internal perceptions of the self and the world and the activity of the self in the world (as objectively experienced and described by others.) In addition, personality describes perceptions and actions that are consistent through time and characterize an individual with both biologic inborn traits and capacities (temperament) and acquired learned responses (character).

Most current understandings of personality suggest that inborn capacities and limitations interact with the accidents of environmental advantages and deficiencies to unfold the internal psychological structures and externally revealed patterns of behavior that we call personality.

2. When do personality traits become a personality disorder?

Constellations of personality traits that assume enduring, rigid patterns of maladaptive response to the stressors of life form the bases of a personality disorder.

3. Describe the salient features of the three major groups of personality disorders.

Ten personality disorders are grouped into three clusters (A–C). Disorders within clusters appear to share common features that suggest relationships among them. The clustering also acknowledges a high degree of overlap in symptomatology.

Cluster A: Persons who are unusual, odd or eccentric in their thinking and appearance

• *Paranoid Personality Disorder*—characterized by a perception of others as motivated by a desire to harm or demean, a questioning of the trustworthiness of others, the bearing of grudges, and a tendency to be easily slighted and to find hidden meanings in the actions or words of others, confirming suspicions and mistrust.

• *Schizoid Personality Disorder*—characterized by a restriction in the capacity for social connection and an inability to feel or express emotions, the choice of solitary lifestyle, denial of the subjective experience of strong emotions, little affect expression, and apparent indifference to social, sexual, and emotional intimacy.

• *Schizotypal Personality Disorder*—characterized by the deficits in interpersonal connection of schizoid personality disorder with the additional features of oddities in thinking and behavior that share common themes with schizophrenia (though not as severe) and paranoid personality disorder, such as suspiciousness, ideas of reference, magical thinking, and additionally displaying quirky modes of speech, dress, and manner.

Cluster B: Persons who are dramatic, highly emotional, and engage in erratic behaviors

• *Antisocial Personality Disorder*—characterized by irresponsible behaviors, beginning in adolescence and carrying through to an adulthood of inconsistent work and social relationships, failure to conform to social norms, disregard for truth, impulsiveness, aggression, reckless behaviors, and lack of remorse for injuries to others.

• *Borderline Personality Disorder*—characterized by unstable moods, relationships, and identity; impulsiveness, with intense emotional reactions leading to reckless self-damaging behaviors, suicide threats and attempts, an impaired ability to regulate moods and mood-dictated expressions of anger and other strongly felt feeling states, and transient paranoid ideation.

• *Histrionic Personality Disorder*—characterized by extreme and inappropriate emotionality, with seductive sexualized interactions with others, fluctuating extremes of feeling states often dramatically demonstrated, low frustration tolerance and preoccupation with immediate gratification, and vague, shallow, impressionistic speech.

• *Narcissistic Personality Disorder*—characterized by imagined or enacted grandiosity in the absence of empathic connection with others, an easily injured and highly overvalued sense of self-importance, an unrealistic sense of uniqueness in a context of interpersonal callousness, entitlement, and demand for attention.

Cluster C: Persons with excessive fearfulness and anxiety

• *Avoidant Personality Disorder*—characterized by social discomfort based on a pervasive fear of being negatively judged, an inability to tolerate disapproval, a need for guarantees of acceptance, and an unwillingness to engage in social and interpersonal engagements that risk exposure to these fearsome situations.

• *Dependent Personality Disorder*—characterized by pervasive dependent behavior and fear of interpersonal loss leading to an unwillingness to take chances, express opinions, make decisions, or undertake projects for fear of severing overvalued connections with others, with attendant feelings of abandonment and loss when even small rifts occur in relationships.

• *Obsessive-Compulsive Personality Disorder*—characterized by inflexible demands for perfectionism that interfere with functioning, demands for submission by others to unreasonable standards, preoccupation with rules, details, right and wrong, and a marked lack of generosity in dealing with others.

Personality disorders under investigation for inclusion

• *Passive-Aggressive Personality Disorder* (Negativistic Personality Disorder)—characterized by a passive opposition to the demands of life, leading to an impaired capacity to work and accomplish goals, with irritable and oppositional responses to authority, deliberate procrastination, protestations of unreasonable expectations and personal misfortune, over-valuation of actual performance, and a concerted critical obstructionist stance to undertakings involving others coupled with feelings of being unappreciated.

• *Depressive Personality Disorder*—characterized by pervasive and nearly continuous feelings of gloom and hopelessness, low self-concept with a critical attacking attitude toward the self; persistent worry, blaming of others and self, and overall harboring a guilty, sad, unhappy view of life.

4. Are children and adolescents diagnosed with personality disorders?

Not usually. Because personality is presumed to be determined only partly by inborn traits or temperament, psychiatrists are wary of applying personality disorder diagnoses to youngsters. As defining criteria, such disorders have maladaptive long-term functioning and inflexible traits. It is the nature of human development over the entire life-span, and perhaps most prominently during the first 20 years of life, to try various methods of responding to and exploiting the world. This process necessarily involves many responses that are less than ideally adaptive and fruitful.

5. Do excessive characteristics in childhood herald adult personality disorders?

Perhaps. Certain childhood disorders, diagnosed in persons under 18 years of age, appear to bear some relationship to the later development of personality disorders.

Disorder of childhood/adolescence	Personality disorder
Conduct disorder	Antisocial personality disorder
Avoidant disorder of childhood	Avoidant personality disorder
Identity disorder	Borderline personality disorder

6. What overall characteristics suggest the possibility of a personality disorder?

One of the hallmarks of a personality disorder is that the patient does not accept personal responsibility for the subjective distress that he or she experiences. A second hallmark is that the disorder is observable within the context of human relationships. The invisibility of the source of the problems to the patient is called ego syntonicity. To the patient, the problem lies not within the self but with others. Thus, the paranoid patient does not see suspicion and mistrust as excessive, out of context, or causing repeated failures in relationships. Such perceptions appear justified and reasonable responses to the measureless potential for injury in everyday life. Similarly, the narcissistic patient does not complain about the relentlessly alienating effects of grandiose and unempathic exploitation of others; rather, the patient complains about the infuriating and hurtful sense of living in a world of persons who do not afford him or her appropriate credit and admiration.

7. What reactions in the caregiver may suggest that the patient has a personality disorder?

Clinicians usually discover the presence of a personality disorder in the context of attempting to provide care for the patient. They find unexpectedly that delivery of care becomes increasingly difficult, apparently troublesome for both physician and patient. Such patients engender powerful responses from the caregivers, as they have from families, friends, and employers; they are irritating, frustrating, and maddening and evoke exaggerated responses from others. In addition, given the symptoms' ego syntonicity, the caregiver may frequently be seen as the source of the patient's distress.

8. Before diagnosing a personality disorder, what common organic causes of abnormal behavior should be considered?

Personality disorders may be mimicked by various organic disorders as well as by other mental illnesses. Three common medical conditions may cause symptoms that appear similar to those described for personality disorders:

1. **Dementias of senile or presenile onset.** Such patients frequently present with behavioral problems, including irritability, paranoia, anger, and impulsiveness. They may demonstrate the exact symptoms of a disordered personality and elicit from family and friends the same

avoidance and anger. The insidious onset masks such dementias, as does the tendency of patients, at least initially, to become exaggerated versions of their former selves. For example, the man who was occasionally irritable and picky gradually becomes an angry, hypercritical caricature of himself, or the sentimental, easily injured woman evolves into a weepy, irrationally inconsolable burlesque of her former self.

2. **Chronic use of certain prescribed medicines.** Chronic changes in mood and attitude may result from certain long-term drug therapies to which both patient and family have become inured. For example, even digitalis may induce chronic depression and paranoia. The differential diagnosis may require subtle questioning about the onset and progression of changes that are nearly invisible to patient or family.

3. **Substance abuse.** Substance abuse, especially alcohol abuse, in a patient or perhaps even in a patient's family may distort personality development and alter long-term patterns. Some research suggests that commencement or cessation of substance use, over time, may radically alter personality style and functioning.

9. What classic patient-caregiver difficulties may occur with patients who have personality disorders or certain personality traits?
Patients with personality disorders can be extremely exasperating to treat. They approach the physician with admixtures of deep-seated fears and suspicions, unbounded wishes for dependency and caretaking, and profoundly distorted views of themselves and their doctors. Although the problems may not be appreciated by the clinician at the onset of the doctor-patient relationship, they soon manifest as characteristic and unwanted feelings and responses from the physician.

The hostile patient. Hostility from a patient is a surprise to clinicians accustomed to grateful and obedient responses. Patients who are paranoid or worried about their vulnerability easily perceive the doctor-patient relationship as unequal (as, in fact, it is) and compromising. They see the physician's ministrations as intrusive and threatening. Such anxiety is rationalized by attacking the physician, devaluing his or her motives, and questioning every decision. This response at first puzzles and later angers the doctor. It flies directly in the face of how physicians see themselves and prefer to be seen by others. Actual care for the patient quickly withers under the barrage of implied or expressed accusation. The doctor soon feels reluctant to pursue appropriate follow-up or to recommend difficult treatments, because he or she no longer wishes to be subjected to hostility and misunderstanding.

The dependent, demanding patient. Dependent patients with powerful wishes for unlimited nurturing initially may be welcomed by the physician, who is perceived as extremely competent and uniquely helpful. The physician responds by returning the patient's admiration and offering more explanations and thoroughness in treatment. Soon, however, such patients reveal an inexpressibly great need for attention. They increase their demands for time, advice, and contact. The physician begins to feel hounded and guilty for not responding wholeheartedly to the increasing demands. Eventually the physician withdraws, puts up barriers, and finds ways to avoid the patient. The patient responds with intensified demands for care and anger at the (accurate) perception of rejection. Thus rigorous medical care falters and fails.

The doctor defeater. Such patients may display paranoia, an exaggerated sense of self-worth, or wildly fluctuating attitudes toward themselves and the caretaker. Some patients seem to choose behaviors obviously in direct opposition to their own best interests. The common thread in their relations with physicians is the unremitting demand for care and the adamant refusal to acknowledge that any treatment is adequate or helpful. The physician becomes increasingly angry at such patients, often expressing the anger as jokes about the patient or benign neglect of the patient's complaints. The wish that the patient "just go away" may be contrary to the physician's ideal self-image and may even result in stubborn attempts to "save" the patient.

In all of these cases—and their many permutations—the patient's mode of interaction is unexpected and misunderstood by the physician. The patient unknowingly frustrates and alienates the physician. The physician, also unknowingly, may take countermeasures in an attempt to proceed with "business as usual," not recognizing that medical reasoning and delivery of care are hampered by the deterioration in the relationship itself.

10. What guidelines should the physician use in caring for the patient with difficult personality traits or a frank personality disorder?
Dealing with patients whose illness manifests in the doctor-patient relationship is not easy. Nor is it easy for the patient, who has a lifetime of failed attempts to relate and to satisfy needs and whose pain over time is enormous. The following guidelines are useful.

1. Recognize the problem by using your own feelings as guides. Take note when you find yourself dreading a patient, imagining the patient on someone else's service, joking about the patient, or arguing with yourself about whether it is necessary to like a patient in order to provide adequate care.

2. Identify what behaviors are affecting the patient's medical care. Discuss the patient with a colleague. Step outside the dysfunctional relationship, and apply diagnostic thinking to the relationship itself. For example, the patient's relentless telephone contact may cause you to pull away, or the insistent demand for ever more and better tests to prove you "wrong" ("I'm sure you're hiding something from me, doctor") or the patient "right" ("I'm just another check in the mail for you, doctor, so I've got to watch out for myself") may force you into practicing defensively and therefore inefficiently.

3. Determine the best way to confront the patient's behavior and spell out its consequences. It is advisable to be consistent with your diagnosis of the problem. For example, the dependent worrier who fears abandonment may be told: "All of these phone calls are making it hard to determine when you really need my help, and they come at times when I cannot think as clearly as I'd like about your problems. I think it best if you save your unscheduled calls for clear medical emergencies, but why don't you give me a call each week when I can make sure that I will have the time to talk with you? Wednesdays after my clinic hours make the most sense."

For the hostile patient whose angry accusations and demeaning attacks betray a fear of dependency and damage, a realistic and reassuring approach that shares control may help the relationship: "It can be very hard to feel that you are putting yourself in someone else's hands when you are ill. I want to make certain that you clearly understand what I'm recommending and that you have as much time as you need to ask questions about how the treatment will work. I want you to feel free to tell me what your worries are. We will need to work together closely on this."

For the self-defeating obstructor, awareness of his or her control and the physician's relative lack of power is essential. The approach to such patients must be both humble and frank with change in behavior couched as a choice rather than a demand: "Drinking as much and as often as you do puts you at great risk. I think that you understand by now how dangerous it is. I can offer some suggestions again for what measures you can take to stop drinking and offer my support, but finally you will have to decide whether or not to do what is best for your health."

11. Is it appropriate for a physician to refer to a colleague the patient who evokes irreconcilable conflict?
Yes. Patients are best treated by physicians who can care about them in a genuine way. This caring may find its highest expression in the ability to tolerate the patient's behavior without becoming personally upset. Each physician has certain strengths and weaknesses in this regard. Part of delivering the best possible care is recognizing limitations and the point at which the ability to offer thoughtful, objective care has become compromised. Just as physicians cannot expect to give good care when they are deprived of sleep, or in the midst of a personal crisis, so they cannot expect to be capable of caring for every sort of problem patient.

If a patient presents impossible conflicts for the physician, it is the physician's right and responsibility to refer the patient to another practitioner from whom the patient may expect medical care uncompromised by negative feelings. This transfer should be undertaken openly, and the physician to whom the patient is referred should be told of the problems in advance. Alternatively, it may be helpful to share the care of such patients in an attempt to dilute the intensity of the conflicts.

12. Is referral to a psychiatrist ever appropriate in the care of patients with difficult personalities?

Yes. Although such patients frequently resent, and recoil from, referral to psychiatrists, it often is profitable to obtain a psychiatric consultation for the patient with a personality disorder or a difficult personality. A psychiatrist may be able to clarify the patterns of the patient's undermining of the relationship and offer suggestions about ways to deal with the conflicts.

BIBLIOGRAPHY

1. Cloninger CR, Svrakic DM, Przybeck TR: A psychobiological model of temperament and character. Arch Gen Psychiatry 50:975–990, 1993.
2. Diagnostic and Statistical Manual of Mental Disorders, 4th ed. Washington, DC, The American Psychiatric Association, 1994.
3. Groves JE: Taking care of the hateful patient. N Engl J Med 298:893–897, 1978.
4. Kaplan HI, Freedman AM, Sadock BJ (eds): Comprehensive Textbook of Psychiatry III. Baltimore, Williams & Wilkins, 1980.
5. Morey L: Personality disorders in DSM-III and DSM-III-R: Convergence, coverage, and internal consistency. Am J Psychiatry 145:573–577, 1988.
6. Nestadt G, Romanoski AJ, Samuels JF, et al: The relationship between personality and DSM-III axis I disorders in the population: Results from an epidemiological survey. Am J Psychiatry 149:1228–1233, 1992.
7. Oldham JM (ed): Personality Disorders: New Perspectives on Diagnostic Validity. Washington, DC, American Psychiatric Press, 1991.
8. Perry JC: Problems and considerations in the valid assessment of personality disorders. Am J Psychiatry 149:1645–1653, 1992.
9. Stone MH: Abnormalities of Personality. New York, W. W. Norton, 1993.
10. Svrakic DM, Whitehead C, Przybeck TR, Cloninger CR: Differential diagnosis of personality disorders by the seven factor model of temperament and character. Arch Gen Psychiatry 50:991–999, 1993.
11. Valliant GE: Adaptation to Life. Boston, Little, Brown, 1977.
12. Widiger TA, Frances A, Spitzer RL, Williams JBW: The DSM-III-R personality disorders: An overview. Am J Psychiatry 145:786–795, 1988.

III. Primary Disorders of the Cardiovascular System

12. HYPERTENSION

David L. Olson, M.D., and Stuart L. Linas, M.D.

1. When is a patient hypertensive?

A patient is considered to be hypertensive when the average of two or more measurements over 4 weeks detects systolic blood pressure of 140 mmHg or greater and/or diastolic blood pressure of 90 mmHg or greater. Patients with systolic blood pressure ≥ 210 mmHg and diastolic blood pressure ≥ 120 mmHg should be evaluated or referred for care immediately.

2. Why should hypertension be treated?

Hypertension is a major risk factor for coronary, cerebral, and renal vascular disease. The Framingham heart study cohort demonstrated a statistically significant, progressive increase in coronary heart disease with increases in either systolic or diastolic blood pressure. Considerable evidence suggests that therapy reduces stroke and renal disease. In addition, hypertension clearly increases the risk of left ventricular hypertrophy (LVH), retinal changes (Keith-Wagener-Barker classification), and central nervous system injury (cerebral infarction and hemorrhage).

3. Does treatment of systolic hypertension alter outcome in elderly patients?

Yes. The Systolic Hypertension in the Elderly Program (SHEP), a large, multicenter, randomized, placebo-controlled, and blinded study, followed patients with a mean age of 72 years, an average systolic blood pressure of 170 mmHg, and diastolic blood pressure less than 90 mmHg. Patients were randomized to treatment aimed at reducing systolic blood pressure to less than 160 mmHg. Results showed a 36% reduction in the incidence of stroke and a 27% reduction in the incidence of nonfatal myocardial infarction and death in the treatment versus placebo groups.

4. What is the combined effect of elevated levels of serum cholesterol, smoking, and hypertension on the rate of death from coronary heart disease (CHD)?

In the 316,099 men screened in the Multiple Risk Factor Intervention Trial (MRFIT), the rate of death from CHD was 230 times greater among smokers with a cholesterol level and systolic blood pressure in the highest quintile than in nonsmokers with a systolic pressure and cholesterol level in the lowest quintile. The study found a strong graded relationship between death due to CHD and an increase in systolic and diastolic blood pressure or cholesterol levels above 4.65 mmol/L (180 mg/dl).

5. Does therapy for hypertension influence LVH?

Yes. Major advances in understanding the relationship between hypertension and LVH have been made. LVH, found in 50% of all hypertensive patients by echocardiography (5% by electrocardiogram), is a major risk factor for adverse cardiovascular outcomes, such as myocardial ischemia and infarction, congestive heart failure, and sudden death. LVH regresses after the use of calcium channel blockers, beta blockers, and angiotensin-converting enzyme (ACE) inhibitors. No regression of LVH has been seen after treatment with diuretic or vasodilator agents.

6. Describe the relationship between hypertension and abnormal carbohydrate metabolism.
Essential hypertension is associated with insulin resistance, glucose intolerance, and hyperinsulinemia; thus, it may be an insulin-resistant state. In addition, hyperinsulinemia is a risk factor for coronary artery disease (CAD). However, depending on the choice of drugs, treatment of hypertension may worsen (diuretics or beta blocker) or have no effect on insulin resistance.

7. When should secondary hypertension be suspected?
At least 95% of hypertensive patients have primary or essential hypertension. Secondary hypertension should be suspected in (1) patients < 35 years of age, (2) patients with no family history of hypertension, and (3) patients with an abrupt onset or unexplained change in hypertension on maximal medical management. In addition, secondary causes should be considered in subjects with resistant hypertension (i.e., poor blood pressure control with maximal drug therapy).

8. How may the history, physical examination, and initial laboratory data provide clues to the possible etiology of secondary hypertension?
A thorough history, physical examination, and laboratory studies should be performed to look for causes of secondary hypertension. Renovascular hypertension should be suspected in patients less than 35 years old or older patients with an abrupt worsening of blood pressure, especially in the presence of an abdominal bruit. Oral contraceptives are the most common cause of secondary hypertension in women. Symptoms in the history may indicate pheochromocytoma (flushing, palpitation), drug-induced hypertension (e.g., cocaine), or hyperthyroidism. Cushing's syndrome is easily identified by centripetal obesity, moon face, and striae. Coarctation of the aorta may be diagnosed through comparison of arm and leg blood pressures. Diminished clearance of creatinine suggests renal parenchymal disease, the most common cause of secondary hypertension in an unselected population of hypertensive adults. Unprovoked hypokalemia suggests aldosteronism.

9. When should the diagnosis of renovascular hypertension be pursued?
The prevalence of renovascular hypertension among a general population of hypertensive patients is 0.5%, a rate much lower than prior estimates of 5%, but rises with increasing clinical suspicion. Six situations suggest renovascular hypertension: (1) severe hypertension (diastolic blood pressure > 120 mmHg), (2) hypertension refractory to treatment, (3) abrupt onset of sustained moderate-to-severe hypertension at an age < 20 or > 50 years, (4) hypertension with an abdominal bruit, (5) elevation of creatinine after initiation of ACE inhibitors, and (6) flash pulmonary edema in patients with occlusive vascular disease. In these subsets of patients the incidence of renovascular hypertension is as high as 15%.

10. How should renovascular hypertension be evaluated?
Noninvasive tests have a high predictive value in diagnosing renovascular hypertension. Plasma renin activity after administration of captopril and captopril renography have a sensitivity and specificity of >90%. Random plasma renin activity (PRA), intravenous pyelography (IVP), and renography have not been shown to be useful.

11. Describe the most cost-effective evaluation of hypertension associated with hypokalemia.
The most common cause of hypokalemia in the hypertensive patient is diuretic therapy. Thus, patients receiving thiazide diuretics or digoxin should receive potassium supplementation if the level falls below 3.0 mmol/L. In patients requiring large amounts of potassium supplementation, diuretics should be discontinued, and serum and urine concentrations of potassium should be determined 4–5 days later. Hypokalemia in the setting of urinary potassium wasting (urine K+ > 30 mEq/L) is highly suggestive of aldosternonism.

The next test is paired measurement of upright plasma aldosterone concentration (PAC) and PRA. The screening is positive if PRA is less than 3.0 ng/ml/hr or if the PAC–PRA ratio is less than 20. Primary aldosteronism is confirmed when plasma aldosterone levels remain increased (> 10 mg/dl) after volume expansion with 2 liters of normal saline given over 4 hours. Subsequent evaluation should be done under the guidance of a nephrologist or endocrinologist.

12. What is the significance of borderline hypertension?

Patients with borderline measurements are at increased risk for developing hypertension in the near future. Patients with blood pressure $< 130/85$ should be rechecked in 2 years, whereas patients whose blood pressure ranges from 130–139 systolic or 85–89 diastolic should be rechecked at 1 year.

13. When and how should one initiate therapy for hypertension?

Treatment of mild-to-moderate hypertension in an ambulatory setting follows a slow, deliberate course. Patients with mild to moderate hypertension should attempt to modify their lifestyle. Important modifications include weight reduction, moderation of alcohol intake to less than 2 drinks/day, regular mild or moderate physical activity 3 times/week, reduction of sodium intake to less than 2000–3000 mg/day, and smoking cessation. If the blood pressure remains at or above 140/90 mmHg over a 3–6-month period or if the patient has an initial systolic blood pressure of 180–210 mmHg and/or diastolic blood pressure of 110–120 mmHg, pharmacologic therapy should be initiated at lower doses and increased as necessary. In geriatric patients approximately one-half of the usual starting dose should be used. Drug treatment should follow an organized regimen of "stepped" care. For each medication that is chosen, the patient should be reevaluated within a few days to months, depending on the stage of hypertension. If the response is inadequate, the dose may be doubled. If control is inadequate, a second agent is added. If the blood pressure is controlled to less than 140/90 mmHg, therapy is continued and assessed at appropriate intervals. At least some therapy for hypertension is usually required for the remainder of the patient's life.

14. What is the single most important cause of inadequate blood pressure control?

The major cause of poor control is patient noncompliance. Fewer than 50% of patients with high blood pressure keep follow-up appointments, and fewer than 60% take their medications as prescribed. Barriers to adequate medical compliance include poor doctor–patient communication, cost of medications, and side effects. Care providers must consider all of these factors to improve the outcome of hypertensive therapy.

15. How do lifestyle modifications improve hypertension?

Lifestyle modifications may be used as primary treatment for mild hypertension. Such approaches have not definitively reduced morbidity or mortality but often lower blood pressure, reduce the number and dosage of medications, and improve the risk profile for cardiovascular disease.

16. Which hypertensive patient requires hospitalization?

When the diastolic blood pressure is > 140 mmHg and/or evidence suggests hypertensive encephalopathy, hypertension should be treated with careful inpatient monitoring, using parenteral therapy when needed.

17. What laboratory evaluation should all hypertensive patients undergo?

All newly diagnosed hypertensive patients should undergo basic laboratory studies, including urinalysis for protein, glucose and blood; assessment of serum levels of creatinine, potassium, glucose, calcium, and uric acid; and a lipid profile. Further studies may be added at a later date either to evaluate the possibility of secondary hypertension or to analyze the effect of therapeutic trials. Electrocardiograms should be performed on all hypertensive patients to exclude CAD, LVH, and other nascent heart diseases and to establish baseline values.

18. How do age and race affect the choice of antihypertensive agents?

Two groups have been well studied: Afro-American men and elderly patients. Afro-American men are responsive to diuretics in major randomized, controlled trials. Diuretics may have added benefits in this population because they are inexpensive and compliance rates are high. Additional small studies suggest that calcium channel blockers also benefit Afro-American men. Hypertension in elderly patients is effectively controlled with low-dose diuretics. Three recent major clinical trials show that diuretics particularly reduce geriatric cardiovascular morbidity and mortality. Beta blockers also reduce hypertension in elderly patients; however, they have not significantly reduced cardiovascular mortality.

19. How do concomitant medical conditions affect the choice of antihypertensive drugs?

Antihypertensive Drugs in Patients with Additional Medical Illnesses

CONDITION	PREFERRED AGENT	NOT RECOMMENDED
Asthma with chronic obstructive pulmonary disease	ACE inhibitor Calcium antagonist Thiazide diuretic	Beta blocker
Coronary artery disease	Beta blocker Calcium antagonist	Vasodilators
Left ventricular dysfunction (systolic)	ACE inhibitor	Beta blocker Calcium antagonist
Left ventricular hypertrophy	ACE inhibitor Calcium antagonist	Vasodilators Thiazide
Diabetes mellitus	ACE inhibitor	Beta blocker Thiazide
Chronic renal failure (creatinine > 3 mg/dl)	Loop diuretics Calcium antagonist	ACE inhibitor
Renovascular hypertension	Calcium antagonist	ACE inhibitor

20. When should diuretics *not* be used in the treatment of high blood pressure?

Diuretics are well tolerated, inexpensive, safe, and effective. However, they may be relatively contraindicated in patients with CAD, arrhythmia, gout, glucose intolerance, dyslipidemia, or neuropathy with orthostasis.

21. When is an ACE inhibitor contraindicated?

Rarely. The primary contraindications include angioedema related to ACE inhibitor treatment, pregnancy, a creatinine level greater than 3 mg/dl, or potassium greater than 5 mmol/L. ACE inhibitors also may be contraindicated in patients with a history of angioedema unrelated to ACE inhibitors, because there may be an increased risk of angioedema while taking an ACE inhibitor. ACE inhibitors may cause fetal or neonatal morbidity or mortality primarily in the second or third trimester. Thus, treatment with ACE inhibitors should be discontinued immediately after a patient learns that she is pregnant. An ACE inhibitor may worsen azotemia or hyperkalemia by reducing the glomerular filtration rate.

22. List indications for ambulatory or continuous blood pressure monitoring.

- Discrepancy between home and office blood pressure readings
- Persistent elevation of blood pressure in the office without target organ disease
- Episodic elevation of blood pressure
- Hypertension resistant to treatment
- End-organ disease in the face of normal office blood pressure
- Evaluation of efficacy of treatment

23. Does smoking cessation influence hypertension?
Smoking cessation does not directly improve hypertension but profoundly reduces cardiovascular mortality.

24. How do calcium antagonists differ in their hemodynamic effects?
Calcium antagonists lower blood pressure by decreasing either cardiac output (CO) or systemic vascular resistance (SVR). Some calcium antagonists reduce SVR with little (isradipine) or no (felodipine, amlodipine) decreases in CO. Others (verapamil, diltiazem) have major cardiac effects, whereas nifedipine and nicardipine are predominantly vasodilators but decrease CO in the presence of underlying systolic dysfunction. Thus, the choice of calcium channel blocker is determined by additional underlying disease and cost effectiveness.

BIBLIOGRAPHY

1. Clark LT: Improving compliance and increasing control of hypertension: Needs of special hypertensive populations. Am Heart J 121:664, 1991.
2. Dunn FG, Burns JM, Hornung RS: Left ventricular hypertrophy in hypertension. Am Heart J 122:312, 1991.
3. Fifth Report of the Joint National Committee on Detection, Evaluation, and Treatment of High Blood Pressure (JNC V). Arch Intern Med 153:154, 1993.
4. Kaplan NM: Management of hypertension. Dis Mon 38:76, 1992.
5. Kaplan NM: Systemic hypertension: Mechanisms and diagnosis. In Braunwald E (ed): Heart Disease: A Textbook of Cardiovascular Disease. Philadelphia, W.B. Saunders, 1992, pp 817–874.
6. McCarron DA, Haber E, Slater EE: Hypertension. Sci Am Med 7:1, 1993.
7. Neaton JD, Wentworth D, for the Multiple Risk Factor Intervention Trial group: Serum cholesterol, blood pressure, cigarette smoking, and death from coronary heart disease. Arch Intern Med 152:56–64, 1992.
8. Schwartz GL: Initial therapy for hypertension-individualizing care. Mayo Clin Proc 65:73, 1990.
9. SHEP Cooperative Research Group: Prevention of stroke by antihypertensive drug treatment in older persons with isolated systolic hypertension: Final results of the Systolic Hypertension in the Elderly Program (SHEP). JAMA 265:3255, 1991.
10. Weinberger MH, Grim CE, Hollifield JW, et al: Primary aldosteronism. Ann Intern Med 55:86, 1979.
11. Young WF, Hogan MJ, Klee GG, et al: Primary aldosternonism: Diagnosis and treatment. Mayo Clin Proc 65:96, 1990.

13. CHEST PAIN

Valerie Ulstad, M.D.

1. What is the most important tool in distinguishing the cause of chest pain?
The history taken by the health care provider is without question the most valuable tool. It is important to have a systematic way in which to obtain the history.

2. What are the important components of the history in the evaluation of chest pain?
The two Cs should be remembered when evaluating chest pain or discomfort—characterize and categorize.

　　1. **Characterize.** You are seeking a thorough description of the pain. This would include: the *quality* of the sensation (crushing, burning, stabbing, tearing), the *location and radiation* of the pain, the *temporal intensity* of the discomfort, including how it begins (starts abruptly, builds up insidiously) and the *duration* (seconds, minutes, hours, days), the sources of *provocation* (exercise, emotional stress, eating, inhalation/exhalation, changing position), the

palliative features (rest, nitroglycerin, food, change of position), and other *associated features* (pallor, diaphoresis, dyspnea, palpitations).

2. **Categorize.** What organ system are you dealing with? Is there more than one type of pain? Is the discomfort cardiac, pulmonary, gastrointestinal, breast, musculoskeletal, neurologic, or psychological?

3. Name the most common cardiovascular causes of chest pain.
Common causes include atherosclerosis manifesting as chronic ischemic heart disease (angina pectoris) and acute ischemic heart disease (myocardial infarction), pericarditis, dissecting aortic aneurysm, valvular heart disease, and hypertrophic cardiomyopathy. A careful history and physical exam are important in differentiating these individual and sometimes coexistent problems.

4. Describe typical angina pectoris.
Angina pectoris is a clinical syndrome characterized typically by a deep retrosternal pressurelike sensation that occurs during physical exercise particularly in the cold, eating, or emotional excitement. Angina may be described as a tight, gripping, squeezing, crushing, or viselike sensation. Patients may in fact protest at the word "pain" and prefer "discomfort" as a suitable descriptor. When the patient places a clenched fist over the sternum to describe the chest discomfort, angina is strongly suggested (Levine sign). The discomfort usually builds up gradually to its peak. Anginal discomfort usually does not radiate, but when it does, it may radiate to a variety of locations: the neck, jaw, teeth, left or right arm, or back. The ulnar aspect of the left arm is a particularly common site of radiation. There may be accompanying symptoms such as pallor, diaphoresis, nausea, dyspnea, and fatigue. The discomfort usually lasts 5–15 minutes and disappears with rest and/or sublingual nitroglycerin. The frequency of discomfort and level of exertion that precipitates the angina are important in determining the urgency for further diagnostic and therapeutic interventions.

5. List the risk factors for atherosclerotic cardiovascular disease.
Hypertension	Family history
Diabetes	Hyperlipidemia
Smoking	Obesity
Male >40 years of age	Type A personality
Postmenopausal female	

6. What physical findings support the presence of coronary artery disease?
The physical examination in a patient with severe angina can be completely normal. Relatively subtle findings such as an S4, a mitral regurgitation murmur, and/or a sustained apical impulse can occur during an ischemic episode. Hypertension may also be present during pain.

7. Does a normal EKG rule out coronary artery disease as the cause of chest pain?
Absolutely not! The EKG can be normal even during an acute myocardial infarction in up to 10% of patients. The history is more sensitive than the EKG. A normal EKG should never dissuade you from pursuing a worrisome history. Certainly evidence of ST-T changes during an episode of pain can support the clinical diagnosis already made by the history, as would Q waves suggesting previous myocardial infarction.

8. How does the chest pain associated with acute myocardial infarction differ from that of angina pectoris?
The only real difference between these two syndromes is that angina pectoris is relieved relatively promptly with rest and/or nitroglycerin as opposed to acute myocardial infarction where the pain may be prolonged (>30 minutes), lasting potentially for hours. The pain of acute myocardial infarction also tends to radiate more widely.

9. What are anginal equivalents?

These are symptoms that may occur in place of typical anginal chest pain but represent the same pathophysiologic process. Examples include dyspnea; discomfort along the ulnar aspect of the left forearm; lower jaw, teeth, neck or shoulder pain; nausea; indigestion; diaphoresis; or the development of gas or belching. The clinician should initially consider ischemic heart disease in the differential diagnosis of these symptoms.

10. When is chest pain called "atypical"?

Patients with atypical chest pain have only two of three of the following characteristics to their pain: (1) pain in substernal location, (2) pain precipitated by exertion, or (3) pain relieved by rest or nitroglycerin in 10 minutes or less.

11. What is Prinzmetal's angina?

Prinzmetal's angina occurs at rest or with ordinary activity and is not precipitated by exercise. The discomfort tends to occur at night or in the early morning. The episodes may be severe and longer in duration than those of typical angina pectoris. This relatively rare situation is thought to be due to coronary spasm. The clinician would be unable to distinguish between Prinzmetal's angina and an acute ischemic syndrome (like unstable angina or acute myocardial infarction) while actually observing a patient having pain. A history that suggests recurrence, particularly at the same time of day, is suggestive of Prinzmetal's angina.

12. How does typical pericardial pain differ from angina?

Pericardial pain is sharper than angina. The patient may describe the pain as stabbing. The discomfort is often located on the left side of the chest and may radiate to the neck and left trapezius ridge. Leaning forward may alleviate pericardial pain by causing the pericardium to fall away from the heart and worsen when the patient lies flat on the back. Breathing, swallowing, and twisting the upper body may increase discomfort. The pain of pericarditis lasts for hours to days and is unaffected by exercise.

13. What physical findings support the diagnosis of pericarditis?

A low-grade fever may be present. High spiking fevers and a toxic-appearing patient should alert the clinician to possible purulent pericarditis that requires urgent drainage. The classic cardiac exam in acute pericarditis is characterized by tachycardia and a friction rub. The rub may come and go. It is more likely to be heard with the patient lying on his or her back. Having the patient exhale and suspend respirations while one quickly listens maximizes the chances that the rub will be heard. One should of course look for evidence of systemic diseases that may be associated with pericarditis.

14. What are the causes of pericarditis?

Most commonly pericarditis is idiopathic. Other etiologies include postviral, post myocardial infarction, in association with aortic dissection rupturing into the pericardium, following blunt chest trauma, malignancy, post radiation, uremia, postoperative, secondary to drugs (procainamide and hydralazine are the most common), and as part of various connective tissue diseases.

15. Is an abnormal cardiac echocardiogram necessary to make the diagnosis of pericarditis?

No. This is a clinical diagnosis. The absence of an effusion on echo means just that. The echo is insensitive to inflammation. On the other hand, the echocardiogram is capable of detecting a very small amount of pericardial fluid.

16. What are the characteristic symptoms of aortic dissection?

The most striking feature of the classic presentation is its abrupt onset with sudden severe pain. The pain is of maximum intensity immediately (as opposed to the crescendo nature of angina) and may be waxing and waning or unrelenting. The pain is frequently described as ripping or tearing in quality. It commonly radiates from the anterior chest to the back, sometimes following the path of the dissection. The patient may also present with neurologic symptoms or limb ischemia, suggesting compromise of vessels leaving the aorta.

17. What are the risk factors for aortic dissection?
Hypertension is present in 70–90% of persons who develop dissection of the aorta. Other risk factors include Marfan's syndrome, pregnancy, coarctation of the aorta, and trauma.

18. What types of valvular heart disease might present with chest pain?
An important valvular cause of chest discomfort is significant aortic stenosis. The pain is typical anginal-type discomfort probably due to inability to augment coronary blood flow to the hypertrophied myocardium. Angina is one of the classic symptoms of severe aortic stenosis.

Chest pain, which may occur in the presence of mitral valve prolapse, is no more frequent than it is in control subjects without this condition. When chest pain is present with documented mitral valve prolapse, it is most commonly stabbing and unrelated to exertion. The discomfort may, however, mimic angina pectoris.

19. How does hypertrophic cardiomyopathy cause chest pain?
This is typical anginal pain related to subendocardial ischemia with or without coexisting coronary artery disease. The demand of the hypertrophied myocardium outstrips the available myocardial oxygen supply, and ischemia results.

20. What features suggest a pulmonary or pleural etiology of chest pain?
An increase in the chest discomfort with inspiration and sharp, well-localized pain with sudden onset of dyspnea should point to the lungs or pleura as the source of chest pain.

21. What features of the history suggest a musculoskeletal cause of the chest pain?
Aggravation by moving or coughing suggests such a cause. Discrete superficial chest pain probably arises from a musculoskeletal injury. Pain lasting constantly for days or weeks suggests a musculoskeletal etiology, although space-occupying malignant processes in the mediastinum should also be considered.

22. What is Tietze syndrome?
This syndrome consists of discomfort localized to swollen costochondral and costosternal joints which are painful on palpation.

23. Describe the chest pain associated with Da Costa syndrome or neurocirculatory asthenia.
This pain is functional or psychogenic chest pain. It is localized in the area of the cardiac apex, is dull and persistent, and lasts for hours with associated intervals of lancinating inframammary pain that lasts seconds. The pain may be associated with palpitations, hyperventilation, light-headedness, dyspnea, weakness, generalized numbness and tingling, and emotional instability.

24. How may gastrointestinal pathology masquerade as cardiac disease?
Esophageal spasm may closely mimic angina pectoris. The discomfort may be substernal, radiate to the back, be brought on by eating, and may be relieved by nitroglycerin. Relief of the discomfort with antacids, a water brash taste in the mouth, or dysphagia help point to the esophagus as the cause. Stooping or bending tend to provoke esophageal reflux. Indigestion due to peptic ulcer disease may imitate angina. Pain due to pancreatitis or cholecystitis can resemble acute myocardial infarction. Generally there is no relationship between exercise and GI causes of chest pain.

25. How often can the clinician determine a specific cause of chest discomfort?
Chest pain or discomfort is a common clinical problem. The priority is to rule out life-threatening causes promptly, realizing that after this is done as much as 50% of the time no definite etiology for chest pain is found. Serial observation in these cases may provide other clues or simply resolution of the discomfort.

BIBLIOGRAPHY

1. Braunwald E (ed): Heart Disease: A Textbook of Cardiovascular Medicine, 4th ed. Philadelphia, W.B. Saunders, 1992.
2. Christie L, Conti CR: Systematic approach to the evaluation of angina-like chest pain. Am Heart J 102:897, 1981.
3. Constant J: The clinical diagnosis of nonanginal chest pain: The differentiation of angina from nonanginal chest pain by history. Clin Cardiol 6:11, 1983.
4. Hurst JW, Logue RB: Angina pectoris: Words patients use and overlooked precipitating events. Heart Disease and Stroke 2:89–91, 1993.
5. Levine HJ: Difficult problems in the diagnosis of chest pain. Am Heart J 100:108, 1980.
6. Markiewicz W, Stoner J, London E, et al: Mitral valve prolapse in 100 presumably healthy young females. Circulation 53:464–473, 1976.
7. Matthews MB, Julian DG (eds): Angina Pectoris. New York, Churchill Livingstone, 1985.
8. Miller A: Diagnosis of Chest Pain. New York, Raven Press, 1988.
9. Norell M, Lythall D, Coghlan G, et al: Limited value of the resting electrocardiogram in assessing patients with recent onset chest pain. Br Heart J 67:53–56, 1992.
10. Sampson JJ, Cheitlin MD: Pathophysiology and differential diagnosis of cardiac pain. Prog Cardiovasc Dis 13:507, 1971.
11. Shima MA: Evaluation of chest pain: Back to the basics of history and physical examination. Postgrad Med 91:155–158, 161–164, 1992.
12. Tibbing L: Issues in the treatment of noncardiac chest pain. Am J Med 92(5A):84S–87S, 1992.

14. EDEMA

Valerie Ulstad, M.D.

1. Name the signs and symptoms of edema.
- Unexplained weight gain
- Tightness of a ring or shoe
- Puffiness in the face and eyelids, especially in the morning
- Swollen extremities
- Enlarged abdominal girth
- Persistence of indentation of the skin following pressure

2. What is the pathogenesis of edema?
Edema is not a disease but rather a sign suggesting abnormal fluid shifts within the body. Edema forms when the production of interstitial fluid exceeds its removal through the lymphatic and/or venous system. The overproduction or decreased removal of fluid from the interstitium results in edema.

3. Classify the pathophysiologic differential diagnosis of edema.
1. Increased fluid accumulation
   - Hypoalbuminemia
     Decreased synthesis
     Increased loss
   - High hydrostatic pressure
     Systemic venous hypertension
   - Increased capillary permeability
     Immunologic injury—vasculitis
     Idiopathic cyclic edema of women
     Postanoxic syndrome

2. Decreased fluid removal
   - Mechanical obstruction
     Clot
     Tumor
   - Poor venous or lymphatic return
     Infection
     Varicosities
     Neuropathy

4. What factors perpetuate the edematous state?

Edema due to abnormal production of interstitial fluid may cause a drop in the effective circulating blood volume. Underperfusion of the kidney triggers retention of salt and water in an attempt to augment tissue perfusion. Thus, despite massive interstitial edema, salt and water are retained.

5. What is lymphedema?

Painless swelling of the lower extremity(ies) due to obstruction of the lymphatic capillaries and larger lymphatic vessels is termed lymphedema. This condition may be primary (congenital) or secondary. Secondary causes include infection (streptococci, tuberculosis, filariasis), inflammation (chronic dermatitis), and obstruction (tumors, especially of the prostate, and lymphoma).

6. List the causes of venous hypertension that result in peripheral edema.

- Congestive heart failure—right ventricular or biventricular
- Constrictive pericarditis
- Tricuspid regurgitation
- Hemodynamically significant pericardial effusion
- Restrictive cardiomyopathy

7. How can one use the pit recovery time as a clue to the cause of edema?

The pit recovery time is the length of time (in seconds) required for the pit made by one's finger to refill. This simple test is a crude measure of the protein content in the edema fluid. Classically this test is performed by applying firm pressure to the bone, usually pretibially. Osmotic forces act quickly to draw the fluid back into the microvasculature of the pit, once pressure is released. In patients with hypoalbuminemia or early lymphedema, the pit recovery time is short (<40 sec); with increased venous pressure or capillary leak of protein, the recovery time is >40 seconds. The protein concentration in the interstitial fluid is lower in hypoalbuminemia than in the other states. Thus, fluid reequilibrates rapidly, and the pit disappears. This test applies only to acute edema (<3 months' duration). Chronic edema causes interstitial scarring and fibrosis and thus results in a prolonged pit recovery time.

8. Distinguish among the terms stasis dermatitis, brawny edema, and myxedema.

Stasis dermatitis results from edema due to venous incompetence. Initially, a mild, pruritic erythema begins over a varicosity, which becomes hyperpigmented with time as blood extravasates and hemosiderin accumulates.

Brawny edema results from chronic stasis dermatitis that has led to dermal fibrosis. Thus, brawny edema does not pit easily and may lead to ulceration.

Myxedema is the dermopathy associated with Graves' disease. It is pretibial and demarcated from normal skin by its thickened "peau d' orange" appearance, hyperpigmentation, and pruritus.

9. What conditions predispose patients to form edema from venous insufficiency?

- History of phlebitis
- Obesity
- Extensive varicosities
- Peripheral neuropathy

10. Should diuretics be used in the edematous patient?

When the primary cause cannot be reversed, diuretics may be used cautiously to help to mobilize the peripheral edema. However, because diuretics block sodium reabsorption, leading to renal compensation in the face of reduced intravascular volume, diuretics may worsen the condition.

11. When are diuretics of no use in edema?

Lymphedema and edema due to mechanical obstruction do not respond to diuretics.

12. What processes should be considered in asymmetric unilateral edema?
Local: allergic reaction, infection, myxedema
Generalized: inguinal or retroperitoneal lymph node or other mechanical obstruction in the deep venous system or a past injury to the extremity

13. What simple advice may help patients with lower extremity edema of any cause?
1. Practice meticulous skin care: emollients, aggressive care of fungal and potential bacterial infections.
2. Avoid prolonged sitting and binding garments.
3. Use mechanical methods to reduce edema: elevation, graduated compression hose.

14. What is an appropriate evaluation for a patient with suspected venous or lymphatic obstruction that results in lower extremity edema?
Abdominal and pelvic ultrasound examinations, along with computerized tomography, are used to clarify the etiology of obstruction. Lymphangiography is rarely indicated.

BIBLIOGRAPHY

1. Anand IS, Ferrari R, Kalra GS, et al: Edema of cardiac origin: Studies of body water and sodium, renal function, hemodynamic indexes, and plasma hormones in untreated congestive cardiac failure. Circulation 80:299–305, 1989.
2. Henry JA, Altmann P: Assessment of hypoproteinemic oedema: A simple physical sign. B M J i:890–891, 1978.
3. Kelley WN (ed): Textbook of Internal Medicine, 2nd ed. Philadelphia, J.B. Lippincott, 1992.
4. Little RC, Ginsburg JM: The physiology basis for clinical edema. Arch Intern Med 144:1661–1664, 1984.
5. Loscalzo J, Creager MA, Dzau VJ (eds): Vascular Medicine: A Textbook of Vascular Biology and Diseases. Boston, Little, Brown, 1992.
6. Milroy WF: Chronic hereditary edema: Milroy's disease. JAMA 182:14–22, 1928.
7. Sapira JD (ed): The Art and Science of Bedside Diagnosis. Baltimore, Williams & Wilkins, 1990.
8. Schirger A, Harrison EG Jr, Janes JM: Idiopathic lymphedema: Review of 131 cases. JAMA 182:124–132, 1962.
9. Schrier R, Gottschalk CW (eds): Diseases of the Kidney, 4th ed. Boston, Little, Brown, 1988.
10. Thorn GW: Approach to the patient with "idiopathic edema" or "periodic edema." JAMA 206:333–338, 1968.

15. AORTIC VALVE DISEASE

Valerie Ulstad, M.D.

1. How does aortic stenosis result in cardiac failure?
Aortic stenosis presents a fixed obstruction to the forward flow of blood. Thus, cardiac output cannot be augmented in times of need, potentially leading to inadequate blood supply to important vascular beds. The left ventricle hypertrophies to normalize the increased wall tension created by the stenosis. The ventricular hypertrophy results in abnormal ventricular filling, since the ventricle is less compliant. Filling pressure must then be elevated to maintain adequate ventricular filling. Finally the ventricle dilates when the muscle fails.

2. What are the common age-related etiologies of aortic stenosis?
In the adult, aortic stenosis is nearly always the result of progressive leaflet calcification. When aortic stenosis becomes apparent in the 30–50 age group, an underlying congenital bicuspid or unicuspid aortic valve is usually present. After age 50, calcification is usually due to

degeneration of the leaflets. The incidence of degenerative aortic stenosis increases with age. Rheumatic aortic stenosis is now relatively uncommon and is almost always accompanied by rheumatic mitral disease.

3. What is the pathophysiology of the symptoms in a patient with severe aortic stenosis?

Patients with severe aortic stenosis are **SAD**. They have Syncope, Angina, and Dyspnea. Syncope occurs due to reduced cerebral perfusion during exercise. Because cardiac output across the obstruction cannot be increased, the vasodilatation of exercise results in systemic hypotension.

Angina occurs because the myocardial oxygen demand of the hypertrophied ventricle can exceed the available oxygen supply available via the coronaries that may themselves be compressed by the hypertrophied myocardium. The subendocardium is the major site of ischemia in patients with thick hypertrophied ventricles.

Dyspnea or other evidence of congestive heart failure can be due to diastolic or systolic ventricular dysfunction. Systolic dysfunction may develop secondary to coexisting coronary artery disease and/or to subendocardial fibrosis from recurrent subendocardial ischemia of the hypertrophied ventricle. Diastolic dysfunction may result from impaired relation to the hypertrophied ventricle.

4. Does chest pain in aortic stenosis always imply associated coronary artery disease?

No. In 50% of patients with critical aortic stenosis, angina occurs in the absence of coronary artery disease.

5. List eight classic physical findings in aortic stenosis.

- Narrow pulse pressure
- Sustained apical impulse. This results from sustained outflow obstruction.
- Parvus et tardus pulse contour. This is a pulse contour that is small in volume and late in peaking. It results in a delayed carotid upstroke.
- Systolic ejection murmur. This murmur is heard best at the right second intercostal space and often at the left sternal border, with radiation to the neck.
- Systolic ejection click. This may be heard at the moment of termination of the abnormal valve opening and is not heard when the aortic valve is no longer mobile.
- Paradoxically split S2. Because emptying of the left ventricle is delayed, the aortic component now comes at the last part of the second heart sound. In inspiration, filling of the right side of the heart is augmented, so that the two heart sounds are concordant.
- Soft S2. This occurs when the valve moves very little.
- S4. This occurs with active diastolic filling into a hypertrophied ventricle.

6. Does the intensity of murmur help in assessing aortic stenosis?

One should not be fooled by the intensity of the murmur, either soft or loud. However, the duration of the murmur and a later peak of intensity suggest more severe aortic obstruction.

7. How will the physician know when aortic stenosis has become critical?

The development of symptoms in a patient with aortic stenosis portends a poor prognosis. After the development of angina or syncope, the average survival of patients with untreated aortic stenosis is 2–3 years, and 1.5 years after congestive heart failure ensues.

The natural history of aortic stenosis is characterized by a long asymptomatic period followed by a much shorter period. Although the rate of progression of aortic stenosis is unpredictable, once the valve is calcified, progression tends to become more rapid.

8. How should the physician follow patients with aortic stenosis?

By Doppler echocardiography. Noninvasive assessment of the severity of obstruction should be carried out after a murmur radiating to the carotids is detected in order to establish the baseline degree of severity. Patients with mild aortic stenosis should have echo-Doppler every 2 years in anticipation of disease progression.

9. What should you tell your patient who has asymptomatic or mild aortic stenosis?
Tell the patient to:
1. Become familiar with the possible symptoms
2. Avoid vigorous physical activity
3. Schedule regular yearly follow-up with the physician, and undergo echocardiography as directed
4. Request subacute bacterial endocarditis (SBE) prophylaxis for invasive and dental procedures

10. What is the Gallavardin murmur?
It is a murmur of aortic stenosis heard best at the apex and left sternal border. Although it is ejection in quality, it has a high-pitched musical sound that may be confused with mitral regurgitation due to its location. It is associated with aortic stenosis in the elderly. It should not radiate to the axilla, as mitral regurgitation classically may do.

11. When is aortic valve replacement indicated in aortic stenosis?
When the patient starts to become symptomatic, aortic valve replacement is indicated. Aortic valve surgery is usually not indicated in asymptomatic patients even when the valve becomes critically stenosed, because the operative risk exceeds the nonoperative risk.

12. List the indications for percutaneous balloon valvuloplasty of the aortic valve.
This technique is of limited value in adults. Restenosis occurs in half of the patients within 6 months. The procedure may have a role in patients with severe aortic stenosis who are not operative candidates, such as for the patient with cardiogenic shock due to critical aortic stenosis as a bridge to eventual surgery; for palliation of symptoms in selected nonoperable patients; or for the pregnant patient with critical aortic stenosis.

13. How does chronic aortic insufficiency cause left ventricular failure?
In aortic insufficiency the entire stroke volume is ejected into a high-pressure system (the aorta). This is accompanied by an increase in diastolic volume due to regurgitation, leading to ventricular dilatation. Ventricular hypertrophy occurs to normalize wall stress. The increased stroke volume causes enlargement of the left ventricle and the aortic root. Ventricular compliance is increased so that end-diastolic pressure does not become elevated until the ventricle can no longer keep up with the extra volume. End-diastolic volume then increases without an increase in the regurgitant fraction, end-systolic volume increases, but ejection fraction and forward stroke volume both decrease. As the compliance of the ventricle falls, diastolic pressure rises and dyspnea occurs.

14. What are the most common causes of chronic aortic insufficiency?
- Cusp abnormality
  Perforation from endocarditis
  Scarring from rheumatic disease
  Bicuspid aortic valve
- Aortic root distortion (aortitis)
  Ankylosing spondylitis
  Syphilis
  Rheumatoid disease
- Loss of valvular support
  Aortic dissection
- Aortic root dilatation
  Marfan's syndrome

15. Describe all the potential physical findings in chronic aortic insufficiency.
1. Hyperdynamic apical impulse displaced laterally and inferiorly
2. Signs associated with the wide pulse pressure of aortic regurgitation (diastolic runoff into the left ventricle)
   Head bobbing—de Musset's sign
   Vigorous collapsing pulse—Corrigan's pulse
   Pulsations in capillary beds of nails—Quincke's pulse
   Systolic pulsations of the uvula—Müller's sign
   Femoral artery murmurs in systole when compressed proximally and diastolic murmur when compressed distally—Duroziez's sign.
3. Murmurs
   High-pitched, blowing, decrescendo diastolic murmur immediately after S2 heard best at the second right intercostal space, on expiration with the patient leaning forward.
   Systolic ejection murmur due to increased flow across the aortic valve
   Mid-diastolic rumble—the Austin Flint murmur, due to vibration of the anterior leaflet of the mitral valve in the regurgitant jet, may be heard at the apex.

16. Once the diagnosis of aortic insufficiency is confirmed, what are the appropriate advice and follow-up?
Aortic insufficiency can be well tolerated for many years. Asymptomatic patients with severe aortic insufficiency and normal left ventricular function have been shown to remain symptom-free for long periods of time. In addition to SBE prophylaxis, patients require serial clinical exams, periodic echocardiographic exams to detect early heart failure or deterioration in left ventricular function, and periodic exercise tests to confirm their asymptomatic status.

17. When should you consider referral for aortic valve replacement in aortic insufficiency?
Asymptomatic patients with depressed left ventricular (LV) function need to be watched closely. If progressive deterioration in LV function is seen, aortic valve replacement should be considered. If LV dysfunction is truly present, most patients will have symptoms. Exercise testing may be useful to unmask the presence of symptoms in a sedentary individual.

Symptomatic patients should undergo valve replacement in order to improve ventricular function and survival. Patients with severe LV dysfunction are very high-risk surgical candidates, but the prognosis is dismal with medical therapy. It is impossible to predict which patients will have persistent LV dysfunction after surgery.

BIBLIOGRAPHY

1. Bonow RO, Lakatos E, Maron BJ, Epstein SE: Serial long-term assessment of the natural history of asymptomatic patients with chronic aortic regurgitation and normal left ventricular systolic function. Circulation 84:1625–1635, 1991.
2. Braunwald E (ed): Heart Disease: A Textbook of Cardiovascular Medicine, 4th ed. Philadelphia, W.B. Saunders, 1992.
3. Elayda MA, Hall RJ, Reul RM, et al: Aortic valve replacement in patients 80 years and older: Operative risks and long-term results. Circulation 88(Pt. 2):11–16. 1993.
4. Greenberg B, Massie B, Bristow JD, et al: Long term vasodilator therapy of chronic aortic insufficiency: A randomized double-blinded controlled trial. Circulation 78:92–103, 1988.
5. Kennedy KD, Nishimura RA, Holmes DR Jr, Bailey KR: Natural history of moderate aortic stenosis. J Am Coll Cardiol 17:313–319, 1991.
6. Lombard JT, Selzer A: Valvular aortic stenosis: A clinical and hemodynamic profile of patients. Ann Intern Med 106:292–298, 1987.
7. Rahimtoola SH: Perspective on valvular heart disease: An update. J Am Coll Cardiol 14:1–23, 1989.
8. Ross J: Afterload mismatch in aortic and mitral valve disease: Implications for surgical therapy. J Am Coll Cardiol 5:811–826, 1985.
9. Selzer A: Changing aspects of the natural history of valvular aortic stenosis. N Engl J Med 317:91–98, 1987.
10. Siemienczuk D, Greenberg B, Morris C, et al: Chronic aortic insufficiency: Factors associated with progression to aortic valve replacement. Ann Intern Med 110:587–592, 1989.

16. MITRAL VALVE DISEASE

Valerie Ulstad, M.D.

1. What causes mitral valve prolapse (MVP)?

MVP occurs when part of a leaflet or both leaflets of the mitral valve extend above the plane of the atrioventricular junction during ventricular systole. The usual cause is an inherent abnormality of the leaflets and supporting chordae. Normal valves may demonstrate prolapse during conditions that make the left ventricle small, such as the Valsalva maneuver, dehydration, atrial septal defect (blood shunted to the right atrium away from the left atrium leads to underfilling of the left ventricle), and hypertrophic cardiomyopathy. Conditions in which the mitral valve is intrinsically abnormal are most likely to produce significant adverse consequences.

2. How common is mitral valve prolapse?

By strict echocardiographic criteria, approximately 2–5% of the population of the United States has MVP. Myxomatous degeneration of the mitral valve is hereditary as an autosomal dominant trait. Gene penetrance is stronger in women than in men, leading to the predominance of MVP in women.

3. What is MVP syndrome?

Most patients with MVP are completely asymptomatic. However, the MVP syndrome applies to patients whose physical examination or echocardiographic findings are consistent with MVP and who complain of atypical chest pain, palpitations, easy fatigability, light-headedness, or postural syncope.

The pathogenesis of the symptoms is poorly understood but probably is related to autonomic dysfunction. Papillary muscle tension from billowing redundant leaflets may play a role in chest discomfort and development of certain arrhythmias. Patients tend to develop MVP syndrome in the second or third decade of life. Anxiety and panic attacks are no more common in patients with MVP than in the general population. Other names for MVP syndrome include Da Costa's syndrome, soldier's heart, effort syndrome, and neurocirculatory asthenia.

4. Does therapy always help patients with MVP syndrome?

Beta blockers slow the heart rate and increase diastolic filling, thereby increasing left ventricular size and reducing the degree of prolapse. The relief of symptoms with beta blockers is variable. Aerobic exercise has been shown to provide symptomatic improvement for some patients.

5. How is the diagnosis of MVP made?

The diagnosis is largely clinical; the hallmark is a midsystolic click with or without a late systolic murmur. The click occurs when the elongated chordae are snapped tight at the maximal excursion of the valve during closure in early systole. The regurgitant murmur most commonly is produced by abnormal coaptation of the leaflet edges. The Valsalva maneuver and the upright standing position make the ventricle smaller and thus may lead to a louder click earlier in systole and a longer, louder murmur. The auscultatory features may vary from day to day, according to changes in ventricular size.

Once the clinical diagnosis is made, an echocardiogram establishes baseline values and assesses the degree of prolapse, extent of leaflet thickening, and degree of mitral regurgitation. The echocardiographic diagnosis of MVP depends on the criteria used by the echocardiographer. Because the mitral annulus is shaped like a saddle, only in certain echocardiographic views can the prolapse be interpreted as genuine.

6. What risks are associated with MVP?

The major potential complications of MVP are (1) endocarditis, (2) development of severe mitral regurgitation, (3) significant arrhythmias, and (4) stroke due to thromboemboli.

Endocarditis is more likely to occur in patients with thickened, deformed valves. The incidence of endocarditis in this subset of patients is 3.5–6%. Antibiotic prophylaxis for subacute bacterial endocarditis is recommended, especially if thick mitral leaflets and mitral regurgitation murmur are present on physical examination or echocardiogram.

Significant mitral regurgitation (MR) develops in 9–12% of patients with severely deformed valves. Progressive mitral regurgitation is related to various combinations of mitral annulus dilatation, chordal elongation, or chordal rupture. The risk of developing severe MR increases with age in men more than in women. Patients who develop significant MR should be followed echocardiographically. Once symptoms develop and the ventricular end-systolic dimension increases, surgery for mitral valve repair or replacement should be considered.

The incidence of **serious arrhythmia** is low enough that screening for arrhythmias is not indicated.

The abnormal surface of the myxomatous valve potentially predisposes to the development of **thromboemboli.** The presence of MVP increases the risk of stroke and transient ischemic attacks in patients under 45 years of age. Aspirin therapy is rational but unproved.

The risk of **sudden death** is slightly higher in patients with MVP than in the normal population. Ventricular fibrillation appears to be the mechanism of death.

7. List the causes of mitral regurgitation.
Primary mechanisms
    Abnormalities of the leaflets
        Rheumatic valvultis
        Endocarditis
        Myxomatous degeneration
    Abnormalities of the chordae tendinae
        Spontaneous rupture from myxomatous degeneration
        Elongation from myxomatous degeneration
        Scarring and fusion from rheumatic inflammation
    Abnormalities of the papillary muscles
        Ischemic dysfunction
            Disruption secondary to infarction
Secondary mechanisms
    Left ventricular dysfunction and dilatation leading to malalignment
      of the mitral apparatus

8. Which cause of chronic MR most commonly requires surgery?
Myxomatous degeneration of the mitral valve.

9. What is the pathophysiology of chronic MR?
In MR a portion of the left ventricular stroke volume is ejected backward into the relatively low-pressure left atrium. This part of the stroke volume is ineffective because it does not perfuse the body and deleterious because it adds work for the left ventricle. Increased diastolic stress produced by volume overload triggers myocyte hypertrophy and thus increases end-diastolic volume. Increased diastolic volume leads to an augmentation of stroke volume with a preservation of net forward flow. Eventually constant severe volume overload leads to left ventricular systolic dysfunction. Reduced emptying of the ventricle leads to pulmonary congestion and symptoms of dyspnea.

10. How does MR manifest itself?
MR presents with symptoms of left-sided heart failure, including dyspnea, orthopnea, and paroxysmal nocturnal dyspnea. In advanced disease right heart failure also may be present.

11. What are the classic physical findings of chronic MR?

1. The apical impulse is diffuse and laterally displaced.

2. The intensity of the first heart sound is reduced, because the leaflets float relatively near the atrioventricular ring just before the onset of isovolumic contraction as a result of the large volume of blood entering the ventricle.

3. The second heart sound may be widely split, because the aortic valve closes early as a result of reduced stroke volume.

4. A holosystolic murmur, heard best over the apex, radiates to the axilla. A click and a late systolic murmur may be present with MVP. Loudness does not correlate with severity.

5. A third heart sound indicates a large left ventricular filling volume propelled into the left ventricle under higher than normal left atrial pressure. The absence of an S3 suggests that the MR is not severe.

12. When is the optimal time for consideration of surgical intervention in patients with MR?

The correct timing for mitral valve surgery is immediately before the ejection fraction begins to fall, which is usually before the patient develops symptoms. It is hard for the clinician to anticipate the exact time. Close follow-up of patients with significant MR is important, because it is easy to wait too long, leaving the patient with heart failure even after surgery. The normal ejection fraction in MR is > 65%, with a hyperdynamic left ventricle emptying into the low-pressure left atrium. A "normal" ejection fraction in such patients is not normal. Regular echocardiographic evaluations are a reasonable way to follow ventricular function.

Regular exercise testing also may be indicated to uncover early symptoms of exercise intolerance. The mildest symptoms of dyspnea on exertion are an indication to consider surgery. It is currently unclear whether vasodilators retard the progression of MR.

13. Why is mitral valve repair preferrable to replacement?

- Better durability
- Lower risk of endocarditis
- Lower incidence of postoperative thromboembolism
- Better postoperative ventricular function
- Anticoagulation may be avoided

14. What is the most common cause of mitral stenosis?

Rheumatic heart disease is the cause of nearly all cases of mitral stenosis in the United States. In patients without a history of rheumatic fever, it is assumed that the acute episode was mild or misdiagnosed. The valvular stenosis results from the initial inflammation of the heart. Thickening of the leaflets and fusion and shortening of the chordae produce the stenosis several decades after the initial insult. The greater the original inflammation of the heart, the more likely the person is to develop significant valvular sequelae.

15. What is the pathophysiology of mitral stenosis?

The narrowed mitral orifice limits inflow into the left ventricle. The resulting elevation of left atrial pressure leads to pulmonary venous congestion and reactive pulmonary hypertension, which in turn may lead to right ventricular pressure overload and clinical right-heart failure.

16. What are the symptoms of mitral stenosis?

- Dyspnea
- Orthopnea
- Paroxysmal nocturnal dyspnea
- Hemoptysis, when high left atrial pressure causes rupture of small brochial veins
- Systemic embolism in patients with atrial fibrillation secondary to atrial dilation
- Hoarseness, when the enlarged left atrium impinges on the left recurrent laryngeal nerve

17. Describe the results of physical examination in patients with mitral stenosis.
- Normal left ventricular apical impulse
- Possible atrial fibrillation
- Loud first heart sound (S1). The pressure gradient across the mitral valve holds the leaflets in a position deep into the ventricle throughout diastole. The leaflets close through a relatively wide excursion, with onset of isovolumic contraction giving a loud S1. S1 may become soft or absent when the valve becomes so diseased that it does not move at all in systole or diastole.
- Opening snap in diastole. The diseased valve reaches its maximal excursion in diastole and is stopped short by the valvular thickening.
- Diastolic rumbling murmur immediately after the opening snap. The murmur may become louder at the end of diastole in the patient still in sinus rhythm. The accentuation of the murmur is due to increased flow secondary to atrial contraction. Such an increase in intensity is not heard in patients with atrial fibrillation.

18. What are the two common complications of mitral stenosis?
   1. **Atrial fibrillation.** With an associated rapid ventricular response, atrial fibrillation is poorly tolerated, because shortened diastole limits the time for blood to cross the stenotic valve. Such patients may experience sudden onset of pulmonary edema, requiring prompt cardioversion. Medical therapy to achieve rate control is needed if the atrial fibrillation becomes chronic.
   2. **Systemic embolization.** Chronic anticoagulation of patients with atrial fibrillation and mitral stenosis is clearly indicated to prevent systemic embolization of atrial mural thrombi. Many experts advocate anticoagulation for all patients with mitral stenosis, regardless of the rhythm, because 25% of nonanticoagulated patients with mitral stenosis suffer a stystemic embolus.

19. What interventions are available for the patient with disabling symptoms due to mitral stenosis?
Patients who are asymptomatic can be managed medically with careful use of diuretics and control of heart rate. Once mild to moderate symptoms occur, three options are available:
   1. **Percutaneous balloon valvuloplasty** is limited to patients with commissural fusion and noncalcified, pliable leaflets without evidence of left atrial thrombi (which may be dislodged during the procedure) or significant MR. Procedural mortality is $< 1\%$. This is a good option in pregnant women.
   2. **Surgical commissurotomy** has the same indications as balloon valvuloplasty. Procedural mortality is $< 1\%$. This option offers the opportunity for valve reconstruction.
   3. **Mitral valve replacement** results in excellent long-term survival rates.

BIBLIOGRAPHY

1. Angell WW, Oury JH, Shah P: A comparison of replacement and reconstruction in patients with mitral regurgitation. J Thorac Cardiovasc Surg 93:665–674, 1987.
2. Ben Farat M, Maatouk F, Betbout F, et al: Percutaneous balloon mitral valvuloplasty in eight pregnant women with severe mitral stenosis. Eur Heart J 13:1658–1664, 1992.
3. Benjamin EJ, Plehn JF, D'Agostino RB, et al: Mitral annular calcification and the risk of stroke in an elderly cohort. N Engl J Med 327:374–379, 1992.
4. Boudoulas H, Kolibash AJ, Baker P, et al: Mitral valve prolapse and the mitral valve prolapse syndrome. Am Heart J 118:796–818, 1989.
5. Carabello BA: Mitral valve disease. Curr Probl Cardiol 18:421–480, 1993.
6. Cohen DJ, Kuntz RE, Gordon SPF, et al: Predictors of long-term outcome after percutaneous balloon mitral valvuloplasty. N Engl J Med 327:1329–1335, 1992.
7. Dajani AS, Bisno AL, Chung KJ, et al: Prevention of bacterial endocarditis: Recommendations by the American Heart Association. JAMA 264:2919–2922, 1990.
8. Devereux RB, Kramer-Fox R, Kligfield P: Mitral valve prolapse: Causes, clinical manifestations, and management. Ann Intern Med 111:305–317, 1989.

9. Farb A, Tang AL, Atkinson JB, et al: Comparison of cardiac findings in patients with mitral valve prolapse who die suddenly to those who have congestive heart failure from mitral regurgitation and to those with fatal noncardiac conditions. Am J Cardiol 70:234–239, 1992.
10. Galloway AC, Colvin SB, Bauman G, et al: Long-term results of mitral valve reconstruction with Carpentier techniques in 148 patients with mitral insufficiency. Circulation 78 (Suppl I):I-97–I-105.
11. Hochreiter C, Niles N, Devereux R, et al: Mitral regurgitation: Relationship of noninvasive descriptor of right and left ventricular performance to clinical and hemodynamic findings and to prognosis in medically and surgically treated patients. Circulation 73:900–912, 1986.
12. Horstkotte D, Niehues R, Strauer BE: Pathomorphological aspects, aetiology and natural history of acquired mitral valve stenosis. Eur Heart J 12:55–60, 1991.
13. Lehman KG, Francis CK, Dodge HT: Mitral regurgitation in early myocardial infarction: Incidence, clinical detection, and prognostic implications. TIMI Study Group. Ann Intern Med 117:10–17, 1992.
14. Llaneras MR, Nance ML, Streicher JT, et al: Pathogenesis of ischemic mitral regurgitation. J Thorac Cardiovasc Surg 105:439–442, 1993.
15. Reyes VP, Soma Raju B, Wynne J, et al: Percutaneous balloon valvuloplasty compared with open surgical commissurotomy for mitral stenosis. N Engl J Med 331:961–967, 1994.
16. Turi ZG, Reyes VP, Raju S, et al: Percutaneous balloon versus surgical closed commissurotomy for mitral stenosis: A prospective randomized trial. Circulation 83:1179–1185, 1991.
17. Wooley CF, Baker PB, Kolibash AJ, et al: The floppy myxomatous mitral valve, mitral valve prolapse, and mitral regurgitation. Prog Cardiovasc Dis 33:397–433, 1991.

17. SUPRAVENTRICULAR ARRHYTHMIAS

Valerie Ulstad, M.D.

1. When does a rhythm fall into the category of a supraventricular tachycardia (SVT)?
When the heart rate is greater than 100 and there is a narrow QRS complex.

2. What are the two most common mechanisms of SVTs?
Abnormal automaticity and reentry.

3. Explain abnormal automaticity.
The sinoatrial (SA) node, elements of the atrioventricular (AV) node, and the His-Purkinje system spontaneously depolarize and thereby are said to demonstrate automaticity. These cells initiate the normal cardiac impulse and provide a hierarchy of subsidiary pacemakers ready to take over if the SA node fails. The SA node fires at the fastest rate and keeps the lower pacemakers suppressed. In certain pathologic situations, such as metabolic disturbances or certain drug toxicities, cells that do not usually exhibit spontaneous depolarization may become automatic and generate impulses that propagate through the heart.

4. What are the prerequisites for a reentry tachycardia?
Reentry is the most common mechanism producing SVTs. A reentrant rhythm develops when a region of the myocardium is reexcited by one electrical impulse that returns to a given area by a circuitous route. There are three requirements for reentry to take place:

 1. Two distinct parts of the heart must have different conduction velocities: two areas within the AV node; the conduction system and an accessory pathway; or two areas of the ventricular myocardium.

 2. The two parts or paths for propagation of an electrical impulse must have the potential to form a circuit. Because they are different, one must conduct more slowly than the other; the path that conducts more rapidly takes longer to recover.

 3. A premature beat enters the potential circuit and finds one path ready to conduct, but the other blocked because it has not yet recovered. The impulse proceeds down one path and

propagates through the tissue. At that point the second path may have recovered and is ready to conduct the propagated impulse. Thus the premature beat is the trigger. Under normal circumstances both pathways would have been ready to conduct the impulse. However, the premature beat exaggerated the difference between the two paths, finding one ready to conduct, the other still refractory. When the impulse comes around to the pathway that was initially refractory and finds it now ready to conduct, the reentrant circuit begins.

5. What are the four common types of SVTs?

Reentrant atrial tachycardias—Atrial tissue provides the reentry tissue.

Reentrant AV nodal tachycardias—Reentry is in the AV node with a slow and fast pathway in the node itself.

Reentrant AV reciprocating tachycardia—A macroreentrant pathway is formed between the atria and the ventricles via an accessory path bypassing the node.

Automatic tachycardias—Altered automaticity from any portion of the atrium or interatrial septum occurs with ischemia or drugs.

6. Give examples of each type of SVT.

Reentrant atrial tachycardia
  Atrial fibrillation
  Atrial flutter
  Intra-atrial reentrant tachycardia
AV Reentrant nodal tachycardia
  Nodal tachycardia
  Accelerated junctional tachycardia

AV reciprocating tachycardia
  Wolff-Parkinson-White syndrome
  Other accessory path tachycardias
Automatic tachycardias
  Multifocal atrial tachycardia
  Unifocal atrial tachycardia

7. What is paroxysmal SVT?

Paroxysmal SVT is a supraventricular rhythm that is regular at 120–130 beats/minute and has sudden onset and termination. The term is confusing, because it does not describe a specific arrhythmia mechanism but rather the clinical characteristics of the tachycardia. Paroxysmal SVT accounts for one-half of all patients with SVT. In the majority of patients, AV nodal reentry is the mechanism of the paroxysmal tachycardia. The second most common mechanism is AV reciprocating tachycardia via an extranodal bypass tract.

8. How may the P wave be helpful in diagnosing the type of SVT?

No discreet P waves
Distinct P waves at rate 250–340 (F waves)
No P waves

Single abnormal P wave, normal PR
Retrograde (downward P before,
  in, or after QRS)
Short PR
Three different morphologies

Atrial fibrillation, rhythm irregular
Atrial flutter
Nodal tachycardia (retrograde P wave
  buried in ventricular depolarization)
Unifocal atrial tachycardia
Accelerated junctional tachycardia

Accessory pathway
Multifocal atrial tachycardia

9. Which rhythms usually have an irregular rate?

Atrial fibrillation, even at a rapid rate
Atrial flutter (which may be regular)
Multifocal atrial tachycardia

10. The QRS is usually narrow in SVTs. When may the QRS be wide?

1. Aberrant conduction, such as preexisting right or left bundle-branch block.

2. When an accessory connection (as in Wolff-Parkinson-White syndrome) conducts antegrade, the AV node conducts retrograde, and the ventricular myocardium is depolarized cell to cell rather than along the conduction system.

11. In evaluating a patient with SVT, what historical and other medical information should be sought?

History of palpitations or syncope

Symptoms of possible hyperthyroidism or pheochromocytoma

Habits and drug use: alcohol, caffeine, inhaled or oral beta agonists, over-the-counter cold medicines, illicit drug use

Effect of a possible SVT on the patient's lifestyle (e.g., airplane pilot)

12. What are palpitations? To what are they due?

Palpitations represent the patient's awareness of his or her own heart beat. The etiology of palpitations can be determined in a majority of patients. One-half of cases are due to cardiac disease, whereas one-third are due to psychiatric causes and a smaller number to other causes (habits, medicines, metabolic causes). Paroxysms of prolonged palpitations suggest a cardiac arrhythmia, either supraventricular or ventricular in origin.

13. How should patients with SVT be evaluated?

After a complete history and physical examination, the patient should have a chest radiograph and electrocardiogram (EKG); thyroid function tests, hematocrit, and echocardiography should be considered to look for mitral valve prolapse or other evidence of valvular disease.

14. How may carotid sinus massage or Valsalva maneuvers aid in the diagnosis and treatment of arrhythmias?

Carotid sinus massage and Valsalva maneuvers may have three major outcomes: abrupt cessation of the arrhythmia, slowing of heart rate during the maneuver, or no effect. Abrupt cessation of the arrhythmia and conversion to sinus rhythms is the most useful outcome. It may be seen when the arrhythmia is supraventricular and originates from an AV nodal reentrant or aberrant pathway mechanism. Sinus tachycardia slows during massage and subsequently regains speed. Other possible outcomes include accentuation of AV block or dissociation, atrial fibrillation in atrial flutter, and transient slowing of the ventricular rate.

15. When is carotid massage contraindicated?

In patients with possible digoxin toxicity, carotid massage may lead to fatal arrhythmias. Additional risks of carotid massage include stroke, syncope, seizures, asystole, or ventricular arrhythmias. Thus carotid massage should be avoided in elderly patients.

16. When should a patient with supraventricular arrhythmias be hospitalized?

Patients who present with hypotension, chest pain, congestive heart failure, or sustained tachycardia should be hospitalized.

17. When should strategies to provide chronic prophylaxis against paroxysmal SVT be considered?

If the episodes are relatively slow, infrequent, and well tolerated, no therapy may be necessary. Patients should be counselled to limit use of caffeine, alcohol, and other drugs. When symptoms are frequent and bothersome, drug therapy and radiofrequency ablation of the arrhythmogenic focus are options. Drugs should slow AV node conduction; the most common choices are beta blockers and calcium-channel blockers.

18. When should drugs that block the AV node be avoided?

Beta blockers, calcium-channel blockers, and digoxin are contraindicated in patients who may have tachycardias due to accessory pathways. In patients with multifocal atrial tachycardia, digoxin may prove harmful.

19. When and why is it important to recognize Wolff-Parkinson-White (WPW) syndrome or accessory pathway arrhythmias?

WPW syndrome should be suspected in the presence of a delta wave on routine EKG or, more importantly, when the patient has atrial fibrillation that is conducted at a rapid rate (faster than the capability of AV node), resulting in a rapid ventricular response > 280. Of patients with WPW syndrome, 50% experience atrial fibrillation, which may deteriorate to ventricular fibrillation or present as sudden death. Thus, recognition of this rare entity is life-saving and requires referral to a cardiologist for appropriate management.

20. Which patients should be referred to a cardiologist for possible electrophysiologic testing?

1. Patients with uncontrolled symptomatic tachycardias of unknown diagnosis after preliminary work-up

2. Patients with symptomatic tachycardias with delta wave or other suspicion of aberrant conduction. The sole finding of delta waves is controversial.

3. Patients who respond poorly to initial medical management

BIBLIOGRAPHY

1. Benditt DG, Goldstein M, Reyes WJ, Milstein S: Supraventricular tachycardias: Mechanisms and therapies. Hosp Pract Aug. 15, 1988, pp 103–127.
2. Calkins H, Sousa J, El-Atassi R, Rosenheck S, et al: Diagnosis and cure of the Wolff-Parkinson-White syndrome or paroxysmal supraventricular tachycardia during a single electrophysiologic test. N Engl J Med 324:1612–1618, 1991.
3. Camm AJ, Garratt: Adenosine and supraventricular tachycardia. N Engl J Med 325:1621–1629, 1991.
4. DiMarco JP, Miles W, Aktar M, et al: Adenosine for paroxysmal supraventricular tachycardia: Dose ranging and comparison with verapamil. Ann Intern Med 113:104–110, 1990.
5. Dreifus LS, Hessen S, Samuels F: Recognition and management of supraventricular tachycardias. Heart Dis Stroke 2:223–230, 1993.
6. Haines DE, DiMarco JP: Current therapy for supraventricular tachycardia. Curr Probl Cardiol 17:415–477, 1992.
7. Josephson ME, Wellens HJJ: Differential diagnosis of supraventricular tachycardia. Cardiol Clin 8:411–442, 1990.
8. Kalbfleisch SJ, El-Atassi R, Calkins H, et al: Differentiation of paroxysmal narrow QRS complex tachycardias using the 12-lead electrocardiogram. J Am Coll Cardiol 21:85–89, 1993.
9. Kastor JA: Multifocal atrial tachycardia. N Engl J Med 322:1713–1717, 1990.
10. Olshansky B, Wilber DJ, Hariman RJ: Atrial flutter: Update on mechanism and treatment. PACE 15:2308–2335, 1992.
11. Waldo AL: An approach to therapy of supraventricular tachyarrhythmias: An algorithm vs. individualized therapy. Clin Cardiol 17(Suppl II):II21–II26, 1994.

18. ATRIAL FIBRILLATION

Valerie Ulstad, M.D.

1. What is the most common cause of atrial fibrillation?

Approximately 40–50% of patients with atrial fibrillation have coronary artery disease. In addition 15% have hyperthyroidism, whereas another 15% are otherwise healthy.

2. What evaluation should be performed in the patient with new-onset atrial fibrillation?

After a thorough physical examination, most patients should have the following tests:

- Assessment of electrolytes
- Assessment of thyroid-stimulating hormone (TSH)
- 12-lead electrocardiogram (EKG)
- Chest radiograph
- Echocardiogram

3. List five clinical consequences of atrial fibrillation.
1. Increased risk of embolic stroke
2. Increased cardiac mortality
3. Increased overall mortality
4. Impairment of ventricular systolic function
5. Cardiac decompensation in patients with diastolic dysfunction

4. What clinical factors are associated with increased risk of stroke in patients with atrial fibrillation?

Advanced age   Severe left ventricular function
Hypertension   Recent clinical congestive heart failure
History of previous thromboembolic event   Enlarged left atrium
Rheumatic heart disease   Previous myocardial infarction

5. What are the major reasons to consider pharmacologic therapy in patients with atrial fibrillation?

Control of the rate of ventricular response   Maintenance of sinus rhythm
Restoration of sinus rhythm (pharmaco-   Potential reduction of stroke risk
logic cardioversion)

6. What does rate control mean?
Cardiac output increases in most patients with atrial fibrillation to a mean rate of about 140 beats/min. At faster rates, cardiac output begins to fall. A resting rate of 90 beats/min is probably ideal, provided that it can be increased during exercise.

7. Which agents are available to control the rate in atrial fibrillation?
Rate control can be achieved with drugs that slow atrioventricular (AV) node conduction, such as beta blockers, calcium-channel blockers, or digoxin. Sometimes combinations are necessary.

8. Which drugs are useful in pharmacologic cardioversion?
Procainamide has been the most frequently studied drug for cardioversion. Quinidine is also commonly used. Patients with recent-onset atrial fibrillation are more likely to be chemically converted. Digoxin does not influence conversion to sinus rhythm.

9. Describe the practical guidelines for pharmacologic treatment of patients with atrial fibrillation.
1. Treat the symptomatic patient.
2. Treat underlying heart failure.
3. Correct metabolic disturbances.
4. The longer the patient has been in atrial fibrillation, the less likely a response to therapy will be seen.
5. The occurrence of proarrhythmia during therapy is impossible to predict.
6. Consider hospitalizing and monitoring the patient when therapy is started.

10. Which drugs are available for maintenance of normal sinus rhythm after conversion of atrial fibrillation?
Quinidine is a good first choice for maintenance of sinus rhythm. It may be poorly tolerated by many patients. When quinidine is ineffective or poorly tolerated, flecainide or propafenone is a good second choice, if left ventricular function is normal and coronary disease is absent. Procainamide is often poorly tolerated as long-term therapy. If first-line drugs fail and treatment is needed to control symptoms and hemodynamics, referral to a cardiologist is appropriate.

11. Will the patient maintained on quinidine after cardioversion stay in normal sinus rhythm?
A meta-analysis of the randomized control trials investigating the role of quinidine in the therapy of chronic atrial fibrillation demonstrated that quinidine was more effective than no

treatment in maintaining normal sinus rhythm at 3, 6, and 12 months after cardioversion. About 50% of quinidine-treated patients were in sinus rhythm at 12 months after cardioversion compared with 25% of controls. Few data are available for procainamide and disopyramide.

CONTROVERSIES

12. Is pharmacologic treatment of atrial fibrillation to maintain sinus rhythm safe?
The quinidine meta-analysis revealed a strong tendency for more deaths among patients treated with quinidine than among controls. Two percent of patients treated with quinidine died during the 1-year follow-up period, suggesting a possible risk in treatment directed at maintaining the patient in sinus rhythm.

Flecainide is at least as effective as quinidine in maintaining sinus rhythm and is generally better tolerated, but it should be considered only in patients with normal left ventricular function. Proarrhythmia has been reported with its use for supraventricular arrhythmias.

Propafenone and sotalol have been shown to have antifibrillatory properties. When either agent is used in patients with symptomatic atrial fibrillation who have failed conventional therapy, 40–50% are in sinus rhythm 6 months after cardioversion. Isolated reports of sudden death in 10% of patients receiving these medications suggest the need for further study of the risk-benefit ratio.

13. Which patients with atrial fibrillation are at highest risk of embolization?
Patients with rheumatic mitral stenosis and atrial fibrillation have the highest risk of embolic strokes (17 times normal compared with 5 times normal for patients with nonrheumatic atrial fibrillation). Warfarin therapy significantly reduces the incidence of embolic disease in both groups.

14. What is meant by the term "lone atrial fibrillation"?
Lone atrial fibrillation refers to atrial fibrillation in the absence of structural heart disease; it carries a stroke risk of 2.5%/yr.

15. Should every patient with nonrheumatic atrial fibrillation receive anticoagulation therapy?
Data accumulated from clinical trials suggest that most, if not all patients, should be considered for anticoagulation. The Boston Area Anticoagulation Trial for Atrial Fibrillation is the only trial that tested the safety and efficacy of low-dose warfarin for the prevention of stroke in patients with nonrheumatic atrial fibrillation. Maintenance of prothrombin times 1.2–1.5 times control or an international normalized ratio (INR) of 1.5–2.7 resulted in significant reduction in the stroke rate in patients receiving warfarin. From the clinical trials it is clear that the individual at intermediate risk of stroke with a low bleeding risk benefits from warfarin.

Patients without structural heart disease (lone atrial fibrillation) under the age of 60 years with no other risk factors for stroke are at low risk for embolism. In such patients the risk of anticoagulation therapy may outweigh the benefits. The role of warfarin in elderly patients (> 75 years) remains unresolved. Aspirin appears to be ineffective in this group.

16. Does reestablishment of sinus rhythm reduce the risk of stroke?
This is unknown.

BIBLIOGRAPHY

1. The Boston Area Anticoagulation Trial for Atrial Fibrillation Investigators: The effect of low-dose warfarin on the risk of stroke in patients with nonrheumatic atrial fibrillation. N Engl J Med 323:1505–1522, 1990.
2. Cairns JA, Connolly SJ: Nonrheumatic atrial fibrillation: Risk of stroke and role of antithrombotic therapy. Circulation 84:469–492, 1991.
3. Connolly SJ, Laupacis A, Gent M: Canadian atrial fibrillation anticoagulation (CAFA) study. J Am Coll Cardiol 18:349–355, 1991.

4. Coplen SE, Antman EM, Berlin JA, et al: Efficacy and safety of quinidine therapy for maintenance of sinus rhythm after cardioversion: A meta-analysis of randomized control trials. Circulation 82:1106–1116, 1990.
5. Ezekowitz MD, Bridgers SL, James KE, et al: Warfarin in the prevention of stroke associated with nonrheumatic atrial fibrillation. Veterans Affairs Stroke Prevention in Nonrheumatic Atrial Fibrillation Investigators. N Engl J Med 327:1406–1412, 1992.
6. Juul-Moller S, Edvardsson N, Rehnquist-Ahlberg N: Sotalol versus quinidine for the maintenance of sinus rhythm after cardioversion of atrial fibrillation. Circulation 82:1932–1939, 1990.
7. Manning WJ, Silverman DI, Gordon SPF, Krumholz HM, Douglas PS: Cardioversion from atrial fibrillation without prolonged anticoagulation with use of transesophageal echocardiography to exclude the presence of atrial thrombi. N Engl J Med 328:750–755, 1993.
8. Pai SM, Torres V: Atrial fibrillation: New management strategies. Curr Probl Cardiol 18:233–300, 1993.
9. Petersen P, Boysen G, Godtfredsen J, Andersen ED, Anderen B: Placebo-controlled trial of warfarin and aspirin for the prevention of thromboembolic complications in chronic atrial fibrillation: The Copenhagen AFASAK Study. Lancet 1:175–179, 1989.
10. Stein B, Halperin JL, Fuster V: Should patients with atrial fibrillation be anticoagulated prior to and chronically following cardioversion? Cardiovasc Clin 21:231–249, 1990.
11. Stroke Prevention in Atrial Fibrillation Investigators: Stroke prevention in atrial fibrillation study: Final results. Circulation 84:527–539, 1991.
12. Waldo AL: Clinical evaluation in therapy of patients with atrial fibrillation or flutter. Cardiol Clin 8(3):479–490, 1990.
13. Alber GW: Atrial fibrillation and stroke. Arch Intern Med 154:1443–1457, 1994.

19. VENTRICULAR ARRHYTHMIAS

Valerie Ulstad, M.D.

1. Describe the electrocardiographic (EKG) characteristics of the premature ventricular contraction (PVC).

A PVC is an early (premature) QRS complex with a bizarre shape and a duration that exceeds the dominant QRS complex duration in the underlying rhythm. The T wave deflection is large and in the opposite direction from the main QRS deflection. There is no preceding P wave.

The PVC is commonly conducted in a retrograde fashion toward the atria, but the sinoatrial (SA) node is rarely reset by the premature ventricular beat (in contrast to the premature atrial beat). A compensatory pause occurs after the premature beat until the next sinus beat arrives. The next sinus beat after the compensatory pause comes in time with the underlying sinus rhythm determined by the SA node. Another SA depolarization occurs simultaneously with the PVC, but its electrical activity is not seen on the EKG because it is hidden by the wide QRS complex.

2. How common are PVCs?

When a simple 12-lead EKG is used for screening, PVCs are documented in fewer than 1% of the population. If 24-hour Holter monitoring is used, PVCs are observed in 50–80% of normal people. The forms seen in normal people are usually single PVCs, but nonsustained ventricular tachycardia (NSVT) may be seen infrequently. The incidence of ventricular arrhythmias increases with age.

3. What is considered a normal number of PVCs?

Fewer than 100 PVCs/day or 5/hour is within normal limits for the healthy population. A higher number of PVCs or repetitive forms (NSVT) suggest electrical heart disease.

4. Which everyday substances should patients with PVCs avoid?

Caffeine, tobacco, and alcohol increase the incidence of PVCs.

5. What is complex ventricular ectopy?
Complex ventricular ectopy consists of more than 10–30 PVCs/hour and multiform or repetitive patterns of ventricular beats.

6. Define nonsustained ventricular tachycardia (NSVT).
NSVT is defined as 3 or more ventricular beats in a row at a rate of at least 100 beats/minute, lasting 15–30 seconds. Longer runs are called sustained ventricular tachycardia (VT).

7. List the three classes of ventricular arrhythmias.
Benign ventricular arrhythmias
Potentially malignant ventricular arrhythmias
Malignant ventricular arrhythmias

8. Why are some ventricular arrhythmias classified as benign?
Benign forms comprise one-third of all ventricular arrhythmias and are associated with a low risk of sudden cardiac death. They include PVCs of low-to-moderate frequency in persons with normal ejection fraction and no organic heart disease. Benign arrhythmias are usually asymptomatic and found on routine examination. Occasionally patients may present with mild dizziness or palpitations. The only indication for treatment is bothersome symptoms that Holter monitoring clearly demonstrates as due to arrhythmia. For bothersome benign ventricular arrhythmias, beta blockers are the drugs of choice.

9. When should potentially malignant ventricular arrhythmias be treated?
Potentially malignant forms are seen in 65% of patients with ventricular arrhythmias and are associated with a low-to-moderate risk of sudden death. They include PVCs of moderate-to-high frequency, common couplets, or NSVT in the presence of organic heart disease and moderately decreased left ventricular function. Potentially malignant arrhythmias may be symptomatic with mild hemodynamic impairment or completely asymptomatic. The only clear indication for antiarrhythmic treatment is patients with NSVT after myocardial infarction, in whom beta blockers have been shown to reduce mortality.

10. What are malignant ventricular arrhythmias?
Malignant forms are seen in 5% of patients with ventricular arrhythmias and are associated with moderate-to-high risk of sudden death. They include PVCs of moderate-to-high frequency, common couplets, NSVT, sustained uniform VT, sustained multiform VT, and ventricular fibrillation in the presence of organic heart disease and markedly reduced left ventricular ejection fraction. Patients with left ventricular ejection fraction less than 30% are at high risk for malignant arrhythmias. They often present with heart failure, myocardial ischemia, palpitations, syncope, or cardiac arrest. Therapy is indicated to control symptoms and to reduce the risk of sudden death. Patients need a thorough cardiac evaluation and careful choice and follow-up of antiarrhythmic therapy.

11. What is the prognosis for the patient with simple or complex ventricular ectopy and a structurally normal heart?
The prognosis in such patients is excellent, even with nonsustained VT. Exercise-induced ectopy is not associated with an increased risk of sudden death in the normal population. The presence of symptoms with the arrhythmia does not alter the prognosis.

12. What does the presence of a PVC on a routine EKG mean?
PVCs may be the first evidence of underlying congenital, hypertensive, ischemic, or myopathic heart disease. Observation of PVCs should prompt an evaluation for cardiac pathology. A thorough history and physical examination are the first steps. Further testing should be done only if certain aspects of the history and physical need clarifying.

13. How does the presense of PVCs in patients with mitral valve prolapse influence prognosis?
Such patients have more simple and complex PVCs than the general population, but the prognosis is excellent in persons with structurally normal hearts. Reassurance is the best therapy. Bothersome symptoms may be treated with beta blockers if other lifestyle modification fails. Class I agents are not advisable because of an unfavorable risk-benefit ratio.

The risk of sudden death is increased in the patient with a highly redundant mitral valve, severe mitral regurgitation, a history of syncope, a family history of sudden death, or a prolonged QT interval. In this small subgroup, runs of NSVT may be a marker of increased risk.

14. What is the risk associated with ventricular ectopy after myocardial infarction?
In the first weeks after an infarction, approximately 90% of patients have frequent PVCs. Complex forms have been documented in 20–40% during this period. Simple PVCs are not associated with an increased mortality, but complex ectopy, particularly runs of NSVT, independently increases the risk of sudden cardiac death 2- to 5-fold. Left ventricular (LV) function is another independent prognostic factor in the postinfarction patient. LV dysfunction increases the risk of sudden death by 2–3-fold. Patients with complex ventricular ectopy and LV dysfunction are at highest risk, with an incidence of sudden death in the first year after infarction as high as 35%.

15. Will treatment of the postinfarction patient at high risk for sudden death improve survival?
No evidence suggests that suppression of arrhythmia reduces risk and improves survival. Data from the CAST trial indicate that antiarrhythmic therapy may be harmful in such patients.

16. What was the CAST study? What did it show?
The Cardiac Arrhythmia Suppression Trial (CAST) was a long-term, multicenter, placebo-controlled study designed to test the hypothesis that antiarrhythmic drugs for suppression of asymptomatic or mildly symptomatic PVCs reduce the risk of sudden cardiac death in post-infarction patients. After a 10-month follow-up, excessive mortality among patients randomized to encainide and flecainide therapy led to the removal of both agents from the trial. Even though the agents were shown to suppress asymptomatic or mildly symptomatic PVCs, suppression was associated with increased mortality. The benefit of antiarrhythmic drugs other than beta blockers after myocardial infarction is unproved. It has not been demonstrated that antiarrhythmic drugs prevent a first episode of sudden cardiac death in any patient population. Amiodarone is the only other antiarrhythmic agent currently undergoing evaluation in postinfarction trials. Alternatives to current pharmacologic therapy clearly are needed for individuals at high risk.

17. Should the patient with NSVT in the presence of dilated cardiomyopathy and congestive heart failure be treated with antiarrhythmic drugs?
We do not know. In patients with cardiomyopathy and clinical congestive heart failure, the 2-year mortality rate may be as high as 50%. Approximately 40% are sudden cardiac deaths, presumably due to a fatal arrhythmia. Ambulatory monitoring has shown that 70–95% of patients have frequent PVCs and 60–80% have NSVT. This group requires further study to determine whether antiarrhythmic agents offer a survival benefit. Unfortunately, no cohort of patients not receiving antiarrhythmic therapy for NSVT has been followed. The excessive mortality may be due to antiarrhythmic therapy rather simply to the presence of the arrhythmia. Current evidence does not support the use of antiarrhythmic agents to suppress the ectopy in such patients. Angiotensin-converting enzyme inhibitors reduce mortality in patients with LV dysfunction and reduce the frequency of ventricular arrhythmias in patients with clinical heart failure. These drugs, therefore, are currently the best antiarrhythmic therapy for such high-risk patients.

18. Can antiarrhythmic therapy improve survival for patients with aborted sudden cardiac death?
Yes. In the patient resuscitated from sudden cardiac death, the reoccurrence rate of sudden cardiac death is approximately 30% in the first year. Such patients require electrophysiologic

evaluation. Several studies have shown improved survival after antiarrhythmic therapy is directed at the spontaneous arrhythmia documented with monitoring or at the induced arrhythmia in the electrophysiology laboratory. This is the only group of patients in whom antiarrhythmic drugs have been reported to prolong life.

19. Should a patient with hypertrophic cardiomyopathy and complex ventricular ectopy be treated?

In such patients complex ventricular ectopy is associated with an increased risk of sudden cardiac death. Data on the efficacy of amiodarone in preventing sudden cardiac death are conflicting. After previous investigators reported that amiodarone therapy reduced the risk of sudden death in such patients, the National Institutes of Health performed a study on a similar group and found an unexpectedly high incidence of sudden death in patients with hypertrophic cardiomyopathy who received amiodarone. This study showed suppression of the arrhythmias on Holter monitoring but failed to show a reduction in the rate of sudden cardiac death.

20. How is the efficacy of antiarrhythmic therapy assessed?

Efficacy is assessed by clinical symptoms and by objective means such as ambulatory monitoring. Because of the marked spontaneous variability in the frequency of ventricular arrhythmias, a 75–80% reduction in the frequency of PVC and a 90–100% reduction in the presence of NSVT is required to declare that the drug is effective in suppression of arrhythmia.

21. What is proarrhythmia?

Proarrhythmia is the appearance of a new arrhythmia or aggravation of an existing arrhythmia. In the broadest sense, the term refers to bradyarrhythmias, supraventricular tachycardias (SVTs), and VTs. Proarrhythmia is potentially seen with all antiarrhythmic agents; the incidence varies from 5–35%. The etiology is unclear, and occurrence is hard to predict. Proarrhythmia may be part of the mechanism of increased mortality in certain patients treated with antiarrhythmic drugs. The potential for proarrhythmia with antiarrhythmic agents must be considered whenever a patient is started on a new agent and each time the dose is adjusted. A fourfold increase in the number of PVCs and a 10-fold increase in repetitive forms fit the criteria for identifying proarrhythmia with ambulatory monitoring.

22. What are the major side effects of antiarrhythmic therapy?

Noncardiac side effects specific to each agent
Organ toxicity specific to each agent
Proarrhythmia
Conduction defects
Precipitation of congestive heart failure

There are many antiarrhythmic drugs in part because they all pose potential problems. No antiarrhythmic drug is perfect. Beta blockers are probably the best. It is important to be completely familiar with the pharmacology of any prescribed antiarrhythmic drug.

23. When the physician is presented with a hemodynamically stable patient with a wide complex tachycardia, what is the likely diagnosis on the basis of statistics alone?

The differential diagnosis centers on VT or SVT conducted aberrantly through the heart. VT is more common by far and thus most likely.

24. What four clues does the electrocardiogram give to help differentiate VT from SVT with aberrancy?

1. Underlying heart disease favors VT.
2. Capture and fusion beats indicate VT.
3. AV dissociation indicates VT.
4. QRS width > 140 msec in the absence of preexisting bundle-branch block or accessory connection suggests VT.

25. What therapeutic considerations are important in patients with wide complex tachycardia?

1. Assume that the problem is VT, which is much more common.

2. Cardiovert the hemodynamically unstable patient.

3. Do not give verapamil, which can lead to profound hypotension and potentially to cardiovascular collapse in a patient with VT.

4. The drug of choice is probably procainamide, administered intravenously (loading dose followed by infusion).

BIBLIOGRAPHY

1. Braunwald E (ed): Heart Disease: A Textbook of Cardiovascular Medicine, 4th ed. Philadelphia, W.B. Saunders, 1992.
2. Brugada P, Brugada J, Mont L, et al: A new approach to the differential diagnosis of a regular tachycardia with a wide QRS complex. Circulation 83:1649–1659, 1991.
3. Chou T: Electrocardiography in Clinical Practice, 2nd ed. Philadelphia, W.B. Saunders, 1986.
4. Echt DS, Liebson PR, Mitchell LB, et al: Mortality and morbidity in patients receiving encainide, flecainide, or placebo. The Cardiac Arrhythmia Suppression Trial. N Engl J Med 324:781–788, 1991.
5. Ewy GA, Bressler R (eds): Cardiovascular Drugs and the Management of Heart Disease, 2nd ed. New York, Raven Press, 1992.
6. Horowitz LN: Current Management of Arrhythmias. Philadelphia, B.C. Decker, 1991.
7. Hsia HH, Buxton AE: Work-up and management of patients with sustained and nonsustained monomorphic ventricular tachycardia. Cardiol Clin 11:21–37, 1993.
8. Rankin AC, Rae AP, Cobbe SM: Misuse of intravenous verapamil in patients with ventricular tachycardia. Lancet 1:472–474, 1987.
9. Richards DA, Byth K, Ross DL, Uther JB: What is the best predicter of spontaneous ventricular tachycardia and sudden death after myocardial infarction? Circulation 83:756–763, 1991.
10. Wellens JJ: The value of the electrocardiogram in the differential diagnosis of a tachycardia with a widened QRS complex. Am J Med 64:27–33, 1978.

20. CORONARY ARTERY DISEASE

Valerie Ulstad, M.D.

1. What causes myocardial ischemia?

Myocardial ischemia is caused by an imbalance between myocardial oxygen supply and demand.

2. How may myocardial ischemia manifest?

Myocardial ischemia may manifest as angina pectoris, as ST-T changes on the electrocardiogram (EKG), and as left ventricular dysfunction due to inadequate supply of myocardial oxygen for normal contractile function.

3. What are the determinants of myocardial oxygen demand?

The need for oxygen delivery to the heart is increased when any of the following four conditions exist: (1) increased heart rate, (2) increased contractility of the heart, (3) increased afterload for the ejecting heart (crudely measured as the systolic blood pressure), and (4) increased preload (filling of the ventricles in diastole)

4. What are the most common clinical presentations of coronary artery disease (CAD)?

Typical angina pectoris, unstable angina pectoris, acute myocardial infarction, and sudden cardiac death.

5. What is the pathophysiology of typical angina pectoris?

In typical exertional angina pectoris, ischemia results when myocardial oxygen demand is increased but supply is relatively reduced because of atherosclerotic obstruction of 50–70% of the coronary lumen. The affected individual has exertional chest discomfort relieved by rest. Because coronary reserve is reduced most in the subendocardium, ischemia occurs first in this region. An EKG during an episode of pain would likely show ST depression, which is indicative of subendocardial ischemia.

Some patients with chronic stable angina develop ischemia because of dynamic coronary vasoconstriction in the setting of fixed atherosclerotic disease. The eccentric lesions of atherosclerosis leave muscle in the neighboring vessel wall; thus spasm in that area may suddenly worsen the stenosis. Such inappropriate coronary vasoconstriction has been shown to occur with cigarette smoking, exposure to cold, and exercise.

6. Describe the management of a patient with typical angina pectoris.

1. **Educate.** The patient needs to understand the disease process to be motivated to modify CAD risk factors and to seek medical attention promptly if symptoms worsen.

2. **Treat.** The patient should be started on therapy to relieve discomfort and to improve exercise tolerance. Sublingual nitroglycerin should be used as necessary.

3. **Evaluate.** An exercise stress test should be done to define objectively the level of exercise that precipitates myocardial ischemia and to provide the clinician with prognostic information. The patient who develops ischemia either clinically or on EKG during the first minutes of exercise has a poor prognosis. Such a patient should be referred for more invasive evaluation by coronary angiography.

7. What are the objectives in the medical treatment of angina?

1. Reduction of myocardial oxygen demand during exercise or stress: nitrates, beta blockers, calcium-channel blockers.

2. Promotion of maximal coronary vasodilation of the coronary arteries: nitrates, calcium-channel blockers.

Severity of disease determines the amount of therapy. Usually nitrates are the first-line treatment, with other drugs added if more than episodic nitroglycerin is required.

Antianginal Therapy

ANTIANGINAL AGENT	ACTION	IMPORTANT CONSIDERATIONS
Nitrates	Dilate coronaries Decrease preload	8–10 hours/day free of drug to avoid tolerance May cause headache

Beta blockers	Decrease heart rate
	Decrease contractility
	Decrease blood pressure
		All agents potentially block beta$_1$
		  and beta$_2$ receptors; selective
		  agents at low dose block beta$_1$
		  receptors more than beta$_2$
		Can precipitate CHF, broncho-
		  spasm, CNS side effects

Calcium-channel blockers	Dilate coronaries Decrease contractility Decrease systolic pressure Decrease heart rate	Heterogeneous group Constipation

CHF = congestive heart failure; CNS = central nervous system.

8. What education should the patient receive about therapy with nitroglycerin?

Sublingual nitroglycerin prescriptions should be refilled every 6 months because the tablets become outdated. A patient who develops flushing or headache with sublingual therapy probably is using active nitroglycerin. Patients who use nitrates (either orally or by patch) to sustain blood levels must have a 10–12-hour nitrate-free period each day. This decreases the incidence of nitroglycerin tolerance and improves efficacy.

9. What is unstable angina?

The following situations suggest that the anginal pattern is unstable:

1. Rest angina or angina occurring with less effort than previously
2. More frequent angina with the same degree of exertion
3. More protracted discomfort that is less responsive to therapy or rest
4. Prolonged pain without evidence of myocardial infarction
5. Recent onset of angina

10. What is the pathophysiology of unstable angina?

Unstable angina is a clinical syndrome that falls between chronic stable angina pectoris and acute myocardial infarction. Studies suggest that there is a further reduction in myocardial oxygen supply. The involved coronary artery in unstable angina tends to have an eccentric plaque with a fissure or crack and superimposed thrombus adherent to the site of the plaque crack or rupture. The precise factors that lead to plaque rupture are unknown. Platelets adhere to the disrupted thrombogenic intima and produce thromboxane A_2, which stimulates further platelet aggregation. The resultant thrombus is responsible for the sudden change in myocardial oxygen supply and subsequent change in symptoms. The thrombus may be intermittently occlusive, leading to waxing and waning discomfort at rest. If the thrombus completely occludes the vessel, a myocardial infarction follows, unless the vessel can be rapidly opened.

11. Describe the EKG in patients with unstable angina.

The majority of patients have transient ST-T changes (elevation or depression) and/or peaking or inverted T waves during pain. An EKG with ST-T segment deviation in two or more leads is highly predictive of adverse clinical events.

12. What therapy is indicated in patients with unstable angina?

Unstable angina is associated with a tendency to develop continually worsening pain, acute myocardial infarction, life-threatening ventricular arrhythmias, or sudden cardiac death. Patients should be promptly hospitalized for observation, monitoring, antianginal therapy (IV nitroglycerin and beta blockers), and antithrombotic therapy (heparin infusion and aspirin) to promote coronary artery patency. The role of thrombolytic therapy in unstable angina is unclear. Because of the high likelihood of adverse future cardiac events, patients should be considered for coronary angiography and possible revascularization.

13. Describe the presentation of the patient with acute myocardial infarction (AMI).

The patient with AMI usually presents with discomfort similar in character to angina pectoris. The discomfort does not resolve promptly with rest and nitroglycerin. Continued discomfort at rest distinguishes AMI from a simple episode of angina. The EKG in patients with AMI typically show ST segment elevation, suggesting transmural ischemia usually due to obstruction of an epicardial coronary artery.

14. What is the pathophysiology of AMI?

An intracoronary thrombus develops because of atherosclerotic plaque disruption and fissure. When the thrombus totally occludes the vessel, myocardial ischemia begins. If the vessel remains closed, myocardial infarction occurs. In more than 85% of patients with AMI, occluding thrombus can be demonstrated angiographically.

15. Why is prompt recognition of AMI so important?

The obstruction of a coronary artery quickly leads to abnormal ventricular wall motion in the distribution of the affected coronary artery. If the vessel remains closed for longer than 20–40 minutes, the ventricular muscle in the distribution of the coronary artery begins to become necrotic (infarction); the deepest layers of the myocardium are affected first.

The highest priority is to open the coronary artery. Thrombolytic therapy to lyse the occluding thrombus should be considered in every patient with AMI as soon as the diagnosis is made; it is now considered standard therapy.

16. What is thrombolytic therapy?

Thrombolytic agents are capable of causing clot lysis directly or indirectly by accelerating the conversion of plasminogen to plasmin. Plasmin is a proteolytic enzyme that acts on fibrin to cause fibrinolysis, which results in thrombolysis and reperfusion. The three agents approved by the Food and Drug Administration for coronary thrombolysis include streptokinase, alteplase (a recombinant tissue-type plasminogen activator [TPA]), and anistreplase (an acylated plasminogen-streptokinase complex [APSAC]).

17. Does thrombolytic therapy work?

Yes. Intravenous thrombolytic therapy reduces early mortality from AMI by 25%, leads to an increase in postinfarction left ventricular ejection fraction, and reduces the likelihood of postinfarction congestive heart failure. Survival rates with various agents have so far been identical, although the role of adjunctive heparin with each has not yet been well studied. The ongoing GUSTO trial compares survival rates after streptokinase and/or alteplase with immediate and continuous heparin infusion.

18. Who is the ideal candidate for thrombolytic therapy?

Ideal patients (who tend to be included in controlled trials) are younger than 75 years, with ST elevation in two or more contiguous leads, and present within 6 hours of the onset of chest discomfort. Many other patients may benefit from thrombolytic therapy, including patients with new left bundle branch block, elderly patients with large infarctions, and patients presenting between 6 and 12 hours after the onset of pain.

19. What is the major side effect of thrombolytic therapy?

With all thrombolytic agents the major adverse effect is bleeding. Hemorrhage requiring transfusion occurs in 1–5% of patients and intracranial bleeding in 0.5–1.5%.

20. What is the role of aspirin in AMI?

Aspirin has been shown to reduce the incidence of reinfarction in patients treated with streptokinase and to double the reduction in mortality observed with streptokinase alone. Aspirin, 160–325 mg/day, should be started in the emergency department at presentation and continued for at least 1 year or longer.

21. Should beta blockers be given after AMI?

Yes. Beta blockers have been shown to reduce mortality when started several days to several months after infarction. Both selective and nonselective forms of beta blockers reduce the incidence of sudden death after infarction.

22. Should beta blockers be started immediately upon presentation with AMI?

Yes. The immediate use of beta blockers, presumably to reduce myocardial oxygen demand by opposing the heightened adrenergic tone associated with AMI, has been shown to lead to a 13% reduction in 1-week mortality and a 19% reduction in nonfatal reinfarctions.

23. What is the role for angiotensin-converting enzyme (ACE) inhibitors in the postinfarction patient?

The Studies of Left Ventricular Dysfunction (SOLVD) and the Survival and Ventricular Enlargement (SAVE) trials suggest that postinfarction patients with an ejection fraction less than 35% have lower mortality, fewer hospitalizations for heart failure, and a lower incidence of recurrent infarction when treated with an ACE inhibitor.

24. What are the major complications of AMI?
Arrhythmias (particularly ventricular)
Systolic heart failure
Mechanical complications (free wall, septal, or papillary muscle rupture)
Left ventricular (LV) mural thrombus with embolization

25. What is the 1-year mortality rate after AMI?
The 1-year mortality rate after discharge is 4–7%. In patients younger than 70 years who are treated with thrombolytic therapy, the mortality rate may be as low as 3–5%.

26. Name the factors associated with a poor prognosis after AMI.

1. Decreased LV ejection fraction—independent factor
2. Advanced age—independent factor
3. Female sex—independent factor
4. Complex or frequent PVCs—independent factor
5. Congestive heart failure
6. Postinfarction angina
7. Prior myocardial infarction
8. Large infarction
9. Atrial fibrillation
10. Extensive coronary artery disease
11. Diabetes
12. Hypertension
13. Continued smoking
14. Elevated serum cholesterol

27. What can be done to minimize the postinfarction risk?
1. Coronary angiography during acute hospitalization if the patient has continued ischemic symptoms in the hospital
2. Predischarge or early (within weeks) limited exercise testing to identify patients with residual ischemia for referral for coronary angiography and possible revascularization
3. Referral of patients with sustained ventricular tachycardia for coronary angiography and electrophysiologic evaluation
4. Smoking cessation (associated with a 40–60% decrease in mortality)
5. Lowering of cholesterol
6. Use of beta blocker
7. Aspirin
8. ACE inhibitor if ejection fraction is ≤ 35%
9. Referral to cardiac rehabilitation (may reduce mortality by 20–25%)

BIBLIOGRAPHY

1. American College of Cardiology/American Heart Association Task Force on Assessment of Diagnostic and Therapeutic Cardiovascular Procedures (Subcommittee to Develop Guidelines for the Early Management of Patients with Acute Myocardial Infarction): Guidelines for the early management of patients with acute myocardial infarction. J Am Coll Cardiol 16:249–292, 1990.
2. Bertolet BD, Dinerman J, Hartke R Jr, Conti CR: Unstable angina: Relationship of clinical presentation, coronary pathology, and clinical outcome. Clin Cardiol 16:116–122, 1993.
3. Braunwald E: Unstable angina: A classification. Circulation 80:410–414, 1989.
4. Chesebro JH, Zoldhelyi P, Fuster V: Pathogenesis of thrombosis in unstable angina. Am J Cardiol 68:2B–10B, 1991.
5. Conti CR, Hill JA, Mayfield WR: Unstable angina pectoris: Pathogenesis and management. Curr Probl Cardiol 14:549–624, 1989.
6. Eisenberg MS, Aghababian RV, Bossaert L, et al: Thrombolytic therapy. Ann Emerg Med 22(2Pt 2):417–427, 1993.
7. Fuster V, Badimon L, Badimon JJ, Chesebro JH: The pathogenesis of coronary artery disease and the acute coronary syndromes: Part 1. N Engl J Med 326:242–250, 1992.
8. Fuster V, Badimon L, Badimon JJ, Chesebro JH: The pathogenesis of coronary artery disease and the acute coronary syndromes: Part 2. N Engl J Med 326:310–318, 1992.
9. Muller DW, Topol EJ: Selection of patients with acute myocardial infarction for thrombolytic therapy. Ann Intern Med 113:949–960, 1990.
10. Popma JJ, Topol EJ: Adjuncts to thrombolysis for myocardial reperfusion. Ann Intern Med 115:34–44, 1991.

11. Pfeffer MA, Braunwald E, Moye LA, et al: Effects of captopril on mortality and morbidity in patients with left ventricular dysfunction after myocardial infarction: Results of the survival and ventricular enlargement trial. The SAVE Investigators. N Engl J Med 327:669–677, 1992.
12. Puleo P, Roberts R: Early biochemical markers of myocardial necrosis. Cardiovasc Clin 20:143–154, 1989.
13. Shah PK: Pathophysiology of unstable angina. Cardiol Clin 9:11–26, 1991.
14. SOLVD Investigators: Effect of enalapril on mortality and the development of heart failure in asymptomatic patients with reduced left ventricular ejection fractions. N Engl J Med 327:658–691, 1992.
15. Topol EJ: Which thrombolytic agent should one choose? Prog Cardiovasc Dis 34:165–178, 1991.
16. Yusuf S, Sleight P, Held P, McMahon S: Routine medical management of acute myocardial infarction: Lessons from overveiws of recent randomized controlled trials. Circulation 82(Suppl II):II-117–II-134, 1990.
17. Yusuf S, Wittes J, Friedman L: Overview of results of randomized clinical trials in heart disease: I. Treatments following myocardial infarction. JAMA 260:2088–2093, 1988.

21. CONGESTIVE HEART FAILURE

Valerie Ulstad, M.D.

1. What is congestive heart failure (CHF)?

CHF is a clinical syndrome related to cardiac dysfunction (systolic and/or diastolic) and characterized by limited exercise tolerance, fluid retention, and reduced life expectancy.

2. What are the incidence and prevalence of CHF?

Three million people in the United States and 15 million people worldwide have CHF. There are approximately 400,000 new cases in the U.S. each year. The incidence is increasing despite the decline in mortality from cardiovascular disease, probably because an aging population has received benefit from improved therapies. CHF is the most common discharge diagnosis in patients 65 years or older.

3. Describe the New York Heart Association (NYHA) classification of heart failure.

Class I: No limitation of physical activity; no dyspnea, fatigue, or palpitations with ordinary physical activity

Class II: Slight limitation of physical activity; patients have dyspnea, fatigue, or palpitations with ordinary physical activity but are comfortable at rest.

Class III: Marked limitation of activity; less than ordinary physical activity results in symptoms, but patients are comfortable at rest.

Class IV: Symptoms are present at rest and any physical exertion exacerbates the symptoms.

4. Characterize low-output cardiac failure.

Low-output failure, the most common form of heart failure, is characterized by reduced stroke volume, peripheral vasoconstriction, reduced pulse pressure, and increased arteriovenous oxygen difference.

5. What are the most important causes of low-output CHF in the United States?

Coronary artery disease—underlying cause in 50–75%
Hypertension
Dilated cardiomyopathy
Valvular heart disease
Hypertrophic cardiomyopathy
Congenital heart disease
Cor pulmonale
Toxins—alcohol, Adriamycin
Infections

6. What is the most common cause of low-output CHF worldwide?
Chagas disease.

7. List five prognostic indicators in CHF.

Ventricular function measured by ejection fraction	Cardiothoracic ratio
	Plasma norepinephrine levels
Peak exercise oxygen consumption	Ventricular arrhythmias

8. What is the mortality rate from CHF?
The 5-year mortality rate in men is 60%. Women seem to do somewhat better, with a 5-year mortality rate of 45%. When the patient has symptoms of heart failure at rest (class IV), the 1-year mortality rate is about 50%. About 40% of the deaths are sudden, presumably due to ventricular arrhythmias.

9. What is high-output cardiac failure?
High-output cardiac failure is characterized by widened pulse pressure, peripheral vasodilation, and an increased arteriovenous oxygen difference.

10. What conditions are associated with high-output heart failure?

Anemia	Paget disease
Hyperthyroidism	Hepatic disease
Systemic arteriovenous fistula	Dermatologic conditions causing
Beriberi	high blood flow in skin

11. Which symptoms of CHF are due to isolated left ventricular dysfunction?

Dyspnea on exertion	Wheezing
Paroxysmal nocturnal dyspnea	Hemoptysis
Orthopnea	Fatigue
Cough	Weakness

12. What are the clinical signs of isolated left ventricular dysfunction?

Hypotension	Cardiomegaly (systolic dysfunction)
Weak pulses	S3 gallop
Peripheral vasoconstriction	Rales
Cachexia	Pleural effusions
Cheyne-Stokes respirations	

13. Which symptoms of CHF are due to isolated right ventricular dysfunction?
Right upper quadrant discomfort
Abdominal distention
Early satiety

14. What are the clinical signs of isolated right ventricular dysfunction?

Elevated jugular venous pressure	Ascites
Hepatomegaly	Peripheral edema
Splenomegaly	

15. What is the most common cause of right-heart failure?
Left-heart failure.

16. Contrast systolic and diastolic dysfunction.
Systolic dysfunction occurs with a defect in the expulsion of blood from the ventricles or a decrease in ventricular contractility. Diastolic dysfunction occurs with abnormal resistance to ventricular filling in diastole.

17. How do the Frank-Starling curves (stroke volume on the Y axis and end-diastolic volume on the X axis) differ for the normal heart and the heart with severe systolic dysfunction?
Note the effect of increasing preload. The normal heart augments its output with increases in preload. The heart with systolic failure is unable to augment its output further by increasing preload. (See figure, below.)

18. How do the function curves (stroke volume on the Y axis and afterload on the X axis) differ for the normal heart and the heart with severe systolic dysfunction?
Note the effect of increasing impedance or afterload. The normal heart tolerates increased impedance well without a drop in stroke volume. The heart with systolic failure fails further (that is, stroke volume falls further) with increased impedance. (See figure, below.)

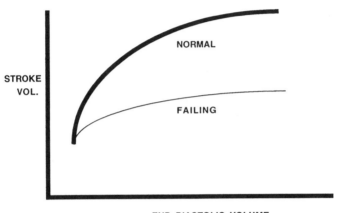

Frank-Starling curves for the normal heart and for the heart with severe systolic dysfunction.

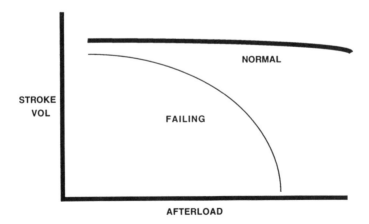

Function curves for the normal heart and for the heart with severe systolic dysfunction.

19. Which is the more common cause of CHF syndrome, systolic or diastolic dysfunction?
Systolic dysfunction is the more common cause. As a result, the terms systolic and CHF syndrome tend to be used synonomously. Such usage is inaccurate.

20. Describe the vicious cycle of heart failure.
A particular cardiac problem causes a drop in cardiac output that leads to activation of the neurohormonal mechanisms, including the sympathetic nervous system, the renin-angiotensin-aldosterone system, and the arginine vasopressin system. The net effects are excessive vasoconstriction and increased sodium and water retention, which lead to increased vascular impedance to the already failing heart. Thus the patient's condition worsens.

21. List the three major goals of therapy for CHF.
Improved quality of life
Prolonged survival
Improved natural history

22. What are the principles of treatment of CHF?
1. Remove or correct the precipitating cause.
2. Correct exacerbating factors.
3. Determine whether the dysfunction is predominantly systolic or diastolic by echocardiography.
4. Treat the syndrome: Improve pump performance in systolic dysfunction with digoxin
5. Reduce the workload:
   - Rest
   - Weight loss for the obese patient
   - Vasodilators
6. Control excessive salt and water retention:
   - Low-sodium diet
   - Diuretics

23. What common causes of cardiac decompensation should be considered in patients with previously stable CHF?
- Myocardial ischemia
- Mitral regurgitation
- Uncontrolled hypertension
- Increased dietary intake of sodium
- Superimposed additional medical illness, especially:
  Poorly controlled diabetes mellitus
  Pneumonia
  Pulmonary embolus

24. When should diuretic therapy be used in the treatment of CHF?
In chronic therapy of **CHF due to systolic dysfunction,** diuretics may not be necessary. Excessive diuresis may result in further activation of the neurohormonal system and intolerance of vasodilators (hypotension).

In chronic therapy of **CHF due to diastolic dysfunction,** diuretics are often needed to decrease pulmonary congestion and to improve dyspnea. Diuretics must be given carefully to avoid an excessive drop in preload, because patients have stiff ventricles with intrinsic resistance to diastolic filling.

Loop diuretics are needed when renal function is abnormal (creatine = > 2.0 mg/dl), because thiazide diuretics are ineffective in such patients. In patients with mild CHF, thiazide diuretics may have a role if renal function is normal. In refractory heart failure a combination of thiazide and loop diuretics may be needed.

25. How should vasodilators be used in CHF due to systolic dysfunction?
In the Studies of Left Ventricular Dysfunction (SOLVD) trial, which enrolled only patients with established heart failure, enalapril was associated with a decrease in overall mortality, although no change in the rate of sudden death was found.

The Digoxin-Captopril Multicenter Research Group, which enrolled patients with mild-to-moderate CHF, showed that captopril improved exercise tolerance and that digoxin improved ejection fraction, whereas treatment with diuretics alone led to increased episodes of hospitalization and emergency department visits as well as increased need for additional diuretics.

In the Cooperative North Scandinavian Enalapril Survival Study (CONSENSUS), enalapril showed improved survival rates compared with placebo in patients with severe CHF.

In the Veterans Administration Cooperative Vasodilator Trial (V-HeFT I) hydralazine and isosorbide dinitrate showed a favorable effect on mortality rates in patients with moderate CHF compared with placebo; prazosin had no effect.

The V-HeFT II study compared hydralazine and isosorbide dinitrate with enalapril in patients with moderate heart failure. Enalapril showed a superior reduction in mortality rates, but exercise tolerance and increase in ejection fraction were superior in patients treated with hydralazine and isosorbide dinitrate.

The above data suggest that angiotension-converting enzyme (ACE) inhibitors should be started in nearly all patients with symptomatic or asymptomatic left ventricular (LV) systolic dysfunction. Hypotension can be prevented by starting with low doses and by avoiding volume depletion before institution of therapy. Marked subsequent increases in blood urea nitrogen (BUN) and creatinine (Cr) suggest renovascular disease, and the ACE inhibitor should be stopped. Hydralazine and isosorbide dinitrate should be tried in patients intolerant of ACE inhibitors or with side effects. Flosequinan can be used as adjunct therapy to digoxin, diuretics, and ACE inhibitors or as primary therapy in patients intolerant of ACE inhibitors.

26. Should the asymptomatic person with LV systolic dysfunction be treated with vasodilator therapy?

Yes. This recommendation is based on the outcome of two major trials. The SOLVD trial showed that enalapril reduced the incidence of heart failure and the rate of related hospitalizations in patients with asymptomatic decreased function (ejection fraction $\leq 35\%$). In the Survival and Ventricular Enlargement (SAVE) study, patients enrolled 3–17 days after infarction with ejection fractions of $< 40\%$ and no clinical heart failure were randomized to captopril or placebo. Captopril improved mortality rates, prevented further reduction in ejection fraction, and reduced the rate of recurrent infarction.

27. How should digoxin and other oral inotropic agents be used in patients with CHF?

In patients with acute decompensation most studies support the use of digoxin. Current data also support its use in patients with chronic heart failure, even those with normal sinus rhythm. Digoxin is a inotrope but also reduces plasma renin activity and plasma aldosterone. Acutely it reduces plasma catecholamines and activity of the sympathetic nervous system.

Other inotropes have a limited role. Dobutamine is the intravenous inotrope of choice in patients with decompensated CHF. Other inotropes, such as amrinone and milrinone, are effective intravenously in patients with acute decompensation, but experience with both drugs is limited. Increased mortality rates have been demonstrated with the oral inotrope enoximine; thus the future use of other oral inotropes must be subject to rigorous scrutiny.

28. What is the difference in approach to treatment of systolic as opposed to diastolic failure?

A patient with systolic dysfunction should be treated with inotropes to improve contractility; with diuretics to decrease congestion due to increased preload; and with vasodilators to decrease afterload or impedance imposed on the left ventricle by vasoconstrictors released by neurohumoral activation.

A patient with diastolic failure should be treated with agents to improve relaxation (negative inotropes), gentle diuresis if congestion exists (because the ventricle does not fill well, excessive diuresis decreases cardiac output precipitously), and agents to slow the heart rate (so that diastole is longer and allows more time to fill). Patients with diastolic dysfunction may tolerate vasodilators poorly.

29. How does one distinguish between systolic and diastolic dysfunction as the cause of the clinical syndrome of CHF?

The clinical syndrome is the same in both types of dysfunction. Echocardiography is a useful test in any patient with new heart failure. This test may demonstrate any important valvular or pericardial disease. Systolic dysfunction is evident with decreased contractility of the heart. If both left and right ventricular systolic functions are normal, restricted ventricular filling or diastolic dysfunction may be the culprit. Echo-Doppler studies may be used to look more carefully for diastolic dysfunction.

30. What endpoints should be evaluated in drug trials for treatment of CHF?

Improved quality of life
Improved exercise capacity
Reversal of neurohormonal abnormalities
Reduction of mortality

31. Describe the common types of cardiomyopathy.

Cardiomyopathy is a condition of varying and frequently unknown etiology in which the dominant feature is cardiomegaly and low-output cardiac failure. Cardiomyopathies are categorized in three groups:

Dilated
- Most common type; dilation of all chambers
- Decrease in systolic function of the ventricles
- Causes include idiopathic factors, alcohol, adriamycin, myocarditis, valve replacement, diabetes, thyroid disease, thiamine deficiency, pheochromocytoma, and peripartum complications
- Chest radiograph shows enlarged heart; echocardiography shows enlarged chambers and reduced contractility; radionuclide ventriculography shows reduced ejection fraction

Hypertrophic
- Less common; thickening of ventricular wall; small ventricular cavity
- Abnormal diastolic function
- Causes include genetic factors, hypertension, and acromegaly
- Chest radiograph shows normal to mildly enlarged heart size, echocardiography shows small ventricular chamber, increased wall thickness, and increased contractility

Restrictive (infiltrative)
- Rare
- Systolic and diastolic function affected; both ventricles affected equally
- Causes include amyloid and sarcoid disorders and hemochromatosis
- Diagnosis often found only with biopsy after hemodynamic evaluation shows equal diastolic filling pattern (square-root sign) on right and left sides of heart

32. Which patients should undergo cardiac transplantation?

Transplantation should be considered in patients who remain severely compromised despite medical therapy. The 5-year survival rate for cardiac transplantation is 70–75%. Donor availability, however, limits widespread application.

33. What factors are associated with increased morbidity or mortality from cardiac transplant?

Obesity
Diabetes with organ damage
Pulmonary hypertension
Previous cardiac or thoracic surgery
Chronic lung disease
Intrinsic hepatic or renal disease

BIBLIOGRAPHY

1. Captopril-Digoxin Multicenter Research Group: Comparative effects of captopril and digoxin in patients with mild to moderate heart failure. JAMA 259:539–544, 1988.
2. Captopril Multicenter Research Group: A placebo-controlled trial of captopril in refractory congestive heart failure. J Am Coll Cardiol 2:755–763, 1983.

3. Cohn JN: Physiological variables as markers for symptoms, risks and interventions in heart failure. Circulation 87 (Suppl VII):VII-110–VII-114, 1993.

4. Cohn JN, Archibald D, Ziesche S, et al: Effect of vasodilator therapy on mortality in chronic congestive heart failure: Results of a Veterans Administration Cooperative Study (V-HeFT). N Engl J Med 314:1547–1552, 1986.

5. Cohn JN, Johnson GR, Shabeti R, et al: Ejection fraction, peak exercise oxygen consumption, cardiothoracic ratio, ventricular arrhythmias, and plasma norepinephrine as determinants of prognosis in heart failure. Circulation 87 (Suppl VI):VI-5–VI-16, 1993.

6. Cohn JN, Johnson GR, Ziesche S, et al: A comparison of enalapril with hydralazine–isosorbide dinitrate in the treatment of chronic congestive heart failure. V-HeFT II. N Engl J Med 325:303–310, 1991.

7. CONSENSUS Trial Study Group: Effects of enalapril on mortality in severe congestive heart failure: Results of the Cooperative North Scandinavian Enalapril Survival Study (CONSENSUS). N Engl J Med 316:1429–1435, 1987.

8. Fletcher RD, Cintron GB, Johnson G, et al: Enalapril decreases ventricular tachycardia in patients with chronic congestive heart failure. Circulation 87 (Suppl VI):VI-49–VI-55, 1993.

9. Francis GS: Development of arrhythmias in the patient with congestive heart failure: Pathophysiology, prevalence, and prognosis. Am J Cardiol 57:3B-7B, 1986.

10. Goldman S, Johnson G, Cohn JN, et al: Mechanism of death in heart failure: The vasodilator-heart failure trials. Circulation 87(Suppl VI):VI-24–VI-31.

11. Lorell BH: Significance of diastolic dysfunction of the heart. Annu Rev Med 42:411–436, 1991.

12. McFate-Smith W: Epidemiology of congestive heart failure. Am J Cardiol 55:3A-8A, 1985.

13. Parmley WW: Pathophysiology and current therapy of congestive heart failure. J Am Coll Cardiol 13:771–785, 1989.

14. SOLVD Investigators: Effect of enalapril on survival in patients with reduced left ventricular ejection fractions and congestive heart failure. N Engl J Med 325:293–302, 1991.

15. SOLVD Investigators: Effect of enalapril on mortality and development of heart failure in asymptomatic patients with reduced left ventricular ejection fractions. N Engl J Med 327:685–691, 1992.

22. CARDIAC TESTING

Valerie Ulstad, M.D.

1. How often is the initial electrocardiogram (EKG) diagnostic of myocardial infarction (MI)?

The initial EKG is diagnostic in 60% of patients. In 25% the EKG is abnormal but not diagnostic. In 15% the EKG is absolutely normal. Therefore decisions about admission to the hospital should be based primarily on the history and current findings.

2. Does an EKG without Q waves rule out a previous MI?

No. A definitive diagnosis of a previous MI depends on the presence of pathologic Q waves. Within 6–12 months after an acute MI, about 30% of EKGs are still abnormal but no longer diagnostic for previous MI because the Q waves are absent. After 10 years 6–10% of EKGs are completely normal.

3. List nine contraindications to exercise testing.

1. Unstable angina
2. Uncontrolled hypertension
3. Critical aortic stenosis
4. Hypertrophic cardio-myopathy with significant obstruction
5. Untreated life-threatening cardiac arrhythmias
6. Decompensated heart failure
7. Advanced atrioventricular (AV) block
8. Acute pericarditis or myocarditis
9. Other acute illness

4. When should a stress test be stopped?

1. **Patient signs and symptoms**
   - Severe fatigue
   - Severe dyspnea
   - Chest pain
   - Marked elevation in systolic blood pressure (> 250 mmHg)
   - Definite drop in systolic blood pressure (≥ 10 mmHg)

2. **EKG changes**
   - ≥ 3-mm ST depression
   - ≥1-mm ST elevation in lead without abnormal Q wave
   - Ventricular tachycardia
   - Paroxysmal supraventricular tachycardia
   - Decrease in heart rate

3. **Noncardiac factors**
   - Patient request
   - Gait disturbance
   - Technical problems interfering with test interpretation

5. In addition to exercise-induced chest pain, what signs and symptoms during an exercise test indicate an adverse prognosis and probable multivessel coronary artery disease (CAD)?

1. Inability to exercise to 6 metabolic equivalents (METS) in an otherwise healthy patient
2. Failure to increase systolic blood pressure to ≥ 120 mmHg
3. Definite drop in systolic blood pressure ≥ 10 mmHg
4. ST depression > 2mm
5. Downsloping ST depression under 6 METS, in 5 or more leads or persisting more than 5 minutes into recovery
6. Exercise-induced ST elevation (excluding lead aVR)
7. Sustained ventricular tachycardia

6. What is the value of a stress test in patients with an uncomplicated MI before hospital discharge?

A low-level exercise test to 5–6 METS or 70–80% of the age-predicted maximal heart rate is frequently performed before hospital discharge to assess the patient's functional capacity and to test for residual provocable myocardial ischemia at a relatively low level of myocardial oxygen demand. A negative submaximal stress test is associated with a 1-year mortality rate of 1–2%. An ischemic response indicates a poorer prognosis. Cardiac catheterization before discharge should be considered in such patients to assess revascularization options.

7. Should an exercise stress test be done after percutaneous transluminal coronary angioplasty (PTCA)?

The restenosis rate after PTCA is 20–30%, usually within 6 months. In the patient who is asymptomatic after PTCA, an exercise test at 6 months allows documentation of important restenosis but also allows the dilated vessel sufficient time to heal. If the patient has had multivessel PTCA, an exercise thallium stress test is ideal to localize the area of significant restenosis.

8. What is a thallium stress test?

The patient exercises as on a regular exercise test. An intravenous line is placed before the exercise begins so that thallium can be administered near peak exercise. Accumulation of thallium in the myocardium is related to coronary blood flow and cellular extraction of the tracer by myocardial tissue. Thallium resembles potassium in that it is actively transported into cells by the sodium-potassium/adenosine triphosphatase system and by facilitated diffusion. Thallium-201 is cyclotron-produced and has a low energy level and a half-life of 72–73 hours; it is relatively expensive but associated with some degree of radiation exposure.

At peak exercise 1.5–2 mCu of thallium-201 is injected intravenously while the patient continues to exercise for another minute. After 5–10 minutes images are obtained in anterior, 60° left anterior oblique, and left lateral projections. Redistribution images in the same views are obtained 2–4 hours later. Normally thallium is distributed homogeneously throughout the myocardium.

9. Describe the findings of an abnormal thallium scan. What do they mean?

Perfusion defects on exercise imaging may be due to scars, ischemic zones, or both.

A **reversible defect** indicates viable myocardium.

A **fixed defect** represents irreversibly damaged tissue or severely ischemic myocardium.

Increased lung uptake of thallium on exercise imaging indicates exercise-induced LV dysfunction of any etiology. An increased lung uptake is seen at rest in patients with a high LV filling pressure. In either case, this finding is a poor prognostic sign.

10. When is exercise thallium testing preferred over exercise electrocardiography for the diagnosis of CAD?

Exercise thallium stress testing is preferable (1) when the baseline EKG is abnormal; (2) when pretest probability of CAD is intermediate (thallium does not add much information when the pretest probability is low or high); or (3) when the localization or extent of ischemia is in question.

11. How much exercise must a patient do to get a reliable result from thallium testing?

Failure to stress patients adequately results in the provocation of less than maximal coronary vasodilation. This compromises the quality of the information. Patients who have exercised to 85% of age-predicted maximal heart rate have exercised adequately.

12. What does SPECT stand for?

SPECT stands for single-photon emission computed tomography, an advance in thallium imaging that allows better regional localization of ischemia by providing tomographic images of the heart in any plane.

13. How does stress echocardiography compare with stress thallium testing in the assessment of CAD?

Stress echocardiography is an inexpensive and sensitive way to assess the distribution and severity of myocardial ischemia; it is as sensitive and specific as exercise SPECT thallium testing. Stress echocardiography is more portable, in many cases cheaper, and more readily available than SPECT thallium testing. Clinicians should use the stress test modality that is done best at their institution. All sophisticated stress tests require significant experience to provide accurate clinical data.

14. Which stress test should be used in patients with left bundle branch block (LBBB)?

Exercise-induced ST depression cannot be used as a diagnostic or prognostic indicator in patients with LBBB. Most patients will have ST depression with exercise, and the extent of ST depression is not meaningful. Thallium stress testing is also problematic. Patients with LBBB frequently have exercise-induced myocardial perfusion defects in the anteroapical and anteroseptal areas and angiographically normal coronary arteries. The altered sequence of depolarization is believed to be the cause of thallium abnormality. Thus, exercise echocardiography is a good option as a diagnostic and prognostic test for the patient with LBBB.

15. How should patients on digoxin be evaluated for CAD?

Digitalis glycosides may produce exertional ST depression even with no evidence of digitalis effect on the resting EKG. Absence of ST depression during an exercise test in a patient on digitalis glycosides is considered a valid negative response. Digitalis should be withheld 1–2 weeks before exercise testing if one plans to rely only on EKG data. Having the patient remain on the drug is an option if one uses thallium perfusion imaging or stress echocardiography instead.

16. What are the options for stress testing in the patient who cannot exercise?

Dobutamine or dipyridamole stress echocardiography is often used for such patients. Dobutamine increases cardiac contractility and heart rate, thereby increasing myocardial oxygen demand and simulating physical stress. Dipyridamole increases coronary blood flow and leads to redistribution of flow, producing a steal phenomenon in the distribution of significant coronary stenosis. Simultaneous echocardiographic imaging allows the detection, grading, and localization of wall-motion abnormalities due to ischemic provocation.

Dipyridamole thallium-201 imaging is also used in patients who cannot exercise. The most extensive experience with this test has been in the assessment of perioperative risk in patients requiring peripheral vascular surgery. Predictive value is greatest when the patient has clinical evidence of CAD, such as angina, previous MI, Q waves on the EKG, S3 gallop, congestive heart failure, or diabetes. The patient with none of the above features has a low perioperative risk, and the patient with three or more has a high risk, no matter what the dipyridamole thallium test shows. Adenosine may be used instead of dipyridamole. It is probably safer in patients with cerebral vascular disease because of its short half-life. Any vasodilator can induce cerebral hypoperfusion.

17. How does antianginal therapy affect the exercise treadmill test?

Nitrates, beta blockers, or calcium-channel blockers prolong the time to the onset of ischemic ST segment depression, and increase exercise tolerance. If the treadmill test is done for diagnostic purposes, cardiac drugs should be withheld for 3–5 half-lives. If the adequacy of drug therapy is being assessed, the test should be done with the patient taking the antianginal medication.

18. What diagnostic test should be ordered after a positive exercise treadmill test in a middle-aged woman with no risk factors and atypical chest pain to eliminate the diagnosis of significant CAD?

In this setting exercise-induced ST depression is more likely to be falsely positive for CAD. Exercise thallium testing improves the diagnostic yield in patients with a suspected false-positive test.

19. What is the best way to assess the severity of aortic stenosis (AS)?

Two-dimensional echocardiography detects a thickened and calcified aortic valve with reduced opening. The LV size and wall thickness also can be assessed. Doppler echocardiography determines the transvalvular gradient and the valve area. AS is severe if the peak aortic flow velocity exceeds 4.5 m/sec, the aortic valve area is < 0.75 cm², and the LV outflow tract/aortic flow velocity is ≤ 0.25. A complete echocardiographic examination gives the clinician the necessary data to interpret the patient's complaints. Echocardiography can be done serially with minimal patient discomfort.

Before the refinement of echocardiographic technology, it was necessary to cross the aortic valve in a retrograde fashion in the catheterization laboratory in order to confirm the presence of severe AS. Now the only reason to catheterize a patient with AS before surgery is to perform coronary angiography when coincident CAD is suspected. Such a patient may receive bypass grafts at the time of valve surgery.

20. Is there a reliable test to assess the presence of left atrial clot before cardioversion of atrial fibrillation?

Successful cardioversion is associated with a 5–7% incidence of embolism among patients who have not received anticoagulant therapy. Atrial thrombi are poorly detected by transthoracic echocardiography. A normal transthoracic echocardiogram does not rule out the presence of left atrial thrombi.

The standard practice is several weeks of oral anticoagulation in patients with atrial fibrillation of unknown duration or duration > 2 days. Cardioversion of an anticoagulated patient carries an embolic rate of < 1.6%.

Transesophageal echocardiography (TEE) is a highly accurate method of detecting atrial thrombi. If TEE excludes the presence of thrombi, early cardioversion probably can be performed safely without preprocedure anticoagulation. However, skeptics point out that small thrombi potentially missed by TEE can have important consequences, that the risk of anticoagulation in most patients is low, and that larger studies are neeeded. Anticoagulation during and after the procedure is still recommended until atrial contractility returns to normal.

21. Which imaging modalities can be used in patients in whom aortic dissection is suspected?
Potential imaging modalities include aortography, CT, magnetic resonance imaging (MRI), and TEE. The choice of test depends on the precise information that is sought by the surgeon and the expertise available in acquiring the images. Potentially available diagnostic information includes presence of dissection, involvement of the aortic root, sites of entry, extent of dissection, branch-vessel involvement, thrombus in the false lumen, aortic insufficiency, pericardial effusion, and coronary artery involvement.

All modalities are similar in specificity, but MRI and TEE tend to be more sensitive. Sensitivity is most important because aortic dissection is a rapidly lethal condition. MRI is probably better at defining the site of the intimal tear and recognizing intraluminal thrombus. Both modalities are noninvasive and easily identify the presence of pericardial effusion; neither require the use of intravenous contrast material. TEE is superior at detecting and quantifying the degree of aortic insufficiency and in detecting involvement of the proximal coronary arteries. TEE tends to be more readily available and more rapid, because it can be performed at the patient's bedside.

22. What is the best test for rapid evaluation of potential cardiac etiologies in a hypotensive patient?
As fluid support is initiated, a simple transthoracic echocardiogram rapidly reveals the status of ventricular function. A hyperdynamic left ventricle suggests hypovolemia or sepsis as a cause of the hypotension. A poorly contractile left ventricle suggests low-output heart failure as the cause. A large pericardial effusion causing right atrial and right ventricular diastolic collapse indicates a hemodynamically significant pericardial effusion that needs emergent drainage. A markedly dilated right ventricle leads to consideration of right ventricular infarction or large pulmonary embolus as the culprit. With such information the physician can begin to tailor therapy. A Swan-Ganz catheter eventually may be in order, but it should not be the starting point.

23. What is a signal-averaged EKG? How is it used?
Signal-averaged EKG is a diagnostic test used to detect delayed, low-amplitude electrical activation in the terminal portion of the QRS complex. The signal-averaged EKG is an amplified representation of the QRS complex. The amplification allows the small late potentials to be seen. The late potential is a moderately sensitive and highly specific indicator for inducible ventricular tachycardia in the electrophysiology laboratory. The clinical application of signal-averaged EKGs is still under study.

24. What does rest radionuclide ventriculography evaluate?
Rest radionuclide ventriculography provides a quantitative measurement of left ventricular ejection fraction. The red blood cells are tagged with a radioactive label, and counts in the left ventricle are obtained by a gamma counter in systole and diastole. The fraction of counts lost from diastole to systole is the ejection fraction. It can be obtained simply and requires no artificial assumptions about geometry of the left ventricle. It is reproducible on serial measurements and is the desired test for accurate measurement of the ejection fraction. The accuracy of the test may be affected by frequent premature atrial or ventricular beats or by atrial fibrillation.

BIBLIOGRAPHY

1. Braunwald E (ed): Heart Disease: A Textbook of Cardiovascular Medicine, 4th ed. Philadelphia, W.B. Saunders, 1992.
2. Bonow RO, Dilsizian V: Thallium-201 and technetium-99m-sestamibi for assessing viable myocardium. J Nucl Med 33:815–818, 1992.

3. Brown KA: Prognostic value of thallium-201 myocardial perfusion imaging: A diagnostic tool comes of age. Circulation 83:363–381, 1991.
4. Cigarroa JE, Isselbacher EM, DeSanctis RW, Eagle KA: Diagnostic imaging in the evaluation of suspected aortic dissection: Old standards and new directions. N Engl J Med 328:35–43, 1993.
5. Eagle KA, Coley CM, Newell JB, et al: Combining clinical and thallium data optimizes preoperative assessment of cardiac risk before major vascular surgery. Ann Intern Med 110:859–866, 1989.
6. Ehman RL, Julsrud PR: Magnetic resonance imaging of the heart. Mayo Clin Proc 64:1134–1146, 1989.
7. Hendel RC, Layden JJ, Leppo JA: Prognostic value of dipyridamole thallium scintigraphy for evaluation of ischemic heart disease. J Am Coll Cardiol 15:109–116, 1990.
8. Kahn JK, Sills MN, Corbett JR, Willerson JT: What is the current role of nuclear cardiology in clinical medicine? Chest 97:442–446, 1990.
9. Kotler TS, Diamond GA: Exercise thallium-201 scintigraphy in the diagnosis and prognosis of coronary artery disease. Ann Intern Med 113:684–702, 1990.
10. Manning WJ, Silverman DI, Gordon SPF, et al: Cardioversion from atrial fibrillation without prolonged anticoagulation with use of transesophageal echocardiography to exclude the presence of atrial thrombi. N Engl J Med 328:750–755, 1993.
11. Nienaber CA, von Kodolistch Y, Nicolas V, et al: The diagnosis of thoracic aortic dissection by noninvasive imaging procedures. N Engl J Med 328:1–9, 1993.
12. Schlant RC, Blomquist CG, Brandenburg RO, et al: Guidelines for exercise testing: A report of the American College of Cardiology/American Heart Association Task Force on Assessment of Cardiovascular Procedures (Subcommittee on Exercise Testing). J Am Coll Cardiol 8:725–738, 1986.
13. Sox HC, Littenberg B, Garber AM: The role of exercise testing in screening for coronary artery disease. Ann Intern Med 110:456–469, 1989.

IV. Disorders of the Eyes, Ears, Nose, and Throat

23. VISUAL IMPAIRMENT

Jon M. Braverman, M.D., and Thomas D. MacKenzie, M.D.

1. How is vision generally measured in the primary care office?

Most patients read an eye chart, which tests central visual acuity. Testing of standard acuity requires the equivalent of a 20-ft Snellen target. However, testing near vision in a patient who is farsighted or presbyopic (over 40 years of age) does not yield accurate results unless a near correction is used.

Peripheral vision can be tested grossly by confrontation. The examiner sits in front of the patient, and each closes the opposite eye to overlap respective fields. The examiner then asks the patient either to count the number of fingers presented within the field or to indicate when a finger is first seen entering the field. Most modern ophthalmologic practices use automated computerized perimeters to assess visual fields more accurately.

Several other components of vision can be measured, including color perception, dark adaptation, and contrast sensitivity. Changes in these parameters may occur secondary to eye disease; however, the tools and techniques required for evaluation are usually beyond the resources of a primary care provider.

2. What three levels of visual processing should be considered in evaluating the possible etiologies of diminished visual acuity?

1. Loss of the ability to form a clear image on the retina
2. Loss of the ability of the retina to process the image (retinal or nerve injury)
3. Loss of the ability to process the information from the retina to higher perceptual centers via the intracranial visual pathway.

3. Which structures of the eye are required to produce a clear retinal image?

A clear retinal image requires three components: a clear cornea with a normal tear film, a clear lens, and a clear vitreous (intraocular) medium.

4. List the three most common causes of visual impairment in adults.

Cataracts, macular degeneration, and chronic glaucoma. Although presbyopia is the most common cause of reduced near acuity in adults, it is not regarded as a disease.

5. How can the ophthalmoscopic exam aid in defining the etiology of decreased visual acuity?

The direct ophthalmoscopic exam is initially all that is necessary to identify the characteristics of the three most common causes of visual loss in adults. If necessary, a 1% tropicamide solution should be used to dilate the pupil in order to optimize visualization. The three major diagnoses may be suggested by the following abnormalities:

Cataract: A developing cataract is suggested by a cloudy view of the optic nerve and retinal vessels, along with loss of brightness of the red reflex.

Chronic open-angle glaucoma: If the view of the optic nerve is clear but the ratio of the optic cup to the entire nerve head area (cup-to-disc) ratio is high, chronic open-angle glaucoma may be the cause.

Macular degeneration: In the presence of central vision impairment and a good view of the fundus that reveals a grossly normal-appearing optic nerve, macular degeneration may be suspected. Subtle changes in the macular microanatomy may be difficult to appreciate.

6. What causes vitreous opacification?

Vitreous opacification, as evidenced by poor visibility of the fundus on ophthalmoscopic exam, is usually due to hemorrhage, although on occasion it may result from inflammatory or infectious processes. Conditions that may cause vitreous hemorrhage include hypertension, coagulation abnormalities, proliferative diabetic retinopathy, sickle-cell retinopathy, and retinal detachment.

7. What causes blurring of the optic disk?

- Papilledema due to increased central nervous system pressure
- Optic neuritis (papillitis)
- Arterial ischemia to the optic disc, resulting in pale color and an edematous disc
- Retinal vein occlusion, which is usually accompanied by hemorrhages and dilated veins.

8. When should cataract removal be considered?

In the United States, 70% of people over age 75 years have an opacification of the lens, referred to as a cataract. The degree of visual acuity loss is directly proportional to the density of the cataract, provided that no other ocular disease is present. However, much controversy surrounds the timing of cataract surgery, and the health care expenditure associated with removal is enormous. Detection of the cataract is not an indication for ophthalmologic surgery. Apparent premature surgery is best avoided by carefully determining the degree to which the cataract impairs the patient's activities and safety.

9. Can a cataract cause serious ocular problems other than visual limitations due to poor light transmission?

Yes. On occasion, cataracts may contribute to various secondary disorders, including intraocular inflammation due to leaking of lens material inside the eye; chronic glaucoma resulting from the inflammatory response to liberated lens material; and acute glaucoma due to the physical apposition of the swollen lens with the iris and subsequent closure of the filtering angle.

10. Which diseases interfere with the ability of the retina to process images?

Senile macular degeneration, retinal detachment, vascular ischemia, trauma, and certain acute infections of the retina (cytomegalovirus, herpes, especially in the immunocompromised host) can interfere with the processing of retinal images.

11. What is the natural history of macular degeneration?

Macular degeneration usually occurs in patients older than 55 years and progresses with time. To date, no preventive or therapeutic strategies have been proved to slow macular degeneration. Current anecdotal reports refer to possible stabilization or slowing of macular changes by dietary supplementation, particularly zinc and antioxidant vitamins. However, subretinal neovascular tissue growth, a complication of macular degeneration, may be treated by lasers to prevent bleeding and scarring. Any acute or subacute change in the eye affected by macular degeneration should be investigated to rule out this complication.

12. Why should patients be screened for glaucoma?

Glaucoma causes end-organ damage (optic atrophy) through increased pressure in the vitreous element. The changes are not perceivable by the patient; moreover, the earliest changes typically result in loss of peripheral vision long before central vision is affected. Thus, early diagnosis and prevention of blindness require routine screening to detect subtle changes in peripheral vision due to increased intraocular pressure. Because measurement of intraocular pressure is a technique prone to error, referral to a provider with special training in ophthalmology usually is required.

13. Who should be screened for glaucoma?

Risks factors for open-angle glaucoma include age (over 40 years), high myopia, diabetes, and family history of glaucoma. The American Academy of Ophthalmology currently recommends routine yearly screening for patients at risk.

14. What is standard therapy for patients with chronic open-angle glaucoma?

Treatment of open-angle glaucoma begins with the use of topical agents to reduce intraocular pressure. Oral carbonic anhydrase inhibitors are second-line agents because of systemic side effects. Laser therapy and intraocular surgery are reserved for patients whose condition is not controlled effectively by medial therapy, although studies to evaluate the efficacy of early surgical intervention in glaucoma are ongoing.

15. What causes floaters?

Opacities in the vitreous element cause patients to complain of floaters, which are particularly noticeable when gazing at a clear background, such as a white wall or blue sky. Floaters, which may be single or multiple, are due to several causes, including acute retinitis, retinal tear, vitreous detachment (as a consequence of aging), or debris consisting of inflammatory cells, red blood cells, or cholesterol crystals.

16. What diagnoses should be considered in a patient who experiences a sudden, painless unilateral loss of vision?

- Central retinal artery occlusion, often due to an embolus or vasculitis
- Giant cell arteritis resulting in central retinal artery occlusion or ischemic optic neuropathy
- Central retinal vein occlusion
- Retinal detachment
- Acute hemorrhage into the vitreous element
- Optic neuritis

17. What diagnoses should be considered in a patient who complains of sudden loss of vision in both eyes?

Sudden loss of vision in both eyes is an extremely uncommon event. If the fundi are normal, one must consider toxic neuritis or a possible conversion reaction (diagnosis of exclusion).

18. What is the classic cause of a bitemporal hemianoptic visual defect?

Lesions, usually pituitary tumors, that involve the optic chiasm.

BIBLIOGRAPHY

1. American Academy of Ophthalmology: 1989–1990 Public and Professional Information Catalog. San Francisco, American Academy of Ophthalmology, 1989, pp 9–13.
2. American Academy of Ophthalmology: Educational Programs 1990. San Francisco, American Academy of Ophthalmology, 1990, pp 16–17.
3. Newell W: Ophthalmology: Principles and Concepts, 5th ed. St. Louis, Mosby, 1992.
4. Sussman EJ, et al: Diagnosis of diabetic eye disease. JAMA 247:3231–3234, 1982.
5. Sweet EH, et al: Eye care by primary care physicians. Ophthalmology 98:1454–1460, 1991.

24. EYE PAIN AND INFLAMMATORY DISEASES

Jon M. Braverman, M.D., and Thomas D. MacKenzie, M.D.

1. What are the usual sources of eye pain?

The eyelid, cornea, conjunctivae and uveal tract (iris, ciliary body, and choroid) are the most richly innervated structures of the eye; thus, lesions affecting these areas are the most painful. Pathology confined to the vitreous element, retina, and optic nerve is likely to be painless. Diseases of the sinuses and orbit also may cause referred pain to the eye.

2. Which diseases are associated with a red eye?

A red eye is the most common ocular complaint in the general population. The presence and severity of pain and visual changes are used to distinguish the many different entities that may account for this finding.

Possible Causes of Red Eye as Determined by Associated Findings

PAIN	VISUAL CHANGES	ETIOLOGY
Yes, severe	Acute loss	Acute glaucoma
Yes	Blurring	Corneal inflammation (keratitis) or ulceration
Yes, with photophobia	Blurring	Uveal tract or scleral inflammation
No	Acute or subacute loss	Vascular or retinal disease
No	No	Conjunctival inflammation (Conjunctivitis)

3. Acute-angle closure glaucoma is an absolute ocular emergency. When should the primary care provider suspect this diagnosis?

Acute elevations in intraocular pressure are far more damaging than slowly and chronically acquired elevations. The clinical presentation relects this basic difference. Acute-angle closure glaucoma presents as an extremely painful eye (unilateral) with loss of vision. The pupil is mid-dilated and nonreactive, and marked conjunctival injection is accompanied by clouding of the cornea due to edema. The fundus is poorly visualized. This constellation of symptoms and findings requires immediate referral to an ophthalmologist.

4. What is the significance of photophobia?

Photophobia, the avoidance of light due to pain, may result from ocular or nonocular processes. Ocular photophobia results from intraocular inflammation or congestion of the structures of the uveal tract, including the iris and ciliary body, and their associated contractile muscles. During exposure to light, pupillary constriction therefore leads to pain. Thus, inflammation in any of these structures (uveitis for all; iritis, cyclitis, choroiditis) is indicated by the complaint of photophobia. Nonocular processes resulting in photophobia include migraine, meningeal irritation, and certain drugs, particularly those that cause pupillary dilation via anticholinergic properties.

5. What are the usual causes of uveitis?

Inflammation of the uveal tract, presenting as photophobia and injection, is usually idiopathic. Abnormal pupils that react poorly to light may result from adhesions, called posterior synechiae, of the iris tissue to the lens surface.

Several systemic diseases also are associated with uveitis or variable inflammation of the components of the uvea, including rheumatoid arthritis, sarcoidosis, lupus erythematosus, ankylosing spondylitis, Reiter's syndrome, inflammatory bowel disease, and juvenile rheumatoid arthritis. Infectious causes include syphilis, herpes simplex, varicella zoster, cytomegalovirus, and Lyme disease.

Treatment ranges from topical cycloplegics to systemic steroids or other immunosuppressive agents. Referral to an ophthalmologist is appropriate for work-up and treatment.

6. What are the most common causes of conjunctivitis?
Bacterial, viral, allergic, and irritant etiologies are possible. Patients usually complain of red eyes and a sticky or watery discharge. Irritation is common, but severe pain and photophobia are not. Bacterial or viral conjunctivitis is usually self-limited, but it may be treated with a topical antibiotic without steroids, such as sulfacetamide (10% 3–4 times/day). Topical aminoglycoside should be reserved for more refractory disease. Allergic conjunctivitis may be effectively treated with a new class of nonsteroidal topical anti-inflammatory agents. Irritant conjunctivitis, including dry eyes, may be treated with topical, nonpreserved lubricants.

7. When are topical steroids contraindicated in the treatment of eye disorders?
Topical steroids are absolutely contraindicated in patients who have a history of herpetic eye disease or who may have herpetic infection at presentation. Such patients require referral to an ophthalmologist.

8. What is ocular medicamentosis?
Ocular medicamentosis refers to an iatrogenic or medication-induced conjunctivitis. Inflammation is a reaction to prescribed medication, any of its components or contaminants, or to over-the-counter medicines or home remedies used by the patient to relieve the original conjunctivitis. This entity is improved by discontinuing all medications and using topical, nonpreserved lubricants if needed.

9. What produces the sensation of a foreign body in the eye with blinking?
   Foreign body
   Corneal abrasion
   Eyelid injury or a turned-in eyelid (which may cause an abrasion)
   Keratitis

10. What are common infectious causes of keratitis?
Herpes simplex infection and zoster dermatomal infection cause keratitis, although other viral and bacterial infections are also possible. Steroids are contraindicated in acute herpes simplex infections. Accurate diagnosis and therapy with the consultation of an ophthalmologist are paramount.

11. What principles should guide therapy for a foreign body?
   1. Attempt removal under topical anesthetic only with a cooperative patient and blunt-tip instruments (a cotton applicator moistened with anesthetic is best).
   2. Ascertain the mechanism of injury. Any circumstance involving high-speed microprojectiles should be further evaluated by the opthalmologist.
   3. Patch the eye after treatment and refer the patient to an ophthalmologist. Topical 10% sulfa ointment is a well-tolerated medication.

12. What is the difference between a sty and a chalazion?
A sty is painful and usually due to a bacterial infection. A chalazion is a mildly painful swelling of the eyelid margin due to granulomatous inflammation and usually resolves spontaneously with warm soaks and time. Both are common inflammations of the sebaceous glands of the eyelid.

13. Name the potential eye diseases associated with acquired immunodeficiency syndrome (AIDS).

Over one-half of all patients with AIDS have ocular complications. Cotton wool spots, due to microvascular disease, are the most frequent physical finding. Ocular complications include the following:

- CMV retinitis, as evidenced by hemorrhage and exudate on funduscopic examination
- Eye infections due to toxoplasmosis and *Pneumocystis carinii*
- Retinal necrosis due to herpetic infections (simplex and zoster), with or without keratitis or iritis
- Kaposi's sarcoma and non-Hodgkin's lymphoma
- Optic neuropathy, sometimes a side effect of anti-tuberculous treatment

14. What causes cotton wool spots in the fundus?

Cotton wool spots represent ischemic injury to the superficial nerve layer of the retina. Although frequently seen in severe hypertensive retinopathy, they are not pathognomonic and also may occur with diabetes mellitus, anemia, leukemia, collagen vascular disease, endocarditis, and AIDS.

BIBLIOGRAPHY

1. American Academy of Ophthalmology: 1989–1990 Public and Professional Information Catalog. San Francisco, American Academy of Ophthalmology, 1989, pp 9–13.
2. American Academy of Ophthalmology: Educational Programs 1990. San Francisco, American Academy of Ophthalmology, 1990, pp 16–17.
3. Newell W: Ophthalmology: Principles and Concepts, 5th ed. St. Louis, Mosby, 1992.
4. Sussman EJ, et al: Diagnosis of diabetic eye disease. JAMA 247:3231–3234, 1982.
5. Sweet EH, et al: Eye care by primary care physicians. Ophthalmology 98:1454–1460, 1991.

25. HEARING LOSS AND TINNITUS

Thomas D. MacKenzie, M.D., and Michael L. Lepore, M.D., F.A.C.S.

1. What percentage of adults over the age of 65 years have a handicapping hearing loss?

Data from the National Health Interview Survey in 1989 indicate that approximately 29% of people over age 65 years and 36% of people over age 75 years have a hearing loss severe enough to interfere with effective conversation. Presbycusis, the most common variety, may be defined as an unexplained, slowly progressive decline in aural sensitivity due to the aging process. The hearing loss is usually symmetric, as is noise-induced hearing loss.

2. Why does hearing loss progress to a severe state before the patient seeks assistance?

The aging process may be accompanied by a number of chronic physical conditions of which the patient is acutely aware. Hearing loss, however, most commonly develops over many years and is therefore overshadowed by the acuity of concurrent conditions. The patient unknowingly develops coping mechanisms and does not notice an acute change in hearing until a severe loss is present.

3. What psychological effects of hearing loss may offer clues to its presence?

Patients often withdraw from their surroundings. They may demonstrate conversational manipulation, phobic behavior, paranoia, and mood disorders. The most frequent symptoms are mood disorders, as manifested by insomnia, loss of appetite, guilt, fatigue, anxiety, and uncontrolled emotional outbursts.

4. How does one evaluate the patient with presbycusis?

A careful history and a high index of suspicion in the particularly susceptible patient group are extremely important to identify warning signs. All elderly patients should undergo evaluation of hearing. Particularly important signs are difficulty with hearing in a room with other people and turning up the sound on the television set. Tinnitus is also an early symptom of hearing loss. A careful history of previous exposure to loud noise is important to ascertain. If hearing loss is suspected, an audiometric evaluation should be performed to determine the type and quality.

5. What level of noise exposure may contribute to hearing loss?

Long exposure to noise over 90 dB SPL (sound pressure level) may cause progressive symmetrical hearing loss. Sources of chronic noise exposure with corresponding db SPL levels are listed below.

Riveting steel tank	130	Boiler shop	100
Automobile horn	120	Hydraulic press	100
Sandblasting	112	Can manufacturing plant	100
Wood-working shop	100	Subway	90
Punch press	100	Average factory	80
Pneumatic drill	100		

6. What is the most common cause of sudden deafness?

The incidence of sudden deafness is reported to be 5–20 per 100,000 persons per year. This figure, however, is probably higher because some patients recover so rapidly that they do not seek medical attention. The common etiology of sudden deafness is idiopathic sudden sensorineural hearing loss. Characteristically approximately one-third of patients develop hearing loss upon awakening in the morning, and about one-half also notice disequilibrium or frank vertigo. The intensity of the vertigo usually corresponds to the severity of the hearing loss. Some of the predisposing factors associated with idiopathic sudden sensorineural hearing loss include changes in the physical environment, such as altitude or atmospheric pressure; emotional disturbances; diabetes; atherosclerosis; pregnancy; use of contraceptive drugs; and stress of surgery, physical exertion, or general anesthesia.

7. What are the specific causes of acute hearing loss?

1. Viral infections may affect the cochlea by causing labyrinthitis or direct inflammation of the cochlear nerve. Measles, mumps, influenza, and adenoviruses have been associated with sudden deafness. Herpes zoster has been shown to produce a viral neuronitis or ganglionitis.

2. Tumors of the cerebellopontine angle may produce sudden deafness.

3. Damage to the organ of Corti may be induced by sneezing, coughing, bending, the Valsalva maneuver, or scuba diving.

4. Rupture of the round or oval window is usually accompanied by positional nystagmus. A positive fistula sign is demonstrated by applying positive pressure to the tympanic membrane, which causes ipsilateral nystagmus.

8. When should aggressive evaluation of a patient with sudden hearing loss be undertaken?

Initial evaluation of all patients should include a careful history, otologic and neurologic examination, audiologic testing, and routine laboratory studies. If hearing does not return in 1 month or if serial audiograms demonstrate progressive loss, then computerized tomography (CT) or magnetic resonance imaging (MRI) with gadolinium of the internal auditory meatus should be performed to rule out the presence of an acoustic tumor.

9. What is the anticipated natural history of idiopathic sensorineural hearing loss?

Age appears to play a significant role in recovery. Patients under the age of 40 years recover normal hearing approximately 50% of the time. The more severe the hearing loss, the less likely the recovery. The presence of vertigo is a bad prognostic sign. Spontaneous recovery may occur within days or weeks; if the loss persists beyond 1 month, there is little likelihood for recovery.

10. Why should patients with an idiopathic sensorineural hearing loss without resolution be tested for syphilis?

In its late phase syphilis may cause sensorineural hearing loss as the only manifestation of disease. Approximately 7% of patients with otherwise unexplained sensorineural hearing loss have a positive treponemal antibody test, as do 7% of patients with Ménière's disease. Thus any patient with a positive treponemal antibody test and unexplained hearing loss should be treated for syphilitic otitis.

11. What other infectious disease may lead to hearing loss?

Tuberculosis may cause sensorineural and conductive hearing loss, although this is unlikely in the absence of pulmonary disease.

12. What commonly used medications may lead to hearing loss?

Aminoglycosides, loop diuretics such as furosemide, salicylates, and antineoplastic agents such as cisplatin.

13. How do the Weber and Rinne tests help in delineating the origin of hearing loss?

Both tests are used to determine whether hearing loss is conductive or sensorineural. The **Weber test** is done by placing the stem of the tuning fork midline on the skull and asking the patient whether the tone is heard in one ear better than in the other. The tone is louder on the side on which the balance of bone (sensorineural) to conductive hearing sensation is greatest. For example, if a patient has wax in the right ear, an ipsilateral conductive hearing loss causes a relative increase in bone (sensorineural) conduction. Thus, the Weber test lateralizes to the right. By contrast, an acoustic neuroma on the right side is accompanied by a relative decrease in bone conduction; thus the Weber test lateralizes to the opposite side.

The **Rinne test** is done by placing the vibrating tuning fork on the mastoid process and asking the patient to acknowledge when the sound is no longer audible (bone conduction). At that point, the vibrating bells of the tuning fork are held at the external auditory canal. The patient normally should hear the tone better by air conduction than by bone conduction.

14. What precautions should be taken before removing impacted ear wax?

Before removing impacted ear wax by irrigation, the patient should be questioned about a previous history of perforated tympanic membrane or of chronic otitis media. Care also must be exercised in the diabetic patient to avoid trauma to the ear canal and secondary external otitis. In patients with perforations or previously draining ears, the cerumen must be removed by using a microscope. To avoid complications, such patients should be referred to an otolaryngologist.

15. What potentially life-threatening disorder is heralded by new-onset tinnitus?

Tinnitus, a common symptom in primary care practice, is characterized by the complaint of ringing or any other abnormal sound in the ear. Most disorders associated with tinnitus are not life-threatening. However, tinnitus may be a prominent manifestation of one medical emergency: salicylate toxicity. Elderly patients who take aspirin chronically, as opposed to patients taking acute overdoses, experience the highest mortality rate from salicylism. One needs to ask specifically about aspirin intake, because many patients do not consider it a prescribed medicine. When in doubt, an aspirin level is appropriate. Other manifestations of salicylism should be sought.

16. What are the most common causes of tinnitus?

Tinnitus can be broadly divided into categories, objective and subjective. **Objective tinnitus** is less common and often can be heard not only by the patient but also by the examiner. Causes of objective tinnitus include vascular abnormalities, such as arteriovenous shunts, arterial bruits, venous hums, and mechanical abnormalities, such as disorders of the eustachian tube and stapedial muscle spasm. This type of tinnitus may be pulsatile in the case of vascular disorders or may change character based on the position of the head, pharynx, or jaw. **Subjective tinnitus** is far more common and most likely arises from damaged cochlear hair cells that discharge continuously. The vast majority of patients with subjective tinnitus have an otologic disorder.

17. Which diseases are associated with unilateral tinnitus?

The majority of subjective tinnitus is bilateral. Unilateral tinnitus is usually due to an otologic disorder, such as chronic suppurative otitis, trauma, or Ménière's disease. In the absence of these diagnoses, work-up should include an MRI scan in search of a central auditory lesion.

18. Who should be involved in the diagnosis and management of the patient with severe tinnitus?

The primary care provider may need assistance from specialists in audiology, otolaryngology, neurology, and occasionally psychiatry. The audiologist localizes the pathology to the ear or to the central nervous system and through special testing detects the pitch and loudness of the tinnitus, the minimal masking level that eliminates the tinnitus, and the residual inhibition. An otolaryngologist or neurologist performs a thorough evaluation of the ears, nose, throat, head, and neck regions to determine the presence of any pathology that may explain the tinnitus. A neurologist may be required for diagnosis if a central lesion is suspected. In patients who are refractory to treatment or who have unexplained tinnitus, associated psychologic disorders may require management.

19. How frequently can tinnitus be controlled?

About 30–40% of patients who report severe tinnitus may be treated, whereas 45–60% respond well to maskers or amplification instruments. Therefore only 10–15% are refractory to therapy. In addition to addressing local otologic problems as an etiology, any eustachian tube dysfunction should be corrected, because it may significantly intensify tinnitus. Adequate ventilation of the eustachian tube and middle ear is achieved through the use of antihistamines and decongestants.

20. What advice should be given to patients with tinnitus?

1. Avoid loud noises, caffeine, drug use, alcohol excess, and tobacco.
2. Maintain an active lifestyle.
3. Join support groups such as the American Tinnitus Association (Portland, OR).

BIBLIOGRAPHY

1. Barker RL, Burton JR, Zieve PD (eds): Principles of Ambulatory Medicine. Baltimore, Williams & Wilkins, 1991.
2. Kohut RI, Hinojosak R: Sudden hearing loss. In Bailey BJ, et al (eds): Head and Neck Surgery—Otolaryngology, vol 2. Philadelphia, J.B. Lippincott, 1993, p 1820.
3. Koopmann CF Jr: Otolaryngologic (head and neck) problems in the elderly. Med Clin North Am 75:1373–1388, 1991.
4. Lavizzo-Mourney RJ, Siegler EL: Hearing impairment in the elderly. J Gen Intern Med 7:191–198, 1992.
5. Lichtenstein MJ: Hearing and visual impairments. Clin Geriatr Med 8:173–182, 1992.
6. Nadol JB: Hearing loss. N Engl J Med 329:1092–1102, 1993.
7. Patt BS, Meyerhoff WL: Aging and auditory vestibular system. In Bailey BJ, et al (eds): Head and Neck Surgery—Otolaryngology, vol 2. Philadelphia, J.B. Lippincott, 1993, p 1843.
8. Schleuning AJ: Management of the patient with tinnitus. Med Clin North Am 76:1225–1237, 1991.
9. Shikowitz MJ: Sudden sensorineural hearing loss. Med Clin North Am 75:1239–1250, 1991.
10. Shulman A: Electrodiagnostics, Electrotherapeutics and Other Approaches to the Management of Tinnitus. The American Academy of Otolaryngology—Head and Neck Surgery Instructional Courses, vol 2. St. Louis, Mosby, 1989, p 137.
11. Vernon J, Schleuning AJ: Tinnitus: Its Care and Treatment. The American Academy of Otolaryngology—Head and Neck Surgery Instructional Courses, vol 2. St. Louis, Mosby, 1989, p 131.

26. EAR PAIN AND INFECTIONS

Thomas D. MacKenzie, M.D., and Michael L. Lepore, M.D., F.A.C.S.

1. What entities cause ear pain?

Otalgia is a frequent complaint with multiple possible causes. Patients may have a pathologic process confined to the ear (primary otaliga), or the pain may be referred to the ear from another source (secondary otalgia). Because most of the ear develops embryologically from the first (mandibular) and second (hyoid) branchial arches, any process in the distribution of the two arches from the larynx and pharynx to the skull base may refer pain to the ear. Some of the common causes of primary otalgia are listed below.

Common Causes of Primary Otalgia

PINNA AND EXTERNAL CANAL	MIDDLE EAR AND MASTOID
Furunculosis	Acute otitis media
External otitis	Acute mastoiditis
Foreign body in the external canal	Acute eustachian tube obstruction
Impacted cerumen	
Acute myringitis and myringitis bullosa	
Trauma to the tympanic membrane	
Perichondritis	

Causes of secondary otalgia include dental pathology, cancer of the larynx and pyriform sinus, tonsillitis, peritonsillar abscess, arthritis of the cricoarytenoid joint, nasopharyngeal pathology, temporomandibular joint disease, and lesions of the esophagus.

2. What is swimmer's ear?

Swimmer's ear is otitis externa, an extremely painful inflammatory process of the external ear canal and auricle. It is often associated with swimming and is a frequent diagnosis in primary care, especially in children. The disease is usually highly responsive to otic antibiotic therapy. However, prevention of recurrence may require the use of ear protection with swimming.

3. Who is at risk for serious complications associated with otitis externa?

Patients over the age of 50 years and patients with diabetes are at risk for severe complications related to simple otitis externa. The disease may progress rapidly to a life-threatening condition of necrotizing (malignant) otitis externa. This syndrome is characterized by severe pain, purulent discharge, and progressive cellulitis of the ear and the base of the skull. If not adequately treated, otitis externa may be complicated by facial and other cranial nerve palsies, meningitis, mastoiditis, parotitis, osteomyelitis of the temporal bone or base of the skull, and death. It is frequently caused by *Pseudomonas aeruginosa*, and treatment requires specific oral antipseudomonal antibiotics. In the more severe forms complicated by cranial nerve involvement, hospitalization with intravenous antibiotics and surgical intervention may be required.

4. What causes otorrhea?

Otorrhea is a discharge from the ear canal associated with disease of both the middle ear and external canal. Disorders of the middle ear that result in otorrhea include acute otitis media with perforation (or the presence of a tympanostomy tube) and chronic suppurative otitis media. Disorders of the external canal that lead to otorrhea include otitis externa and necrotizing otitis externa.

5. How is otitis media classified?

For purposes of treatment and evaluation, otitis media is classified as acute (< 3 weeks' duration), subacute (3 weeks–3 months), and chronic (> 3 months) otitis media.

6. Name the four most commonly identified pathogens associated with acute otitis media.

Streptococcus pneumoniae (most common)   Group A Streptococcus
Haemophilus influenzae   Moraxella catarrhalis

7. What is the most important factor in the pathogenesis of middle ear disease?

Abnormal function of the eustachian tube appears to be the most important pathogenic factor. The normal eustachian tube serves three functions: (1) it provides protection from nasopharyngeal secretions and sound pressure; (2) it acts to clear middle ear secretions by its mucociliary activity; and (3) it provides a ventilatory function for the middle ear. This function depends on gas absorption and on the characteristics of the mastoid air-cell system of the middle ear.

8. What is the most reasonable treatment approach in a patient with an acute episode of otitis media?

Uncomplicated otitis media should be treated with oral antimicrobials. Amoxicillin should be considered the drug of first choice; additional considerations include trimethoprim-sulfamethoxazole, erythromycin, sulfisoxazole, amoxicillin-clavulanate, and cefaclor. Clinical improvement should be evident in 72 hours, and a 10-day course is usually adequate. If no significant improvement is seen with amoxicillin, a beta-lactamase-producing organism should be suspected and antibiotic therapy should be changed. In refractory acute cases, tympanocentesis with or without myringotomy relieves pain, and culture of the middle ear effusion may yield the causative organism.

9. How does otitis media in neonates or young infants differ from otitis media in older children or adults?

In neonates and young infants, the incidence of unusual organisms, particularly gram-negative bacilli and Staphylococcus aureus, is higher.

10. What is the incidence of persistent middle ear effusion after a 10-day course of antibiotics?

Up to 50% of patients are clinically well but have a persistent middle ear infection after a full course of antibiotics. Several options should be considered, because persistent effusions may lead to hearing loss with speech and language delay as well as provide a medium for bacterial growth. The patient should be treated for a longer time with the same antimicrobial agent, and systemic decongestants and/or antihistamines should be used to encourage evacuation of the eustachian tube. The Valsalva maneuver may be performed in the physician's office to inflate the eustachian tube.

A middle ear effusion may persist for approximately 3 months after an acute episode of otitis media resolves. However, if the patient is asymptomatic, watchful waiting is a reasonable approach. If the patient is continuously symptomatic, a more aggressive approach is necessary. In children with multiple episodes of acute otitis media with or without persistent middle ear effusions, speech and language delays may result from hearing loss.

11. What considerations must be given to adults who fail to resolve otitis media or a middle ear effusion?

In adults the nasopharynx must be examined carefully and repeatedly for pathology. Nasopharyngeal carcinoma and lymphoma may cause intermittent or persistent middle ear problems.

12. How is recurrent otitis media managed?

The development of recurrent otitis media should be considered an indication for intervention. Initially diseases that have a role in the etiology of recurrent episodes must be considered, including sinusitis, nasal allergy, immune deficiency, nasopharyngeal pathology, cleft palate, and submucosal palate. A child with recurrent episodes of otitis media and persistent middle ear effusion may be treated more aggressively. Chemoprophylaxis with chronic antibiotics may be used. Myringotomy, which may decrease the frequency of episodes and possible complications, should be considered carefully.

13. What are the consequences of untreated or inadequately treated acute otitis media?

Because of the widespread use of antimicrobial therapy, the incidence of complications from acute otitis media has decreased dramatically. However, because of the potential for serious morbidity, complications must be recognized early. Intracranial complications include lateral sinus thrombophlebitis, extradural abscesses, subdural abscesses, brain abscess, and meningitis. Local complications include conductive or sensorineural hearing loss; perforation of the tympanic membrane; chronic suppurative otitis media with or without cholesteatoma; atelectasis with retraction pockets and adhesions of the tympanic membrane; and erosion of the incus with ossicular discontinuity, labyrinthitis, and facial nerve paralysis.

14. What is Gradenigo's syndrome?

Gradenigo's syndrome is the triad of otalgia, otorrhea, and paralysis of the abducens nerve. It occurs as a complication of otitis media and requires immediate referral to an otolaryngologist.

15. How is chronic otitis media manifested?

Chronic otitis media is an indolent inflammatory process involving the eustachian tube, middle ear, and mastoid air-cell system. Two varieties are commonly recognized: chronic suppurative otitis media (CSOM) and chronic otitis media with effusion (COME). Both conditions begin in childhood, usually in patients with a history of recurrent otitis media. In CSOM, hearing loss, painless otorrhea, and tympanic perforation are common. In COME, the hallmark is a 24–40 dB conductive hearing loss.

16. What is the most serious complication of chronic otitis media?

The development of cholesteatoma is the most serious complication of chronic otitis media. In the presence of chronic otitis media, retraction pockets or cysts form in the middle ear and are lined by skin. Desquamation leads to a build-up of keratin. Keratin-containing cysts, called cholesteatomas, invade the surrounding bone, leading to facial nerve paralysis, vertigo, and meningitis. As they grow in the middle ear, the cysts may cause destruction of the incus, stapes and malleus leading to severe conductive hearing loss. Cholesteatomas are often visible as a white ball in the middle ear. Their presence is usually an indication for surgery.

BIBLIOGRAPHY

1. Barker RL, Burton JR, Zieve PD (eds): Principles of Ambulatory Medicine. Baltimore, Williams & Wilkins, 1991.
2. Bartoshuk LM, Kveton JF, Karrer T: Taste. In Bailey BJ, et al (eds): Head and Neck Surgery— Otolaryngology, vol 1. Philadelphia, J.B. Lippincott, 1993, p 520.
3. Hirsh BE: Infections of the external ear. Am J Otolaryngol 13:(3):145–155, 1992.
4. Jahn AF: Chronic otitis media: Diagnosis and treatment. Med Clin North Am 75:1277–1291, 1991.
5. Kenna MA: Otitis media with effusion. In Bailey BJ, et al (eds): Head and Neck Surgery— Otolaryngology, vol 2. Philadelphia, J.B. Lippincott, 1993, p 1592.
6. Paparella MM: Otalgia. In Paparella MM, et al (eds): Otolaryngology, vol 2. Philadelphia, W.B. Saunders, 1980, p 1354.
7. Pelton SI, Klein JO: The draining ear. Otitis media and externa. Infect Dis Clin North Am 2:117–129, 1988.
8. Rubin J, Yu VL: Malignant external otitis: Insights into pathogenesis, clinical manifestations, diagnosis, and therapy. Am J Med 85:391–398, 1988.

27. SORE THROAT AND HOARSENESS

Andrew Steele, M.D., M.P.H.

1. What are the main causes of sore throat?

About 50% of cases of sore throat are caused by viruses. The most common viruses include adenovirus, influenzavirus, parainfluenza virus, coxsackievirus, rhinovirus, coronavirus, and respiratory syncytial virus.

About 20% of cases are caused by bacteria. Group A beta-hemolytic streptococcus (GABHS) is the most common cause, accounting for about 10–20% of pharyngitis in adults. Other bacterial causes for pharyngitis include non-group A streptococci, *Neisseria gonorrhoeae*, *Haemophilus influenzae*, *Corynebacterium diphtheriae*, *Mycoplasma pneumoniae*, and *Chlamydia trachomatis*. In about 30% of cases, no cause is found. The etiologies in such cases are believed to be a combination of environmental factors, allergies, and mouth-breathing. Common causes in the immunocompromised host include *Candida albicans* (thrush), herpes simplex virus, and cytomegalovirus (CMV).

2. What presenting clinical features help to distinguish viral from bacterial pharyngitis?

Etiologies of Pharyngitis

SYMPTOM	VIRAL	BACTERIAL
Cough	Common	Rare
Fever	Occasional	Common
Exudate	Occasional	Common
Tender anterior cervical nodes	Occasional	Common
Enlarged tonsils	Occasional	Common

3. Why should the primary care provider treat streptococcal pharyngitis?

1. Treatment shortens the course of illness with decreased fevers and decreased pain by 24–48 hours.
2. Treatment prevents suppurative complications.
3. Treatment prevents rheumatic fever.
4. Treatment decreases person-to-person spread of the disease.

4. What is the probability that a person with streptococcal pharyngitis will develop acute rheumatic fever?

The probability of developing acute rheumatic fever depends on whether the patient has epidemic or endemic pharyngitis. For epidemic GABHS, the probability of developing acute rheumatic fever is about 3%. In endemic areas the probability is about 0.3%.

5. Will treatment for GABHS pharyngitis protect against poststreptococcal glomerulonephritis?

Most studies have not shown a protective effect of treatment on the development of poststreptococcal glomerulonephritis.

6. How often do patients with acute rheumatic fever develop cardiac disease?

Assuming that patients with acute rheumatic fever receive appropriate prophylactic antibiotic therapy, about 1% subsequently develop severe cardiac disease (class IV rheumatic heart disease) and 4% develop debilitating rheumatic heart disease.

7. To what degree does antibiotic treatment lower the risk of developing acute rheumatic fever?
Treatment has been shown to decrease the risk of subsequent acute rheumatic fever by 90%. This effect may occur even if antibiotics are started later than 9 days after the onset of symptoms. To be fully effective, antibiotics should be given for 10 days.

8. What are the main local suppurative complications of GABHS?
The main complications are peritonsillar abscess and retropharyngeal abscess. Less common complications include suppurative otitis media and cervical lymphadenitis.

9. What is the recommended treatment for acute streptococcal pharyngitis?
The drug of choice is penicillin VK, 250 mg 4 times daily for 10 days. Benzathine penicillin G, given intramuscularly in a dose of 1.2 million units, is also effective. For penicillin-allergic patients, the first choice is erythromycin, 250 mg 4 times daily for 10 days. Azithromycin, clarithromycin, oral second- or third-generation cephalosporins also may be used, although they have not yet been proved in clinical trials to prevent acute rheumatic fever. The length of treatment is crucial; failure rate decreases when treatment is increased from 7 to 10 days.

10. What is the probability of an allergic reaction to penicillin therapy?
Overall, the probability of an allergic reaction is less than 1%. About one-half of allergic reactions are serious (moderate-to-severe anaphylaxis or serum sickness) and one-half are mild (urticaria and maculopapular eruptions). The probability of an allergic reaction depends in part on whether the drug is administered intramuscularly or orally. Serious allergies are more common with benzathine penicillin than with oral penicillin.

11. How should the care provider decide when empirical treatment for suspected GABHS is appropriate in a patient with sore throat?
   1. Determine the clinical probability that the patient has GABHS on the basis of the history and physical examination. The probability (%) of group A streptococcal pharyngitis based on prevalence and clinical findings is determined by the "strep score" which is derived by giving 1 point for each of the following: tonsillar exudate, anterior cervical lymphadenopathy, absence of cough, and presence of fever.

	PREVALENCE	
STREP SCORE	In Most Office Practices (%)	In Emergency Departments (%)
0	1	3
1	4	8
2	9	18
3	21	38
4	43	63

Adapted from Centor RM, Meier FA.[2]

   2. Use the predicted probability of GABHS in the following evaluation and treatment algorithm.

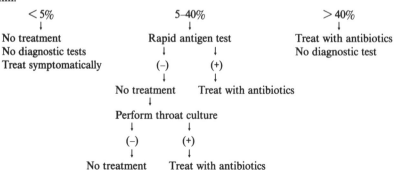

12. What are the most common causes of hoarseness?

Hoarseness is due to abnormal vibration of the vocal cords, which may result from local disorders or from paralysis of the laryngeal nerve. The most common cause of hoarseness is local inflammation of the vocal cords due to viral laryngitis or voice abuse. Other local causes result from laryngeal carcinoma, papillomas and polyps, trauma, or irritants. The common causes of laryngeal nerve paralysis in adults are carcinoma (20%); nerve injury from cardiomegaly, chest trauma, or other factors (23%); surgical damage (23%); and inflammatory lesions or lesions of the central nervous system such as stroke (14%).

13. What is the best medical treatment for hoarseness?

The patient with hoarseness should rest the voice and stop smoking (if this applies). Humidifiers at home and work may help. Underlying etiologic diseases should be treated when possible (e.g., antibiotics for bacterial infections and thyroid hormone replacement for myxedema).

14. When should a complaint of hoarseness undergo more aggressive evaluation?

Hoarseness that persists for 6–8 weeks, especially in a smoker, or that is accompanied by other symptoms suggestive of malignancy (mass, neck or chest pain, weight loss, shortness of breath, and aspiration) should be evaluated immediately.

15. What systemic medical diseases may be associated with hoarseness?

Hypothyroidism, rheumatoid arthritis (cricoarytenoid arthritis), and diabetes mellitus.

16. What is the initial evaluation of hoarseness?

After the history and physical examination, indirect laryngoscopy should be performed to evaluate voice quality, vocal cord mobility, and the presence or absence of masses.

BIBLIOGRAPHY

1. Centor RM, Meier FA, Dalton HP: Throat cultures and rapid tests for diagnosis of group A streptococcal pharyngitis. Ann Intern Med 105:892, 1986.
2. Centor RM, Meier FA: Sore throat. In Dornbrand L, Hoole A, Pickard C (eds): Manual of Clinical Problems in Adult Ambulatory Care. Boston, Little, Brown, 1992.
3. Hillner BE, Centor RM: What a difference a day makes: A decision analysis of adult streptococcal pharyngitis. J Gen Intern Med 2:242, 1987.
4. Komaroff AL, Pass TM, Aronson MD, et al: The prediction of streptococcal pharyngitis in adults. J Gen Intern Med 1:1, 1986.
5. Koster F: Respiratory tract infections. In Barker LR, Burton JR, Zieve PD (eds): Principles of Ambulatory Medicine. Baltimore, Williams & Wilkins, 1991, pp 303–320.
6. Maragos ND: Hoarseness. Prim Care 17:347, 1990.
7. Randolph MF, Gerber MA, DeMeo KK, Wright L: Effect of antibiotic therapy on the clinical course of streptococcal pharyngitis. J Pediatr 106:870, 1985.
8. Tompkins RK, Burnes DC, Cable BS: An analysis of the cost-effectiveness of pharyngitis management and acute rheumatic fever prevention. Ann Intern Med 86:481, 1977.

28. ORAL LESIONS

Thomas D. MacKenzie, M.D., and Michael L. Lepore, M.D., F.A.C.S.

1. What is the most common cause of xerostomia (dry mouth)?

Medications are the most common cause of oral dryness, especially in older persons. In fact, increased use of medications in the geriatric population may explain the widely believed myth that salivary gland dysfunction is part of the normal aging process. The mechanisms by which medications may cause xerostomia include salivary gland hypofunction, mucosal dehydration, total body dehydration, altered sensory function, and cognitive disorders. Medications that frequently decrease salivary flow rates by blocking cholinergic activity are tricyclic antidepressants; antipsychotics; centrally acting antihypertensives such as clonidine; diphenhydramine; and the belladonna alkaloids, such as atropine, scopolamine, and hyoscyamine.

2. What medical conditions are commonly associated with xerostomia?

The two most common medical conditions associated with xerostomia are Sjögren's syndrome and radiation-induced salivary gland dysfunction. In its primary form Sjögren's syndrome is characterized by lymphocytic infiltration of the salivary and lacrimal glands, thus leading to dry mouth and dry eyes. It also may occur in association with another major rheumatologic disease, such as rheumatoid arthritis, systemic lupus erythematosus, primary biliary cirrhosis, or scleroderma. The vast majority of patients with radiation-induced salivary gland dysfunction have received ionizing radiation for head and neck carcinoma. A number of other disorders may lead to dysfunction of one or more of the major salivary glands (parotid, submandibular, and sublingual). Patients are rarely symptomatic because salivary flow must decrease by approximately 50% before xerostomia develops.

3. Why should salivary gland hypofunction raise concern?

Saliva contains various polypeptides and glycoproteins that have antimicrobial activity. In the absence of these elements, the patient is prone to recurrent oral candidiasis and dental decay.

4. What is the most common cause of recurrent painful mouth sores?

Aphthous ulcers are the most common type of nontraumatic mouth sores. In the general population, the incidence is 10–20%. Among professionals and upper socioeconomic groups the incidence is higher.

5. What causes aphthous ulcers?

The cause of aphthous ulcers is still unknown, but possibilities include (1) viral agents (herpes simplex virus), (2) bacteria (*Streptococcus sanguis*), (3) nutritional deficiencies (B_{12}, folate, iron), (4) hormonal alterations, (5) stress, (6) trauma, (7) food allergies (nuts, chocolate, gluten) and (8) immunologic abnormalities.

6. Describe the various types of aphthous ulcers.

Three types of aphthous ulceration are recognized: minor, major, and herpetiform. In the minor variety, the patient usually notices a tingling or burning sensation before the ulcer appears. The ulcerations usually measure less than 1.0 cm and are localized to the freely movable keratinized gingiva. They are white in the center surrounded by a red border. They are extremely painful and usually resolve in approximately 7–10 days.

The major variety may occur on the movable mucosa, soft palate, tongue, and tonsillar pillars. They are much more painful than the minor ulcers and also much larger, measuring 1–3 cm. From 1–10 ulcers may be present.

Herpetiform ulcers are similar to herpetic lesions. Usually 10–100 ulcers are present, measuring 1–3 mm in diameter. The small ulcers may coalesce, forming larger ulcers. The minor and major types generally do not leave a scar, whereas the herpetiform variety may leave a scar if the ulcerations coalesce.

7. What is the current treatment for aphthous stomatitis?

Treatment includes both medical management and cauterization, if necessary. The ulcer bed may be cauterized either chemically or electrically. Silver nitrate is commonly used for chemical cauterization. After the application of silver nitrate the area should be swabbed with a cotton-tip applicator impregnated with sodium chloride, which converts the silver nitrate to silver chloride, thereby preventing a deep burn. Medical treatment includes oral antibiotics, anti-inflammatory agents, or immunosuppressants. Local measures include the use of an oral suspension of tetracycline or topical steroids such as 0.5% fluocinonide ointment or a betamethasone solution.

8. What is the significance of the presence of creamy white, curdlike lesions on the tongue and buccal mucosa?

Creamy white, curdlike lesions are likely due to oral candidiasis (thrush). These are considered the same entity and therefore should be represented as such. *Candida* species are present in normal oral flora in 40–60% of the population. In certain immunocompromised states, overgrowth of candida may lead to thrush. The lesions represent patches of *Candida albicans* with leukocytes and desquamated epithelial cells. Common conditions that lead to thrush include inhaled corticosteroid use for reactive airways disease; debilitating systemic illnesses, such as cancer; and other immunocompromised states, such as acquired immunodeficiency syndrome (AIDS) and neutropenia. Less common etiologies include diabetes, pregnancy, adrenal insufficiency, systemic antibiotic or steroid use, nutritional deficiencies, and poor oral hygiene. The differential diagnosis includes leukoplakia and hyperkeratosis. Patients who have thrush for no obvious reason should be evaluated for infection with the human immunodeficiency virus (HIV).

9. How is thrush diagnosed?

The diagnosis can be made easily by scraping the lesions, which are easy to remove and have an erythematous base, and examining the scrapings in potassium hydroxide under the microscope. Characteristic hyphae and blastospores are easily recognized.

10. What is desquamative gingivitis?

Desquamative gingivitis, which affects women over the age of 30 years, is characterized by diffuse erythematous desquamation, ulceration, and at times bullae formation involving the free and attached gingiva. Associated conditions include lichen planus, cicatricial pemphigoid, bullous pemphigoid, pemphigus vulgaris, dermatitis herpetiformis, and drug reactions. Incisional biopsy is frequently necessary for diagnosis. Immunofluorescent studies may aid in differentiating the various entities.

11. How can one differentiate between the various white lesions of the oral cavity?

Lesions of the oral cavity may present acutely as red lesions, but during the course of the disease white elements appear and may predominate. White lesions of the mouth are often benign; however, 5–10% of oral malignancies present as white lesions. Thus the examining physician must always be concerned that the lesion in question is a possible malignancy. White lesions of the mouth may be separated into two broad clinical categories: keratotic and nonkeratotic. The most important clinical feature distinguishing the two groups is the ability of the lesion to adhere to the surface epithelium. Leukoplakia, carcinoma, and primary skin diseases are usually keratotic. Infectious and bullous skin diseases usually present as nonkeratotic lesions.

Keratotic and Nonkeratotic Factors

KERATOTIC	NONKERATOTIC
Firmly adherent	Removed relatively easily
Usually of long duration	Usually of short duration
Usually change slowly	Frequently change rapidly
Surface is usually elevated and may be smooth, roughened, or even verrucous	Usually erosive or ulcerative

12. What are characteristically premalignant lesions?

Leukoplakia refers to a white patch or plaque of the mouth that cannot be removed by rubbing and cannot be ascribed to other apparent skin diseases, such as lichen planus. The incidence of malignancy may be as high as 30% in patients with leukoplakia; thus a biopsy is necessary. Asymptomatic, velvety red lesions of the mouth may be even more suspect for carcinoma in situ and should be biopsied.

13. What is "geographic" tongue?

Loss and regrowth of papillae lead to red patches on the tongue. This "geographic" appearance is asymptomatic and results from an idiopathic inflammatory condition.

14. What are the most common locations of squamous cell carcinoma of the mouth?

The most common locations are the lower lip, floor of the mouth, and tongue. Painless ulcers not healing in 1–2 weeks are highly suspect and should be biopsied.

15. What is the major differential diagnosis of an oral pigmented lesion?

The most worrisome diagnosis is malignant melanoma, but other possibilities include nevi and benign macules, lesions of Peutz-Jeghers disease, or Addison's disease. Any new suspicious lesion should be followed and biopsied early.

16. Who develops hairy leukoplakia?

White painless lesions that appear "hairy" are often found in patients with AIDS, usually on the lateral aspects of the tongue. They are caused by the Epstein-Barr virus and may temporarily respond to high-dose acyclovir.

17. What is the difference between loss of taste (ageusia) and loss of flavor?

Smell and taste are separate senses. The combination of both produces the sensation of flavor, which is distinct from either sense alone. If the olfactory neurons are damaged (by head trauma or viral invasion) or if the nasal passages are blocked (by polyps or edema), the only sensation is produced by the taste buds. This loss of flavor is perceived by the patient as a loss of taste.

18. How can taste and olfactory problems be differentiated?

If the patient can differentiate table salt, sugar, the sour taste of lemon juice, or the bitter taste of dark chocolate or coffee, the taste system is intact. Patients who lack the ability to smell state that they can taste the above but nothing else. Hence the problem is olfactory.

19. A 42-year-old woman presents with the chief complaint that sweet beverages taste bitter. Does this dysgeusia (abnormal taste) represent a true pathologic condition?

The effect of taste pleasure and displeasure is present at birth. Sugar produces a pleasurable response, whereas quinine produces a displeasurable response. Some patients may suffer from a chronic bitter taste in the mouth (bitter dysgeusia). To determine the possible origin of the dysgeusia, the mouth may be anesthetized with a topical anesthetic for 60 seconds. If a strong taste solution is given, the patient should not be able to taste. If the dysgeusia is not abolished, it does not originate in the mouth. Most patients usually complain that a sweet beverage, such as cola, tastes bitter. If topographic testing reveals that the patient has lost the ability to taste sweet, the residual taste of the cola is genuinely bitter. Various substances can alter taste because they affect the taste membrane:

1. **The orange juice effect**: Sodium laurel sulfate, the detergent in toothpaste and mouthwash, decreases the intensity of sweet tastes (orange juice) and adds bitter taste to acids.

2. **The artichoke effect**: If the tongue is exposed to artichoke, which contains chlorogenic acid, beverages such as milk, water, or wine taste as if they have been sweetened.

3. **Acetazolamide**, which is used to treat glaucoma, also may make substances taste bitter.

20. A 69-year-old man who drinks and smokes heavily presents with the chief complaints of difficulty in tasting food and numbness on the anterior two-thirds of the tongue. What are the possible causes and sites of lesions?

Taste sensation in the anterior two-thirds of the tongue is supplied by a branch of the facial nerve called the chorda tympani nerve. This nerve travels along the posterior wall of the middle ear to the infratemporal fossa and the submandibular gland region, where it joins the lingual nerve to innervate the ipsilateral anterior two-thirds of the tongue. Pathology involving these regions must be carefully ruled out. Possible pathologic processes include neoplastic lesions in the floor of the mouth, submandibular gland region, or infratemporal fossa; acute and chronic otitis media; Bell's palsy; and Lyme disease.

21. How should severe toothaches be managed by the primary care provider?

Toothaches are most commonly a manifestation of inflammation of the pulp (pulpitis). They generally occur in the presence of large dental caries or large restorations (fillings). Management depends greatly on the clinical presentation:

1. In the absence of fever and intraoral or extraoral swelling, patients can be managed with analgesics (acetaminophen with or without codeine) and a dental referral within 24 hours.

2. In patients with intraoral or extraoral swelling or with a low-grade fever, antibiotics (penicillin or erythromycin for penicillin-allergic patients) also should be given.

3. For patients with a fever above 101°F or with edema that causes facial asymmetry, an urgent dental referral is mandatory. Complications may include full-blown facial cellulitis or destruction of the alveolar bone that supports the teeth.

BIBLIOGRAPHY

1. Aragon SB, Jafek BW: Stomatitis. In Head and Neck Surgery—Otolaryngology, vol 1. Philadelphia, J.B. Lippincott, 1993, p 531.
2. Atkinson JC, Fox PC: Salivary gland dysfunction. Clin Geriatr Med 499–508, 1992.
3. Barker RL, Burton JR, Zieve PD (eds): Principles of Ambulatory Medicine. Baltimore, Williams & Wilkins, 1991.
4. Epstein JB: The painful mouth: Mucositis, gingivitis, stomatitis. Inf Dis Clin North Am 2:183–200, 1988.
5. Krull EA, Fellman AC, Fabian LA: White lesions of the mouth. Ciba Clin Symp 25(2):1–32, 1973.
6. Lucente FE: Otolaryngologic aspects of acquired immunodeficiency syndrome. Med Clin North Am 75:1389–1398, 1991.
7. Mandell GL, Douglas RG, Bennett JE (eds): Principles and Practice of Infectious Disease. New York, Churchill Livingstone, 1990.

V. Endocrine and Metabolic Disorders

29. DIABETES MELLITUS

Christina Bryan, M.D., and Fred D. Hofeldt, M.D.

1. What end-organ damage is associated with diabetes mellitus?

Diabetes mellitus, a frequently occurring chronic disease, is associated with blindness, renal failure, myocardial infarction, amputation, stroke, and coma. Quality of life is diminished by impotence, bowel and bladder dysmotility, peripheral neuropathy, and neuropathic arthritis.

2. When is a person considered to be diabetic?

According to national guidelines, the diagnosis of diabetes in nonpregnant adults is made in any of the following scenarios: (1) plasma glucose > 200 mg/dl in patients with classic symptoms of polyuria, ploydipsia, polyphaghia, and weight loss; (2) fasting plasma glucose > 140 mg/dl on two occasions; and (3) two 75-gm oral glucose tolerance tests with fasting plasma glucose < 140 mg/dl, 2-hour plasma glucose ≥ 200 mg/dl, and one intervening value ≥ 200 mg/dl.

3. Describe and characterize the three types of diabetes mellitus.

In **type I diabetes,** endogenous insulin secretion is diminished. Type I diabetes has an autoimmune etiology and is associated with human leukocyte antigen (HLA) markers. Islet cell antibodies are present. Typically, type I diabetes has its onset during childhood, presenting with ketoacidosis. Patients always require exogenous insulin, (insulin-dependent diabetes mellitus [IDDM]). They are usually lean and make up 10% of the diabetic population.

In **type II diabetes** endogenous insulin is produced but cells are resistant to insulin action. Alterations in the insulin receptor or postreceptor function prevent normal cellular uptake of glucose. Persons with type II diabetes may not be prone to ketosis without insulin. Type II diabetes usually presents after age 30 years in genetically predisposed families. Often patients can be treated with diet alone or diet plus oral hypoglycemics, but exogenous insulin may be required to control hyperglycemia and associated microvascular complications. Type II disease is termed non–insulin-dependent diabetes (NIDDM). Such patients comprise 90% of diabetics and usually are obese.

A **third type of diabetes** is secondary to pancreatic compromise, drugs, or disease. Resection of the pancreas and recurrent bouts of pancreatitis in alcoholics are frequent causes of secondary diabetes. Drugs that induce diabetes include thiazides, hydantoins, and steroids.

4. Which syndromes include diabetes as part of their clinical presentation?

Hemochromatosis	Acromegaly	Glucagonoma
Cushing's disease or syndrome	Pheochromocytoma	Somatostatinoma

All of the above conditions are secondary causes of diabetes mellitus.

5. Who should be screened for diabetes?

Approximately 6% of the American population is diabetic. In addition, about 6 million adults with diabetes are undiagnosed. Although screening of the general population is not indicated, screening is of value in high-risk individuals with the following characteristics:

1. Obesity (> 20% over ideal body weight)
2. Family history of diabetes
3. American Indian, African-American, or Hispanic ancestry
4. Age > 40 years plus one other high-risk condition
5. Previously identified impaired glucose tolerance
6. Hypertension and hyperlipidemia, cholesterol $\geq$ 240 mg/dl, or triglycerides $\geq$ 250 mg/dl
7. History of gestational diabetes or delivery of infant weighing over 9 lbs
8. Classic symptoms—polyuria, polydipsia, fatigue, weight loss
9. Recurrent skin, genital, or urinary tract infections

6. Describe the process of screening for diabetes.

In screening nonpregnant adults with a high-risk profile, plasma glucose is measured after a 3-hour fast. Normal values are up to 115 mg/dl. If the patient has eaten within the past 3 hours, a value $\geq$ 160 mg/dl is abnormal. After a patient has a positive result, diagnosis must be made by further testing.

All pregnant women should be screened between 24–28 weeks' gestation with 50 gm of oral glucose at any time of day, followed by venous glucose sampling 1 hour later. If the plasma value is $\geq$ 140 mg/dl or $\geq$ 7.8 mM/dl, the 100-gm oral glucose tolerance test is performed. Diagnosis is based on two or more readings equal to or greater than the following values:

Fasting	105 mg/dl	(5.8 mM/dl)
1 hr	190 mg/dl	(10.6 mM/dl)
2 hr	165 mg/dl	(9.2 mM/dl)
3 hr	145 mg/dl	(8.1 mM/dl)

7. How should a patient newly diagnosed with diabetes be evaluated?

1. **History.** The initial history should include the date of onset of diabetes and presenting symptoms. It is also important to learn whether the patient has had ketoacidosis, hypoglycemia, or infections and with what frequency. The patient's attitude toward the disease should be evaluated. The history also should determine whether other endocrine, renal, or cardiovascular problems coexist and what medications are taken. In addition, the patient should be questioned about smoking, impotence, family planning, and a family history of diabetes.

2. **Laboratory evaluation.** Baseline laboratory studies should include a fasting glucose, fasting lipid profile, glycosylated hemoglobin, urinalysis, creatinine, electrolytes, thyroid-stimulating hormone (TSH), and electrocardiogram (EKG) in patients over 40 years of age. For patients over 30 years old at onset of diabetes, microalbumin should be measured annually. Physical examination must include height, weight, blood pressure, vision measurement, and examination of eye grounds. Baseline neurologic and cardiovascular examinations should be obtained. The foot examination should include peripheral pulses, sensation, and search for skin lesions and deformities.

3. **Follow-up.** Frequency of follow-up depends on the degree of hyperglycemia and related secondary problems, especially hyperlipidemia and hypertension. Hyperglycemic diabetic patients are seen at 1–2 week intervals until control is achieved.

4. **Education.** All patients must receive formal education about diabetes. The patient's education must include glucose monitoring, diet, exercise, foot care, sick-day rules, hypoglycemic reaction, use of insulin, and need for annual examination.

8. What are the goals of diabetic therapy, as suggested by the Diabetes Control and Complications Trials (DCCT)? Why?

In view of the DCCT results, improved glucose control must be the goal in all diabetic persons, with the expectation that long-term outcome will be measurably improved. In patients with type I diabetes, the method of intensive insulin therapy implies at least 3 injections of insulin daily and 4 measurements of glucose/day. In these patients with type I diabetes, intensive insulin therapy improves hemoglobin A_1C and reduces the first appearance of retinopathy by

27%; severe nonproliferative and proliferative retinopathy requiring laser treatment by 45%; and expected progression of clinically meaningful retinopathy by 34–46%. Intensive insulin therapy reduces the development of microalbuminuria by 35%, clinical grade albuminuria by 56%, and clinical neuropathy by 60%.

9. What are the risks of intensive insulin therapy?
Drawbacks of intensive insulin therapy include a 3-fold increase in severe hypoglycemia and weight gain. However, major macrovascular events, worsened neurobehavioral status, or diminished quality of life were not found.

10. Which patients may be at greater risk for an adverse outcome during intensive therapy?
The risk-benefit ratio for use of intensive insulin therapy may be less favorable in the following groups: children under 13 years of age, patients with known coronary artery or cerebrovascular disease, patients with far-advanced complications, such as renal failure, and patients with recurrent severe hypoglycemia or hypoglycemic unawareness.

11. Which patients have the greatest risk of severe hypoglycemia?
Elderly patients on longer-acting oral hypoglycemics may experience episodes of hypoglycemia, especially in the setting of renal insufficiency or acute illness. The diabetic patient with loss of glucose counterregulatory hormone response or autonomic neuropathy and patients on intensive insulin therapy also are at increased risk of hypoglycemia. Patients with hypoglycemic unawareness do not have warning symptoms or reflex hormonal mechanisms to stimulate glucose production to reverse the hypoglycemia.

12. What advice should be given to patients about hypoglycemia?
At all times, diabetic persons must carry glucose snacks to treat hypoglycemic symptoms. Identification cards help to direct treatment if the individual is found unconscious.

13. Describe the process of screening for and monitoring diabetic retinopathy.
Diabetes is the leading cause of adult blindness. Screening examinations for diabetic retinopathy should begin in patients with type I diabetes after 5 years of disease or after puberty. In patients with type II diabetes, retinal screening should begin at the time of diagnosis. Examinations should be repeated annually by an ophthalmologist. The 7-field stereophotography of the retina is one method, but annual dilated retinal examination by an ophthalmologist is most often done. The use of panretinal photocoagulation in proliferative retinopathy or severe nonproliferative retinopathy has been shown to save vision, as has focal argon laser therapy in patients with macular edema.

14. What are the basic principles for screening and follow-up of diabetic nephropathy?
Screening for diabetic nephropathy includes taking a family history for hypertension, measuring blood pressure, and checking urinalysis and serum creatinine. If these screens are normal, only an annual urinalysis is required. After 5 years of disease, a 24-hour urine specimen can be collected to assess microalbumin in patients who remain urine protein negative.

15. Characterize the three types of diabetic neuropathy.
Focal neuropathies involve sensory or motor loss of a particular nerve; for example, wrist or foot drop or diplopia due to cranial nerve palsy.

Distal symmetric polyneuropathy is most commonly manifest as stocking/glove paresthesias.

Autonomic neuropathy manifests as distal anhydrosis with compensatory increased sweating on face and trunk; gastrointestinal dysmotility; bladder overfilling with incomplete emptying; impotence; impaired glucose counterregulation; hypoglycemic unawareness; orthostatic hypotension; and loss of cardiac rate deceleration.

16. What are the macrovascular complications of diabetes? What can be done about them?
Diabetic persons are at increased risk for myocardial infarction, stroke, peripheral vascular disease, and amputation. They should be screened for arteriosclerotic disease at presentation with a vascular and cardiac history, physical examination for pulses and blood flow, a fasting lipid profile, and an EKG if $\geq$ 40 years of age. Proteinuria should be assessed, because it may indicate increased cardiovascular risk. Aggressive control of weight, physical activity, and treatment of hypertension and dyslipidemia are mandatory. Above all, smoking cessation reduces the morbidity of macrovascular complications. To prevent amputation, the high-risk foot should be identified. All feet must be examined annually, but the high-risk foot demands careful examination at each visit. Any of the following characteristics result in a high-risk foot: abnormal gait, neuropathy, peripheral vascular disease, structural deformity, history of foot ulcers, abnormal skin or nails, and history of skin infections.

17. How can the level of glycemic control be determined?
The level of glycemic control is best measured by using the hemoglobin A_1C or the fructosamine assay. The fructosamime assay, which reflects glucose control during the previous 3–6 weeks, is useful in monitoring glycemic control in pregnant women and patients on intensive insulin therapy. The patient's education must include glucose monitoring, diet, exercise, foot care, sick-day rules, hypoglycemic reaction, use of insulin, and need for annual examination.

18. What is included in the annual evaluation of a patient with diabetes?
Secondary morbidity from renal, ocular, neurologic, and cardiovascular sources should be monitored annually. British authorities suggest the following as a comprehensive list for annual review:

1. Weight
2. Hemoglobin A_1C
3. Blood pressure
4. Smoking
5. Visual acuity and optic fundi
6. Feet
7. Lipid assessment
8. Proteinuria
9. Creatinine
10. Peripheral neuropathy, vibratory sense, light touch, pain
11. Impotence
12. Family planning advice about glycemic control during conception
13. Annual review of educational concepts

Patients need ready access to their health care team (e.g., physician, nurse, diabetes educator, dietician, podiatrist).

19. What are current recommendations for a diabetic diet?
In general, the diet should contain 25–30 kcal/kg of nonobese body weight or the number of calories needed to achieve normal body weight. Thirty percent or less of the calories should be in the form of fat with 8–10% saturated fat, as stated in the guidelines of the National Cholesterol Education Program (NCEP). The proportion of fat and carbohydrate calories depends on dietary goals. Fat calories are restricted for weight loss and hypercholesterolemia, while a moderate carbohydrate intake is required for treatment of associated hypertriglyceridemia. Simple carbohydrates can be substituted for more complex carbohydrates. Cholesterol should be < 200 mg/day. Meals and snacks should be eaten at the same time each day and contain the same proportion of total daily calories. Patients need education from a professional to implement this diet in practical and inexpensive terms.

20. What are the beneficial effects of exercise? What advice should be given to patients?
Exercise has beneficial effects on insulin receptor function and glycemic control. It increases cardiovascular fitness, decreases risk for macrovascular complications, helps to maintain ideal body weight, and complements dietary compliance. Patients with well-controlled diabetes should avoid hypoglycemia by snacking before exercise. Runners should be advised to use the abdomen rather than the legs as the injection site, because the leg muscle group does the largest amount of exercise, which increases the absorption and bioavailability of insulin.

Patients with poorly controlled diabetes and plasma glucose values in the range of 300–400 mg/dl should not exercise. Because of insufficient bioavailable insulin, exercise may worsen their condition by increasing hyperglycemia and promoting ketosis. Exercise can be undertaken after glycemic control is improved.

21. What is the initial therapy for patients with type II diabetes?

Diet is the cornerstone of treatment for diabetes mellitus. Mild type II diabetes is often controlled with diet alone. Weight loss of as little as 10 pounds improves metabolic control in type II diabetes; therefore, normal weight must always be stressed as a therapeutic goal.

If type II diabetes is not controlled by diet, the second line of treatment includes oral agents that stimulate beta cells to produce insulin in a more timely response to eating and increase the number and efficiency of insulin receptors, thereby improving peripheral insulin resistance. With the use of oral agents, hepatic glucose production is decreased and fasting hyperglycemia improves.

22. Compare the oral hypoglycemic agents currently available.

It is important to note the individual characteristics of hypoglycemic agents before prescribing them. They differ in site of metabolism, half-life, activity of hepatic metabolites, and side effects. Chlorpropamide may cause the syndrome of inappropriate secretion of antidiuretic hormone (SIADH or hyponatremia) and has antiabuse-like effects. Of the second-generation agents, glyburide is best at suppression of hepatic glucose production. Glipizide is most efficient at increasing postprandial insulin levels and enhancing peripheral glucose uptake.

Comparison of Oral Hypoglycemic Agents

FIRST GENERATION	HALF-LIFE	HEPATIC METABOLISM
Chlorpropamide	36 hr	No
Tolbutamide	4 hr	Yes
Tolazamide	7 hr	Yes—active metabolites
Glyburide	10 hr	Yes—weak metabolites
Glipizide	4 hr	Yes

23. Which agents are safest in elderly patients?

Tolbutamide and glipizide. They have inactive metabolites (see table in question 22).

24. How is insulin therapy initiated in patients with type II diabetes?

Patients with type II diabetes who need exogenous insulin may begin with a morning injection that combines neutral protamine hagedorn (NPH) and regular insulin. A second injection can be added before supper, if needed. It is best to adjust the dose with patients at their usual level of physical activity while consistently following their diet and doing home glucose monitoring (HGM). Intervals of 2–4 days between dosage changes are best. Rarely the addition of a small dose of second-generation oral agent may improve insulin sensitivity. Such a program may consist of an oral agent at breakfast with administration of insulin before supper. Establishing normoglycemia may temporarily improve insulin secretion and insulin action so that the need for exogenous insulin is reduced and the patient's condition improves.

25. How should patients with type I diabetes be treated?

Insulin is needed in all patients with type I diabetes. The total insulin dose is lower than in patients with type II diabetes, who are more insulin-resistant.

Two insulin regimens are recommended in IDDM: (1) two injections (in the morning and before supper) of combined NPH/regular insulin (starting ratio = 70/30) with a third injection of regular insulin before lunch; (2) Ultralente insulin in the morning or evening with Semilente insulin before breakfast, lunch, and dinner. An arbitrary starting dose of a total of 24 U/day can be divided into separate doses, with two-thirds given before breakfast and one-third before supper. Some physicians start insulin at 0.5 U/kg as a total daily insulin dose. Adjustments are best done every 2–4 days on an outpatient basis in patients who have a consistent diet and exercise pattern. Decisions about dosage changes initially can be managed by the doctor or nurse specialist, but once the patient is educated and confident, the patient can make the decisions.

26. What is the approach to diabetic dyslipidemia?
　　1. Patients with diabetic dyslipidemia should avoid drugs that aggravate the dyslipidemia, such as beta blockers and thiazides, and choose lipid-neutral antihypertensive agents. Typically diabetics have a combined hyperlipidemia with elevated levels of total cholesterol, low-density lipoprotein, and triglycerides and low levels of high-density lipoprotein.
　　2. Glucose must be controlled aggressively through optimal diet, exercise, oral agents, or insulin.
　　3. A low cholesterol diet, combined with increased physical activity, should be tried aggressively for 6 months before the addition of lipid-lowering drugs.
　　4. Because diabetes and hypothyroidism often coexist, TSH should be checked in the dyslipidemic diabetic in good glycemic control.
　　5. Lipid values not meeting NCEP guidelines will require appropriate lipid-lowering therapy.

BIBLIOGRAPHY

1. Baker JR, Metcalf PA, Holdaway M, Johnson RN: Serum fructosomine concentrations as a measure of blood glucose control in type I (insulin dependent) diabetes mellitus. BMJ 290:352–355, 1985.
2. Diabetes Control and Complications Trial: Update and Implications. Indianapolis, IN, Boehringer-Mannheim.
3. Diabetes mellitus. In Wilson JD, Foster DW (eds): Williams' Textbook of Endocrinology. Philadelphia, W.B. Saunders, 1992, pp 1255–1333.
4. Hofeldt F: The office management of diabetes mellitus. Mod Med 58:36–58, 1990.
5. Howard L: Diabetes management guidelines. Bristol, UK [unpublished].
6. Screening for diabetes. Diabetes Care 16(2):8, 1993.
7. Summary of the NCEP Adult Treatment Panel II Report. JAMA 269, 1993.

30. ABNORMALITIES OF LIPIDS

Raymond Estacio, M.D., and Robert H. Eckel, M.D.

1. Name the two major classes of lipoproteins.
Lipoproteins are carrier vehicles for the solubilization and subsequent transport of lipids in plasma. All lipoproteins consist of cholesterol (ester and unesterified), triglyceride (TG), phospholipid, and apoprotein (the protein component). The two major classes of lipoproteins are distinguished by a change in the relative proportion of these components as the lipoprotein becomes progressively smaller and more dense:
　　1. TG-rich lipoproteins: chylomicrons and very-low-density lipoproteins (VLDL)
　　2. Cholesterol-rich lipoproteins: low- and high-density lipoproteins (LDL and HDL, respectively). Intermediate-density lipoproteins are present in very small quantities in fasting plasma; however, they may be related to the pathogenesis of atherosclerosis.

2. Which lipoprotein is most important in the pathogenesis of atherosclerosis?

LDL. Current evidence suggests that when LDL moves into the subintimal space, it becomes oxidized and thus is no longer recognized by the normal LDL receptor. As part of this process, circulating monocytes and T lymphocytes are attracted, and the oxidized LDL is taken up by tissue macrophages to form foam cells. Subsequently, arterial wall injury induced by smoking, hypertension, and hypercholesterolemia leads to platelet aggregation and release of mitogens, such as platelet-derived growth factor. Ultimately, smooth muscle cell proliferation and fibrosis occur.

3. What is the importance of HDL in atherosclerosis?

There appears to be an inverse relationship between the levels of HDL cholesterol and atherosclerosis. Although HDL may be important in the early reversibility of LDL-induced damage, the mechanism explaining the inverse relationship between levels of HDL cholesterol and atherosclerosis remains unclear. One theory is that HDL mediates the process of reverse cholesterol transport. Although this theory is not entirely consistent with known biochemical data, it suggests that when HDL binds to cell surfaces, it is not internalized and degraded like LDL. In addition, HDL may promote cellular efflux of cholesterol and diminish the extra-hepatic tissue burden of excessive cholesterol.

4. What is the definition of significant hyperlipidemia?

As defined by the National Cholesterol Education Program Adult Treatment Panel II Recommendations for Consideration of the Diagnosis of Hyperlipidemia, the following levels, when consistently determined after a 12-hour fast, should be considered for treatment:

Total cholesterol > 200 mg/dl
LDL cholesterol > 130 mg/dl
TG > 250 mg/dl

5. Who should be screened for hyperlipidemia?

All adults over 20 years of age and children of dyslipidemic parents should be evaluated at least every 5 years. Screening may occur without fasting and should include a total cholesterol and HDL cholesterol.

6. What are the caveats of screening for nonfasting cholesterol?

1. False-positive result: the increased level of cholesterol may be secondary to increases in VLDL or HDL rather than LDL.

2. False-negative result: individuals with reduced levels of HDL may be missed by this procedure. Thus, adequate evaluation and work-up before therapy requires several determinations of cholesterol, triglycerides, and HDL cholesterol after a 12-hour fast.

7. How does the provider determine the level of LDL cholesterol?

Currently, tests for cholesterol, triglycerides, and HDL cholesterol are readily available in standard laboratories. When triglyceride levels are less than 400 mg/dl, VLDL cholesterol is well approximated by the total triglycerides divided by 5. When the triglycerides are higher than 400 mg/dl, VLDL becomes TG-enriched and the denominator becomes larger. Thus, when triglycerides are less than 400 mg/dl, one may easily calculate LDL from these measurements as follows:

Cholesterol = (LDL + HDL + VLDL) cholesterol
LDL cholesterol = cholesterol – (HDL cholesterol + TG/5)
LDL cholesterol may be measured, but the available laboratory test
is timely and costly.

8. How can the physical manifestations of the dyslipidemias be more easily remembered?

Relating the physical manifestations of dyslipidemia to the lipoproteins important in normal metabolism may help to recall physical abnormalities more easily.

Physical Manifestations of Dyslipidemias

METABOLISM	ABNORMALITY OF METABOLISM	ELEVATED LEVELS	PHYSICAL MANIFESTATION
TG-rich particles (chylomicrons from dietary fat and VLDL synthesized from liver) from the plasma are presented to peripheral tissues for utilization. Lipoprotein lipase at the capillary endothelium removes some TG and other surface components.	Increased chylomicrons (+VLDL)	Severe hypertri-glyceridemia Mild hypercho-lesterolemia	Eruptive xanthomas Lipemia retinalis Pancreatitis Hepatosplenomegaly (LPL deficiency)
After TG removal, remnants of chylomicrons and VLDL are taken up by the liver. Chylomicron remnants are completely metabolized by the liver, whereas some VLDL remnants give rise to LDL.	Increased remnants	Both hypertri-glyceridemia and hypercho-lesterolemia (usually TG > cholesterol)	Plantar xanthomas Tuberous xanthomas Atherosclerosis
LDL are formed only from the metabolism of VLDL (mostly small remnants.)	Increased LDL	Hypercho-lesterolemia	Tendinous xanthomas Xanthelasma Arcus cornealis Atherosclerosis
HDLs are secreted by the liver and intestine Cholesterol ester transfer protein (CETP), which facilitates this movement of cholesterol from HDL to other lipoproteins, also controls HDL composition and metabolism.	Decreased HDL	Hyperrcho-lesterolemia	Atherosclerosis (decreased HDL)

9. What conditions cause hypertriglyceridemia?

Hypertriglyceridemia may result from an increase in VLDL production, or a decrease in triglyceride (TGL) metabolism. Severe hypertriglycidemia may occur when two disorders are simultaneously present and fat remains in the diet.

Increased VLDL production
   Acquired
      Insulin resistance
      Alcohol
   Inherited
      Autosomal dominant familial
        disorders

Decreased VLDL (and chylomicron) metabolism
   Acquired
      Insulin deficiency
   Inherited
      LPL deficiency
      Deficiency of apo-CII activator

10. Why might an alternate approach to the historical classification (Types I–V) of the five types of dyslipidemias be desirable?

- The historical classification is too difficult to retain in memory.
- The historical classification does not reflect the pathophysiologic mechanisms responsible for the lipid elevations.
- The historical classification does not allow easily for combinations of more than one pathophysiologic defect.
- The historical classification of patterns may change in each individual patient, depending on complicating secondary diseases, medications, and diet.

11. Which single disease causes abnormal lipid remnant catabolism?

Abnormal lipid remnant catabolism is caused by familial dysbetalipoproteinemia (broad beta disease), which results in part from abnormalities in the apo E gene. Although this genetic predisposition occurs in 1% of the population, it becomes clinically expressed only when acquired forms of VLDL metabolism are also present. Lipoprotein electrophoresis is indicated to distinguish this disease from combined defects of VLDL and LDL.

12. Which diseases or medications cause a combined hyperlipidemia (increases in cholesterol and triglycerides)?

Disease	**Medications**
Hypothyroidism	Diuretics
Nephrotic syndrome	Glucocorticoids
Diabetes mellitus	
Liver disease (parenchymal or obstructive)	

13. What is the beneficial effect of estrogen on lipid profiles?
Although oral estrogens increase triglycerides, they have a beneficial effect by decreasing LDL and augmenting HDL.

14. Name the two autosomal dominant inherited defects in cholesterol metabolism that lead to premature cardiac death.
1. Increased cholesterol (LDL) production: **familial combined hyperlipidemia**. This disorder of VLDL production results in a threefold increase in the risk for coronary artery disease. Despite the abnormality in VLDL, the disease often presents as isolated LDL elevation.
2. Decreased LDL catabolism: **familial hypercholesterolemia**. This disorder occurs from complete or partial absence of or defects in the LDL receptor. An increase in LDL production is also present. Patients have a twofold (heterozygotes) or fourfold (homozygote) increase in cholesterol levels; premature death from atherosclerosis is common (even before age 20 years in homozygotes).

15. When do defects in HDL occur?
Defects in HDL may occur because of alterations in the composition of HDL due to other dyslipidemias or because of a reduction in HDL particle number. Most defects are acquired; the factors that decrease HDL cholesterol are listed below:

Genetic	Male gender (rare: hypoalphalipoprotenemia, CETP deficiency)
Acquired	Diet—decreased fat (high carbohydrate), obesity
	Drugs—beta blockers, diuretics, progestins, androgens
	Others—hypertriglyceridemia, sedentary lifestyle, smoking

16. Provide three lines of clinical evidence that support the treatment of hyperlipidemia for the prevention, arrest, and reversibility of atherosclerosis.
1. The incidence of morbid and mortal coronary artery disease is decreased in men at high risk of atherosclerosis due to high LDL cholesterol levels when LDL cholesterol is lowered by lifestyle modification and/or cholesterol lowering medication. The benefit in outcome is directly related to the magnitude of LDL reduction (Lipid Research Clinics Coronary Prevention Trial, Helsinki Heart Study, Coronary Drug Project).
2. Coronary atherosclerosis ceases to progress and may reverse in patients with hypercholesterolemia who are treated for hyperlipidemia, even over a short duration (2.5 years). (Cholesterol Lowering Atherosclerosis Study, FATS Study).
3. The number of coronary events is diminished in men who demonstrate a decrease in LDL cholesterol and an increase in HDL cholesterol after 5 years of intervention for hypercholesterolemia (Helsinki Heart Study).

17. How should treatment goals be determined for the patient with hypercholesterolemia?
According to the Adult Treatment Panel II Recommendations of the National Cholesterol Education Program, treatment of hypercholesterolemia is based on targeted LDL cholesterol levels determined by the presence of additional risk factors for coronary artery disease.

Positive Risk Factors
   Age: Male > 45 years
        Female > 55 years or premature menopause without estrogen replacement
   Familial history of premature coronary artery disease (CAD) (defined as myocardial
        infarction or sudden death before age 55 years in the father or other first-degree male
        relatives or before 65 years in the mother or other first-degree female relatives)
   Current cigarette smoking
   Hypertension (blood pressure > 140/90 mmHg or prescription of antihypertensive
        medication)
   Low HDL cholesterol (< 35 mg/dl)
   Diabetes mellitus
Negative Risk Factors
   High HDL cholesterol (> 60 mg/dl)

Targeted LDL levels
   Without CAD and < 2 risk factors   < 160 mg/dl
   Without CAD and ≥ 2 risk factors   < 130 mg/dl
   With CAD   < 100 mg/dl

---

18. Should hypertriglyceridemia be aggressively treated?

The prevention of pancreatitis in patients at risk for severe hypertriglyceridemia is a clear indication for lipid-lowering therapy. However, the relationship between hypertriglyceridemia and atherosclerosis is much less clear. Because hypertriglyceridemia is often accompanied by increases in cholesterol and diseases with risk factors for atherosclerosis, the question is less easily answered. In patients with familial hypertriglyceridemia (and increased VLDL), no increased risk of atherosclerosis is found. In patients with familial combined hyperlipidemia or diabetes mellitus, hypertriglyceridemia is a risk factor for cardiovascular disease. Evidence of benefit from lowering of triglycerides, however, is lacking.

19. What sequential recommendations for the treatment of hyperlipidemia should be followed by the primary care provider?

The following sequential recommendations may prevent the patient from appearing prematurely **DEAD** in the emergency room:

   Discontinue or reduce dosage of all drugs that may contribute to hyperlipidemia and treat any specific etiologies (e.g., thyroid disorder)

   Exercise aerobically. Lipoproteins appear to be altered in proportion to the level of exercise; usually VLDL is decreased, HDL is increased, and LDL is not affected.

   Abstain from excessive calories and from bad calories in the form of dietary saturated fats.

Disorder	Restriction
Chylomicronemia	Fat < 20% of calories; alcohol
Hyperlipidemia, obesity	Calories, ± alcohol
Hypertriglyceridemia	± Alcohol
Hypercholesterolemia	Cholesterol, saturated fat (< 10% calories)

   Drugs may be used to treat specific lipid abnormalities; however, the anticipated outcome and the known side effects must be carefully monitored.

20. What is the expected response to dietary management of hyperlipidemia?

1. For severe hypertriglyceridemia, dietary fat restriction leads to remission within days.

2. With weight reduction maintained over several months, triglycerides decrease and HDL cholesterol rises; LDL cholesterol is unaffected.

3. Dietary restriction of cholesterol (300 mg) accompanied by restriction of saturated fat (< 10% of calories) produces a maximal decrement in LDL cholesterol of 25%. However, the decrement is usually much less (5–10%).

21. Does increasing fiber in the diet reduce cholesterol?

Soluble fiber has a dose-dependent effect on lowering total and LDL cholesterol. However, the reduction is usually insignificant when cholesterol ($<$ 300 mg) and saturated fat ($<$ 10% calories) are already restricted.

22. Why has gemfibrozil replaced clofibrate as the drug of choice to lower triglycerides?

Although both gemfibrozil and clofibrate lower triglycerides and increase HDL cholesterol, gemfibrozil has become the drug of choice because it has not proved to produce the major side effect of clofibrate: cholelithiasis. Whether both drugs cause an increase in cancer is still open to question. Fish oils also lower triglycerides, but they do not increase HDL cholesterol or lower LDL cholesterol, and high doses are associated with a fishy odor.

23. When is nicotinic acid the preferred drug for therapy?

Because nicotinic acid lowers VLDL apo-B synthesis, it is the drug of choice for familial combined hyperlipidemia. Its use is otherwise limited by its side effects and the need for careful monitoring: flushing, gastrointestinal symptoms, glucose intolerance, transaminasemia, and hyperuricemia. Only the rapidly absorbed form should be used, and patients with prior hyperuricemia should be pretreated. Other side effects may be diminished by slow escalation of dose and/or aspirin.

24. How is pharmacologic therapy of LDL cholesterol optimized?

An HMG CoA reductase inhibitor (e.g., lovastatin, 10 mg at night to 40 mg twice daily or others, depending on cost) can lower LDL cholesterol by 35–40%. Transaminases are monitored every 3 months. A second lipid-lowering drug—usually a bile acid-binding resin (cholestyramine), which may lower LDL cholesterol by an additional 25%—may be instituted to reach target levels.

25. When should levels of creatine phosphokinase (CPK) be monitored in lipid therapy?

Patients on an HMG CoA reductase inhibitor and a second lipid-lowering drug (gemfibrozil, nicotinic acid) or cyclosporin are at risk for the development of myositis. Thus, a careful history and CPK determination should be regularly determined.

26. What options are available for patients with homozygous familial hypercholesterolemia?

Patients with homozygous familial hypercholestrolemia respond poorly to pharmacologic management. The decision to treat more aggressively with plasmapheresis or liver transplantation is difficult and must be individualized.

27. What guidelines should be followed in treating dyslipidemia in the elderly?

Because no convincing evidence indicates that aggressive control in the elderly, among whom dyslipidemia is more common, will alter outcome, individualized therapy is warranted. The principle of "do no harm" with drug toxicity, strenuous exercise, and overly restricted diets should be followed. Realistic goals and correction of secondary factors (e.g., smoking, obesity, hypertension) should be pursued.

BIBLIOGRAPHY

1. Criqui MH, et al: Plasma triglyceride level and mortality from coronary heart disease. N Engl J Med 328:1220, 1993.
2. Grundy SM, et al: The place of HDL in cholesterol management. A perspective from the National Cholesterol Education Program. Arch Intern Med 149:505, 1989.
3. Kreisberg RA: Low high-density lipoprotein cholesterol: What does it mean, what can we do about it, and what should we do about it? Am J Med 94:1, 1993.
4. Report of the National Cholesterol Education Program Expert Panel on Detection, Evaluation, and Treatment of High Blood Cholesterol in Adults. The Expert Panel. Arch Intern Med 148:36, 1988.

5. Summary of the Second Report of the National Cholesterol Education Program (NCEP) Expert Panel on Detection, Education and Treatment of High Blood Cholesterol in Adults (Adult Treatment Panel II). JAMA 269:3015, 1993.
6. Hunninghake DB, et al: The efficacy of intensive dietary therapy alone or combined with lovastatin in outpatients with hypercholesterolemia. N Engl J Med 328:1213, 1993.
7. Manninen V, et al: Joint effects of serum triglyceride and LDL cholesterol and HDL cholesterol concentrations on coronary heart disease risk in the Helsinki Heart Study. Implications for treatment. Circulation 85:37–45, 1992.

31. INFERTILITY

Julie Rifkin, M.D.

1. What defines an infertile couple?

Normal couples are generally able to conceive within 9 months. Failure to conceive after 1 year of unprotected intercourse is highly suggestive of a fertility problem. Infertility affects 10–15% of all couples in the United States. Unfortunately, 15% of such couples receive no diagnosis to explain their inability to conceive. Approximately 1 in 7 couples is infertile at age 30–34 years; 1 in 5 at age 35–39 years; and 1 in 4 at age 40–44 years. The risk of infertility is doubled for women aged 33–44 years compared with women aged 30–34 years. Up to 50% of infertile couples may conceive spontaneously in the second year of unprotected intercourse.

2. How can the history aid in uncovering clues to infertility?

It is critical to confirm a history of sexual intercourse. Sometimes simple layman's terms are required. Both partners require a thorough medical history. Poorly controlled systemic disorders may contribute to lower fertility rates (e.g., hypothyroidism, diabetes mellitus, ulcerative colitis). The following questions provide important clues to diagnosing infertility:

1. Has the woman been pregnant before? If so, what was the outcome?
2. Has the man fathered children before?
3. Has the couple previously used any birth control methods?
4. How long has the couple been together?
5. How long have they attempted to conceive?
6. Has the woman ever menstruated?
7. Are the menstrual cycles regular? (Ovulatory dysfunction or anovulation is suggested by cycles shorter than 21 or longer than 35 days.)
8. Is there a recent onset of dysmenorrhea (which may suggest endometriosis)?
9. How often does the couple have intercourse?
10. Is there a history of an abnormal pelvic exam or Papanicolaou smear?
11. Is there a history of prior abdominal or pelvic surgery?
12. Is either partner taking medications? (Minor tranquilizers, phenothiazines, or antihypertensives may interfere with ovulatory function.)
13. Is there a history of excessive smoking, caffeine intake, or excessive alcohol consumption?
14. Is there a history of pelvic inflammatory disease (PID), septic abortion, use of intrauterine devices (IUDs), ruptured appendix, or ectopic pregnancy? (Positive history alerts physician to possible tubal damage.)

3. What are common medical causes of infertility?

1. Ovulatory dysfunction	4. Subclinical hypothyroidism
2. Inadequate luteal phase	5. Asymptomatic genital infection
3. Subclinical hypoprolactinemia	6. Antisperm antibodies

4. What is the first step in evaluating male infertility?

Carefully performed semen analysis is a useful first step. The specimen is best collected by masturbation. Three specimens should be evaluated at least 2 weeks apart. At least 2 specimens must contain 1 ml of semen and $> 20 \times 10^6$/ml total sperm concentration. At least 50% of the sperm must demonstrate normal morphology, and 60% must show progressive movement.

5. Can the postcoital test substitute for a semen analysis?

No. The postcoital test (PCT) may determine whether a specific interaction takes place between a patient's sperm and his partner's cervical mucus. Although most physicians recommend PCT as an important step in infertility evaluation, it is a poorly standardized, nonspecific, and insensitive test. The PCT should occur 1–2 days before ovulation and 8–12 hours after coitus. A sample of the vaginal pool and samples from the ectocervix are aspirated into syringes and placed on slides. Microscopic examination provides information on spinnbarkeit (stretchability of cervical mucus), ferning, amount of cervical mucus, cellularity, and viscosity. Normal mucus characteristics are indicative of ovulation. The number and movement of sperm are also recorded. Oligoasthenospermia or abnormal cervical mucus is suspected when less than 5 sperm/hpf are found.

6. What is the simplest way to assess the presence of ovulation in the majority of women?

Ovulation disorders account for 10–24% of female infertility. Thus assessment of ovulatory function is important; the simplest method is to obtain a menstrual history. A history of uterine bleeding at 21–36-day intervals, accompanied by midcycle mittelschmerz, premenstrual symptoms, and dysmenorrhea, indicates ovulation in 90% of women. Other methods include the following:

Basal body temperature. Charting of basal body temperature (BBT) is a noninvasive, inexpensive method to detect ovulation. The patient records her oral temperatures each morning while still in bed after 6–8 hours of uninterrupted sleep. The preovulatory phase averages 97.5° F, and the luteinizing hormone (LH) surge results in an increased temperature 2 days following the LH peak. A biphasic BBT indicates ovulation, although less frequently a monophasic BBT may also be normal.

Serum progesterone in mid luteal phase. A progesterone level of 5 ng/ml 4–7 days before the next predicted menstrual cycle is a reliable indicator of ovulation.

Transvaginal ultrasound. Although expensive and time-consuming, transvaginal ultrasound can track a follicle to pinpoint the time of ovulation.

7. How can a woman predict when ovulation will occur?

1. Basal body temperature, as described above.
2. Urine LH. Quick and reliable enzyme-lined immunosorbent assays that measure the LH surge are commercially available. Ovulation occurs approximately 32–38 hours after the onset of the LH surge.

8. When should a patient undergo an endometrial biopsy?

An endometrial biopsy performed in late luteal phase is the standard clinical test for diagnosing luteal phase defects. The corpus luteum must function normally for implantation to occur and persist. Thus, both infertility and recurrent abortion may result from defects in the luteal phase. Because endometrial biopsy is painful and expensive, infertility specialists may proceed directly to ovulation induction if this type of defect is suspected.

9. How does an inadequate luteal phase affect infertility?

The corpus luteum (ruptured follicle from the ovary) must function normally to allow implantation and to maintain early pregnancy. Infertility and recurrent abortion may be caused by luteal phase defects (inadequate amounts of progesterone produced by the corpus luteum). Serum progesterone levels drawn during the luteal phase are not useful in establishing defects. Endometrial biopsy in the late luteal phase is the standard clinical test for diagnosing luteal phase defects. Populations at infertility clinics demonstrate a 5–10% incidence of luteal phase dysfunction. It is usually an idiopathic disorder.

Treatment regimens that enhance folliculogenesis are helpful, including therapy with clomiphene, human menopausal gonadotropin (hMG), human chorionic gonadotropin (hCG), or progesterone vaginal suppositories.

10. When should a hysterosalpingogram and/or laparoscopy be considered?

Hysterosalpingography is useful in infertile patients with a history of PID, septic abortion, tubal surgery, or ectopic pregnancy. No history of tubal damage is obtained from about one-half of patients with an abnormal examination. Hysterosalpingography is performed to rule out uterine and/or tubal defects, usually before ovulation induction therapy. The test is performed by a radiologist who injects iodine-based contrast media into the external cervical os. Radiographs record the movement of the contrast liquid through the uterus and tubes. This examination does not detect endometriosis or periadnexal adhesions. The hysterosalpingogram is a screening procedure that provides the first clue to the possibility of a uterine anomaly.

11. What is the final diagnostic procedure of an infertility evaluation?

Laparoscopy is the final diagnostic procedure of an infertility work-up. It is useful in detecting pelvic adhesions and endometriosis. Such abnormalities may be treated through the laparoscope by lysis of the adhesions or fulguration of endometriosis implants.

12. Which tests should be ordered to evaluate amenorrhea and oligomenorrhea?

Beta chorionic gonadotropin (βCG)—to rule out pregnancy
Prolactin—to screen for pituitary adenoma
Thyroid-stimulating hormone (TSH)—to screen for hypothyroidism
Follicle-stimulating hormone (FSH)—to screen for primary ovarian failure

13. What is the purpose of a progesterone withdrawal test?

A progesterone withdrawal test is used to evaluate amenorrhea when the tests described above are normal. Withdrawal bleeding that occurs 4–14 days after 7–10 days of medroxyprogesterone (Provera) confirms an intact hypothalamic-pituitary-ovarian axis and patency of the reproductive tract. This test also confirms the adequacy of circulating estrogen to sustain a proliferative endometrium. In the absence of response, the patient is given estrogen (Premarin, 1.25 mg orally) for 25 days, followed by progesterone for 16–25 days; subsequent bleeding eliminates the uterus as a cause of amenorrhea.

14. When and how should ovulation be induced?

Ovulation induction may be used to treat infertile women with oligomenorrhea or amenorrhea without ovarian failure (i.e., the ovaries are able to produce estrogen). Clomiphene is the agent of choice to induce ovulation in most patients. By competing with endogenous estrogens for estradiol binding sites in the hypothalamus, clomiphene blocks the normal negative estrogen feedback and leads to increased pulse frequency of gonadotropin-releasing hormone (Gn-RH). Ovulation is achieved in approximately 90% of patients using clomiphene. The overall pregnancy rate is roughly 50%.

15. What are the risks of stimulated ovulation?

Severe ovarian hyperstimulation is the most significant complication of gonadotropin therapy. The ovaries may become massively enlarged with development of ascites, hydrothorax, renal failure, and thromboembolic phenomenon. The exact pathogenesis of this syndrome is unknown.

16. How often does stimulated ovulation result in pregnancy when the cause of infertility is unknown?

Ovulation eventually can be induced in 99% of patients, with a 50% pregnancy rate. Multiple gestations result in 10% of patients.

17. Can women with secondary amenorrhea or polycystic ovary disease be treated?
Yes. Gn-RH is the treatment of choice for amenorrhea secondary to pituitary or hypothalamic dysfunction. It is delivered subcutaneously by a pump in a pulsatile fashion. The pregnancy rate is 30–35% per treatment cycle. Repetitive treatment yields near normal pregnancy rates. Referral to a specialist should not be denied to such patients.

18. What are assisted reproductive techniques (ARTs)?
   1. **In vitro fertilization** (IVF). IVF allows conception in patients with surgically uncorrectable fallopian tube disease, endometriosis, or unexplained infertility. Pregnancy rates are highly variable. The 1990 pregnancy rate for IVF as reported by the American Fertility Society is 19% per retrieval.
   2. **Gamete intrafallopian transfer** (GIFT). This method uses IVF protocols to obtain oocytes. The oocytes and spermatozoa are then placed directly into the fallopian tube via laparoscopy. GIFT pregnancy rates averaged 29% with 22% deliveries in 1990.
   3. **Zygote intrafallopian transfer** (ZIFT). The technology and pregnancy rate are similar to IVF. The embryo is placed in the fallopian tube 24 hours after fertilization.
   4. **Oocyte donation.** This procedure may be considered for women with ovarian failure whose endometrium is capable of responding to gonadal steroids. The patient's endometrium is prepared with an artificial steroid regimen. The donated oocytes are fertilized with the partner's sperm and placed into the patient's uterine cavity. One program has reported a live birth rate of nearly 50% per embryo transfer. Oocyte donation may be the most successful method of achieving pregnancy in older patients.

CONTROVERSY

19. Should embryos and oocytes be cryopreserved?
Cryopreservation has the potential to produce a new life and great joy for an infertile couple. It also has the potential to be exploited and improperly used. Perhaps such techniques create more questions than answers. If the partners separate, is oocyte or embryo custody an issue? If both partners die, who becomes guardian of the embryos? Does freezing produce genetic changes after months or years? These questions and many more require collection of extensive data and intense ethical consideration.

BIBLIOGRAPHY

 1. Alexander NS, Sampson JH, Fulgram DL: Pregnancy rates in patients treated for antisperm antibodies with prednisone. Int J Fertil 28:63, 1983.
 2. Collins JA: Diagnostic assessment of the ovulating processes. Semin Reprod Endocrinol 8:145, 1990.
 3. Corsan GH, Ghazi D, Kemmann E: Home urinary luteinizing hormone assays: Clinical applications. Fertil Steril 53:591, 1990.
 4. Dodson WC, Hughes CL, Whitesides DB, Riley AG: The effect of leuprolide acetate on ovulation induction with human menopausal gonadotropins in polycystic ovary syndrome. J Clin Endocrinol Metab 65:95, 1987.
 5. Kerin JF, Liu JH, Phillipai G, et al: Evidence for a hypothalamic site of action of clomiphene citrate in women. J Clin Endocrin Metab 61:265, 1985.
 6. Lobo RA: Unexplained infertility. J Reprod Med 38:241–249, 1993.
 7. Sauer MV, Paulson RJ: Human oocyte and pre-embryo donation: An evolving method for the treatment of female infertility. Am J Obstet Gynecol 163:1421, 1990.
 8. Sauer MV, Paulson RJ, Lolo RA: A preliminary report on oocyte donation extending reproductive potential to women over forty. N Engl J Med 323:1157, 1990.
 9. Seigal MS: The male infertility investigation and the role of the andrology laboratory. J Reprod Med 38:317–334, 1993.
10. Wong PC, Asch RH: Induction of follicular development with luteinizing hormone-releasing hormone. Semin Reprod Endocrinol 5:399, 1987.

32. THYROID DISEASE

Daniel H. Bessesen, M.D.

1. How is the secretion of thyroid hormone regulated?
As with a number of other endocrine systems, the hypothalamus works with the pituitary gland to regulate the production of bioavailable thyroid hormone. The hypothalamus secretes thyrotropin-releasing hormone (TRH) into the pituitary portal system. TRH stimulates the production of thyroid-stimulating hormone (TSH) by the pituitary gland. In addition, dopamine and indirect effects of cortisol inhibit pituitary secretion of TSH. TSH, which is produced in a pulsatile manner with 2–3 peaks/day, stimulates the production of thyroid hormone (T4) by the thyroid gland; 99.8% of T4 is bound to proteins in the plasma compartment. The primary proteins that bind thyroid hormone are thyroid-binding globulin (TBG), thyroid-binding prealbumin, and albumin. T4 may be peripherally deiodinated to the more bioactive T3; 98% of T3 is protein-bound in the circulation. T4 also may be peripherally deiodinated to the bioinactive reverse T3. Circulating levels of free T4 and T3 provide negative feedback for pituitary production of TSH and hypothalamic production of TRH. This system maintains constant levels of circulating free T4 and T3.

2. Which tissues are affected by thyroid hormone?
Thyroid hormone diffuses through the cell membrane of all cells and acts through an intranuclear receptor present in many tissues. The hormone and receptor complex then bind to DNA-regulatory elements to mediate the effects of thyroid hormone. As a result, thyroid hormone has important effects on virtually all tissues of the body. Among other effects, T4 and T3 increase metabolic rate, gastrointestinal motility, cardiac contractility and heart rate, body temperature, and anxiety levels; decrease body weight; and change skin texture.

3. What is the most important laboratory test for evaluating the hypothalamic–pituitary–thyroid (HPT) axis?
Assessment of serum TSH is the most important test in evaluating the HPT axis. Because most thyroid disease results from dysfunction of the thyroid gland rather than pituitary or hypothalamic disease, the TSH level is usually the first parameter to become abnormal during the course of thyroid disease. Older radioimmunoassays (RIA) were unable to differentiate between low and normal levels of TSH. When assessed by these older RIAs, the TSH level was useful only in the differentiation of hypothyroidism, which results in elevated levels. Newer immunoradiometric and chemoluminescence assays also differentiate between normal and low levels of TSH and thus between thyroid gland hyperfunction (low levels) and hypofunction (high levels).

4. What must be considered in the interpretation of a serum T4 level?
A number of tests are available for assessing serum T4 levels. The most common test assesses total serum T4. However, because over 99% of serum T4 is bound to proteins, some assessment of protein-binding must accompany any measurement of total T4. The most common test for assessing T4 protein-binding is a T3 resin uptake (T3RU), which measures the protein-binding capacity for thyroid hormone in the plasma. If both T4 and T3RU are elevated, hyperthyroidism is the likely diagnosis. If both T4 and T3RU are decreased, hypothyroidism is the likely diagnosis. However, if T4 and T3RU move in opposite directions, a protein-binding abnormality is the likely diagnosis. Alternatively the level of free T4 can be assessed directly either by radioimmunoassay or by equilibrium dialysis. Measurements of free T4 obviate the need for T3RU.

Assessment of Serum Levels

CONDITION	T4	T3RU	FTI	THYROID-BINDING PROTEINS
Hyperthyroidism	↑	↑	↑	NL
Hypothyroidism	↓	↓	↓	NL
Binding-protein excess	↑	↓	NL	↑
Binding-protein deficiency	↓	↑	NL	↓

FTI = free thyroxine index; NL = normal.

5. List the signs and symptoms of hyperthyroidism.

In the ambulatory setting, most patients with hyperthyroidism present with a single complaint. Deeper questioning, however, identifies a more broadly positive review of systems.

Symptoms
- Heat intolerance
- Weight loss
- Nausea
- Hyperdefecation
- Amenorrhea
- Goiter
- Discomfort in the eyes
- Headache
- Psychic disturbances (e.g., anxiety irritability or nervousness)
- Tremulousness

Physical signs
- Tachycardia
- Widened pulse pressure (but not hypertension)
- Atrial fibrillation
- Warm, moist skin
- Stare
- Lid lag
- Onycholysis
- Goiter

6. What is the most common cause of hyperthyroidism?

The most common cause of hyperthyroidism is Graves' disease, in which autoantibodies stimulate the TSH receptor and cause autonomous production of thyroid hormone by the thyroid gland. Graves' disease is associated with proptosis from retro-orbital inflammatory infiltration and occasionally with pretibial myxedema. The second most common cause of biochemical hyperthyroidism in most clinics is the use of thyroid-hormone medication. Less common causes of hyperthyroidism include an autonomously functioning (hot) nodule, toxic multinodular goiter, and thyroiditis.

7. Describe the three most common varieties of thyroiditis.

The most common variety of thyroiditis is **subacute thyroiditis**, which usually follows a viral illness and presents with a painful, tender goiter and signs and symptoms of hyperthyroidism. **Postpartum thyroiditis** is usually painless and associated with mild enlargement of the thyroid gland; it tends to recur with subsequent pregnancies.

Hashitoxicosis, the third common form, occurs in association with lymphocytic infiltration of the thyroid gland. The hyperthyroidism associated with thyroiditis is caused by injury to the thyroid gland and release of stored thyroid hormone. The hyperthyroid period is therefore short, lasting 2–3 months; it is followed by a hypothyroid period, which may last for 6–18 months. Approximately 50% of patients eventually become euthyroid.

8. Define apathetic hyperthyroidism.

Apathetic hyperthyroidism is an atypical presentation of hyperthyroidism in elderly patients. The placid or even depressed presentation may be more suggestive of hypothyroidism than hyperthyroidism. Weight loss is often a striking feature, as are cardiovascular manifestations such as atrial fibrillation and congestive heart failure. Many patients also manifest a proximal myopathy. The thyroid gland often is only minimally enlarged and may be multinodular. Eye findings typical of Graves' disease are minimal or absent.

9. How may the specific cause of hyperthyroidism be determined?
The physical examination often provides clues to the cause of hyperthyroidism. Graves' disease usually presents with a diffusely enlarged thyroid gland in association with proptosis. Autonomously functioning nodules form within the thyroid gland, the remainder of which is suppressed (small or absent). A toxic multinodular goiter is usually palpable. Subacute thyroiditis is suggested when the thyroid gland is tender.

The most definitive method for determining the cause of hyperthyroidism, however, is the thyroid scan. In Graves' disease, the thyroid gland shows diffuse, homogeneous, increased uptake of radioactive iodine. An autonomously functioning nodule shows increased radioactive iodine uptake in the nodule, but the remainder of the gland shows no uptake. With a toxic multinodular goiter, multiple areas of autonomous uptake may be identified. With thyroiditis or hyperthyroidism caused by ingestion of thyroid hormone medication, radioactive iodine uptake is suppressed or absent.

10. List the available treatments of Graves' disease.
Antithyroid medications, radioactive iodine, and surgery.

11. When is surgery indicated to treat Graves' disease?
Surgery is rarely used to treat Graves' disease because the other treatment modalities are highly effective. Because very few surgeons have adequate experience in operating on patients with Graves' disease, complications, including hypoparathyroidism and recurrent laryngeal nerve palsy, are unacceptably high.

12. What are the risks and benefits of radioactive iodine therapy for Graves' disease?
Radioactive iodine (I^{131}) is a highly effective therapy for Graves' disease. A single dose successfully treats hyperthyroidism in 95% of patients. The dose is adjusted in accordance with the size of the gland (the larger the gland, the larger the dose) and the avidity of the gland for the radionucleotide (the higher the percentage of uptake, the lower the dose). Many patients may be concerned that treatment with I^{131} increases the risk of cancer, but 35 years of experience have produced no supportive evidence. Several potential problems, however, are associated with I^{131}. Approximately 60% of patients become hypothyroid within 2 years after treatment and must take thyroid hormone supplementation for the rest of their lives. A second complication is potential worsening of Graves' ophthalmopathy. This issue is controversial, but some authors believe that active ophthalmopathy is a relative indication for antithyroid drug therapy.

If I^{131} is administered to a woman of reproductive age, the clinician must be certain that she is not pregnant. The most effective approach is to administer I^{131} within 10 days of the last menstrual period and to document a negative serum pregnancy test on the day of administration. I^{131} has the potential of destroying the fetal thyroid gland. Studies have shown that the fetus does not develop a thyroid gland until 12–15 weeks of gestation; therefore, if I^{131} is administered in the first trimester, the risk to the fetus is relatively small. However, it is prudent to be aggressive in ensuring that I^{131} is not given to a pregnant woman.

13. What two types of medical therapy may be used in the treatment of Graves' disease?
Symptomatic treatment. Beta blockers reduce the tremulousness and tachycardia associated with hyperthyroidism. Propranolol is the most widely used drug, but metoprolol or atenolol also alleviate symptoms.

Antithyroid drugs. Two antithyroid drugs are commonly used: propylthiouracil (PTU) and methimazole. Both drugs are effective at inhibiting production of thyroid hormone. PTU has the added benefit of inhibiting peripheral conversion of T4 to T3 and the disadvantage of requiring administration 3 times/day. Both drugs also may have an immunomodulating effect in Graves' disease. Antithyroid drugs are typically advocated for patients with mild hyperthyroidism and relatively small goiters. The goal of therapy is to maintain a euthyroid state until the Graves' disease spontaneously remits. The rates of spontaneous remission, however, vary widely in the literature. Some authors suggest that only 20–30% of cases spontaneously remit, whereas other authors report remission rates of 65–70%. Antithyroid drug therapy has the advantage of achieving a euthyroid state within several weeks, whereas I^{131} may take 2–3 months.

14. When should a patient with Graves' disease be hospitalized?

The indications for hospitalization include altered mental status, fever, congestive heart failure, new atrial fibrillation, and intractable nausea and vomiting. Patients with atrial fibrillation from Graves' disease should be treated with beta blockade and anticoagulation; digoxin alone is generally not effective in slowing the ventricular response rate.

15. How is Graves' eye disease evaluated and managed?

Graves' disease is associated with inflammatory infiltration of the extraocular muscles, which usually causes mild proptosis and a sensation of dry eyes. The patient should lubricate the eyes with eyedrops (daytime) or lubricating ointment (nighttime) and wear sunglasses. If the eyes remain open during sleep, cornea ulceration may result; thus some patients may benefit from taping the eyes shut at night. Elevating the head of the bed and taking low doses of a thiazide diuretic also may help. Rare patients may experience diplopia from extraocular muscle dysfunction or decreased visual acuity due to compression of the optic nerve; therefore, visual acuity and eye movements should be documented at each visit. If diplopia or decreased visual acuity develops, the patient should be referred to an ophthalmologist with experience in treating Graves' eye disease.

16. What are the signs and symptoms of hypothyroidism?

Hypothyroidism may cause weight gain, fatigue, cold intolerance, constipation, and, in women, menstrual irregularities. Physical signs include periorbital puffiness; diastolic hypertension; cold, dry skin; delayed relaxation phase of the reflexes; and bradycardia. The diagnostic biochemical test is assessment of serum TSH level, which is elevated in the presence of primary thyroid gland failure.

17. What causes hypothyroidism?

The most common cause of hypothyroidism is autoimmune destruction of the thyroid gland, which may be associated with increased circulating levels of antimicrosomal antibodies or antithyroglobulin antibodies. A less common cause is secondary destruction of the pituitary gland, which may be associated with a pituitary tumor or previous cranial irradiation. The least common cause of hypothyroidism is glandular destruction from neck irradiation used to treat Hodgkin's disease or head and neck cancer. Lithium therapy for manic depressive illness may unmask underlying hypothyrodism.

18. What populations are at special risk for hypothyroidism?

Biochemical hypothyroidism is present in up to 8% of individuals over the age of 65 years. It is more common in people with diabetes, adrenal insufficiency, and autoimmune hypogonadism and should be considered in the evaluation of dementia in elderly patients.

19. How is hypothyroidism treated?

Levothyroxine (LT4) is the treatment of choice for hypothyroidism. The half-life of LT4 in a euthyroid individual is 7 days. Thus the clinician should wait 6 weeks after beginning a daily replacement dose before checking the TSH level to document adequacy of therapy. The goal of therapy is to normalize the TSH level. The physician needs to check only the TSH level when following a patient with primary hypothyroidism on hormone replacement therapy. The average dose required is 1.6 μg/kg of ideal body weight. Levothyroxine requirements increase by an average of 45% during pregnancy. A number of recent studies have shown that excessive thyroid hormone replacement (suppressed TSH) is quite common. Overreplacement carries a risk of inducing osteoporosis and therefore should be avoided.

20. Describe the treatment of the patient with an elevated level of TSH but a normal level of T4.
The patient with an increased level of TSH but normal T4 level presents a special problem. This condition is known as subclinical hypothyroidism. Treatment is advisable for two reasons. The first is that patients eventually may become frankly hypothyroid. A number of prospective studies have shown, however, that only a minority of patients progress to overt hypothyroidism; such patients have high titers of antimicrosomal antibodies (>1:1000) and higher values of TSH (>15). The second reason is potential metabolic dysfunction, which may be manifested by depression, heart failure, abnormal lipids, or hypertension. Randomized prospective trials report subjective or objective improvement in approximately 60% of patients with subclinical hypothyroidism after treatment with levothyroxine. In practice it is reasonable to place the patient on a dose of levothyroxine that normalizes TSH for 12 months and to monitor for subjective or objective improvement. If no improvement is evident, if the initial TSH was less than 15, and if antimicrosomal antibodies were less than 1:1000, therapy could be discontinued.

21. How common are thyroid nodules?
The prevalence of thyroid nodules is a function of the method used for identification. In several series in which thyroid glands were palpated by experienced endocrinologists, 3–5% of normal adults were found to harbor thyroid nodules. In a study in which 2-mm sections of thyroid glands were obtained at autopsy, nodules were found in 50% of cadavers.

22. Which nodules are likely to be benign?
Nodules with autonomous function (i.e., nodules that are hot on radioactive iodine thyroid scan) are virtually never malignant. Simple, thin-walled cysts also are unlikely to be cancerous.

23. How should a solitary thyroid nodule be evaluated?
Thyroid cancer usually presents as a solitary thyroid nodule. However, only 3–5% of thyroid nodules are malignant. The goal is to identify and remove the subset of nodules that are malignant.

After assessment of TSH to ensure normal thyroid hormone levels, there are two approaches to the work-up of a solitary thyroid nodule: thyroid scan and fine-needle aspiration (FNA). If the initial scan reveals a hot nodule, no further evaluation is necessary. If the nodule is warm, the patient is placed on suppressive doses of levothyroxine, and the scan is repeated. If the nodule still takes up the radioactive iodine, it is autonomous; no further work-up is necessary, and suppressive therapy is of no benefit. If the nodule is cold or is not seen, referral to an endocrinologist for FNA is indicated.

An alternative approach to the work-up is to perform an initial FNA on all thyroid nodules. The FNA, which is performed with a 23–25-gauge needle, is a safe well-tolerated procedure. The FNA biopsy categorizes nodules into one of several groups. A minority (5–10%) are suggestive of cancer; most (60–70%) are benign; and 15–20% are "suspicious." Because the risk of cancer in suspicious nodules is 20–30%, most authors recommend surgical removal. Even experienced hands fail to obtain adequate material for biopsy in 10–15% of aspirated nodules. If the FNA is performed first and it suggests cancer, a thyroid scan should then be performed. If the nodule is cold on scan, it should be removed. If it is hot, the cytology should be ignored and the patient does not require surgery.

CONTROVERSY

24. How should a solitary thyroid nodule be managed?
If the FNA is either suspicious or suggests malignancy, the patient should be referred for surgical excision. If the nodule is hot or autonomous, thyroid function tests should be obtained every 6–12 months, because such nodules tend to grow and eventually to cause hyperthyroidism. If the nodule appears to be a benign adenoma, management is controversial. In the past the usual approach was to administer suppressive doses of levothyroxine with the hope that

reduction of TSH concentration would shrink the nodule and prevent malignant conversion. However, recent randomized, controlled trials suggest that suppressive therapy has no effect on the size of solitary nodules. In addition, suppressive therapy with levothyroxine may predispose to osteoporosis. The proper therapy for solitary thyroid nodules is currently controversial. A reasonable middle course is to place the patient on levothyroxine with a goal of suppressing TSH to the intermediate level of 0.1–0.5 m U/L. If the nodule does not shrink within 6–12 months, therapy should be discontinued to minimize the risk of osteoporosis. The nodule is then measured periodically, and FNA is repeated if the nodule grows.

BIBLIOGRAPHY

1. Gharib H, Goellner JR: Fine needle aspiration biopsy of the thyroid: An appraisal. Ann Intern Med 118:282–289, 1993.
2. Greenspan FS: Thyroid diseases. Med Clin North Am 75:1–239, 1991.
3. Hashizume K, Ichikawa K, Sakurai A, et al: Administration of thyroxine in treated Graves' disease. N Engl J Med 324:947–953, 1991.
4. Hay ID, Klee GG: Thyroid dysfunction. Endocrinol Metab Clin North Am 17:473–501, 1988.
5. Helfand M, Crapo LM: Screening for thyroid disease. Ann Intern Med 112:840–849, 1990.
6. Ladenson PW: Treatments for Graves' disease. N Engl J Med 324:989–991, 1991.
7. Mandel SJ, Brent GA, Larsen PR: Levothyroxine therapy in patients with thyroid disease. Ann Intern Med 119:492–502, 1993.
8. Ridgway EC: Clinician's evaluation of a solitary thyroid nodule. J Clin Endocrinol Metab 74:231–235, 1992.
9. Stall GM, Harris S, Sokoll LJ, Dawson-Hughes B: Accelerated bone loss in hypothyroid patients overtreated with L-thyroxine. Ann Intern Med 113:265–269, 1990.

33. OSTEOPOROSIS

Fred D. Hofeldt, M.D.

1. Distinguish metabolic bone disease from localized bone disease.

In metabolic bone disease all the bone metabolic units throughout the skeleton are equally affected by the generalized disease process. Examples include osteoporosis, osteomalacia, osteitis fibrosis cystica, osteogenesis imperfecti, and osteopetrosis. Localized bone disease, on the other hand, may be unifocal or multicentric. Examples include Paget's disease, fibrous dysplasia, bone cysts, healing fractures, Sudeck's atrophy, other limb injury, and disuse osteoporosis.

2. What is osteoporosis?

Osteoporosis is a systemic metabolic skeletal disease characterized by low bone mass and microarchitectural deterioration of bone tissue, which results in increased bone fragility and fracture susceptibility. This process may involve loss of both cortical and trabecular bone. **Type I osteoporosis** is postmenopausal and usually presents with type A fractures (i.e., fractures of trabecular bone, which is found in vertebrae and the wrist). **Type II osteoporosis** is senile osteoporosis that involves loss of cortical and trabecular bone and presents with type B fractures (hip). Osteoporosis may be due to high or low turnover states.

3. What leads to osteomalacia?

Osteomalacia is abnormal bone mineralization, frequently due to defects in substrate availability (i.e., calcium and/or phosphate). It also may be due to alterations in vitamin D metabolism or certain drugs that cause abnormal mineralization, such as sodium fluoride or bisphosphonates.

Causes of Osteomalacia

Vitamin D deficiency
- Diet plus decreased sunlight
- Gastrointestinal disorders (malabsorption, gastrectomy, pancreatitis, sprue, celiac, small-bowel resection)
- Drugs (bile-binding resins [cholestyramine, colestipol], laxative abuse)

25-Hydroxyvitamin D deficiency
- Liver disease
- Anticonvulsive drugs (diphenylhydantoin, barbiturates)
- Antituberculosis drugs (rifampin, isoniazid)

1,25-Dihydroxyvitamin D deficiency
- Renal failure
- Advanced age
- Vitamin D-dependent rickets, type I
- Familial sex-linked hypophosphatemia (also sporadic and acquired)
- Oncogenic osteomalacia
- Drugs (ketoconazole, isoniazid)

1,25-Dihydroxyvitamin D-resistant syndrome
- Vitamin D-dependent rickets, type II

Hypophosphatemia
- Deficiency of phosphate (diet, antacids)
- Renal tubular defects (Fanconi syndrome and its variants)
- Familial sex-linked hypophosphatemic vitamin D-resistant rickets (phosphate diabetes)
- Sporadic hypophosphatemia
- Acquired hypophosphatemia (including oncogenic osteomalacia)

Miscellaneous
- Fluoride, diphosphonates
- Fibrogenesis imperfecta ossium
- Hypophosphatasia
- Parenteral nutrition, ureterosigmoidostomy

4. What does osteopenia mean in a radiologist's report?

Osteopenia is a descriptive radiologic diagnosis suggesting that the bone mass is reduced by standard radiographic techniques. This interpretation usually is based on radiographs of the chest and/or lumbar spine. Before bone loss is evident, approximately 30–40% of the skeleton has demineralized.

5. What is the most common cause of osteopenia?

The most common cause is age-related idiopathic osteoporosis. Other specific causes of osteopenia are listed below.

Causes of Osteopenia

Idiopathic age-related osteoporosis
1. Juvenile
2. Young adults
3. Postmenopausal (type I)
4. Senile (type II)

Secondary to disease states
1. Metabolic conditions
   - Calcium deficiency
   - Vitamin D–deficient states
   - Malnutrition
   - Idiopathic hypercalciuria
   - Renal tubular acidosis and other systemic acidosis
   - Scurvy

(Table continued on following page.)

Causes of Osteopenia (Continued)

Secondary to disease states *(Cont.)*

2. Endocrine conditions
   - Thyrotoxicosis
   - Cushing's syndrome
   - Male and female hypogonadal states
   - Hypoamenorrheic female runners
   - Prolactinoma
   - Hyperparathyroidism
3. Renal disease
4. Gastrointestinal-liver disease
5. Hereditary connective tissue disease
   - Osteogenesis imperfecta
   - Homocystinuria
   - Ehlers-Danlos syndrome
   - Marfan syndrome
6. Bone marrow infiltration
   - Multiple myeloma
   - Lymphoma
   - Leukemia
7. Drugs
   - Diphenylhydantoin
   - Phenobarbital
   - Thyroid hormone
   - Corticosteroids
   - Chronic heparin therapy
8. Lifestyle
   - Nutrition
   - Alcohol
   - Smoking
   - Inactivity
   - Immobilization
   - Excessive coffee, soft drinks
9. Miscellaneous
   - Rheumatoid arteritis
   - Systemic mastocytosis

6. What risk factors need to be assessed in the osteoporotic patient?

Risk factors for osteoporosis include positive family history; life-long history of poor dietary calcium intake, particularly during adolescent years; physical inactivity or immobilization; smoking; malnutrition; hypogonadal state; and ingestion of substances of high phosphate intake, such as soft drinks or large portions of red meats. Coffee is a calciuretic substance. Because fat cells can act as an endocrine organ and convert adrenal androgens to estrogens, lean body mass is a risk factor for osteoporosis, especially in Asian or Caucasian females.

7. Which laboratory tests help to evaluate an osteopenic patient?

The initial tests are a complete blood count with sedimentation rate and routine chemistry panel that includes assessment of electrolytes, calcium, phosphate, and alkaline phosphatase as well as liver and renal function tests. A 24-hour urine collection is analyzed for calcium, phosphate, and creatinine. Calcium and phosphate measurements help to assess calcium-phosphate balance. In the osteopenic patient with anemia and elevated sedimentation rate, multiple myeloma should be considered, and serum protein electrophoresis and/or urine protein electrophoresis should be performed.

Abnormalities of liver and kidney function define secondary causes of osteopenia. The electrolytes are helpful in identifying patients with renal tubular acidosis. Serum alkaline phosphatase is a marker of bone osteoblast function and helps to identify patients with high-turnover osteoporosis or osteomalacia. A 24-hour urine collection for measurement of calcium excretion identifies patients with renal hypercalcuria (i.e., urinary calcium greater than 4 mg calcium/kg body weight) or hypocalciuria, which suggests a calcium-deficient state. An extremely low urine phosphate value may identify a patient who is phosphate-depleted, consuming phosphate-binding antacids, or vegetarian.

Other more specific but expensive laboratory tests may be selectively indicated, including measurement of parathyroid hormone, serum osteocalcin, vitamin D metabolites [25 (OH) D_3 and 1,25 $(OH)_2D_3$], urine hydroxyproline, or hydroxypyridinium. Osteocalcin is a marker of osteoblast function, whereas urinary hydroxyproline or hydroxypyridinium reflects osteoclast function.

8. When are bone density measurements medically indicated?

The National Osteoporosis Foundation and the National Institutes of Health have established that bone measurements are warranted for the evaluation of (1) female patients for whom estrogen replacement is being considered; (2) hypoamenorrheal runners; (3) patients with radiographic evidence of osteopenia; (4) hyperparathyroid patients who are candidates for surgery; (5) in steroid-treated patients; and (6) patients on various treatment programs for osteopenia.

9. How can a bone biopsy help to evaluate patients with metabolic bone disease?
The bone biopsy is useful in evaluating high- and low-turnover osteoporosis, osteomalacia, primary and secondary hyperparathyroidism, osteogenesis imperfecti, and aluminum toxicity.

10. Is a bone biopsy similar to a bone marrow biopsy?
No. A bone biopsy is performed after administration of tetracycline, 250 mg 3 times/day for 3 days, followed by a 10-day period without medication and readministration of tetracycline, 250 mg 3 times/day for an additional 3 days. Three days after tetracycline labeling, an iliac crest bone biopsy may be performed. The biopsy shows the amount of trabecular bone volume, supporting the diagnosis of osteopenia. The amount of unmineralized matrix is measured and expressed as osteoid surface and osteoid seam thickness. The amount of tetracycline-labeled surface defines the amount of active mineralization by osteoblasts and determines rates of bone formation. Specific stains determine osteoclast counts and aluminum toxicity.

11. What preventive measures should be recommended to patients at risk for osteoporosis?
   1. An adequate calcium intake of at least 800–1,000 mg of elemental calcium/day can be ingested in food substances; however, because of hypercholesterolemic issues and the recommendation to avoid foods high in saturated fats, patients may need calcium supplementations. If calcium supplementations are prescribed, they are best taken with meals.
   2. Outdoor activities should be encouraged; minimal erythremic sunlight exposure provides 400–1,200 units of vitamin D from synthesis in the skin. The recommended daily allowance of vitamin D is 400 units, which is contained in a multivitamin capsule.
   3. Weight-bearing exercises stimulate bone remodeling and inhibit osteolysis. Inactivity is discouraged.
   4. Male or female hypogonadism needs evaluation.

12. What are the drug treatment protocols for osteoporosis?
Patients with known osteoporosis should be ingesting 1500 mg of elemental calcium per day. Currently, the Food and Drug Administration recommends only two protocols for treating osteoporosis: (1) estrogens alone or estrogens plus progestin and (2) thyrocalcitonin. The minimal dose of conjugated estrogens to stabilize bone density is 0.625 mg. The transdermal estradiol patch, which provides 0.05 mg/day when applied twice weekly, also prevents postmenopausal bone loss. Thyrocalcitonin is given as subcutaneous injections, starting with initial doses of 100 IU/day for 5 of 7 days/week for 3–6 months, after which it may be given in doses of 100 IU 3 times/week for 2–3 years. At this time other protocols are considered investigational, including the cyclic use of etidronate.

13. Should vitamin D be used to treat osteoporosis?
No. Vitamin D and vitamin D metabolites are not recommended for the treatment of osteoporosis and should be reserved for treatment of vitamin D deficiency.

14. What are the benefits of estrogen therapy?
Estrogens are the most effective agents for treating and preventing osteoporosis. They stabilize bone density, prevent both vertebral and hip fractures, and have protective effects in hypogonadal women of all ages. Estrogens also have a cardioprotective effect by lowering low-density lipoprotein (LDL) and raising high-density lipoprotein (HDL) cholesterol. Some patients on oral estrogen therapy may show an increase in serum triglycerides. When this occurs, the estrogen patch should be substituted; its use may not adversely affect serum triglycerides. Hence, a fasting lipid profile should be checked 4–6 weeks after initiating estrogen therapy. In addition to the cardioprotective effects on lipids, estrogen increases

calcitonin-related peptide, a potent vasorelaxer, and stabilizes abnormal vasomotion in patients with established atherosclerosis and hypercholesterolemia.

15. When is estrogen therapy for prevention of osteoporosis contraindicated?
Estrogen therapy is contraindicated in suspected or known pregnancy, in patients who have estrogen-related neoplasms, and in patients with active thromboembolic disease. Relative contraindications include patients with previous thrombotic disease, estrogen-related headaches, or hypertension.

BIBLIOGRAPHY

1. Civitelli R, et al: Bone turnover in postmenopausal osteoporosis: Effect of calcitonin treatment. J Clin Invest 82:1268–1274, 1988.
2. Consensus development conference diagnosis prophylaxis and treatment of osteoporosis. Am J Med 94:646–650, 1993.
3. Hahn TJ: Physiology of bone: Mechanisms of osteopenic disorders. Hosp Pract Aug:73–90, 1986.
4. Hofeldt FD: Proximal femoral fractures. Clin Orthop Rel Res 218:12–18, 1987.
5. Horsman A, et al: The effect of estrogen dose in postmenopausal bone loss. N Engl J Med 309:1405–1407, 1983.
6. Hutchinson TA, et al: Relative contributions of aging and estrogen deficiency to postmenopausal bone loss. N Engl J Med 311:1273–1275, 1984.
7. Lukert BP: Osteoporosis—A review and update. Arch Phys Med Rehab 63:480–487, 1982.
8. Riggs BL, et al: Evidence for two distinct syndromes of involutional osteoporosis. Am J Med 75:899–901, 1983.

VI. Problems of the Gastrointestinal Tract

34. HEARTBURN AND DYSPHAGIA

Thomas V. Davis, D.O., and Stephen Steinberg, M.D.

1. What is gastroesophageal reflux disease (GERD)?
GERD is the spectrum of signs and symptoms related to the reflux of acid (or alkaline) secretions from the stomach into the esophagus. Examples include heartburn, noncardiac chest pain, and symptoms related to chronic injury, such as esophageal inflammation and ulceration. Symptoms often occur in the absence of even histologic evidence of inflammation; conversely, even severe esophagitis and its complications may be present without associated symptoms. Physicians should suspect GERD when patients complain of frequent or difficult-to-control heartburn, dysphagia, nocturnal wheezing, atypical chest pain, chronic cough or sore throat, or hoarseness.

2. How common is GERD? What effect does it have on national health care spending?
Up to 36% of healthy Americans experience heartburn at least once a month, and an estimated 7% experience heartburn daily. Two to three million dollars are spent each year on over-the-counter and prescription medications to treat symptoms of acid reflux. Furthermore, reflux esophagitis may lead to complications, such as strictures, bleeding, ulceration, and perforation, that require hospitalization and/or invasive interventions.

3. What pathophysiologic factors influence GERD?
1. Reflux of gastric acid into the esophagus as a result of decreased resting amplitude of the lower esophageal sphincter, combined with the effects of gravity in the supine position.
2. Impaired esophageal luminal clearance of acid caused by ineffective peristaltic activity (low-amplitude, aperistaltic, retrograde, or spastic esophageal contractions). Decreased salivation (a source of bicarbonate) on occasion may contribute to impaired acid clearance.
3. Decrease in the mucosal protective mechanisms, such as the unstirred mucus layer and epithelial bicarbonate secretion.
4. Increased pain sensitivity of the esophageal mucosal receptors to acids.

4. List foods and medications that may contribute to GERD.
The following foods and medications have been shown to increase esophageal reflux by diminishing lower esophageal sphincter pressure or diminishing peristaltic activity.

Foods	Medications
Fatty foods	Xanthines (including caffeine)
Oils (including peppermint, onion and garlic)	Beta-adrenergic antagonists
	Calcium channel blockers
Chocolate, alcohol, and nicotine	Anticholinergics

5. What is waterbrash?
It is the spontaneous and abrupt onset of salivary secretions followed by a bitter or acid taste in the mouth. This symptom is believed to be initiated by esophageal acid and often precedes overt regurgitation. Other common symptoms of GERD include pyrosis (heartburn),

dysphagia (difficulty swallowing), odynophagia (painful swallowing), and gastrointestinal bleeding (in the case of severe erosive esophagitis).

6. Which esophageal disorders result in an increased incidence of cancer?
   1. **Barrett's esophagus.** In this condition, also known as intestinal metaplasia of the mucosa, columnar epithelium replaces the normal squamous epithelium, possibly as a result of continuous irritation and inflammation. Because 10–15% of patients with Barrett's epithelium may develop adenocarcinoma of the esophagus, frequent endoscopic surveillance with mucosal biopsy and brushings is warranted.
   2. **Plummer-Vinson syndrome.** This syndrome, which consists of intermittent solid food dysphagia (from a cervical esophageal web) and iron deficiency anemia, may be associated with glossitis, stomatitis, and achlorhydria as well as an increased incidence of squamous cell carcinoma of the esophagus.
   3. **Post-caustic ingestion.** In addition to the immediate injury and subsequent complications resulting from alkaline and acid substances, the risk of malignancy is significantly increased in subsequent years.

7. What causes the "steakhouse" syndrome?
Meat impaction of the lower tubular esophagus caused by a distal esophageal mucosal ring (B ring) or Schatzki's ring is referred to as "steakhouse" syndrome. Symptomatic dysphagia occurs when the diameter of the ring is 13 mm or less; mucosal rings are often asymptomatic until challenged with a large bolus of food.

8. What diagnosis should be considered in a patient who complains of dysphagia with regurgitation of undigested food?
Zenker's diverticulum is a mucosal herniation formed by the protrusion of the posterior hypopharyngeal mucosa between the oblique fibers of the inferior pharyngeal constrictor and the transverse fibers of the cricopharyngeus. Zenker's diverticulum is proximal to the esophagus and is not a true diverticulum because it has no muscular wall. The typical history includes dysphagia and occasional regurgitation of undigested food. It is often associated with bad breath, from putrifaction of food remaining in the pouch. An upper GI series (cine-swallow) is the best way to establish the diagnosis. Surgical resection, the definitive treatment, is usually reserved for markedly symptomatic cases.

9. List the major types of dysphagia and their common causes.
Dysphagia is the subjective sensation of impairment in the transit of a food bolus through the esophagus. A history of greater impairment to solids than to liquids generally implies a mechanical obstruction such as a stricture, whereas equal impairment or impairment to liquids implies a functional abnormality. Dysphagia can be subdivided into three categories:
   1. **Oropharyngeal disorders** of the neuromuscular components of the proximal esophagus and distal pharynx may be caused by cerebrovascular accidents, multiple sclerosis, amyotrophic lateral sclerosis, and Parkinson's disease.
   2. **Mechanical obstruction** is caused by a structural abnormality that results in obstruction of food bolus transport. Such abnormalities include strictures (benign and malignant), rings, webs, and Zenker's diverticulum.
   3. **Esophageal motility disorder** is caused by motor dysfunction of the peristaltic mechanism of the esophagus. Etiologies include achalasia, scleroderma, diabetic neuropathy, amyloidosis, and medications.

10. What swallowing problems do patients with scleroderma or CREST syndrome experience?
Progressive systemic sclerosis (scleroderma) and CREST syndrome (subcutaneous calcinosis, Raynaud's phenomenon, esophageal dysmotility, sclerodactyly, and telangiectasia) are associated with impaired or absent lower esophageal sphincter function and esophageal peristalsis due to involvement of esophageal smooth muscle. The result is often free reflux of

acid into the esophagus, the effect of which is worsened by the inability to clear the acid (absent peristalsis). Reflux symptoms are often severe, and complications such as Barrett's esophagus, ulcerative esophagitis, and strictures are frequent.

11. What are the steps in evaluation and management of GERD?

When patients have symptoms of reflux more than 3 times/week, medical intervention is warranted.

Mechanical measures should always be implemented first. Because gravity is one of the most important factors in the reduction of esophageal reflux, elevating the head of the bed 6 inches is especially useful for patients with nocturnal reflux symptoms. Efficacy is equivalent to histamine (H_2) blockers. Other mechanical measures include avoiding tight-fitting clothing and weight loss for obese habitus.

Dietary alterations also should be implemented. Avoiding offending foods or medications when possible may decrease the frequency and duration of reflux episodes.

If a patient fails conservative measures, acid suppression therapy is indicated. Acid suppression may be achieved by using H_2 receptor antagonists (cimetidine, ranitidine, famotidine) or proton pump inhibitors (omeprazole). Medications need to be tailored to each patient and titrated to symptomatic relief. Cost effectiveness also should be evaluated. It may be less expensive, for example, to change a patient from twice daily standard doses of H_2 to once daily omeprazole.

Finally, in patients who are refractory to the above measures or who may require extended pharmacologic therapy (as young patients), aggressive evaluation and antireflux surgery should be considered.

12. What tests are commonly used to evaluate GERD? What are their strengths and limitations?

1. **Esophagoscopy** is the gold standard for evaluating esophageal mucosal and structural abnormalities that result from GERD. Biopsies are taken at the esophagogastric (EG) junction to look for microscopic evidence of inflammation. Endoscopy cannot, however, quantitate the frequency or duration of esophageal reflux.

2. A **barium esophagogram** is useful in defining intraluminal lesions that may result as complications of acid reflux. It is poor overall in evaluating mucosal inflammation and, like endoscopy, does not aid in quantitation of reflux episodes.

3. **Esophageal manometry** is helpful in evaluating the resting pressure of the lower esophageal sphincter and esophageal peristalsis (acid clearing), but provides little information on the actual extent of reflux. It is helpful as a preoperative evaluation to confirm that a procedure that tightens the lower esophageal sphincter (e.g., Nissen fundoplication) is likely to be helpful and that peristalsis is adequate to overcome the surgically increased pressures. It is also useful in evaluating noncardiac chest pain, which is occasionally related to motility abnormalities.

4. **24-Hour esophageal pH testing** is the gold standard for documenting and quantitating the number and extent of reflux episodes in a given unit of time, usually 24 hours. It also helps define which episodes are symptomatic; the patients' symptom diary may be correlated to the esophageal probes pH data. In the patient whose symptoms do not respond to empiric therapy and in whom endoscopy does not demonstrate evidence of inflammation, it is the best test to confirm that reflux is indeed present and that symptoms are associated.

5. The **acid perfusion test**, also known as the Bernstein test, involves dripping 0.1N solution of hydrochloric acid alternated (unknown to the patient) with normal saline into the distal esophagus. A positive test reproduces the patient's symptoms with the acid infusion phase of the test. This qualitative test is rarely used today.

13. Do all complaints of dysphagia warrant evaluation?

All complaints of persistent dysphagia warrant investigation. Single episodes of dysphagia may be followed if the event is minor (such as having a pill stuck in the esophagus) and does not affect the patient greatly (as in occlusion of the esophagus with a meat bolus). Weight loss is the most significant associated finding. The following tests can be used to evaluate the cause of dysphagia, each with its own diagnostic and therapeutic strengths and weaknesses:

1. **Endoscopy** is the gold standard for evaluating esophageal lesions such as rings, webs, strictures, masses, and esophagitis. Biopsy can be performed to establish benignity of the lesion. Dilation of the obstruction via through-the-scope (TTS) balloon dilators or esophageal bougienage also may be performed.

2. The **cine-esophagogram** is useful in investigating the swallowing mechanism and in evaluating patients with oropharyngeal dysphagia. A tailored barium study also may be performed, in which barium "foods" with various consistencies are administered to evaluate the patient's ability to initiate swallowing.

3. An **esophageal motility study** helps to determine the general contraction profile of the esophagus. It provides amplitude and duration of the esophageal contraction wave and sphincter pressure.

14. A patient presents to the emergency department with symptoms consistent with esophageal food impaction. The patient is unable to handle secretions and is drooling. What should or should not be done to resolve the impaction?

Medications that may help to relax the esophageal obstruction and thus relieve the impaction may be administered, including intravenous glucagon, sublingual nitroglycerin, or a calcium-channel blocker, such as nifedipine. Meat tenderizers such as papain should be avoided, because they may induce esophageal perforation. Endoscopy should be used if conservative measures fail. Endoscopy is both diagnostic and therapeutic; the offending object may be removed and the type of esophageal obstruction identified. Barium swallow studies should be avoided in patients who are unable to handle secretions. The barium study provides no therapy; pulmonary aspiration of barium may result; and barium mixed with food and secretions in the esophagus makes subsequent endoscopy more difficult.

15. What is the most common cause of dysphagia or odynophagia in patients with acquired immunodeficiency syndrome (AIDS)?

Candida esophagitis is the most frequent cause of difficult or painful swallowing in patients with AIDS. Thus an appropriate anticandidal agent should be initiated empirically early in the course of symptoms. Common agents include nystatin, ketoconazole, and fluconazole. Ketoconazole, however, needs an acid environment for optimal absorption. Many patients with AIDS are achlorhydric or take acid-suppressing medications that may reduce the effectiveness of ketoconazole.

Anticandidal therapy relieves symptoms in more than 50% of patients. However, if the patient's symptoms persist or progress after several days of anticandidal therapy, endoscopy with biopsy and brushing should be performed to evaluate the esophagus for lesions from cytomegalovirus, herpes simplex virus, or idiopathic ulcerations due to human immunodeficiency virus (HIV). Barium studies miss a significant number of lesions, and definitive diagnosis is difficult to obtain from esophageal contrast studies.

BIBLIOGRAPHY

1. Boyce GA, Boyce WB Jr: Esophagus: Anatomy and structural anomalies. In Yamada T (ed): Textbook of Gastroenterology. Philadelphia, J. B. Lippincott, 1991.
2. Castell CO: Approach to the patient with dysphagia. In Yamada T (ed): Textbook of Gastroenterology. Philadelphia, J.B. Lippincott, 1991.
3. Jaffin B: Disorders of the esophagus. In Sachar DB, Waye JD, Lewis BS (eds): Pocket Guide to Gastroenterology. Baltimore, Williams & Wilkins, 1991.
4. Orlando RC: Reflux esophagitis. In Yamada T (ed): Textbook of Gastroenterology. Philadelphia, J.B. Lippincott, 1991.
5. Pope CE II: Heartburn, dysphagia, and other esophageal symptoms. In Sleisenger MH, Fordtran JS (eds): Gastrointestinal Disease, 4th ed. Philadelphia, W.B. Saunders, 1989.
6. Wilcox CM: Esophageal disease in the acquired immunodeficiency syndrome: Etiology, diagnosis, and management. Am J Med 92:412–421, 1992.

35. DYSPEPSIA AND PEPTIC ULCER DISEASE

Thomas E. Trouillot, M.D., and Stephen E. Steinberg, M.D.

1. What is dyspepsia?

Dyspepsia is a vague constellation of upper GI or biliary tract symptoms that may include epigastric discomfort or pain, nausea, vomiting, heartburn, bloating, belching, and dysphagia. Dyspepsia may represent organic disease, such as peptic ulcers, gastritis, or esophagitis. The more common term is nonulcer dyspepsia, which refers to the above constellation of findings in the absence of peptic ulcers or other mucosal pathology (i.e., after a negative endoscopy).

2. What is the history pertinent to peptic ulcer disease (PUD)?

1. Does the patient use aspirin or nonsteroidal anti-inflammatory drugs (NSAIDs)? These agents interfere with the normal mucosal defense mechanisms, which utilize prostaglandins. NSAIDs also may cause a topical irritation that directly damages the mucosa. Symptoms correlate poorly with NSAID-induced ulceration.

2. Does the patient smoke cigarettes? Smokers have an increased incidence of ulcer recurrence as well as impaired healing and require higher doses of histamine (H_2) blockers to achieve the same degree of acid suppression.

3. Are other risk factors present? Although the evidence is controversial, psychological stress, alcohol consumption, and caffeine have been implicated in ulcer formation and/or impaired healing.

3. Do all patients with PUD have characteristic symptoms?

Abdominal pain, primarily in the epigastrium, that radiates to the back is suggestive of PUD. Although the pain is not continuous, it usually occurs on a daily basis. Ingestion of food (an excellent antacid) or antacids may relieve the pain, although it recurs 1–3 hours after meals; it often awakens patients at night but is absent before breakfast. However, studies show PUD may be asymptomatic in 15–44% of cases, especially in the elderly.

4. Describe the relationship between upper GI bleeding and PUD.

Significant bleeding occurs in approximately 25% of cases. Patients may present acutely with orthostatic hypotension, hematemesis, and melena. When the bleeding is sudden, the anemia is often normocytic. A chronic bleed from an ulcer may present more subtly with minimal dyspeptic symptoms and microcytic anemia that, on further evaluation, is found to be an iron deficiency anemia often associated with hemoccult-positive stools.

5. Why is careful observation necessary after an upper GI bleed?

Careful observation is necessary because the "rebleed" rate in the first 48 hours may be as high as 50%, depending on the endoscopic findings.

6. What complications other than GI bleeding may occur with PUD?

Scarring may result in obstruction, most often at the pylorus or in the duodenal bulb, that usually is associated with recurrent vomiting and weight loss. Severe esophagitis may result from impaired emptying of gastric contents. Perforation of an ulcer into the peritoneal cavity or penetration of the ulcer into adjacent structures, most commonly the pancreas, also may occur. In either instance, pain often is accompanied with an elevated level of amylase. Surgical repair is recommended when such complications occur.

7. How is the diagnosis of PUD best made?

Endoscopy provides a safe means of diagnosis as well as an opportunity to obtain mucosal biopsies to confirm or eliminate the presence of *Helicobacter pylori* or malignancy. Endoscopic inspection of the mucosa also identifies esophagitis, gastritis, or duodenitis, which often are missed radiographically. In cases complicated by acute bleeding, endoscopy provides therapeutic intervention by various modalities that may result in hemostasis. The major complications from endoscopy, although rare (0.001–0.01), include perforation, bleeding, aspiration, and those associated with the anesthetics used for conscious sedation.

Compared with endoscopy, an upper GI series has lower morbidity, is less expensive, and may have a sensitivity approaching 80–90% with an air-contrast study. However, direct comparisons between an upper GI series and endoscopy reveal a sensitivity of 54% vs. 92%, respectively, when other gastroduodenal lesions are included.

8. How can benign and malignant ulcers be distinguished?

A benign-appearing ulcer has a smooth, regular rim with a smooth, flat base when evaluated endoscopically or radiologically. Folds radiating from the edge of the ulcer crater are usually symmetrical. In contrast, the malignant ulcer may have an irregular raised margin surrounded by clubbed gastric folds that suggest local tumor invasion. Large (>2 cm), recurrent, or malignant-appearing gastric ulcers should be biopsied and brushed for cytologic evaluation to rule out cancer. Follow-up endoscopy may be required after 4–6 weeks.

9. What is the role of *Helicobacter pylori* in PUD?

H. pylori has been associated with antral (type B) gastritis, duodenal ulcers (>85%), and, to a lesser degree, gastric ulcers (>65%). It should now be considered the most common cause of non–NSAID-related peptic ulcers. The presence of *H. pylori* can be confirmed either histologically from an antral biopsy or by the cod liver oil test, which detects the urease enzyme contained in the organism. Treatment with bismuth and antibiotics and/or omeprazole has been shown to eradicate *H. pylori* colonization, thus promoting ulcer healing and resolution of gastritis.

10. What are the pharmacologic options in treating PUD?

First, medications or habits that impair ulcer healing, including aspirin, NSAIDs, cigarettes, and alcohol, should be discontinued. H_2 antagonists, the mainstay in PUD treatment before recognition of the role of *H. pylori*, bind to histamine receptors on the basolateral membrane of parietal cells and thus impair gastric acid secretion. Omeprazole has the same effect by inhibiting the hydrogen-potassium ATPase pump on the luminal surface of parietal cells. Compared with H_2 antagonists, omeprazole shortens the healing rates of duodenal ulcers, although it is more costly when used for more than 8 weeks. Sucralfate provides local cytoprotection by enhancing mucosal defenses, and has healing rates similar to those of H_2 blockers, although the relapse rate was lower in one study. Misoprostol inhibits acid secretion by blocking histamine stimulated cyclic adenosine monophosphate in the parietal cell. Misoprostol and H_2 antagonists are the only agents with proved efficacy in preventing NSAID-induced mucosal injury.

11. How does treatment affect the natural history of duodenal ulcer disease?

Although the complete healing rates for antacids (>80%), H_2 blockers (85–90%), and omeprazole (>90%) are high, each has a high recurrence rate once therapy is discontinued (>50% in the first year). Studies have shown that eradication of *H. pylori* appears to alter the natural history and markedly reduces the relapse rate.

12. What are the indications for surgical management of PUD?

The primary indication for surgery is an ulcer that fails to heal, although with currently available agents this indication is uncommon. Recurrent disease is a more common indication, particularly when the cost of long-term medical management is considered. Ulcer disease complicated by bleeding, perforation, penetration, and gastric outlet obstruction is usually managed surgically. Lastly, giant duodenal ulcers (>5 cm) are usually resected because of the high complication rate.

13. What are the surgical options for treatment of PUD?
Vagotomy is the basis of all peptic ulcer operations. Proximal gastric vagotomy (highly selective vagotomy, parietal cell vagotomy), has become the most popular routine surgical procedure for the management of duodenal ulcer disease. The operation is designed to denervate the parietal (acid-secreting) cells in the stomach while preserving vagal innervation to the antropyloric region to allow near-normal gastric emptying of solids. The recurrence rate is 5–20%. Truncal vagotomy/antrectomy is the best operation in terms of ulcer recurrence (<1%), however, the incidence of postoperative problems is greater.

14. What is the difference between a Billroth I and a Billroth II operation?
In a Billroth I operation, after resection of a portion of the stomach and the duodenal bulb, the cut ends are reanastomosed. After a similar resection, a Billroth II operation is completed by oversewing the duodenal remnant and anastomosing the cut edge of the stomach to the jejeunum.

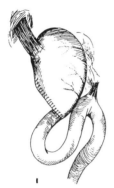 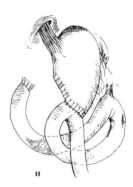

I   II

15. What problems result from ulcer surgery?
Virtually all ulcer operations result in the more rapid emptying of liquids from the stomach or gastric remnant and delayed emptying of solids, which may be so severe as to result in formation of a "bezoar," a mass of fiber and food material that does not leave the stomach. The rapid movement of hypertonic liquid nutrients from the stomach into the small intestine may result in large volumes of intestinal fluid secretion (at the expense of blood volume) as well as elevation of various hormones (e.g., serotonin, bradykinin, substance P, vasoactive intestinal peptide). The patient may experience flushing, light-headedness, diaphoresis, tachycardia, and postural hypotension as well as cramping and diarrhea. This constellation is referred to as "dumping syndrome." Other problems include alkaline gastritis, when bile refluxes into the stomach and injures the gastric mucosa; ulcers at the gastrointestinal anastomosis; weight loss; and iron deficiency, particularly with Billroth II anatomy, in which blood loss at the anastomosis (small ulcers) is common.

16. In a patient with recurrent ulcers, routine screening tests reveal an elevated level of serum calcium. In addition, she reveals a family history of pituitary tumor. What is the suspected etiology of her PUD?
Zollinger-Ellison syndrome is due to an endocrine tumor that secretes gastrin, which results in gastric acid hypersecretion. Such gastrinomas result in recurrent PUD that is refractory to conventional therapy. Gastrinomas, which are usually found in the duodenum or pancreas, are diagnosed most specifically by an elevated gastrin level, which paradoxically increases after an infusion of secretin. Approximately 25% of patients with gastrinomas have the multiple endocrine neoplasia (MEN I) syndrome, like the above patient. MEN I syndrome includes gastrinoma, hyperparathyroidism, and pituitary gland hyperplasia or tumor. The gastrinomas are often difficult to identify when they are solitary and rarely resectable when associated with the MEN I syndrome, because such tumors are often multifocal.

BIBLIOGRAPHY

1. Gilbert G, Chan CH, Thomas E: Peptic ulcer disease: How to treat it now. Postgrad Med 89(4):91–93,96,98, 1991.
2. Hixson LJ, Kelley CL, Jones WN, Tuohy CD: Current trends in the pharmacotherapy for peptic ulcer disease. Arch Intern Med 152:726–732, 1992.
3. Rosen SD, Rogers AI: Clinical recognition and evaluation of peptic ulcer disease. Postgrad Med 88(5):42–47,51,55, 1990.
4. Silverstein F: Nonsteroidal anti-inflammatory drugs and peptic ulcer disease: An overview. Postgrad Med 89(7):33–40, 1991.
5. Sleisenger MH, Fordtran JS: Gastrointestinal Disease: Pathophysiology, Diagnosis, Management, 5th ed. Philadelphia, W.B. Saunders, 1993, pp 580–678.
6. Soll AH: Pathogenesis of peptic ulcer and implications for therapy. N Engl J Med 322:909–916, 1990.
7. Soll AH, Weinstein WM, Kurata J, McCarthy D: Nonsteroidal anti-inflammatory drugs and peptic ulcer diseases. Ann Intern Med 114:307–319, 1991.

36. ABDOMINAL PAIN

*Leonard Berry, Jr, M.D., Roshan Shrestha, M.D.,
and Stephen E. Steinberg, M.D.*

1. Distinguish between visceral (splanchnic) and parietal pain.

Visceral pain is associated with tension or stretching of a hollow viscus such as the intestine. Pain is diffuse and tends to be poorly localized. It is frequently associated with autonomic responses such as vomiting, tachycardia, bradycardia, diarrhea, hypotension, and muscle rigidity. Uncomplicated small bowel obstruction provides an example of visceral pain.

Parietal pain results from irritation or inflammation of a parietal surface. As a result, the pain is sharp and more localized. It is associated with voluntary muscular rigidity called guarding. Parietal pain also may be associated with cutaneous hypesthesia. Severe acute appendicitis and peritonitis, in which parietal surfaces are inflamed and irritated, provide examples of parietal pain.

2. Describe rebound and referred pain.

Both types of pain are due to irritation of serosal surface. **Rebound tenderness** occurs when the palpating hand pushes deep into the abdomen; upon its rapid withdrawal, the inflamed surfaces of the peritoneum rub one against each other, and the patient experiences sharp pain. **Referred pain** occurs at a site distant from the location of the inciting process. A patient with a subphrenic abscess following splenectomy or a bile leak following laparoscopic cholecystectomy may experience shoulder pain. The pain is referred to the shoulder as a result of irritation of a branch of the phrenic nerve in the diaphragm.

3. What physical exam maneuvers are helpful in assessing the retroperitoneal area?

Percussion of the paravertebral areas and a search for positive psoas or obturator signs are helpful in assessing the retroperitoneal area. The **psoas sign** is right or left lower quadrant pain resulting from psoas muscle irritation. To evaluate the right psoas, the patient lies on the left side and the right leg is passively extended at the hip. The test is positive if extension produces pain, suggesting a focal inflammatory process on the psoas muscle. The sign is frequently positive in retroperitoneal (psoas muscle) abscesses, which usually occur on the right side and are related to Crohn's disease; it may be positive with acute appendicitis, particularly when the appendix is in the retrocecal location. The **obturator test** involves passive internal rotation of a flexed thigh with the patient in the supine position. A positive obturator sign indicates irritation at that site, often related to an abscess.

4. List the medical and surgical differential diagnosis of acute abdominal pain.

Surgical

Perforated viscus (stomach, duodenum, colon)   Volvulus
Ruptured spleen   Ovarian torsion
Dissecting or ruptured abdominal aortic aneurysm   Strangulated hernia
Bowel obstruction   Acute cholecystitis
Appendicitis   Ruptured pancreatic
Mesenteric infarction   pseudocyst

Medical

Biliary disease (colic, cholangitis, bile   Mesenteric lymphadenitis
leak)   Nongastrointestinal causes
Pancreatitis   Pneumonia
Pseudocyst   Diabetic ketoacidosis
Crohn's disease   Sickle-cell crisis
Intermittent small bowel obstruction   Porphyria
Endometriosis   Vasculitis

5. What is postcholecystectomy syndrome?

Ten to 15% of patients who undergo cholecystectomy continue to experience the same pain postoperatively, which is referred to as the postcholecystectomy syndrome. In some patients, retained common duct stones are identified; much less commonly the sphincter of Oddi (the muscle at the opening of the bile and pancreatic ducts into the small intestine) is found to be hypertensive. Such patients usually have intermittently elevated liver function tests and/or amylase, which may be associated with progressive dilation of the bile duct. Other patients with this syndrome have irritable bowel, esophagitis, or peptic ulcer disease. For many, no explanation will be uncovered.

6. How may the chest radiograph be helpful in the diagnosis of a patient with abdominal pain?

The radiologic technique used for a chest radiograph may allow identification of free air under the diaphragm, which is not easily seen with an abdominal series. Occasionally, pleural effusions may be associated with subdiaphragmatic processes such as pancreatitis and abscesses. Lastly, pneumococcal pneumonia may present as abdominal pain in the absence of abdominal pathology.

7. What is the sentinel loop sign?

In the setting of a localized inflammatory process such as pancreatitis, a loop of bowel adjacent to the lesion may become distended with gas, thus becoming more apparent on radiographs. This is described as a sentinel loop, because it heralds an underlying process.

8. What is McBurney's point?

The pain of acute appendicitis typically originates as poorly localized periumbilical visceral pain; it then changes to a more localized right lower quadrant (RLQ) parietal pain that is frequently associated with guarding and rebound. The location in the RLQ midway between the symphysis pubis and the iliac crest where the pain settles is referred to as McBurney's point.

9. How may the location of abdominal pain be helpful?

Visceral pain tends to be poorly localized and diffuse. Pain produced by irritation of parietal peritoneum is confined to the area involved by the disease. The pain in biliary, duodenal, or pancreatic disease is often referred to the back. Pain of upper GI tract etiology tends to localize above the umbilicus, whereas pain of colonic origin is more likely to be suprapubic.

10. How should the duration of abdominal pain help in the assessment of etiology?

Pain that lasts 6 hours or longer suggests a surgical problem.

11. Why is biliary colic a misnomer?
Although biliary tract pain is described as "biliary colic," it is most often constant, lasting from a few minutes to several hours. It is impossible to distinguish gallbladder pain from stones that intermittently obstruct the common bile duct.

12. When should ischemic small bowel be considered as a cause of abdominal pain?
Mesenteric ischemia is probably the most difficult and dangerous entity to be considered in the patient with acute abdominal pain. It is most difficult because the clinical and laboratory findings do not provide clues to the significance of the problem. The abdomen may be tender and bowel signs diminished, but early in the process the examination is not impressive. Likewise, the radiographs show a nonspecific bowel gas pattern. Only when injury has progressed to bowel necrosis and the likelihood of patient survival is markedly diminished does the seriousness of the situation become apparent. Ischemic bowel should be considered when persistent mid- or migratory abdominal pain occurs in a patient with risk factors, such as embolic events, atherosclerotic cardiovascular disease, and diabetes. An elevated white blood cell count or acidosis may be clues. An angiogram should be performed. Even when the condition is diagnosed early, mortality exceeds 60%.

13. Describe the difference between ischemia of the large and small bowels.
Because of its blood supply (the superior mesenteric artery), small-bowel ischemia frequently involves the entire bowel from the ligament of Treitz (proximal jejunum) to the caecum, with dire consequences. In contrast, the collateral circulation to the large bowel usually means that compromise, which takes the form of ischemic colitis with pain and bloody diarrhea, is self-limited. It does not often progress to full-thickness injury and perforation.

14. How does the physician prove that abdominal pain in a patient with chronic pancreatitis is related to the pancreatitis?
No proof is possible. Such patients frequently have exacerbation with no change in amylase or lipase and no evidence of acute disease activity by radiographic studies. This difficulty frequently results in the labeling of patients as "drug-seeking."

15. How does abstinence from alcohol affect the pain of chronic pancreatitis?
Unfortunately, chronic pancreatitis is a process that, once initiated by chronic alcohol ingestion, progresses even in the absence of ongoing alcohol intake.

16. Describe the treatment for the pain of chronic pancreatitis.
An empirical trial of pancreatic enzyme supplementation is usually the first option. An early study suggested that it may be effective, and there are few if any side effects. Results are usually disappointing. It is often helpful to manage analgesics through a pain clinic. Percutaneous celiac axis block may predict a beneficial effect to surgical ablation of the celiac axis. Endoscopic retrograde cholangiopancreatography may be helpful in identifying a mechanical lesion (stone or stricture) that can be managed endoscopically or surgically. The most radical step, pancreatectomy, improves pain in 70–90% of patients. The pain of chronic pancreatitis "burns out" in many patients over the years.

17. How should the patient with chronic undefined abdominal pain be managed?
Serious and/or identifiable processes are eliminated by negative radiographic and laboratory studies, absence of constitutional findings, and passage of time (the most important test). Patients should not be told that nothing is wrong or that they are not having pain, but rather that by the means available today, it is impossible to identify the cause. They should be reassured that under such circumstances an undiscovered serious problem would be rare. Therefore attention should be turned to quality of life. Patients may be referred to the pain clinic to manage the real pain that the physician has not been able to elucidate. Most patients do not have the pain 1 year later.

37. CONSTIPATION

Stephen E. Steinberg, M.D.

1. How does the care giver determine whether the patient is constipated?
Constipation is diagnosed by the patient, not the physician; it is a subjective symptom, particularly in American culture. Most surveys suggest that a daily stool is common in healthy populations, but the frequency is quite variable and related to dietary intake. Of healthy persons, 5% report two or fewer stools per week. Consistency is also an aspect of constipation; hard, pelletlike stools, even if daily, often are considered to represent constipation. It is often best to use the patient's baseline pattern and to consider a decrease in frequency and/or an increase in hardness as constipation.

2. Can any test objectively assess constipation?
In addition to the history and a rectal examination that provides information about stool consistency, a test of colonic transit time may be helpful. The patient ingests radiopaque markers ("sitzmarks"), and daily flat plates are used to evaluate transit through the colon. This technique provides an objective test for a symptom that is often highly subjective. In normal individuals, without a diet excessively high in fiber, stool transit time is about 3 days with a great deal of variability.

3. Is constipation more common with increasing age?
Depending on the definition, the prevalence of constipation is 5–20%. With increasing age, 3–5 times more women than men have complaints of constipation. Although the elderly often complain of constipation (23% in one study), one-half of the same individuals report daily bowel movements, and over 90% report at least 3 bowel movements per week.

4. What is the most common gastrointestinal (GI) condition that causes patients to visit a health care provider?
Irritable bowel syndrome (IBS) is characterized by bowel habits alternating between constipation and diarrhea, accompanied by abdominal pain. It is the most common GI condition for which help is sought. It appears to be a motor disorder that is affected by stress and food intake. Concomitant psychiatric illness is more common in patients with IBS.

5. How are patients with IBS managed?
The management of IBS usually consists of eliminating other significant pathology (chronicity with absence of weight loss, fever, other constitutional signs); high-fiber diet or supplements; identification of specific dietary intolerances; antispasmodic, antidiarrheal, antiflatulent, and analgesic medications; and attention to contributing psychological factors.

6. What mechanical problems should be considered with new-onset constipation?
Strictures related to tumors, inflammation (e.g., diverticulitis, ischemic colitis), or surgery
Perianal disease (e.g., fissures, abscesses)
Volvulus
Hernias

7. Which metabolic and endocrine disorders may be associated with constipation?
Diabetes (acidosis, neuropathy)   Hypothyroidism
Uremia   Panhypopituitarism
Hypokalemia   Pheochromocytoma
Hypercalcemia (of any etiology)

8. List the drugs that may be associated with constipation.

Analgesics	Antiparkinsonian agents
Anesthetic agents	Ganglionic blockers
Antacids (calcium, aluminum)	Iron
Anticholinergics	Antihypertensives
Anticonvulsants	Laxative addiction
Antidepressants	Monoamine oxidase inhibitors
Barium sulfate	Heavy metals
Bismuth	Opiates
Diuretics	Psychotropic agents

9. How is constipation managed?
After eliminating mechanical, metabolic, endocrine, systemic, and drug etiologies, attention is turned to symptomatic management. Deficiency of dietary bulk is probably the most common cause of constipation in western countries. This problem is addressed by an increase in dietary fiber (wheat bran, oatmeal, fruits, root vegetables) and supplementation with psyllium-containing compounds. Behavioral modification to varying degrees may be helpful in patients who frequently suppress the urge to defecate because of busy lifestyle or lack of facilities. Exercise also appears to enhance colonic motility. Often reassurance is the most important therapy.

10. What disorder should be considered in a young adult with a history of chronic constipation and a dilated sigmoid on flat-plate radiography of the abdomen?
In addition to considering the above factors, the patient should be evaluated for Hirschsprung's disease. In this disorder, the absence of neurons in the diseased segment of the internal anal sphincter results in failure of reflex relaxation during defecation. The result is chronic constipation. Although more common in children, it is occasionally seen in young adults. Anal manometry documenting the sphincter disorder and biopsies showing the absence of neurons suggest the need for surgical correction.

11. What other neurologic problems are associated with constipation?
   Peripheral: autonomic neuropathies; various disorders that affect the ganglions
   Central: medulla and cord lesions and injuries (e.g., cauda equina tumor, tabes dorsalis, multiple sclerosis); cerebral lesions such as cerebrovascular accidents, parkinsonism, and tumors.

12. Describe the six different types of laxatives.
   1. Bulk-forming agents are high in fiber (natural foods, psyllium). They increase stool volume by absorbing water and require water ingestion (without water, obstruction has been reported).
   2. Emollient laxatives (dioctyl potassium sulfosuccinate) are surfactants that may increase water secretion into the gut and facilitate the mixture of water and fatty substances into the stool, thus softening it.
   3. The most common lubricant laxative is mineral oil, which decreases the colonic removal of water from the stool and lubricates it for easier passage.
   4. Magnesium, sulfate, phosphate and citrate-based laxatives exert an osmotic effect to draw water into the colon; they also promote motility.
   5. Stimulant laxatives (anthraquinone derivatives such as cascara and phenolphthalein) enhance motility by neurologic stimulation and may alter fluid secretion and absorption as well.
   6. Hyperosmotic laxatives include glycerin and lactulose.

13. When should laxative abuse be suspected?
The patient may complain of abdominal pain, nausea, vomiting, weight loss, muscle weakness, and lassitude. Hypokalemia and abnormalities on barium enema and rectal biopsy may be

noted. Diagnosis requires a high degree of suspicion. With alkalization of the stool and urine, phenolphthalein (the most commonly abused laxative) changes from colorless at pH 8.5 to pink or red above pH 9.0.

14. Are there potential risks for patients who experience chronic constipation?
Yes. The frequency of urinary tract infections appears to increase in women with constipation. Several controlled studies have also shown a link between colorectal cancer and constipation, particularly in women. This association may be related to low dietary fiber intake, which leads to smaller stool volumes and slower colonic transit time. Potential carcinogens may spend more time in contact with the colonic mucosa.

BIBLIOGRAPHY

1. Connell AM, Zfass AM: Constipation. In Bayless TM (ed): Current Therapy in Gastroenterology and Liver Disease. Toronto, B.C. Decker, 1986.
2. Devroede G: Constipation. In Sleisenger MH, Fordtran JS (eds): Gastrointestinal Disease. Philadelphia, W.B. Saunders, 1989.

38. DIARRHEA

Marcelle Owens, M.D., and Stephen E. Steinberg, M.D.

1. What is diarrhea?
Diarrhea is defined as an increase in the weight of stool (normal = < 200 grams) produced per day. It is important to make this distinction, because many patients complain of "diarrhea" when they experience loose stools, increased frequency of small amounts of stool, fecal incontinence, tenesmus, or urgency, all of which have distinct differential diagnoses.

2. What 10 elements should be included in the evaluation of a patient with diarrhea?

Character of the stool	Weight loss
Timing of bowel movements	Medications
Duration of symptoms	Past medical and surgical history
Abdominal pain	Travel history
Fever	Relationship of diarrhea to food

3. What is the significance of nocturnal diarrhea?
Nocturnal occurrence suggests that the diarrhea is likely to have an identifiable pathologic etiology. For example, patients with irritable bowel syndrome frequently complain of diarrhea, but it occurs most often early in the morning and rarely awakens the patient from sleep. On the other hand, patients with diarrhea associated with diabetes frequently are awakened from sleep.

4. How does the duration of diarrheal symptoms affect the evaluation?
Most cases of acute diarrhea (typically less than 2 weeks' duration) are infectious in etiology and are self-limited; usually they require only symptomatic management. Chronic diarrhea (typically lasting more than 2 weeks) is more difficult to characterize and may be more diagnostically challenging. Common causes of chronic diarrhea include irritable bowel syndrome, inflammatory bowel disease, lactose intolerance, medications, and various infections.

5. How does the symptom of weight loss in a patient with diarrhea help with the differential diagnosis?
Not all patients with diarrhea have weight loss. When present, weight loss is suggestive of malabsorption, inflammation (enteritis or colitis), hyperthyroidism, or malignancy.

6. What food history is helpful in the evaluation of diarrhea?
Diarrhea may be caused by milk (lactase deficiency), soft drinks (sucrose intolerance) or gluten-containing foods (celiac sprue). In addition, heavy alcohol consumption may lead to episodes of diarrhea through its effect on the intestinal mucosa.

7. When do symptoms of food poisoning occur in relationship to ingestion?
Staphylococci grow in poorly refrigerated foods, producing an exotoxin. The exotoxin produces symptoms in most people shortly after ingestion of the contaminated food. In contrast, coliforms produce symptoms through actual invasion of the host by endotoxins as well as some exotoxins. The toxins are passed vertically and require an incubation time (24–48 hours).

8. What kinds of surgery may be associated with subsequent diarrhea?
Surgery for peptic ulcer disease involving a drainage procedure (Billroth I or II or Roux-en-Y gastroenterostomy) may result in diarrhea associated with dumping. If blind loops are created (Billroth II), bacterial overgrowth may be the etiology. Finally, if part of the terminal ileum is removed (or diseased), malabsorption may allow bile acids (which induce fluid secretion) into the colon.

9. What information in the patient's history may help to distinguish between secretory and osmotic diarrhea?
If the patient fasts, osmotic diarrhea diminishes, but secretory diarrhea persists unchanged. Therefore, a history of bowel movements after the patient has gone to bed may be helpful in distinguishing between secretory and osmotic diarrhea. Causes of osmotic diarrhea include lactose intolerance, laxative abuse (lactulose), and excessive use of antacids. Causes of secretory diarrhea include enterotoxins (e.g., cholera, *Shigella sp.*, and *Escherichia coli*), laxative abuse (phenolphthalein), bile acids, fatty acids, and tumor elaboration of secretagogues (i.e., vasoactive intestinal peptide).

10. What does the symptom of tenesmus indicate?
Tenesmus is the sensation of incomplete rectal emptying. Tenesmus indicates rectal involvement in the pathologic process. Examples include proctitis (inflammatory bowel disease, infectious), anorectal fissures, and anorectal carcinoma.

11. How is the rectal examination helpful in a patient with diarrhea?
The identification of anorectal fistulas may point to the diagnosis of Crohn's disease; a rectal mass may indicate the presence of an anorectal carcinoma or villous adenoma.

12. What routine examinations should be done in the evaluation of diarrhea?
Unless the etiology of diarrhea is obvious, stool should be examined for white blood cells and blood (occult or gross), which suggest inflammatory disease (usually colonic). A positive stool clinitest suggests carbohydrate malabsorption, usually related to proximal small bowel injury, as does a stool pH $<$ 5.5. A sample of stool for assessment of fat content may suggest fat malabsorption.

13. Is flexible sigmoidoscopy useful in the evaluation of a patient with diarrhea?
Most patients with *chronic* diarrhea should undergo flexible sigmoidoscopy for evidence of colitis (infectious or inflammatory) or tumors. In addition, the typical lesions of antibiotic-associated

diarrhea or amebiasis (pseudomembranes and typical ulcerations, respectively) may be observed and biopsied during sigmoidoscopy.

14. Which parasitic diseases are most likely to cause diarrhea, usually following a trip to the outdoors?

Amebiasis and giardiasis. Three separate fresh stool specimens should be examined for ova and parasites, but examination for giardia cysts or trophozoites may be positive only 50% of the time. Examination of small bowel fluid or small bowel biopsy may be necessary for diagnosis of giardiasis. Microscopic examination of the stool for amebae has a higher yield (approximately 90%). Sigmoidoscopy may be done to evaluate the possibility of colitis due to amebiasis.

15. How is the diagnosis of antibiotic-associated colitis established?

Antibiotic-associated colitis is caused by a toxin produced by *Clostridium difficile*, which overgrows in the bowel after a patient has been treated with antibiotics or, occasionally, chemotherapy. Definitive diagnosis can be established by the use of endoscopy (sigmoidoscopy or colonoscopy) or by identification of *C. difficile* toxin in the stool. The distal colon is involved in most cases of pseudomembranous colitis, but up to one-third of patients have findings limited to the right colon and thus require colonoscopy for diagnosis. Typical lesions seen at endoscopy are multiple elevated yellowish-white plaques of varying sizes with adjacent mucosa either normal or exhibiting hyperemia and edema.

16. What is the most likely cause of bloody diarrhea in an otherwise healthy individual? How is it treated?

Infection with *Campylobacter jejuni* is the most common cause. In most cases the disease is self-limited (3–5 days), and no treatment is required. For particularly severe cases, erythromycin is the usual first choice.

17. Should antibiotics be given to patients with documented bacterial diarrhea?

No. In most cases of bacterial diarrhea, the patient is spontaneously recovering by the time the results of the stool culture are available. Antibiotic therapy may not change the disease course for several infections *(Salmonella, Yersinia,* and *Campylobacter)* after 3 days of symptoms; therefore, the potential risks of antibiotic therapy may outweigh the potential benefits. In fact, in patients with *Salmonella enteritidis* infection, the rate of intestinal carriage of the organism may actually increase with antibiotic treatment.

18. What advice and treatment should be given to patients to prevent travelers' diarrhea?

Travelers' diarrhea generally occurs in people who have traveled from an industrialized country to a developing country. It is defined as three or more loose stools per day or any loose stool accompanied by abdominal cramping, fever, or vomiting. The majority of cases of travelers' diarrhea are caused by bacterial pathogens, the most common being enterotoxigenic *E. coli.* Prevention of travelers' diarrhea can be attempted in two ways. First, travelers should avoid eating and drinking risky foods such as unpeeled fruits, nonbottled water, and salads. Second, pharmacologic agents may be taken to reduce the incidence of travelers' diarrhea, although some authorities caution against their use because of the risk of adverse side effects, emergence of drug resistance, and relative cost. Appropriate antimicrobial agents include bismuth subsalicylate, trimethoprim-sulfamethoxazole, trimethoprim alone, mecillinam, norfloxacin, and ciprofloxacin. Protective efficacy is variable, correlating with site of travel, length of stay, and choice of antimicrobial agent.

19. Which viral pathogens frequently cause diarrhea?

Rotavirus
Norwalk agent
Enteric adenovirus

BIBLIOGRAPHY

1. Gorback S (ed): Infectious Diarrhea. Boston, MA, Blackwell, 1986.
2. Jinich H, Hersh T: Physicians' Guide to the Etiology and Treatment of Diarrhea. Oradell, NJ, Medical Economics Books, 1982.
3. Miskovitz PF, Rochwarger AM: The Evaluation and Treatment of the Patient with Diarrhea. Stoneham, MA, Andover, 1993.
4. Okhuysen PC, Ericsson CD: Travelers' diarrhea: Prevention and treatment. Med Clin North Am 76:1357–1373, 1992.
5. Sleisenger MH, Fordtran JS (eds): Gastrointestinal Disease, 4th ed. Philadelphia, W.B. Saunders, 1989.

39. ANORECTAL DISEASES

Louis A. Morris, M.D., and Stephen E. Steinberg, M.D.

1. What is the difference between internal and external hemorrhoids?

Internal hemorrhoids, which arise from the superior hemorrhoidal cushion above (internal to) the dentate line and occur in the right anterior, right posterior, and left lateral positions, are lined with columnar rectal mucosa. External hemorrhoids, which occur below (external to) the dentate line and arise from the inferior hemorrhoidal venous plexus, are lined by perianal squamous epithelium. Because of the many pain receptors in the squamous epithelium, thrombosis of external hemorrhoids causes a significant amount of pain.

2. Are hemorrhoids more common in patients with portal hypertension?

The incidence of hemorrhoids is not increased in patients with portal hypertension. Hemorrhoidal bleeding may be a significant problem in patients with liver disease because of accompanying thrombocytopenia and coagulopathy. Hemorrhoids and anorectal varices, however, are separate entities. Hemorrhoids have no connection to the portal system; although the distinction can be difficult, anorectal varices span the dentate line and may bleed from either the squamous or the rectal side.

3. What are the usual presenting complaints of internal hemorrhoids?

Internal hemorrhoids may be associated with discomfort, pruritus, prolapse, fecal soiling, and, most commonly, hematochezia. Bright red blood usually is seen on toilet paper or dripping into toilet water at the end of defecation. Blood may coat the stool.

4. When is it appropriate to attribute occult bleeding to hemorrhoids?

Hemorrhoids should not be presumed to be the source of bright red or occult bleeding until other, more significant sources have been excluded.

5. What are the choices in the treatment of internal hemorrhoids?

Treatment is based on the severity of the hemorrhoids. Internal hemorrhoids are classified by the degree of protrusion. First-degree hemorrhoids bulge into the rectal lumen but not out of the anus; second-degree hemorrhoids protrude into the anal canal with straining but reduce easily; third-degree hemorrhoids require manual reduction; and fourth-degree hemorrhoids are not reducible and are at risk to strangulate. Treatment of first- and second-degree hemorrhoids is usually conservative, consisting of high-fiber diet, sitz baths, and anal hygiene. Definitive therapies, which result in thrombosis of the hemorrhoidal vessels, include photocoagulation, electrocoagulation, rubber band ligation, and cryosurgery. For third- and fourth-degree hemorrhoids the treatment of choice is hemorrhoidectomy, in which both the vessel and redundant tissue are removed.

6. What triad of findings occur with anal fissures?

Anal fissures are linear ulcers in the anal canal that cause pain and bleeding. The classic triad of a chronic anal fissure includes the fissure, a proximal hypertrophic anal papilla, and the "sentinel pile," a fibrotic piece of skin just distal to the fissure.

7. When should a search for a secondary cause of anal fissures be undertaken?

Ninety percent of anal fissures are located in the posterior midline. If a fissure is found in the lateral position, a search for a secondary cause, such as Crohn's disease, tuberculosis, carcinoma, or syphilis, should be undertaken. A history of anal intercourse also should be sought.

8. How are anorectal abscesses related to the development of anorectal fistula?

The anal glands arise from the anal canal at the level of the crypts of Morgagni. Both anorectal abscesses and fistulas appear to begin with an infection in an occluded gland. Acutely infected anal glands result in anorectal abscess, whereas chronically infected glands give rise to anorectal fistulas. Approximately two-thirds of perirectal abscesses evolve into anal fistulas or recurrent abscesses.

9. Which patients should avoid surgical treatment for rectal fistulae?

In the majority of patients without underlying problems, fistulas should be managed surgically. However, the fistulas that develop in patients with Crohn's disease present a difficult problem. A rectal ulcer may give rise to fistulas that open into the perianal skin, scrotum, vulva, or groin. The management of such fistulas requires optimal treatment of the underlying Crohn's disease. Asymptomatic fistulas do not require treatment. A commonly used medical regimen is metronidazole, 20 mg/kg/day. Partial and complete healing is seen in up to 68% of patients, but therapy with metronidazole is hampered by a high rate of paresthesias with prolonged use and recurrence of fistulas after discontinuation of the antibiotic. Surgical management is considered only after medical treatments have failed.

10. Who is at risk for rectal prolapse?

Rectal prolapse is more common in women than men and is associated with straining at stool, fecal incontinence, poor pelvic muscle tone, and pelvic trauma (including childbirth). The three types of rectal prolapse are complete, occult, and mucosal. **Complete rectal prolapse** occurs when all layers of the rectum descend through the anal canal. Clinically one sees red concentric folds that protrude with double thickness with straining. In **occult rectal prolapse** no protrusion is visible; the intussusception occurs internally and is best seen with defecography. **Mucosal rectal prolapse** occurs when a short segment of rectum, not circumferential, protrudes through the anus. Instead of concentric rings, as in complete rectal prolapse, one sees radial folds.

11. Describe the solitary rectal ulcer syndrome.

The solitary rectal ulcer syndrome is usually associated with disordered defecation. The term is a misnomer because there may be multiple ulcers or none at all (a localized erythematous or nodular lesion may be all that is seen). More common in women, the syndrome is related to prolonged straining at stool and difficulty in the initiation of defecation. Mucosal rectal prolapse is seen in 90% of patients and, combined with the high transmural pressures generated during defecation, is thought to be the cause of the ulceration, which usually occurs anteriorly in the rectum. Treatment is conservative with avoidance of straining and addition of fiber to the diet. Surgical excision is often associated with recurrence, because the underlying problem has not been corrected.

12. What causes pruritus ani?

Pruritus ani (chronic perianal itching) most often occurs without obvious explanation. Toilet papers with perfumes, dyes, or cleansing agents may be identified as the irritant. Patients are advised to cleanse the area fastidiously with water only and to use absorbent cotton or plain white facial tissue for wipes.

13. What is the differential diagnosis of anorectal pain?
The various causes of anorectal pain include acute proctitis, tumor (e.g., cauda equina and pelvic tumors), anal fissure, intersphincteric abscess, prostatitis, endometriosis, trauma or arthritis of the coccyx, and idiopathic factors such as proctalgia fugax and levator syndrome. Proctalgia fugax is characterized by severe, short-lived (less than 1 minute) attacks of rectal pain that occur infrequently. Most patients do not seek medical attention. Although the cause is unknown, it appears to be associated with the irritable bowel syndrome. Levator syndrome is a chronic aching pain of the levator ani muscles, usually precipitated by defecation or prolonged sitting. Rectal exam reveals tenderness and spasm of the levator ani muscles, usually left-sided, as the examining finger sweeps forward from the coccyx.

14. What is the differential diagnosis of acute proctitis (rectal pain, discharge) in the immuno-competent gay man?
The differential diagnosis includes four major etiologies: *Neisseria gonorrhoeae*, *Chlamydia trachomatis*, herpes simplex virus (HSV), and *Treponema pallidum*. The symptoms of gonorrhea infection include rectal discharge, bleeding, and anal dyspareunia. Asymptomatic infections are quite common. Constipation is more common than diarrhea. Acute chlamydial infection may cause bloody diarrhea, tenesmus, discharge, and, on rare occasions, fistula formation. It is associated with tender, enlarged inguinal lymph nodes that harbor the intracellular organism. Infection with HSV causes anal pain, constipation, urinary symptoms (e.g., retention), sacral paresthesias, and buttock and thigh pain. Many patients have no visible mucocutaneous lesions. Finally, arorectal syphilis may be associated with pain, discharge, and tenesmus. The chancre of primary syphilis is present on the squamous epithelium of the anal canal, and inguinal adenopathy is often present.

15. What are the risk factors for the development of anal carcinoma?
Anal carcinoma is associated with male homosexual behavior and a history of genital warts, which suggests a role for human papillomavirus as a causal agent. Other factors associated with increased risk include smoking, other sexually transmitted diseases, Crohn's disease, and renal transplantation. Recent studies suggest that the standard practice of wide excision for noninfiltrating anal carcinoma has been supplanted by radiation therapy and combination chemotherapy. Tumor regression occurs in most cases, and normal anal function is retained.

BIBLIOGRAPHY

1. Barnett JL, Raper SE: Anorectal diseases. In Yamada T (ed): Textbook of Gastroenterology. Philadelphia, J.B. Lippincott, 1991, pp 1813–1835.
2. Brandt LJ, Bernstein LH, Boley SJ, et al: Metronidazole therapy for perineal Crohn's disease: A follow-up study. Gastroenterology 83:383, 1982.
3. Daling JR, Weiss NS, Hislop TG, et al: Sexual practices, sexually transmitted diseases, and the incidence of anal cancer. N Engl J Med 317:973–977, 1987.
4. Lowry AC, Goldberg SM: Internal and overt rectal procidentia. Gastroenterol Clin North Am 16:47–69, 1987.
5. Salvati EP: The levator syndrome and its variant. Gastroenterol Clin North Am 16:71–77, 1987.
6. Smith LE: Hemorrhoids: A review of current techniques and management. Gastroenterol Clin North Am 16:79–91, 1987.

40. ACUTE LIVER DISEASE

Bahri Bilir, M.D., and Stephen E. Steinberg, M.D.

1. What are the causes of yellow skin discoloration aside from hyperbilirubinemia?

Yellow skin discoloration may be caused by ingestion of foods rich in carotene and lycopene (e.g., carrots and tomatoes) or use of antimalarial drugs (e.g., quinacrine, chloroquine), busulfan, or dinitrophenol.

2. How is the ratio of the hepatic transaminases AST to ALT useful in differentiating alcoholic hepatitis from viral and stone related liver disease?

Alcohol represses the synthesis of alanine aminotransferase (ALT) more than aspartate aminotransferase (AST). With hepatic injury (alcoholic hepatitis), the released enzymes reflect this effect. Thus a serum AST/ALT ratio > 2 is characteristic of acute alcoholic hepatitis (when the AST is < 300). Elevations in AST are modest, rarely exceeding 300–400 IU/L, regardless of the severity of the hepatic injury. In contrast, patients with acute common duct obstruction (e.g., gallstones) may have a transient (sharp) increase in the transaminases, occasionally to very high levels (and usually with associated elevation of the alkaline phosphatase). However, the AST/ALT ratio is less than 1. In acute viral or drug-induced hepatitis, enzymes typically exceed 1,000 if the injury is moderate or severe; the AST/ALT ratio is again less than 1.

3. What problems are associated with cholestasis of pregnancy?

Premature birth, increased fetal distress, and a high perinatal mortality.

4. Which serologic tests are useful in evaluating acute hepatitis of possible viral etiology?

IgM antibodies to hepatitis A virus are the best test for diagnosing acute hepatitis A. For acute hepatitis B the appropriate tests are hepatitis B surface antigen and hepatitis B surface Ab and IgM-Ab to HB_c antigen. For hepatitis C the first screening test is the enzyme-linked immuno-sorbent assay (ELISA) for the hepatitis C antibody. In the acute phase (and occasionally in the chronic phase) of hepatitis C infection, the antibody may not be positive despite active viral infection. In this case, hepatitis C virus RNA detection by polymerase chain reaction (PCR) is the most sensitive test.

5. What is the range of incubation periods for hepatitis A, B, and C viruses?

It is easiest to remember the incubation periods by the "2 to 6" rule:

    Hepatitis A: 2 to 6 *weeks*
    Hepatitis B: 2 to 6 *months*
    Hepatitis C: 2 *weeks* to 6 *months*

6. Which virus(es) is spread by sexual contact?

Hepatitis B has been shown to be transmitted by sexual contact, whereas this route has not been clearly established for the hepatitis C virus. Hepatitis A and E viruses are spread by the fecal-oral route. Hepatitis B, C, and D viruses are spread by serum. In addition, another "non-A, non-B, non-C, non-E" hepatitis virus appears to be transmittted by the fecal-oral route.

7. What is the mode of transmission of hepatitis C?

Of 500 million persons worldwide believed to be infected with hepatitis C, only 25% give a history of blood transfusion, and in 50% the mode of infection is uncertain. Likewise, the route of infection in community-acquired cases is unknown. Whereas body secretions from patients who test positive for RNA of the hepatitis C virus do not seem to contain the virus, both dentists and oral surgeons appear to be at increased risk of infection. The virus may be passed in blood product concentrates, but this method of transmission can be prevented by vapor heating.

8. What recommendations should be given to persons traveling to areas endemic for hepatitis?
For **hepatitis A:** strict sanitation (hand-washing, avoiding local water, peeling fruit); avoiding known vectors (e.g., oysters); immunoglobulin (there is no "hyperimmune" globulin); and vaccination when prolonged stays are planned.

For **hepatitis B:** vaccination and avoidance of high-risk activities (any activity that provides exposure to blood or body fluids). Endemic areas include southeast Asia.

For **hepatitis C:** no current recommendations.

9. What advice should be given to casual, household, and sexual contacts of patients with hepatitis A, B, and C?

HEPATITIS TYPE	CASUAL/HOUSEHOLD CONTACTS	SEXUAL CONTACTS
A	Strict sanitation practice Immunoglobulin	Strict sanitation practice Immunoglobulin
B	Avoid contact with blood and body secretions Vaccination	Hepatitis B immunoglobulin Vaccination
C	Simple hygiene principle (transmission rate is very low)	Controversial (some suggest immunoglobulin after exposure)

10. How risky is hepatitis B vaccination?
Fewer than 0.1% of 43,618 persons immunized for hepatitis B experienced an adverse reaction other than transient fever or sore arm. Serious reactions (e.g., Guillain-Barré syndrome) did not occur, nor did transmission of the human immunodeficiency virus (HIV). All health care workers, family members, and sexual contacts of HbsAg-positive individuals, prison guards, and other persons with likelihood of exposure should be vaccinated.

11. Who should receive hyperimmune globulin to prevent hepatitis?
Hyperimmune globulin is used only in the prophylaxis of hepatitis B infection. It should be given in the following situations:

1. After homosexual or heterosexual contact with an HBsAg-positive partner
2. After a percutaneous puncture (e.g., in health care workers or in drug abusers sharing needles)
3. In neonates who are born to HBsAg-positive mothers. Such individuals (except neonates) also should be started on hepatitis B vaccine.

12. Can patients be reinfected with hepatitis viruses?
It is extremely unlikely. Patients with chronic hepatitis C often have exacerbations that should not be confused with reinfection.

13. Which patients with viral hepatitis may be treated with interferon?
Interferon does not have a proven role in the treatment of acute viral hepatitis. Chronic hepatitis due to B, C, or D viruses may be treated with interferon. Preliminary results from the treatment of acute hepatitis C exposure (e.g., needlesticks) with interferon are encouraging.

14. When should a patient with acute viral hepatitis be hospitalized?
Patients who are severely debilitated and, in particular, unable to maintain adequate oral intake should be hospitalized. In addition, any patient whose clinical features suggest the

possible development of acute liver failure (encephalopathy and coagulopathy) should be hospitalized immediately.

15. What syndromes other than liver disease are associated with viral hepatitis?

Atypical manifestations of hepatitis A include immune complex deposition causing leuko-cytoclastic vasculitis, cryoglobulinemia, arthritis, and acute oliguric renal failure. All resolve spontaneously.

An acute illness that resembles serum sickness—with symptoms of fever, rash, urticaria, arthralgias, and on occasion acute arthritis—occurs in 10–20% of patients during the incubation period of hepatitis B. HBsAg-anti-HBs complexes apparently play a role in the pathogenesis. With persistent hepatitis B infection, immune complex glomerulonephritis may occur, and 30–50% of patients with polyarteritis nodosa have evidence of hepatitis B infections.

Hepatits C appears to be causal in some cases of aplastic anemia. Viral antibodies are highly prevalent in the serum and cryoprecipitate of patients with essential mixed cryoglobu-linemia. Hepatitis C also has been associated with Sjögren's syndrome.

16. What is the clinical course of acute liver failure?

Initially, nonspecific symptoms such as malaise and nausea develop in a previously healthy individual; jaundice develops shortly thereafter, followed by the rapid onset and progression of altered mental status (hepatic encephalopathy) and coagulopathy. Death occurs within 2–10 days.

17. How often is acute liver failure viral in etiology?

Viral hepatitis accounts for about 40–70% of all cases, including hepatitis A (rare), B (most common identifiable virus), C (rare), D (common with B), and E (rare, but occurs in epidemics with a high incidence of fulminant hepatitis, particularly in pregnant women). Cytomegalovirus, Epstein-Barr virus, and herpesviruses are occasionally implicated; herpes viruses affect immunosuppressed patients and at times pregnant women. The remaining cases are accounted for by (1) drugs and toxins, including fluorinated hydrocarbons (trichloroethylene and tetrachloroethane), *Amanita phalloides* (death-cap mushroom), and acetaminophen; (2) vascular causes (low flow states); and (3) various other disorders, including Wilson's disease, acute fatty liver of pregnancy, and Reye's syndrome. In 40% of all cases of acute liver failure, the etiology is unclear and attributed to an unknown hepatitis virus (non A–non B–non C).

18. What is the significance of a "flap" in acute liver disease?

A "flap," or asterixis, is a manifestation of progressive hepatic encephalopathy, but it is not specific to liver disease. It also may be seen with other instances of metabolic toxicity, such as uremia and carbon dioxide narcosis, as well as after cerebrovascular events. Evaluation for a "flap" consists of having the patient extend the arms and pronate the hands (with fingers spread and extended). If the patient has asterixis, he or she is unable to maintain tonic extension. The sudden relaxation results in a quick drop of the hand and slower restoration to the extended position.

19. What causes death in fulminant liver failure?

Cerebral edema is the usual cause of death. Less commonly, sepsis and metabolic complications, including hypoglycemia and multiorgan failure, are responsible.

20. What is the treatment of fulminant liver failure?

The most effective treatment is liver transplantation. Although some patients with acute liver failure recover spontaneously with supportive therapy, the mortality rate without transplantation approaches 80%. Progressive increase in prothrombin time, development of encephalopathy, and progressive renal failure are indications for transplantation. Such patients are best cared for in an intensive care setting by specialists with access to liver transplantation. Because the transport of patients with advancing encephalopathy is hazardous, consideration should be given to early transfer of any patient with altered mentation; bleeding, decrease in liver size, or precipitous fall in transaminases predicts a poor prognosis.

21. What is the success rate of orthotopic liver transplantation in acute liver failure?
The 1-year survival rate exceeds 60%.

BIBLIOGRAPHY

1. Carre G, Schiff ER: Viral, bacterial, and parasitic causes of liver disease. Curr Opin Gastroenterol 9:349–354, 1993.
2. Martin P, Pappes SC: Fulminant hepatic failure. Dig Dis Sci 8:138–151, 1990.
3. Muraca M, Fevery T, Blancheart N: Analytical aspects and clinical interpretation of serum bilirubin. Semin Liver Dis 137–138, 1988.
4. O'Grady JG, Alexander GJM, Hugler KM, Williams R: Early indicators of prognosis in fulminant liver failure. Gastroenterology 97:439–445, 1989.
5. Reichling TT, Kaplan MM: Clinical use of serum enzymes in liver disease. Dig Dis Sci 31:1601–1633, 1988.
6. Sherlock S: Viral hepatitis C. Curr Opin Gastroenterol 9:341–349, 1993.
7. Stolz A, Kaplowitz N: Approach to the patient with cholestatic jaundice. N Engl J Med 308:1515–1518, 1983.

41. CHRONIC LIVER DISEASES

Bahri Bilir, M.D., and Stephen E. Steinberg, M.D.

1. At what point should a patient be evaluated for chronic hepatitis?
Chronic hepatitis is defined as persistence of elevated transaminases for at least 6 months. Because enzyme levels may fluctuate (particularly with hepatitis C), occasional normal values do not exclude the diagnosis of chronic hepatitis.

2. What disorders should be considered in a patient with chronic hepatitis?
The differential diagnosis includes viral hepatitis (B, C, and D), drug-induced hepatitis, autoimmune hepatitis, Wilson's disease, and alpha-1 antitrypsin deficiency. Alcoholic hepatitis, steatohepatitis, and primary biliary cirrhosis also should be considered.

3. Describe the proper use and interpretation of hepatitis B serology.
Of the widely available serologic tests, hepatitis B surface antigen is the most useful marker of chronic infection and/or carrier state. Antibody to surface antigen is found in patients who have cleared the infection or who have been immunized. Core antibody can be useful in identifying early hepatitis B infections (before tests for surface antigen become positive). Because it is long-lived, core antibody is also useful in epidemiologic studies to identify individuals infected with hepatitis B in the past.

4. Describe the test for chronic hepatitis C.
Hepatitis C antibody identifies patients whose chronic hepatitis may be due to C virus. Because of the 5–10% false-negative rate, antibody-negative patients may be evaluated by the more sensitive "RIBA" assay. Identification of hepatitis C virus RNA by PCR is very sensitive but is not yet widely available.

5. When is it appropriate to test for hepatitis A and D viruses and cytomegalovirus (CMV) as etiologies for chronic hepatitis?
Hepatitis A virus does not cause chronic hepatitis. The hepatitis D virus is incomplete and requires the presence of the hepatitis B virus for infectivity; therefore the test for delta antigen

should be performed only in patients with B infections. CMV cultures should be considered in the immunocompromised patient.

6. What is the likelihood of chronicity for hepatitis B and C?
Of acute hepatitis B infections, 10–15% ultimately progress to chronicity; for hepatitis C infections, the rate is 50% or more.

7. What tests should be ordered to screen for hemochromatosis?
Transferrin saturation (greater than 61%) and serum ferritin level are the primary screening tests for hemochromatosis. The gold standard for the diagnosis of hemochromatosis is quantitation of iron in the liver biopsy specimen. Magnetic resonance imaging and computed tomography may be suggestive but are not diagnostic of hemochromatosis. Family members of affected individuals should be screened.

8. When should Wilson's disease be considered?
Wilson's disease should be considered in children or young adults with chronic elevation of transaminases. The disease is almost always diagnosed before the age of 30 years. Patients with classic Wilson's disease show both liver and neurologic involvement and a positive family history; often, however, only one organ is affected initially. Initial tests include serum copper (high), 24-hour urine copper (high), ophthalmologic examination (for Kayser-Fleischer rings), and ceruloplasmin levels (low). If the screening tests are abnormal, the diagnosis is established by quantitation of copper in the liver biopsy specimen.

9. How are patients screened for alpha-1 antitrypsin deficiency?
Alpha-1 antitrypsin is a protease inhibitor synthesized by the liver. Individuals who are homozygous for a variant of the normal protein are predisposed to the early onset of chronic active hepatitis, liver cirrhosis, and emphysema. Screening for alpha-1 antitrypsin is done by routine serum protein electrophoresis (SPEP). A normal alpha-1 peak on serum protein electrophoresis helps to rule out alpha-1 antitrypsin deficiency. The diagnosis is established by measuring the serum alpha-1 antitrypsin level and phenotyping. Because expression is variable, some patients with the deficiency may not develop hepatitis or may do so only with additional insults (alcohol, hepatitis C).

10. Which patients are at risk for the development of hepatocellular carcinoma?
Chronic hepatitis that results in cirrhosis is a significant risk factor for the development of hepatoma; chronic hepatitis B infection confers an additional risk, independent of cirrhosis. Hepatic ultrasonography and alpha-fetoprotein have been successfully used as screening modalities in high-risk patients.

11. What three laboratory findings suggest the diagnosis of primary biliary cirrhosis?
Increased levels of alkaline phosphatase, gammaglobulins (mostly IgM type), and antimitochondrial antibody titers are highly suggestive of primary biliary cirrhosis. Bilirubin is elevated late in the disease, which occurs with greatest frequency in middle-aged women.

12. List five findings in the extremities that are associated with chronic liver disease.
Palmar erythema	Dupuytren's contracture (most often
Spider angiomata	seen in alcoholic cirrhosis)
White nails	Thenar and hypothenar atrophy

13. When is caput medusae seen?
Caput medusae is a name given to engorged veins surrounding the umbilicus. The direction of blood flow is away from the umbilicus. This physical finding is most commonly seen in portal hypertension due to cirrhosis, but it may occur with thrombosis of the inferior or superior vena cava.

14. Should asymptomatic esophageal varices be treated prophylactically to prevent bleeding?
Prophylactic eradication of incidentally discovered varices by sclerotherapy or variceal ligation banding is not recommended. Sclerotherapy has proved ineffective and ligation has not yet been evaluated. Some data suggest that one can delay the time to initial bleeding by treating nonbleeding varices with beta-adrenergic blockade.

15. What is the role of endoscopy in the initial management of acute variceal hemorrhage?
After resuscitation, patients should undergo endoscopic evaluation with sclerosis or banding of varices. This approach controls the initial bleeding in more than 90% of patients.

16. Why should acetaminophen be avoided in patients with alcoholic liver disease?
Chronic alcohol intake increases the activity of the cytochrome P450 system, normally a minor pathway of acetaminophen metabolism. A larger fraction of the acetaminophen is metabolized through the P450 system, resulting in increased amounts of toxic metabolites, which ordinarily are detoxified by glutathione. Alcoholics also have low amounts of glutathione in the liver because of concomitant poor nutrition. As a result, the increased levels of toxic metabolites cannot be detoxified, and hepatocyte necrosis results, occasionally even with modest amounts of acetaminophen (3–6 gm/day).

17. Describe the management of the patient with moderate ascites.
The majority of patients with mild ascites can be managed with salt restriction (< 2 gm/day). Moderate ascites (visible, but not tense) usually requires a potassium-sparing diuretic (spironolactone or amiloride), occasionally in combination with a loop diuretic (furosemide or bumetanide). The combination is synergistic in patients with liver disease. If ascites is still refractory, large-volume paracentesis or placement of a LeVeen shunt may be tried.

BIBLIOGRAPHY

1. Berg PS, Klein R, Lindenborn-Fotmos T: Antimitochondrial antibodies in primary biliary cirrhosis. J Hepatol 2:123, 1986.
2. Edwards CQ, Kushner JP: Screening for hemochromatosis. N Engl J Med 328:1616–1620, 1993.
3. Hollinger FB, Lemon SM, Margolis HS: Viral hepatitis and liver disease. In Proceedings of the 7th International Symposium. Baltimore, Williams & Wilkins, 1991.
4. Madden WC: Chronic hepatitis. Dis Mon 2:53–126, 1993.
5. McIntyre N: Symptoms and Signs of Liver Disease. Oxford Textbook of Clinical Hepatology, vol. 1. Oxford, Oxford University Press, 1991.
6. Rowdley KV, Smanik EJ, Tavill AS: Metabolic liver diseases. Curr Opin Gastroenterol 2:466–473, 1992.
7. Runyon BA: Care of the patient with ascites. N Engl J Med 330:337–342, 1994.
8. Runyon BA: Bacterial infection in patients with cirrhosis. J Hepatol 18:271–272, 1993.
9. Wong F, Blendi LM: Ascites and porto-systemic encephalopathy as complications of cirrhosis. Curr Opin Gastroenterol 9:391–395, 1993.

42. BILIARY TRACT DISEASE

Louis A. Morris, M.D., and Stephen E. Steinberg, M.D.

1. A 40-year-old obese white woman on estrogen replacement therapy has gallstones. What is the most likely composition of the stones?
In the United States 80% of gallstones are composed of cholesterol. Cholesterol stones are extremely common and occur more frequently in women and with advancing age. By age 75 years, 20% of men and 35% of women have gallstones.

2. List the risk factors for cholesterol gallstones.

- Age: 50 years and over
- Gender: female
- Diet: high fat
- Genetics: siblings
- Obesity > 20% above ideal body weight
- Pregnancy
- Rapid weight loss
- Drugs: Clofibrate, oral estrogens, contraceptives
- Ethnic groups: American Indians
- Total parenteral nutrition

3. A 30-year-old black man with sickle-cell anemia has gallstones. What type of gallstone is the patient most likely to have?

The patient most likely has pigment stones, which are formed in the presence of unconjugated bilirubin and precipitate with calcium to form calcium bilirubinate stones. Amounts of unconjugated bilirubin are increased in hemolytic anemia and cirrhosis. Pigment stones come in two varieties: brown and black. Black stones are radiopaque and hard, whereas brown stones are soft and radiolucent. Brown stones are common in Asia as a result of infection by bacteria and parasites that deconjugate bilirubin.

4. Distinguish between cholecystolithiasis, choledocholithiasis, and biliary colic.

Cholecystolithiasis and **choledocholithiasis** are the descriptions for stones in the gall-bladder and in the bile duct, respectively. Both often occur without symptoms. In reality, biliary pain is not colicky, but rather a steady (not fluctuating) pain localized to the epigastrium or less commonly the right upper quadrant. It may last from 1–6 hours and often occurs at random, with no relation to meals. Pain frequently radiates to the right scapula or shoulder or into the back. Because it is related to obstruction rather than infection, it usually occurs without constitutional signs (e.g., fever, chills). The **biliary colic** of a typical "gall-bladder attack" is indistinguishable from that of transient obstruction of the bile duct with a stone.

5. What are the complications of choledocholithiasis?

In addition to biliary colic, bile duct stones may cause cholangitis, pancreatitis, and, less commonly, strictures or secondary biliary cirrhosis.

6. What is the most common cause of pancreatitis in nondrinkers?

Gallstone-related pancreatitis is the most frequent type in nondrinkers. It typically occurs in patients with smaller rather than larger stones, presumably because small stones are able to migrate to the end of the bile duct at its junction with the pancreatic duct. The mechanisms by which the stones cause pancreatitis are unclear. Biliary sludge and crystals are also associated with pancreatitis. Biliary sludge occurs when cholesterol or calcium bilirubinate precipitates in bile and may be a precursor to gallstone formation. Studies have shown that after gallstones and alcohol, biliary sludge is the third most common etiology of acute pancreatitis. Sphincter of Oddi dysfunction, pancreas divisum, or unsuspected stones are less common. Ceftriaxone, a third-generation cephalosporin, has been implicated as a cause of biliary sludge; it may precipitate with calcium to form crystals and sludge. The crystals and sludge dissolve when the drug is discontinued; thus symptoms rarely require surgical intervention.

7. What is the current recommendation for patients with an incidental finding of gallstones?

The majority of patients with gallstones are asymptomatic. Several studies have followed patients with initially asymptomatic stones and recorded the incidence of symptoms or complications. In a study of 123 faculty members of the University of Michigan who were followed for 24 years, the rate of development of biliary pain was 1.3% per year. At 20 years of follow-up only 18% were symptomatic. Other studies have confirmed the development of symptoms in 1–2% per year. These studies show that the majority of patients with gallstones have a benign course; therefore no prophylactic therapy is required.

8. Once symptoms develop, does the natural history of gallstones change?
Probably. Patients who develop biliary pain are likely to have recurrent attacks, although up to 30% of patients have no further episodes. The rate of recurrence may be as high as 30–50% per year in the first few years. Acute complications in patients who present with biliary pain occur at a rate of approximately 1–1.5% per year.

9. Is fatty food intolerance related to gallstone disease?
It is commonly believed that fatty foods cause increased biliary pain; however, studies using test meals in a blinded fashion have shown no correlation between fat content and symptoms. In addition, gallbladder contractility does not change significantly when fatty foods or nonfatty foods are ingested. Symptoms such as belching, bloating, and fatty food intolerance are not caused by gallstones.

10. What is the appropriate treatment for gallstones in diabetic patients?
Early autopsy studies purported to show an increased risk for gallstones in diabetic patients, but the studies were not controlled for confounding risk factors such as obesity and hyperlipidemia, disorders that are common in the diabetic population. Studies that controlled for these factors have not shown an increased risk of gallstone formation. In addition, previous studies appeared to show a significantly greater morbidity and mortality for cholecystectomy in diabetic patients than in the general population. More recent data indicate that biliary surgery in diabetic patients is not associated with an increased morbidity and mortality. Therefore, diabetic patients should be managed no differently from other patients.

11. What radiologic studies are useful in the diagnosis of patients with suspected gallstones?
Ultrasonography has high specificity and sensitivity for the diagnosis of gallstones and is usually the first test. The false-negative rate is approximately 5%. Ultrasound is also useful in detecting fluid around the gallbladder, thickening of the gallbladder wall, and dilation of the biliary tree. However, it is not helpful in excluding stones in the common bile duct; the false-negative rate is high unless the bile duct is markedly dilated. Oral cholecystography is useful when nonsurgical methods of gallstone treatment are considered. Contrast tablets are administered to the patient on the night before the study, and films are obtained to assess the size and number of stones, patency of the cystic duct, and function of the gallbladder.

12. What is the best test to order when acute cholecystitis is suspected?
Hepatobiliary scintigraphy is highly useful in the diagnosis of acute cholecystitis. After a 2–4 hour fast the patient is given a radiolabeled agent, which is taken up by the liver and excreted into the biliary system. Images of the gallbladder, common bile duct, and small bowel should appear within 45 minutes. Failure to image the gallbladder by 90 minutes is strongly suggestive of cystic duct obstruction, but false-positive scans may result from prolonged fasting or total parenteral nutrition. The false-negative rate of this test is less than 5%.

13. When should a common duct stone be suspected? What test should be ordered?
The most reliable way to confirm the clinical suspicion of common bile duct stones is with serial liver function tests, including assessment of direct bilirubin, transaminases, and alkaline phosphatase. When a stone obstructs the duct, the transaminases rise abruptly, occasionally to very high levels. Within a few hours they begin to fall (even if the obstruction persists), and the levels of direct bilirubin and alkaline phosphatase rise at a moderate pace. When the obstruction is alleviated (by passage, movement of the stone back into the duct, or removal), all abnormalities rapidly return toward normal. Cholecystitis is associated with only minimal changes in liver function tests, and hepatitis does not demonstrate rapid fluctuations. Although the finding of a dilated common duct on ultrasound or computed tomographic (CT) scan may be suggestive, both modalities often fail to find common duct stones, especially when the duct is of normal caliber. Neither test is required to make or act on the diagnosis of common bile duct stone.

14. What is Charcot's triad?
Stones within the common bile duct are usually associated with infected bile, and cholangitis often results if obstruction occurs. Charcot's triad consists of upper abdominal pain, fever secondary to bacteremia, and jaundice from extrahepatic obstruction. Reynold's pentad is the addition of hypotension and mental confusion in more severe suppurative cases. The most common organisms include *Escherichia coli, Klebsiella* sp., *Pseudomonas* sp., enterococci, and anaerobes.

15. What nonsurgical options are available for the management of gallstones?
The medical management of symptomatic gallstones includes oral bile acids, contact dissolution therapy, and extracorporeal shock wave lithotripsy. Oral bile acids such as ursodeoxycholic acid work by increasing the solubility of cholesterol in bile; therefore, they are effective only for cholesterol stones. Stones dissolve at a rate of 1 mm/month and must be less than 1.5 cm. The best stones for this therapy are smaller than 0.5 cm and float on oral cholecystography (indicating that the density of the stone is less than that of bile). The negative aspect is that the drug must be taken for 2 years; in addition, recurrence rates of up to 50% at 5 years have been reported. Candidates for oral dissolution therapy include older patients who are at high risk for surgery and patients on a rapid weight-loss program, who are at increased risk for developing gallstones.

16. What is the role of extracorporeal shock wave lithotripsy (ESWL)?
Although ESWL has been approved by the FDA for the treatment of kidney stones, it has not received approval for gallstones. Shock waves are focused on the gallstones and fragment them into small particles. Appropriate candidates are patients with 1–3 radiolucent stones (i.e., no calcification) with a diameter $\leq$ 3 cm. In addition, it is believed that oral dissolution agents must be used to clear the gallbladder of the resulting fragments. The clearance rate diminishes with the number of stones in the gallbladder. Contraindications to ESWL include use of anticoagulation; presence of a coagulopathy, pregnancy, aneurysms, or cysts in the path of the shock waves; and complications related to the gallstones.

17. Which procedure is associated with more complications—laparoscopic or open cholecystectomy?
Open cholecystectomy is one of the safest surgical procedures with mortality rates of less than 1%, although the rate increases with age and for urgent procedures. The incidence of bile duct injury is 0.1–0.2%. Recovery time after open cholecystectomy may take months because of the extensive abdominal incision. Laparoscopic cholecystectomy has gained popularity since its introduction in 1989. The advantages include minimal incisions, decreased postoperative pain, improved recovery time with discharge from the hospital in 1–2 days, and unrestricted activity at 8 days. The disadvantages of laparoscopic cholecystectomy include longer anesthesia time and increased rate of complications, which are likely to improve as experience with the procedure increases. The rate of bile duct injury is approximately 0.5%; 5% of patients require conversion to open cholecystectomy.

18. What are the contraindications to the performance of laparoscopic cholecystectomy?
Contraindications to laparoscopic cholecystectomy include generalized peritonitis, severe acute pancreatitis, cirrhosis with portal hypertension, unresponsive coagulopathy, and carcinoma of the gallbladder. Pregnancy in the third trimester is a contraindication because of potential injury to the uterus. Patients with chronic obstructive pulmonary disease need to be monitored carefully because the CO_2 used to insufflate the abdominal cavity may cause hypercarbia and acidosis. Obesity is generally not a problem unless the abdominal wall is so large that the instruments cannot reach the gallbladder.

19. What percentage of patients with pancreatitis secondary to gallstones will pass the gallstone?
It is postulated that the lodging of a gallstone at the duodenal papilla is the precipitant of an attack of acute gallstone pancreatitis. In approximately 80–90% of patients with gallstone

pancreatitis; the stones pass into the gastrointestinal tract. This estimate is based on studies that found stones in the stool of patients within 8 days of the attack of pancreatitis. There appears to be no relation between stone size (1–12 mm) and severity of the pancreatitis.

20. What is the role of endoscopic retrograde cholangiopancreatography (ERCP) in acute gallstone pancreatitis?
A recent study found that ERCP with papillotomy performed within 24 hours of the onset of symptoms resulted in a decrease in incidence of biliary sepsis. There was no change in mortality or other complications, such as pseudocyst. ERCP is indicated in episodes of gallstone pancreatitis that are deemed to be severe, that do not resolve with conservative measures, or that are associated with possible acute cholangitis.

21. What is the association between gallstones and gallbladder carcinoma? Does cholecystectomy have a role in the prevention of gallbladder cancer?
The incidence of gallbladder cancer in the United States is low. Despite a definite association with gallstones (70–90% of patients with gallbladder cancer have gallstones), the incidence of gallbladder cancer in patients with gallstones is low (0.5–3%). A causal role has not been proved. In general, cholecystectomy is not recommended for the prevention of gallbladder carcinoma, with the possible exception of very large stones.

BIBLIOGRAPHY

1. Aucott JN, Cooper GS, Bloom AD, et al: Management of gallstones in diabetic patients. Arch Intern Med 153:1053–1058, 1993.
2. Carey MC: Pathogenesis of gallstones. Am J Surg 165:410–419, 1993.
3. Fan ST, Lai ECS, Mok FPT, et al: Early treatment of acute biliary pancreatitis by endoscopic papillotomy. N Engl J Med 328:228–232, 11993.
4. Goldschmid S, Brady PG: Approaches to the management of cholelithiasis for the medical consultant. Med Clin North Am 77:413–426, 1993.
5. Lai ECS, Mok FPT, Tan ESY, et al: Endoscopic biliary drainage for severe acute cholangitis. N Engl J Med 326:1582–1586, 1992.
6. National Institutes of Health Consensus Development Conference Statement on Gallstones and Laparoscopic Cholecystectomy. Am J Surg 165:390–396, 1993.
7. Ransohoff DF, Gracie WA: Treatment of gallstones. Ann Intern Med 119:606–619, 1993.
8. Strasberg SM, Calvien PA: Overview of therapeutic modalities for the treatment of gallstone disease. Am J Surg 165:420–426, 1993.

43. ENDOSCOPY: INDICATIONS AND OUTCOMES

Nuray Bilir, M.D., Randall Lee, M.D., and Stephen E. Steinberg, M.D.

1. When should colonoscopy be performed instead of a double-contrast barium enema?
Colonoscopy is the preferred method for evaluation of symptoms of hematochezia, for surveillance after resection of colon cancer or polyps, and for surveillance of inflammatory bowel disease. For these indications, the ability to perform hemostasis therapy, to obtain biopsies, and to remove polyps during colonoscopy outweighs the cost savings of the purely diagnostic double-contrast barium enema.

2. What is the recommended surveillance interval after colonoscopic removal of a few benign adenomatous polyps?

According to data from the National Polyps Study, after an initial high-quality colonoscopy during which all synchronous adenomas were removed, a follow-up colonoscopy should be performed in 3 years. The purpose of this surveillance is to check for adenomas which may have been missed on the first colonoscopy (synchronous lesions) and for adenomas which may have formed in the interim (metachronous lesions). If the examination at the 3-year interval is unremarkable, the subsequent intervals may be extended to 5 years. Because it takes 3–6 years for a polyp to grow to visibility and another 4–6 years for the small proportion that will become malignant to do so, a long screening window is possible.

3. What is the diagnostic accuracy of colonoscopy?

The sensitivity of colonoscopy varies with the size of the lesion. Colonoscopy has a detection rate of greater than 95% for lesions larger than 1.0 cm, of 85–90% for lesions between 0.5–1.0 cm, and of 70–80% for lesions less than 0.5 cm in diameter.

4. What are the usual indications for esophagogastroduodenoscopy (EGD)?

An EGD is usually indicated to evaluate upper abdominal symptoms that have not responded to an appropriate trial of therapy or that are associated with anorexia and weight loss, complaints of dysphagia or odynophagia, or persistent nausea and vomiting. Additionally, EGD is recommended to biopsy lesions detected by radiographs, to treat upper gastrointestinal (GI) bleeding, and to assess mucosal injury after ingestion of a corrosive agent.

5. How effective is endoscopic therapy of bleeding peptic ulcers?

Endoscopic therapy with an Nd:YAG laser, thermal probe, bipolar electrical probe, or injection of a sclerosant induces acute hemostasis in an actively bleeding peptic ulcer in approximately 90% of patients. When compared with conservative medical therapy, endoscopic hemostasis significantly reduces the cost of hospitalization, the need for transfusions, and the requirement for emergency surgery.

6. What are the advantages of early upper endoscopy for acute gastrointestinal bleeding?

In addition to controlling hemorrhage in many situations, early endoscopy can be used to assess the risk of ongoing or additional bleeding. This assessment may allow a decision for early discharge in the patient with a Mallory-Weiss tear (low risk of rebleed), esophatitis, or low-risk ulcer disease; it also affects decisions about which patients need monitoring in an intensive care setting and for how long.

7. Should EGD be performed for a complaint of bright red blood per rectum (BRBpr)?

Melena, or black, tarry stools and "coffee grounds" results from the action of acidic blood in the stomach or proximal small bowel. In patients with massive upper GI bleeding, there may not be enough time (or acid) for this action to occur because of the effect of blood in intestinal transit. Any patient who is hemodynamically unstable or who has an uncertain source of BRBpr should undergo upper endoscopy. A nasogastric tube, even if it returns bile, does not exclude an upper GI source.

8. Why is EGD essential to the evaluation of a patient who may have swallowed a corrosive substance?

An EGD offers a better assessment of the extent and severity of the chemical burn than a history and physical examination or an upper GI barium radiograph and this allows better therapeutic management decisions. Minor mucosal burns may be managed conservatively. Severe mucosal burns should prompt consideration of urgent surgical resection before perforation develops. Small-caliber, flexible endoscopes do not increase the risk of perforation.

9. What are the usual indications for endoscopic retrograde cholangiopancreatography (ERCP)?

ERCP is usually indicated to evaluate and treat symptoms that suggest disorders of the biliary system and pancreas. Examples include jaundice that is possibly obstructive; cholangitis; acute or recurrent pancreatitis; recurrent upper abdominal pain associated with transient liver function test abnormalities; and, less commonly, steatorrhea. Specific disorders that may be diagnosed and treated by ERCP include choledocholithiasis, benign or malignant bile duct stricture, bile duct leak, pancreatic pseudocyst, and pancreatic duct disruption.

10. What is the role of ERCP in suspected acute cholangitis?

Acute cholangitis is usually caused by biliary obstruction from a gallstone. When severe, it is associated with a high mortality rate ($> 30\%$), whether managed conservatively or surgically. Endoscopic drainage is safe and effective and should be used as early as possible in the course of the disease.

11. What is the role of ERCP in the evaluation of recurrent acute pancreatitis?

In approximately 30% of patients with recurrent pancreatitis of uncertain etiology, ERCP yields an explanation. Possible findings include previously unsuspected common duct stones; anatomic abnormalities (pancreas divisum, choledochocele); sphincter of Oddi dysfunction; and, rarely, pancreatic malignancy.

12. What is the significance of post-ERCP hyperamylasemia?

Salivary amylase is often elevated after any form of upper endoscopy. An asymptomatic rise in serum amylase may be present after 40–75% of ERCPs that image the pancreatic duct. The incidence of post-ERCP pancreatitis varies according to which study is quoted and how pancreatitis is defined. Clinically significant pancreatitis occurs after only about 1% of all ERCPs. The performance of sphincter of Oddi manometry during an ERCP increases the incidence of acute pancreatitis.

13. What are the indications for placement of a percutaneous endoscopic gastrostomy tube (PEG)?

A PEG should be considered when a patient with a functional GI tract is not expected to ingest orally for several weeks. Examples include patients with oropharyngeal dysphagia due to neurologic injury and patients with obstructing oropharyngeal tumors. In addition, PEG should be considered as a palliative decompression device for patients with chronic bowel obstruction due to peritoneal carcinomatosis.

14. Describe the management of suspected esophageal foreign body impactions.

If the suspected foreign body is radiopaque, it is helpful to search for it with a plain radiograph of the neck or chest. Endoscopy should be performed for evaluation and removal; the prior performance of a barium study makes endoscopy more difficult and should be avoided.

15. How does endoscopic ultrasound (EUS) compare with computed tomography (CT) in the evaluation of carcinoma of the mediastinal area?

EUS detects mediastinal lymph node involvement with an accuracy of 70–80%, whereas CT detects only 20–50% of such lesions. In addition, EUS is more sensitive than CT for detecting malignant invasion into the diaphragm, aorta, and pericardium. Mounting data suggest that an EUS examination should be performed on all candidates for curative resection of esophogeal carcinoma.

16. What is the role of laser therapy in the treatment of GI malignancies?

Use of the laser through the endoscope may offer effective palliation for patients with obstructing lesions of the esophagus or rectosigmoid and for patients with bleeding. It may be curative for small lesions, when the patient is not a surgical candidate.

17. How does endoscopic management of malignant biliary tract lesions compare with surgical or percutaneous palliation?

The endoscopic placement of biliary stents is safer and more effective than percutaneous placement of similar stents and allows shorter hospital stays than surgical decompression. Surgery, however, is preferred when the tumor threatens to obstruct the bowel.

BIBLIOGRAPHY

1. Bond JH: Colonoscopy and neoplastic disorders of the colon. Gastrointest Endosc Clin North Am 3(4):585–776, 1993.
2. Bond JH: Polyp guideline: Diagnosis, treatment, and surveillance for patients with nonfamilial colorectal polyps. Ann Intern Med 119:836–843, 1993.
3. Jensen DM: Severe nonvariceal upper GI hemorrhage. Gastrointest Endosc Clin North Am 1(2):209–433, 1991.
4. Kozarek RA: Endoscopic approach to biliary stones. Gastrointest Endosc Clin North Am 1(1):3–208, 1991.
5. Yamada T (ed): Textbook of Gastroenterology. Philadelphia, J.B. Lippincott, 1991.

VII. Gender-specific Care

44. BREAST MASSES AND PAIN

Elizabeth Brew, M.D.

1. What is one of the more difficult aspects of evaluating a woman with a palpable breast mass?

Determining whether an actual mass is present in the breast can be very difficult. Discrete and dominant describe a mass that needs to be biopsied. Suspicious masses are three-dimensional, distinct from surroundng tissues, and generally asymmetrical in relation to the other breast. Only 10–20% of breast masses are initially discovered by the physician; therefore, an area that the patient feels is abnormal must be evaluated thoroughly. The examining physician must always err on the side of caution.

2. What aspects of the history are important in the evaluation of a breast mass?

Duration of the mass
Related and referred pain
Change in physical characteristics with menstrual cycle variations
Preexisting breast cancer risk factors (menstrual and family history, previous breast disease)

3. What characteristics of a breast mass are suggestive of cancer?

Masses that are firm, nontender, irregular with indistinct borders, immobile, and fixed due to skin or deep fascial attachments are suggestive of cancer. Skin dimpling and nipple retraction are also suspicious for carcinoma. Bloody nipple discharge and palpably enlarged lymph nodes are other worrisome findings.

4. What is the likely diagnosis in an adolescent with a discrete breast mass?

The mass is most likely a fibroadenoma. After fine-needle aspiration confirms the diagnosis, surgical removal should be considered, because the lesion is likely to enlarge.

5. What is fibrocystic disease of the breast?

Unclear. The term should not be used, because it does not refer to a specific disease or entity.

6. What causes breast pain or tenderness?

1. Cyclical breast tenderness in women of reproductive age that is related to the menstrual cycle
2. Breast abscess
3. Inflammatory breast carcinoma

7. What clue suggests inflammatory breast carcinoma as opposed to an infection?

Erythema completely surrounding the areola suggests malignancy until proved otherwise. This finding is virtually absent in breast infection.

8. What organisms are responsible for breast infections?
Staphylococci and anaerobic organisms (peptostreptococci).

9. What is the gold standard in the diagnosis of a palpable solid breast mass?
The gold standard is excisional biopsy: "Perfection in diagnosis will require the removal of every solid mass. This can be expected to result in the biopsy of many benign lesions, but removal of many of them is desirable on other grounds. Although in some instances the probability of cancer may be exceedingly small, it is never zero. If biopsy is not recommended, the probability of cancer should be estimated so the patient can decide whether the level of risk is acceptable to her."[1]

Other biopsy techniques include **fine-needle aspiration** (see question 13), which aspirates cells that are then smeared on a slide for cytologic analysis. **Core-needle biopsy** withdraws a core of tissue for pathologic evaluation. **Incisional biopsy** removes part of the mass, whereas **excisional biopsy** excises the entire mass.

10. What role does mammography play in the evaluation of a woman with a palpable breast mass?
It is absolutely critical to have mammography in its proper perspective. The purpose of mammography is not primarily to characterize the mass but to evaluate the breasts for clinically occult lesions. A normal mammogram adds no information to the evaluation of a palpable breast mass. An abnormal mammogram may or may not be of any value, and even when a suspicious lesion is seen on a mammogram, it may not coincide with a palpable mass. Therapeutic decisions should **not** be based on a negative mammogram in a woman with a palpable breast mass.

11. Are mammograms necessary in evaluating a woman with a palpable breast mass?
Mammography is part of the examination of a woman with a breast mass but its limitations must be kept in mind. One study reported that when both palpation and mammography suggest that a mass is benign, the error rate is 3.7%—far too high to be acceptable to patients and physicians.[3]

12. What are the sensitivity and specificity of mammography, physical examination, and a combination of both?

	SENSITIVITY (%)	SPECIFICITY (%)	OVERALL ACCURACY
Combination mammography and physical examination	95	—	77
Mammography alone	94	55	73
Physical examination alone	88	71	81

From Van Dam PA, Van Goethem MLA, Kersschot E, et al: Palpable solid breast masses: Retrospective single and multimodality evaluation of 201 lesions. Radiology 166:435–439, 1988.

13. What is the role of fine-needle aspiration (FNA) in the evaluation of a solid breast mass?
Fine-needle aspiration of breast masses has become popular in recent years, but it is not always a substitute for open biopsy. However, the use of FNA has markedly diminished the need for open surgical biopsy of lesions that ultimately turn out to be benign. The false-negative rate (negative aspiration cytology in a patient with cancer) varies with the cytopathologist and ranges from 1–35%. This false-negative rate is the Achilles' heel of FNA; therefore, a negative FNA in the presence of a suspicious mass does **not** exclude cancer. The combination of physical examination, mammography, and FNA has a diagnostic accuracy approaching 100%.

The use of fine-needle aspiration in the diagnosis of cancer and subsequent determination of surgical therapy is controversial. However, an excisional biopsy can be done immediately before the operation to confirm a positive FNA.

14. What is a triple negative diagnostic test?

"Triple negative" refers to the combination of a "not suspicious" physical examination, a normal mammogram, and fine-needle aspiration cytology that is not suspicious for cancer. When all three tests are negative, the chance that the lesion is cancerous is reduced to less than 1%. This reduction from the higher false-negative rate of FNA alone is important to justify the use of aspiration cytology. In a combined positive diagnostic test, the physical exam, mammogram, and FNA are suspicious for breast cancer.

15. What technique is used to determine whether a palpable breast mass is a cyst?

Needle aspiration can be both diagnostic and therapeutic. Ultrasound may be necessary first if the patient will not permit aspiration or if the mass is too small and deep for reliable aspiration. Even the most experienced examiner cannot distinguish a cystic from a solid lesion on physical examination.

16. What should be done with the fluid from a cyst aspiration?

The fluid may be discarded if it is not bloody, if the mass disappears, and if the mammogram is normal. Cytologic analysis of cyst fluid is recommended if the fluid is bloody or aspirated from a cyst in a postmenopausal woman. A follow-up mammogram is important to visualize tissue surrounding the collapsed cyst. If a residual mass remains, either fine-needle aspiration or biopsy is recommended.

17. What should be done with a cyst that reappears after the first aspiration?

A cyst may be aspirated one or two times after the initial aspiration. With each repeat aspiration, the physician must review whether the mammogram is normal and the mass completely disappears. Statistically, less than 20% of cysts require repeat aspirations, and less than 9% reappear after two or three aspirations.

18. What is the role of stereotactic-guided core needle biopsy in a woman with a palpable breast mass?

Once again, the management of a palpable mass must not be confused with the management of a mammographic lesion. A palpable mass can be evaluated without stereotactic or other radiologic guidance. If a mammographic lesion is present in the same breast, one must be careful to ensure that the mammographic lesion is coincident with the palpable mass.

19. Can a woman under the age of 30 years develop breast cancer?

Yes. A substantial number of women under the age of 30 years develop breast cancer; however the chance that a breast mass is malignant in women less than 25 years of age is essentially zero.

20. List the pitfalls in the management of palpable breast masses.

1. Assuming that mammography is diagnostic.

    Mammography seldom defines a mass well enough to avoid further diagnostic evaluation (FNA or excisional biopsy). Thus the value of mammography in managing a palpable breast mass is minimal (detection of occult or multifocal disease).

2. Assuming that the radiographic lesion seen on mammography is the same as the palpable lesion.

    If there is any question about this correlation, further evaluation is essential. A follow-up mammogram should be obtained 3 or 4 months after biopsy of all mammographically diagnosed lesions to determine that the suspicious mass was actually excised. The follow-up mammogram also serves as a new baseline, showing the changes after biopsy.

3. Letting a negative or nonsuspicious mammogram influence the judgment of whether a palpable mass needs to be biopsied.

    The decision to biopsy or aspirate should be made on physical examination criteria.

4. Assuming that a benign aspiration cytology is definitive.

BIBLIOGRAPHY

1. Bland KI, Copeland B, Copeland EM III (eds): The Breast: Comprehensive Management of Benign and Malignant Diseases. Philadelphia, W.B. Saunders, 1991.
2. Donegan WL: Evaluation of a palpable breast mass. N Engl J Med 327:937–942, 1992.
3. Layfield LF, Glasgow BJ, Cramer H: Fine-needle aspiration in the management of breast masses. Pathol Annu 24(Pt 2):23–62, 1989.
4. Van Dam PA, Van Goethem MLA, Kersschot E, et al: Palpable solid breast masses: Retrospective single and multimodality evaluation of 201 lesions. Radiology. 166:435–439, 1988.
5. Zitarelli J, Burkhart LL, Weiss SM: False negative breast biopsy for palpable mass. J Surg Oncol 52:61–63, 1993.

45. DYSFUNCTIONAL UTERINE BLEEDING

Julie Rifkin, M.D.

1. Define dysfunctional uterine bleeding.
Loss of the coordinated cyclic hormonal changes that govern the normal menstrual cycle leads to abnormal uterine bleeding. Abnormal uterine bleeding is the most common complaint presented to a gynecologist. Most causes of dysfunctional uterine bleeding fall into the following categories:
  1. Dysfunctional bleeding, with no evidence of organic lesions
  2. Pregnancy
  3. Pelvic lesions—benign or malignant
  4. Extragenital problems: coagulopathies, endocrinopathies

2. What is a normal menstrual cycle?
The normal menstrual cycle ranges from 25–35 days. Day one of the cycle is the first day of bleeding. The average amount of blood lost is 30 ml per cycle; less than 80 ml is considered normal. Many women flow for as few as 2 days or as many as 8 days.

3. What may cause mid-cycle spotting?
Mid-cycle (ovulatory) spotting may occur because ovarian estrogen production is inhibited by the high levels of luteinizing hormone (estrogen withdrawal bleeding).

4. Define these 10 terms that refer to abnormal bleeding patterns.

Amenorrhea	Absent menstrual flow for more than 90 days
Hypermenorrhea	Excessive uterine bleeding occurring during a *regular* menstrual duration
Hypomenorrhea	Decreased menstrual flow, usually with a decrease in duration
Menometrorrhagia	Irregular intermenstrual bleeding with prolongation of menstrual flow
Menorrhagia	Excessive bleeding during a menstrual period either in number of days, amount of blood, or both
Metrorrhagia	Irregular bleeding between menstrual cycles
Oligomenorrhea	Menstrual bleeding at intervals greater than 35 days
Polymenorrhea	Menstrual cycles of less than 22 days duration
Postmenopausal bleeding	Bleeding that occurs 12 months after the cessation of menses
Premenstrual spotting	A frequent variant of metrorrhagia limited to the few days before the beginning of menses

5. What are the common causes of genital bleeding in a young girl?

Menses before the age of 9 years is abnormal. The patient and family should be questioned about maternal use of diethylstilbestrol during pregnancy, possible patient ingestion of birth control pills, and family history of bleeding problems or sexual precocity.

Sexual molestation is the most tragic cause of genital bleeding in a young girl. Known or suspected cases of sexual trauma must be reported to appropriate child protection authorities. Abdominal perforation or rectal entry should be ruled out with examination under anesthesia. All significant hematomas should be followed for enlargement.

Urethral prolapse may cause bleeding as a result of congenital weakness or external trauma. Genital neoplasms are rare in young girls but should be considered. Benign growths include vaginal or cervical polyps and genital hemangiomas. Malignant tumors include sarcoma botryoides, ovarian tumors, and adenocarcinoma of the cervix or vagina.

6. What causes abnormal perimenarcheal bleeding?

The most common cause of abnormal bleeding in perimenarcheal girls is anovulatory cycles. An immature hypothalamic–pituitary–ovarian axis is usually a factor. Most girls enter menarche at 12–13 years of age. During the first year, 80% of the menstrual cycles are anovulatory. When menorrhagia is present, a coagulation defect is the cause in up to 20% of patients. Pregnancy and genitourinary infections (chlamydia and gonorrhea) should be ruled out.

7. Describe the management of abnormal perimenarcheal bleeding.

If the history, physical examination, and pertinent laboratory data reveal no underlying pathology, the treatment of choice is oral contraceptives. With each successive cycle of the pill, the menses become lighter. After several cycles the pill can be stopped, and the patient may be observed for onset of regular menses. Oral medroxyprogesterone, 10 mg/day for 7–10 days, also may be used. The withdrawal bleeding is heavy. The patient must be advised that withdrawal bleeding does not represent treatment failure. Intravenous Premarin, 25 mg intravenously every 4 hours for up to 3 doses, may be required for the patient with profuse, persistent bleeding. After the bleeding stops, oral contraceptives or progesterone is started immediately. Failure to control bleeding with intravenous Premarin calls for further investigation and may require curettage.

8. What causes dysfunctional uterine bleeding in a woman of reproductive age?

The most common cause of abnormal uterine bleeding in women ages 18–40 years is pregnancy and its complications. Beta-human chorionic gondadotropin (β-hCG) is assessed (serum pregnancy test). If the test is positive, the differential diagnoses include threatened, incomplete, or missed abortion; ectopic pregnancy; or gestational trophoblastic disease. If the β-hCG test is negative, then anovulation, uterine leiomyomas, and pelvic inflammatory disease are likely causes. Anovulation with metromenorrhagia may be seen more frequently in women who undergo rapid weight changes and is more common in very thin or obese women.

9. What type of menstrual flow is abnormal for the perimenopausal or postmenopausal woman?

Any bleeding occurring 12 months after the cessation of regular menstrual flow is defined as postmenopausal bleeding. Perimenopausal women often have irregular anovulatory bleeding that may make it difficult to determine when the menopause actually started. The older the patient, the higher the likelihood that the bleeding is related to malignancy. Endometrial carcinoma causes approximately 5% of perimenopausal and 20% of postmenopausal abnormal bleeding. Thus, the differential diagnosis of abnormal bleeding in women 50 years or older is malignancy until proved otherwise. Anovulatory bleeding, atrophic endometrium, and benign etiologies are diagnoses of exclusion.

10. When should a work-up for primary amenorrhea be initiated?

A 16-year-old girl without pubic or axillary hair (adrenarche) and without breast development (thelarche) requires evaluation. Failure to begin menstruation by age 18 years is considered delayed menarche. Primary amenorrhea is uncommon. Abnormal fetal development of the müllerian and wolffian systems or external genitalia accounts for two-thirds of cases. Pituitary–hypothalamic disorders and insensitive follicles account for most of the remaining cases.

The physical examination includes the patient's stature (a height of 60 in suggests gonadal dysgenesis), breast development, hair distribution, inguinal or labial masses, and cutaneous lesions (multiple pigmented nevi, gonadal dysgenesis, acanthosis nigricans, sclerotic ovary syndrome). If the patient appears to have definite pubertal development, a serum pregnancy test should be obtained before any evaluation. Management of primary amenorrhea is guided by the correct diagnosis. Initial evaluation includes measurement of pituitary gonadotropins (follicle-stimulating hormone and luteinizing hormone) and serum prolactin. Further assessment with estrogen and progesterone withdrawal, along with anatomic and chromosomal assessment, may then be undertaken.

11. How is secondary amenorrhea evaluated?
Secondary amenorrhea is defined as the loss of regular menstrual cycles for 3 months. The evaluation includes a serum pregnancy test. If the test is negative, the levels of prolactin and thyroid-stimulating hormone (TSH) are assessed. If the levels are normal, the next step is a progestational challenge. If withdrawal bleeding is noted, anovulation is confirmed. If withdrawal bleeding does not occur, the patient is challenged with oral estrogen on days 1–25 and progesterone on days 16–25. Absence of bleeding indicates a defect in the endometrium or uterine outflow tract. Destruction of the endometrium, referred to as Asherman's syndrome, is generally caused by overzealous postpartum curettage. Multiple synechiae are found on hysterogram. Dilatation and curettage may break up the adhesions.

12. What is the most common presentation of patients with polycystic ovarian disease?
Over 50% of patients with polycystic ovarian disease present with secondary amenorrhea. The diagnosis is strongly supported by the onset of symptoms in adolescence (irregular menses and varying degrees of hirsutism). Serum free testosterone, adrostenedione and LH are usually somewhat elevated; however, the levels overlap considerably with normal values. In many cases the ovaries are not palpably enlarged. Ovarian ultrasound or biopsy is not indicated. Anovulatory amenorrhea may be treated with oral contraceptives or monthly progesterone if the patient does not desire fertility.

13. When should patients with dysmenorrhea be referred to a gynecologist?
Dysmenorrhea, or "difficult monthly flow," is characterized by crampy lower abdominal or pelvic pain that may radiate to the back and thighs. Associated symptoms often include nausea, vomiting, diarrhea, bloating, weakness, fatigue, headaches, and, rarely, syncope. Such symptoms may occur before and during menstruation.

Primary dysmenorrhea begins shortly after menarche and is **not** caused by pelvic pathology. It affects 50–60% of all women in some form. Secondary dysmenorrhea begins later in life. Causes of secondary dysmenorrhea include endometriosis, pelvic inflammatory disease, postsurgical adhesions, myomas, polyps, and use of an intrauterine device. Because secondary dysmenorrhea is usually associated with pelvic pathology, referral to a gynecologist is appropriate.

14. Describe the management of dysmenorrhea, more commonly known as premenstrual syndrome (PMS).
High levels of endometrial prostaglandins are the most likely causes of dysmenorrhea. The pain may be related to prostaglandin-mediated, high-intensity uterine contractions or prostaglandin-induced sensitivity of nerve terminals.

Nonsteroidal anti-inflammatory drugs (NSAIDS) are the treatment of choice for primary dysmenorrhea. The following medications are approved for use:
- Motrin, Advil, Nuprin, Rufen: 400–600 mg 4 times daily
- Naprosyn (naproxen): 250 mg 4 times daily

• Anaprox (naproxen sodium): 275 mg 4 times daily
• Ponstel (mefenamic acid): 250 mg 4 times daily to 500 mg 3 times daily.

There is no advantage to beginning treatment before the onset of menses unless symptoms begin premenstrually. Gastrointestinal upset is a common side effect of NSAIDs. A patient may require a trial of two or more medications to find the one that gives the best pain relief. Most women have good pain relief with NSAIDs.

An alternative regimen for the woman not desiring pregnancy is an oral contraceptive. Because of the inhibition of ovulation, oral contraceptives prevent the development of a lush endometrium and the associated high levels of prostaglandin. If both NSAIDs and oral contraceptives fail, nifedipine (a calcium channel blocker), 10 mg 3 times daily, may be helpful. Oral nifedipine may cause headaches, facial flushing, palpitations, and moderate increases in heart rate. Failure to respond to any treatment modality suggests secondary dysmenorrhea, and the patient should be referred to a gynecologist.

BIBLIOGRAPHY

1. Anderson KE: Calcium antagonists and dysmenorrhea. Ann N Y Acad Sci 522:747–756, 1988.
2. Barnes R, et al: The polycystic ovary syndrome: Pathogenesis and treatment. Ann Intern Med 110:386, 1989.
3. Centers For Disease Control: Sexually transmitted disease treatment guidelines. MMWR 38:85, 1989.
4. Darwood MY: Nonsteroidal anti-inflammatory drugs and changing attitudes toward dysmenorrhea. Am J Med 84(5A):23–33, 1988.
5. Abnormal uterine bleeding. In Droegemueller W, et al (eds): Comprehensive Gynecology. St. Louis, Mosby, 1987, pp 953–964.
6. Klingmuller D, Deves W. Krahe T, et al: Magnetic resonance imaging of the brain in patients with anosmia and hypothalamic hypogonadism (Kallmann's syndrome). J Clin Endocrino Metab 65:581, 1987.
7. Riddick DH: Disorder of menstrual function. In Scott JR, et al (eds): Danforth's Obstetrics and Gynecology, 6th ed. Philadelphia, J.B. Lippincott, 1990, pp 747–771.
8. Weingold AB: Abnormal bleeding. In Kase HG, Weingold AB, Gershenom DM (eds): Principles and Practice of Clinical Gynecology. New York, Churchill Livingstone, 1990.
9. Zimmerman R: Dysfunctional uterine bleeding. Obstet Gynecol Clin North Am 15:107, 1988.

46. MENOPAUSE AND ITS COMPLICATIONS

Julie Rifkin, M.D.

1. What is the climacteric?

The climacteric is the period in which a woman's ovarian function gradually fails. With each menstrual cycle fewer follicles are recruited in the estrogen-producing phase of folliculogenesis. Circulating estrogen begins to decrease. Variations in the menstrual cycle may begin to occur after age 35 but usually not until age 45 years. Menstrual irregularity lasts roughly 2–8 years before the onset of menopause. Women may experience oligomenorrhea and/or hypermenorrhea. Fertility during this time is unpredictable, because not all cycles are ovulatory.

2. What causes hot flashes?

Vasomotor symptoms (hot flush or flash) may occur during the perimenopausal years. The flush may occur sporadically or recur every 10–30 minutes. It is rare for a flush to last an hour. Hot flashes seem to be worse at night. Generalized vasodilation occurs throughout the body and skin temperature rises. Pulsatile release of gonadotropin-releasing hormone (GNRH) from the hypothalamus is responsible for the flush. Stimuli that trigger hot flashes include caffeine, alcohol, spicy foods, hot weather, warm rooms, and emotional distress.

3. What other symptoms may occur as a result of the normal changes associated with the climacteric?

A variety of other estrogen-dependent changes also occur. The vaginal and vulvar epithelium thins. Dyspareunia, pruritus, and abacterial urethritis or cystitis may occur. Other bothersome symptoms during the climacteric include anxiety, tension, depression, irritability, headaches, insomnia, myalgias, and libido changes.

4. What is menopause?

Menopause is the absence of menses for 6–12 months. A level of serum follicle-stimulating hormone (FSH) above 40 IU/L is diagnostic of ovarian failure. Levels of estradiol and luteinizing hormone (LH) are not routinely used to diagnose menopause. No one can predict which menstrual period will be the last.

5. What causes premature menopause?

The average age of menopause is 50 years with a range of 48–55 years. Menopause before the age of 40 is considered premature. Patients with rheumatoid arthritis or diabetes may experience premature menopause. Previous abdominal hysterectomy is also associated with early menopause. This association is believed to be due to compromise of the ovarian vasculature.

6. How is hormone replacement therapy (HRT) used?

HRT is used to treat women with any stigmata of hormone deprivation. Most authorities advocate HRT as prophylaxis against osteoporosis and cardiovascular disease. The decision to use estrogen belongs to the patient once the risks and benefits have been explained. HRT may be used for as long as the patient desires. Vasomotor symptoms that begin before the cessation of menstrual bleeding may be treated with estrogen. If the patient has not had a hysterectomy, a progestational agent is added to prevent endometrial hyperplasia.

7. What type of evaluation is performed before HRT is used?

After a definitive reason to use HRT is established and discussed with the patient, the following evaluation is generally performed:

    1. Examination and laboratory tests
- A complete physical, including breast and pelvic examinations
- Stool guiac analysis
- Papanicolaou smear
- Mammogram
- Fasting lipid profile
- Fasting glucose level
- Liver function tests (with past history of liver disease)

    2. Conditions that contribute to the development of osteoporosis are evaluated in each patient (see chapter 33). Patients unsure about estrogen therapy may be better able to reach a decision if there is evidence of or high risk for osteoporosis. HRT can be prescribed when causes of secondary osteoporosis have been excluded.

8. How do the various regimens of HRT differ, especially for women who have not had a hysterectomy?

Commonly used estrogen-progesterone combinations are described below. Each regimen affords benefit for vasomotor symptoms and osteoporosis. The usual dose of conjugated estrogen is much lower than the dose of synthetic estrogen (ethinyl estradiol) commonly used in oral contraceptives. The usual dose of conjugated estrogen (Premarin) is 0.625 mg. Oral contraceptives usually contain 30–50 μg of ethinyl estradiol.

5 mg of conjugated estrogen = 50 μg of ethinyl estradiol

HRT Regimens

1. Women who have had a hysterectomy are treated with estrogen alone.
   - The usual dose of conjugated estrogen (Premarin, Ogen, Estratab) is 0.625 mg–1.25 mg/day orally.
   - The estrogen patch (Estraderm) is prescribed as 0.05–0.1 mg patches that are applied twice weekly.
   - Injectable estrogen is not recommended for routine use. The peak estrogen level, which is often supraphysiologic, is reached days to weeks after injection. The level then declines over several more weeks. Such patients are most prone to marked fluctuations of estrogen and may seek frequent injections.
2. Women who have **not** had a hysterectomy require a progestin in addition to the estrogen.
   - Oral conjugated estrogen, 0.625 mg–1.25 mg, may be given daily, with the addition of Provera, 10 mg orally on days 1–12 of each month. Withdrawal bleeding usually occurs after the Provera is finished.
   - Both conjugated estrogen, 0.625 mg–1.25 mg, and Provera, 2.5–5.0 mg orally, may be used daily. This regimen is associated with irregular bleeding during the first 4–6 months. After 6 months nearly all patients are amenorrheic.
   - All of the above regimens may be used with the estrogen patch instead of oral estrogen. Pills and patches containing both hormones may be available in the future.

9. What are the side effects of HRT?

Patients usually note breast tenderness and on occasion breast enlargement. Estrogen increases the risk for developing gallbladder disease that requires cholecystectomy. Less common problems include headache, nausea, fluid retention, weight gain, and chloasma. These symptoms are related to estrogen. The progestin component also contributes to breast tenderness and fluid retention and, less commonly, may produce some degree of depression. Unscheduled breakthrough bleeding is the most serious side effect. Prompt investigation (endometrial biopsy) is performed to rule out endometrial cancer.

10. When is HRT contraindicated?

Absolute contraindications:
- Pregnancy
- Undiagnosed dysfunctional uterine bleeding
- Active thrombophlebitis or thromboemboli disorders
- Suspected breast or uterine cancer
- Active liver disease

A history of venous thrombosis is **not** an absolute contraindication to estrogen replacement. Caution is recommended for the following patients:
- Patients who are obese and/or have diabetes are at increased risk for endometrial cancer.
- Patients with a history of migraine headaches may not be able to tolerate HRT.
- Patients with uterine myomata or gallbladder disease may experience worsening of these conditions.
- There is no clear consensus regarding HRT for women with a past history of breast cancer who have been disease-free for several years.

11. What is the association between HRT and endometrial cancer?

The use of estrogen alone in a woman who has not had a hysterectomy significantly increases the risk of developing endometrial cancer. Endometrial hyperplasia, which is believed to be a precursor to endometrial cancer, occurs in 20–40% of women taking unopposed estrogens. Endometrial hyperplasia may be prevented by the addition of a progestin. Currently available studies suggest that the addition of a progestin prevents the increased risk of endometrial cancer associated with the use of estrogen alone.

12. Is an endometrial biopsy required before HRT is prescribed?

A baseline endometrial biopsy is not required before prescribing an estrogen-progestin regimen. The exceptions are patients without evaluation of dysfunctional perimenopausal bleeding and postmenopausal patients with vaginal bleeding. Routine surveillance endometrial biopsies are not required. Unscheduled breakthrough bleeding, however, must be promptly evaluated.

13. What is the currently perceived relationship between estrogen replacement therapy and breast cancer?

Data suggest that estrogen levels most likely influence the risk of developing breast cancer in postmenopausal women. The risk of breast cancer is increased in women with early menarche, late menopause, and obesity. The following statements reflect current information regarding the association of estrogen use and breast cancer risk:

- Women currently using estrogen may have an increased incidence of breast cancer, but the relationship to mortality is unknown.
- Long-term estrogen use (> 10 years) may lead to a small increase in risk of breast cancer.

The small increased risk among current and long-term estrogen users may be misleading. Such patients must see a physician regularly to renew their prescriptions and are therefore screened for breast cancer on a regular basis. Withholding estrogen therapy because of fear of increasing the risk of breast cancer is not well justified.

The risk for breast cancer among estrogen users is not influenced by the dose, the addition of a progestin, or the type of menopause (surgical vs. natural). In addition, the risk of breast cancer is not influenced by a family history of breast cancer or a personal history of benign breast disease.

14. Does HRT reduce a woman's risk of coronary heart disease?

Current data suggest a significant decrease in coronary heart disease among postmenopausal women who use estrogen. Estrogen lowers serum levels of low-density lipoprotein cholesterol about 10–15% and increases serum levels of high-density lipoprotein cholesterol about 10–15%. The reduced risk of coronary disease, however, may not be due to estrogen-induced lipid profile modications. Estrogen receptors are found in the muscularis of coronary arteries, and a direct hormonal influence on vascular tone may be important. Estrogen may alter thrombotic mediators such as endothelium-derived prostacyclin and platelet-derived thromboxane A_2.

The addition of a progestin to estrogen replacement therapy may attenuate estrogen's beneficial effects on lipoproteins. Few good studies are available to analyze the results. Recent studies, however, indicate that users of a combined estrogen-progestin regimen have favorable lipid profiles and receive cardiovascular protection. It is currently suggested that women who use an estrogen-progestin regimen have a lower risk of coronary heart disease compared with women who do not take estrogen.

15. When should HRT be prescribed to prevent or treat postmenopausal osteoporosis?

Any time, but the sooner the better. The benefit of estrogen increases with duration of therapy. The optimal benefit of HRT is seen when estrogen is prescribed within 3 years of menopause. However, estrogen therapy may be prescribed at any time after menopause to prevent additional bone loss. Benefit has been demonstrated even for older women with established osteoporosis.

16. How may vasomotor symptoms be treated if the patient cannot use estrogen?

Several agents may provide relief from vasomotor symptoms in patients who are unable to use estrogen. The therapy should be determined by the severity of the symptoms. Possible therapies include the following:

- **Progestins alone**
  Depomedroxyprogesterone acetate (DMPA), 150 mg intramuscularly each month
- **Alpha-2 adrenergic agonists**
  Clonidine, 0.1 mg orally twice daily
  Methyldopa, 250–500 mg orally twice daily
- **Bellergal-S** (contains 40 mg of phenobarbital, 0.6 mg of ergotamine tartrate, and 0.2 mg of bellafoline alkaloids of belladonna)
- **Natural remedies**

B vitamin supplements	Ginseng tea
Vitamin C	Bee pollen
Zinc	Fenugreek
Vitamin E	Sarsaparilla
Licorice root	

- **Avoidance of stimuli that trigger vasomotor symptoms**

Caffeine	Hot weather
Alcohol	Warm rooms
Spicy foods	Emotional distress

BIBLIOGRAPHY

1. American College of Physicians: Guidelines for counseling postmenopausal women about preventive hormone therapy. Ann Intern Med 117:1039, 1992.
2. Bewley S, Bewley TH: Drug dependence with estrogen replacement therapy. Lancet 290–339, 1992.
3. Carr BR, Dauson-Hughes B, Ettinger B: A real-world approach to osteoporosis. Patient Care April 30, 1993, pp 31–56.
4. Colditz GA, Egan KM, Stampfer MJ: Hormone replacement therapy and risk of breast cancer: Results from epidemiologic studies. Am J Obstet Gynecol 168:1473, 1993.
5. Grady D, Rubin SM, et al: Hormone therapy to prevent disease and prolong life in postmenopausal women. Ann Intern Med 117:1016, 1992.
6. Jones KP: Estrogens and progestins: What to use and how to use it. Clin Obstet Gynecol 35:871, 1992.
7. Lufkin EG, Wahner HW, et al: Treatment of postmenopausal osteoporosis with transdermal estrogen. Ann Intern Med 117:1, 1992.
8. Nabulsi AA, Folsom AR, White A, et al: Association of hormone-replacement therapy with various cardiovascular risk factors in postmenopausal women. N Engl J Med 328:15, 1993.
9. Voda A: Menopause: A normal view. Clin Obstet Gynecol 35:923, 1992.
10. Watts ND, Harris ST, Genant HK, et al: Intermittent cyclical etidronate treatment of postmenopausal osteoporosis. N Engl J Med 323:73, 1990.
11. Wenger NK, Speroff L, Packard B: Cardiovascular health and disease in women. N Engl J Med 329:247, 1993.

47. CONTRACEPTION

Julie Rifkin, M.D.

1. What contraceptive methods are available to women in the United States?
Currently women in the U.S. have several contraceptive methods from which to chose. Concern for efficacy and safety as well as the user's age, general health, and future childbearing plans influence the choice.

Hormonal contraceptives are available as a synthetic estrogen combined with one of several C-19 progestational steroids or as a progestational agent alone. Barrier methods include the diaphragm, sponge, cervical cup, spermicide, and condoms. Hormone-impregnated intrauterine devices (IUDs) use both biochemical and barrier protection. Fertility awareness (rhythm, basal body temperatures, cervical mucus method) and coitus interuptus are not predictably effective. Surgical contraception may be achieved with tubal ligation or vasectomy.

2. How effective are the various contraceptive methods?
The table below lists the first-year failure rates of contraceptive methods per 100 users in 1 year of use.

METHOD	% OF WOMEN EXPERIENCING AN ACCIDENTAL PREGNANCY WITHIN THE FIRST YEAR OF USE		% OF WOMEN CONTINUING USE AT ONE YEAR
	TYPICAL USE	PERFECT USE	
Chance	85	85	
Spermicides	21	6	43
Periodic abstinence	20		67
Calendar		9	
Ovulation method		3	
Symptothermal		2	
Postovulation		1	
Withdrawal	19	4	
Cap			
Parous women	36	26	45
Nulliparous women	18	9	58
Sponge			
Parous women	36	20	45
Nulliparous women	18	9	58
Diaphragm	18	6	58
Condom	12	3	63
Pill	3		72
Progestin only		0.5	
Combined		0.1	
IUD			
Progestasert	2.0	1.5	81
Copper T 380A	0.8	0.6	78
LNg 20	0.1	0.1	81
Depo-Provera	0.3	0.3	70
Norplant (6 capsules)	0.09	0.09	85
Female sterilization	0.4	0.4	100
Male sterilization	0.15	0.10	100

3. How do oral contraceptives work?
Oral contraceptives contain a synthetic estrogen plus a synthetic progestin or a synthetic progestin alone. Oral contraceptives prevent ovulation by suppressing pituitary and hypothalamic hormones and by altering the endometrial lining.

4. Are users of oral combined contraceptives at a higher risk for future development of cancer?
No convincing evidence links oral contraceptives with increased risk of breast cancer. Women who have taken an oral contraceptive for more than 5 years have a small increase in the risk of squamous carcinoma of the cervix. This type of neoplasm, however, is also associated with a woman's level of sexual activity. There appears to be no increase in the risk of cervical cancer for users of oral contraceptives once difference in sexual activity is accounted for. Women taking oral contraceptives have a small risk of developing hepatocellular carcinoma after 8 years of use. Hepatitis B infection is also strongly linked with hepatocellular carcinoma. Oral contraceptives protect against uterine and endometrial cancers.

5. What complications are associated with the use of oral contraceptives?

Severe complications are rare. They are usually related to the cardiovascular system. Adverse reactions include thrombophlebitis, pelvic vein thrombosis, pulmonary embolism, cerebrovascular accidents, myocardial infarction, hepatic ademona, hypertension, gall-bladder disease, retinal vein thrombosis, vascular headache and depression. Other side effects include nausea, weight gain, fluid retention, breast tenderness or fullness, and menstrual irregularities.

6. What group is at greatest risk of cardiovascular complications from oral contraceptives?

Contraceptive users over the age of 35 who smoke are at highest risk for cardiovascular morbidity and mortality. The five danger signs are summarized by the mnemonic **ACHES.**

A = Abdominal pain
C = Chest pain or shortness of breath
H = Headaches
E = Eye problems (blurred vision, flashing lights, blindness)
S = Severe leg pain

7. Are oral contraceptives safe for adolescents?

Oral contraceptives can be safely prescribed for adolescents. Because oral contraceptives offer no protection against acquired immunodeficiency syndrome (AIDS), regular use of a condom **in addition to the pill** is advised until a long-term relationship with one partner is established. The estimated risk of death from oral contraceptive use is 1.3 per 100,000 adolescent users. The estimated risk of death in childbirth is 11.1 per 100,000 adolescent pregnancies.

8. How does the prescription for oral contraceptives differ if the patient is over age 35 years of age?

Women who do not smoke and have no associated risks for premature cardiovascular disease may use oral contraceptives into the fourth and fifth decades. Women over 35 years of age should be prescribed an oral contraceptive containing 35 μg of estrogen or less and a low-potency progestin.

9. Do oral contraceptive users need to be concerned about efficacy when other medications are prescribed?

Yes. Many medications may reduce the efficacy of oral contraceptives. A partial list includes rifampin, dilantin, phenobarbitol, and possibly ampicillin and tetracyclines. Oral contraceptives may alter the activity of the other drugs. A thorough medication list must be obtained before prescribing oral contraceptives. Likewise, careful thought must be given to prescribing additional medications for oral contraceptive users.

10. Is a woman's infertility altered after discontinuing oral contraceptives?

About 25% of women have some delay in establishing ovulatory cycles after stopping oral contraceptives. Most women, however, immediately resume ovulation. Three months after discontinuing oral contraceptives the conception rate returns to normal. The pregnancy rate for oral contraceptive users and users of other methods is the same after 42 months.

11. Why may a care provider recommend that a patient use a nonhormonal contraceptive method after discontinuing oral contraceptives?

Many care providers recommend using a nonhormonal contraceptive method for at least 2 or 3 cycles before attempting to conceive. This advice allows a woman's natural cycle to reestablish itself, thereby providing more accurate pregnancy dates. No evidence suggests an increased risk of spontaneous abortion or birth defects in women who have used oral contraceptives. Any woman who has not resumed menstrual function after 12 months should be evaluated for secondary amenorrhea.

12. Are oral contraceptives safe for nursing mothers to use?

No. Contraceptive steroids have been identified in small amounts in breast milk. In rare instances, jaundice and breast enlargement may occur in infants consuming such milk. The quantity and quality of breast milk is altered by oral contraceptives. Nonhormonal contraceptives are recommended for nursing mothers until the child is weaned.

13. What types of oral contraceptives are available?

Combination, biphasic, triphasic, and progestin-only oral contraceptives are available. Combination oral contraceptives use fixed doses of estrogen and progestin. In biphasic and triphasic oral contraceptives the progestin dose is varied to resemble more closely the natural menstrual cycle. Progestin-only oral contraceptives (mini-pills) are taken continuously and contain no estrogen. The progestin dose in most combination oral contraceptives is 1 mg or less. Progestin-only preparations contain 0.075–0.35 mg of progestin. The estrogen dose does not need to exceed 50 μg.

There is no difference in failure rates among oral contraceptives using 20, 30, 35, or 50 μg of estrogen. The failure rate with a progestin-only pill is somewhat higher (up to 1.1%) than that of combination preparations.

14. What is the "morning-after" pill?

After unprotected intercourse, two tablets of Ovral (ethinyl estradiol and norgestrel) may be taken within 72 and preferably 24 hours. Two more tablets are taken 12 hours after the first dose. Postcoital treatment reduces the pregnancy rate to 1–2%. A pregnancy test is mandatory if menses do not begin within 21 days.

15. What is Norplant?

The Norplant system consists of six silastic capsules that are placed under the skin of the upper arm. Each capsule contains 36 μg of levonorgestrel. The progestin prevents conception by suppressing ovulation and thickening the cervical mucus to inhibit sperm penetration. Approximately one-third of women have prolonged and irregular bleeding with Norplant, whereas 10% may become amenorrheic. Most women resume regular menses after 6–12 months.

The typical first-year pregnancy rate with Norplant is 0.09%. The 5-year cumulative pregnancy rate is 3.9%. Norplant is not acceptably effective after 5 years. The average cost of Norplant is $450–$750. Fertility returns almost immediately when the system is discontinued. Norplant is an excellent contraception system for women who have chronic disease and/or require teratogenic medications. It is also safe for women over the age of 35 years who smoke. Antiseizure medications and rifampin may reduce levels of serum levonorgestrel and decrease the efficacy of the system.

16. List the absolute contraindications to Norplant.

Known or suspected pregnancy
Benign or malignant liver tumors
Active thrombophlebitis or thromboembolic disease
Undiagnosed vaginal bleeding
Known or suspected breast cancer

17. What is the current status of the IUD?

The Dalkon Shield (manufactured by A. H. Robins Company) was removed from the market in 1975 because of its association with high rates of pelvic inflammatory disease and an increased incidence of septic abortion. A large settlement was paid to over 100,000 women who had claims of problems related to the shield. Several companies removed IUDs from the market, because they were no longer a profitable item. Less than 1% of women in the U.S. chose the IUD for contraception.

Two modern IUDs are more effective than oral contraceptives and all of the barrier methods: the copper T380A (ParaGard) and the progesterone-releasing IUD (Progestasert). The copper T380A is effective for 8 years. The Progestasert is replaced annually and is not quite as effective (especially in preventing ectopic pregnancies). Medically, an IUD is not a good contraceptive choice for a nulliparous woman. If the patient is unable to conceive after its removal, she may blame the device.

The IUD's mechanism of action is still poorly understood. It prevents fertilization by several mechanisms. The patient needs to know that the IUD is **not** an abortifacient. Side effects of IUDs include spotting, bleeding, anemia, cramping, and pain. A woman with more than one sexual partner is not a good candidate for the IUD because she is at increased risk for sexually transmitted diseases (STDs).

18. How effective are barrier methods?

All barrier methods are comparable in efficacy. The first-year failure rate ranges between 18 and 22%. Barrier methods include condoms, the cervical cap, the contraceptive sponge, spermicides, and the diaphragm. All barrier methods provide significant protection from STDs. Barrier methods are associated with a decreased risk of developing cervical dysplasia.

Synthetic condoms have been available since the 1840s. Condoms for men should be made of latex to protect against STDs. They must not be used with petroleum-based lubricants, and they must be applied before any genital-to-genital contact. Morning-after hormone treatment should be offered to couples who use condoms.

The **female condom** was approved for use in May 1993. The condom is manufactured as a prelubricated polyurethane sheath. One end is open, and the other is closed. Both ends are fitted with flexible rings. The upper ring aids as an insertion guide and an anchor during use. The outer ring remains outside of the vagina and fits over the labia.

The **cervical cap** is a soft thimble-shaped cup that fits over the cervix and is held in place by suction. The cap is partially filled with spermicide before application. The cap with spermicide provides contraception protection for 48 hours, no matter how many times intercourse occurs.

The **contraceptive sponge** is moistened with water and placed over the cervix. It must be left in place for at least 8 hours after intercourse and should not be worn for more than 24 hours. The sponge is used in conjunction with a spermicide.

Nearly two million women use the **diaphragm**, which was first described in 1880. Diaphragms are prescribed in various sizes and are used with a spermicide. The diaphragm is a dome-shaped rubber cup with a flexible rim that is inserted into the vagina. The rubber dome covers the cervix and the rim (flat, coil, or arching spring) tucks behind the symphysis pubis and fits snugly in the posterior vaginal fornix. The diaphragm must be left in place at least 6 hours after intercourse but should not be left in place for more than 24 hours.

Spermicides kill sperm after immobilizing them. They are available as foam, gels, or creams and contain octoxynol or nonoxynol 9.

Allergic reactions to latex and spermicides may occur. For the woman recurrent cystitis and vaginal discharge also may be troublesome. Toxic shock syndrome may occur if a barrier method is left in place longer than the recommended time.

19. What is fertility awareness?

Fertility awareness requires a woman to chart the most likely days during which she may conceive. Charting involves use of a calendar, recording basal body temperature, and following changes in the cervical mucus. Intercourse is avoided during the periovulatory days. The life span of an ovum is estimated to be 72 hours. Sperm are viable in the female reproductive tract for 2–7 days. The span of fertility may be from 7 days before ovulation to 3 days after ovulation. Approximately 20% of users experience failure during the first year. The most effective way to use fertility awareness is to postpone intercourse until after ovulation has been clearly documented.

20. What is the most commonly used form of birth control in the United States?

Sterilization is the treatment of choice for more than 16 million couples. The failure rate for tubal ligation is 0.2–0.4% in the first year. The failure rate for vasectomy is similar to that for tubal ligation. Vasectomy is simpler, safer, and less expensive than tubal ligation.

21. What is mifepristone?

Mifepristone (RU 486) is a progestin antagonist. Mifepristone may be used as a postcoital contraceptive within 72 hours of unprotected intercourse. The drug is given as a single oral dose of 600 mg. It is highly effective in preventing pregnancy. Mifepristone (600 mg orally) given with a prostaglandin 48 hours later results in a complete abortion rate approaching 100%. The combination is highly effective in women with pregnancy-induced amenorrhea for up to 9 weeks. Side effects are uncommon but may include heavy bleeding, nausea, vomiting, abdominal pain, and fatigue.

BIBLIOGRAPHY

1. Albertson BD, Sinaman MJ: The prediction of ovulation and monitoring of the fertile period. Adv Contracept 3:263, 1989.
2. Cohall AT, Cullins VE, Darney PD, Nelson AL: Contraception in the 1990s: New method and approaches. Patient Care July 15, 1993 (Suppl), pp 1–12.
3. Dickey RP: Managing Contraceptive Pill Patients, 7th ed. Durant, Essent. Med. Infl Sys. Inc., 1993.
4. Harens CS, Sullivan ND, Tilton P: Manual of Outpatient Gynecology, 2nd ed. Boston, Little, Brown, 1991, pp 162–163.
5. Hatcher R, et al: Contraceptive Technology 1990–1992, 15th ed. New York, Irvington, 1984, pp 159–225.
6. Romieu I, Berlin JA, Colditz G: Oral contraceptives and breast cancer: Review and meta-analysis. Cancer 66:2253, 1990.
7. Sivin I, Schmidt R: Effectiveness of IUDs: A review. Contraception 36:55, 1987.
8. Speroff L, Darney PD: A Clinical Guide for Contraception. Baltimore, Williams & Williams, 1992.
9. Sptiz IM, Bardin CW: Mifepristone (RU 486): A modulator of progestin and glucocorticoid action. N Engl J Med 329(6):404, 1993.

48. VAGINAL DISCHARGE AND PELVIC INFLAMMATORY DISEASE

Susan J. Diem, M.D., M.P.H.

1. What is a "normal" vaginal discharge? What are the characteristics of an "abnormal" discharge?

Some degree of vaginal discharge is normal. Normal discharge consists of desquamated vaginal epithelial cells and secretions from cervical glands, sebaceous glands, sweat glands, Bartholin's glands, and Skeene's glands. Transudate through the vaginal wall also contributes to the composition of a normal discharge. Normal secretions are usually clear or white, odorless, and viscous. Polymorphonuclear leukocytes are rare. The amount of discharge varies with the menstrual cycle, age, sexual arousal, pregnancy, and use of oral contraceptives.

An abnormal discharge is usually accompanied by a change in odor, a change in color, or an increase in the amount of the discharge. In addition, patients may note pruritis, dysuria, or staining of underwear.

2. What causes an abnormal vaginal discharge?

1. Infections of the vagina, vulva, cervix, or upper genital tract.

2. Atrophic vaginitis due to estrogen deficiency, which causes thinning and fragility of the vaginal and vulvar epithelium. Hence the epithelium is more vulnerable to injury and inflammation, producing desquamation of cells and stimulation of glandular secretions from the cervical area. In addition such changes may elevate the pH in the vagina and thus result in a change in the bacteria.

3. Foreign bodies such as tampons or diaphragms, if left in the vagina for a prolonged period
4. Irritation from frequent douching
5. Neoplasms of the cervix and uterus.

3. List the infectious causes of a vaginal discharge.

Bacterial vaginosis	Chlamydial cervicitis and pelvic inflammatory disease
Trichomonas vaginosis	Gonococcal cervicitis and pelvic inflammatory disease
Candidal vulvovaginitis	Herpes cervicitis

4. What is bacterial vaginosis (BV)?

Also known as nonspecific vaginitis, BV is the most common cause of vaginal infection. Although its etiology has been debated for years, it is believed to represent an alteration in the microbial flora of the vagina, with an increase in anaerobes and gram-negative bacilli and a decrease in the endogenous *Lactobacillus* flora.

The presence of *Gardnerella vaginalis* also has been implicated in the pathogenesis of BV, but its role is not clearly elucidated. It is cultured commonly in patients with BV but may be found in up to 50% of healthy, asymptomatic women. Most authors believe that *Gardnerella vaginalis* may be necessary but not sufficient alone to cause BV.

Patients with BV often present with a vaginal discharge associated with a change in odor, described as musty or fishy. The odor is due to the production of aromatic amines by the bacteria. The discharge is usually thin, white-yellow, homogeneous, and moderately increased in volume over the patient's normal discharge.

5. How is the diagnosis of BV made?

The diagnosis of BV requires three of the following four findings:

1. The pH of the vaginal discharge should be greater than 4.5. The normal pH of vaginal secretions, ranging from 3.8–4.4, is raised by the production of aromatic amines in the altered microbial environment.

2. "Clue" cells are seen on wet mount. Clue cells are epithelial cells with a granulated surface due to adherence of bacteria. They can be seen under high-dry magnification after a drop of the discharge is mixed with a drop of saline.

3. The "sniff test" is positive. A fishy odor is often produced when a drop of discharge is mixed with 10% potassium hydroxide. The alkalinization is thought to volatilize amines, producing the characteristic fishy odor.

4. The discharge is consistent with BV.

6. Describe the treatment of BV.

Metronidazole is the drug of choice for the treatment of BV. The standard regimens include 500 mg twice daily for 7 days and two 2-gm doses on days 1 and 3. Other options include intravaginal clindamycin cream, metronidazole vaginal gel, and oral clindamycin at a dose of 300 mg twice daily for 7 days. Patients in the first trimester of pregnancy should be treated with one of the alternatives because of risks of teratogenicity from metronidazole.

7. Why is it important to diagnose and treat trichomonas vaginitis?

Trichomonas vaginitis is caused by *Trichomonas vaginalis,* a protozoan usually transmitted by sexual contact. Infection with *T. vaginalis* is associated with an abnormal discharge that ranges in color from white to yellow, gray, or green. Other manifestations can include vaginal itching, dysuria, and dyspraeunia. As many as 50% of infected women are asymptomatic, as are the majority of infected men.

Diagnosis is made by microscopic examination of a drop of the vaginal discharge mixed with saline. The sensitivity of this procedure in symptomatic women is approximately 50–75%, and the specificity approaches 100%. Cultures for *T. vaginalis* have a sensitivity of approximately 90%. In addition, monoclonal antibody tests are available with sensitivities and specificities that approach those of culture.

The standard treatment for trichomoniasis is a single dose of 2 gm of metronidazole. Partners also should be treated. Other dosing regimens may be tried for treatment failures. Alternatives to metronidazole are limited; topical therapy with clotrimazole suppositories or vinegar douches have less success but may be useful options in the first trimester of pregnancy.

8. What infection is suggested by a "strawberry cervix"?

Cervicitis due to *Trichomonas vaginalis,* although rare, is characterized by a "strawberry cervix."

9. What infection is suggested by a white, cheesy discharge?

Candidal vulvovaginitis is caused by the fungi *Candida albicans* and *Candida glabrata.* Infection with *Candida* may cause vulvar and vaginal irritation and inflammation, resulting in burning, itching, dysparenia, and dysuria. Many women have an abnormal discharge, often thick and clumpy. These fungi also are found as part of the normal flora of up to 50% of women.

The diagnosis is made by examining the discharge with a Gram stain or 10% potassium hydroxide solution for the fungal forms. Culture is a more sensitive method for detecting the yeast, but since many women without symptoms have positive yeast cultures, the usefulness of cultures is unclear.

10. What factors predispose to candidal vaginitis?

Predisposing factors for candidiasis include diabetes, acquired immunodeficiency syndrome, recent antibiotic use, pregnancy, corticosteroids, and immunosuppressants.

11. What is the role of oral agents in the treatment of candidal vaginitis?

Candidiasis can be treated with several topical agents, including miconazole, clotrimazole, and butoconazole; all have cure rates of 85% or higher. Oral agents include ketoconazole, fluconazole, and itraconazole. The risk of side effects of oral agents restricts their use to resistant or recurrent candidal vulvovaginitis. They do not appear to be significantly more effective than topical treatments.

12. What is chlamydial cervicitis? How is it treated?

One common cause of cervicitis, *Chlamydia trachomatis,* is transmitted through sexual contact. Symptoms include a mucopurulent discharge, lower abdominal discomfort, fever, and dysuria. However, many patients infected with *C. trachomatis* are asymptomatic.

On examination the cervix is red, edematous, and friable. The diagnosis can be made by culture, a technique that is expensive and technically difficult. Fluorescent antibody testing and enzyme-linked immunoassays are easier to perform and have good sensitivity and specificity.

The mainstay of treatment for chlamydial infection is doxycycline, 100 mg b.i.d. for 7 days, or tetracycline, 500 mg q.i.d. for 7 days. Erythromycin should be used in pregnant patients because the tetracyclines pose a risk to the fetus. Partners also should be treated.

13. When should patients be treated for presumed chlamydial infection?

Patients should be treated for presumed chlamydial infection in the presence of gonococcal cervicitis. Infection with *Neisseria gonorrhoeae* may cause a purulent vaginal discharge due to cervicitis or pelvic inflammatory disease. The discharge may be accompanied by pruritis, dyspareunia, dysuria, and lower abdominal discomfort. The diagnosis of gonococccal cervicitis is made by Gram stain of the discharge, demonstrating gram-negative intracellular diplococci. Cultures are usually performed to confirm the diagnosis.

First-line treatment for gonococcal cervicitis consists of ceftriaxone, 250 mg intramuscularly in a single dose, followed by a 7-day course of doxycycline, 100 mg b.i.d., to treat undiagnosed chlamydial infection. Spectinomycin, 2 gm intramuscularly, can be used for patients allergic to cephalosporins. Alternatives include ciprofloxacin, norfloxacin, and other cephalosporins, although these agents have not been studied as rigorously as the other regimens. Partners also should be treated.

14. What is herpes cervicitis? How is it treated?

Infection with the herpes simplex virus may cause cervicitis with painful, vesicular lesions on the cervix and a vaginal discharge. Diagnosis is made by observing the characteristic lesions, and confirmation is obtained with viral culture, direct immunofluorescence, and enzyme-linked immunoassays.

Treatment consists of acyclovir, 200 mg q.i.d. for 5–10 days, usually orally. This treatment has been shown to decrease the length of viral shedding, to improve symptoms, and to speed healing within 1–2 days. It does not prevent recurrences.

15. Describe the approach to a patient with a vaginal discharge.

History, physical examination, and a few simple laboratory tests can identify the cause of many cases of vaginal discharge.

The history should focus on the nature of the discharge, associated symptoms, sexual history, and other medical conditions.

The physical examination should include inspection of the vulva, vagina, and cervix, noting any erythema, atrophy, abnormal lesions, or foreign bodies. Characteristics of the discharge, such as color and consistency, also should be noted. A bimanual examination should be performed to evaluate cervical motion tenderness, adnexal masses, and uterine masses.

Laboratory studies should include a wet-mount preparation to look for clue cells and trichomonads. A 10% solution of potassium hydroxide added to a sample of discharge facilitates identification of *Candida*. A Gram stain of the discharge should be performed if gonococcal infection is suspected. In addition, pH testing of the discharge may be of some help.

Cultures of the discharge for *N. gonorrhoeae* should be performed if mucopurulent cervicitis is seen on physical examination. Infection with *C. trachomatis* can be evaluated with direct immunofluorescent testing or with cultures. Other tests to consider include a urinalysis, particularly if dysuria is present, and a complete blood count if pelvic inflammatory disease is a diagnostic consideration.

16. Define pelvic inflammatory disease (PID).

PID is an infection of the upper genital tract in women and may include salpingitis, tubo-ovarian abscess, endometritis, and pelvic peritonitis.

17. Which organisms are responsible for PID?

PID is caused by a variety of bacteria, most importantly *N. gonorrhoeae* and *C. trachomatis*, both of which are sexually transmitted. Other organisms that may play a role either in the initial development of PID or as secondary pathogens include aerobes, such as *Streptococcus* sp., *Escherichia coli*, and *Haemophilus influenzae*, and anaerobes, such as *Bacteroides* sp., *Peptostreptococcus* sp., and *Peptococcus* sp. *Actinomyces israelii*, a gram-positive anaerobic organism, is seen in PID related to the use of intrauterine devices.

18. Describe the pathogenesis of PID.

C. trachomatis and *N. gonorrhoeae* initially infect the endocervical canal and cause cervicitis. The infection then ascends the cervix and spreads into the uterus and fallopian tubes. Factors that promote ascension include damage to the endocervical canal by the bacteria, extension of endocervical columnar epithelium beyond the endocervix,and hormonal changes during the menstrual cycle that affect characteristics of the cervical mucus.

19. How is the diagnosis of PID made?

The diagnosis can be difficult to make clinically, because no clinical criteria are universally accepted. In general, the diagnosis requires adnexal tenderness and cervical motion tenderness, often associated with an abnormal vaginal discharge and fever. Nonspecific markers of inflammation, such as sedimentation rate and c-reactive protein, may be elevated.

Further testing is warranted if the diagnosis is in question. Serum levels of beta human chorionic gonadotropin (hCG) should be assessed to exclude a complication of pregnancy. Ultrasonography should be considered if ovarian cyst or ectopic pregnancy is suspected. Endometrial biopsy and culdocentesis are possible options if the diagnosis remains unclear.

The gold standard for the diagnosis of PID is laparoscopy. Laparoscopy should be considered if the diagnosis is unclear, if the patient fails to respond to conventional treatment, or if an unexplained pelvic mass is present.

20. List the possible complications of PID.

Infertility	Chronic pelvic pain
Ectopic pregnancies	Pyosalpinx
Tubo-ovarian abscess	Pelvic adhesions

21. What is the Fitz-Hugh and Curtis syndrome?

The Fitz-Hugh and Curtis syndrome is acute perihepatitis seen with the spread of *N. gonorrhoeae* or *C. trachomatis* from the fallopian tube through the peritoneal cavity to the liver capsule. Patients usually present with right upper quadrant pain and often have clinical evidence of PID.

22. When should patients with PID be hospitalized?

Mild cases of PID can be treated in the outpatient setting. Common regimens include cefoxitin, 2 gm intramuscularly, plus probenecid, 1 gm orally, and doxycycline, 100 mg orally twice daily for 10–14 days. Ceftriaxone, 250 mg intramuscularly, with doxycyline, 100 mg orally twice daily, is an alternative. Erythromycin, 500 mg orally 4 times/day for 10–14 days, can be substituted for doxycycline.

Patients with PID who do not respond to outpatient therapy, whose pain cannot be controlled, or whose diagnosis is in question should be hospitalized. Inpatient antibiotic regimens include cefoxitin, 2 gm intravenously every 6 hours, or cefotetan, 2 gm intravenously every 12 hours, along with doxycycline, 100 mg intravenously or orally every 12 hours. Some third-generation cephalosporins also may be used instead of cefoxitin or cefotetan. Another alternative is clindamycin plus gentamicin intravenously.

Surgery usually is required only for patients with abscesses that do not respond to antibiotics.

BIBLIOGRAPHY

1. Centers for Disease Control: 1989 Sexually transmitted disease treatment guidelines. MMWR 38(Suppl 8): 1–43, 1989.
2. Eschenback D, Hillier S: Advances in diagnostic testing for vaginitis and cervicitis. J Reprod Med 34(Suppl):555–564, 1989.
3. Kahn J, et al: Diagnosing pelvic inflammatory disease: A comprehensive analysis and considerations for developing a new model. JAMA 266:2594–2604, 1991.
4. McCue J: Evaluation and management of vaginitis: An update for primary care practitioners. Arch Intern Med 149:565–568, 1989.
5. Morgan R: Clinical aspects of pelvic inflammatory disease. Am Fam Physician 43:1725–1732, 1991.
6. Moran J, Zenilman J: Therapy for gonococcal infections: Options in 1989. Rev Infect Dis 12(Suppl 6):S633–S644, 1990.
7. Peterson H, Galaid E, Zenilman J: Pelvic inflammatory disease: Review of treatment options. Rev Infect Dis 12(Suppl 6):S656–S664, 1990.
8. Peterson H, et al: Pelvic inflammatory disease: Key treatment issues and options. JAMA 266:2605–2611, 1991.
9. Reed B, Eyler A: Vaginal infections: Diagnosis and management. Am Fam Physician 47:1805–1816, 1993.
10. Rice P, Schacter J: Pathogenesis of pelvic inflammatory disease. What are the questions? JAMA 266:2587–2593, 1991.
11. Sargent S: The "other" sexually transmitted diseases: Chlamydial, herpes simplex virus, and human papillomavirus infections. Postgrad Med 91:359–377, 1992.

12. Sparks J: Vaginitis. J Reprod Med 36:745–752, 1991.
13. Sweet R, et al: Use of laparoscopy to determine the microbiologic etiology of acute salpingitis. Am J Obstet Gynecol 134:68–74, 1979.
14. Toomey K, Bartnes R: Treatment of Chlamydia trachomatis genital infection. Rev Infect Dis 12(Suppl 6):S645–S655, 1990.

49. PROSTATE DISEASE

Norman Peterson, M.D.

1. What are the most common disorders affecting the prostate?
Prostatitis, benign prostatic hypertrophy, and prostatic cancer.

2. What are the typical clinical manifestations of benign prostatic hypertrophy (BPH)?
BPH is manifested by any combination of the following symptoms: slowing of the size and force of the urinary stream, urinary frequency or urgency, sensation of incomplete bladder emptying, and nocturia. Usually symptoms are gradually progressive and therefore may be tolerated until they reach an extreme form. Examination may reveal varying levels of residual urine. Digital rectal examination typically discloses homogeneous, symmetric enlargement of the prostate. Urodynamic evaluation may demonstrate uninhibited detrusor contractions, which are often corrected by relief of outflow obstruction and also may be relieved by anticholinergic medication. Symptoms of prostatic obstruction (prostatism) may be exaggerated by coexiting urinary infection or by disorders that deleteriously influence bladder function, such as diabetes or chronic vesicle overdistention.

3. List the complications of BPH.
Obstruction may culminate in acute urinary retention that requires catheter relief. Less common complications include urinary incontinence, infection, stone formation, and hematuria.

4. Can patients present with prostatism and a clinically normal-sized gland?
Younger patients (early 50s) presenting with prostatism frequently demonstrate an unenlarged, clinically benign gland. Incongruously severe voiding dysfunction is produced by a small fibrous prostate or median bar hypertrophy of the posterior vesicle neck. Management is the same as for BPH. Decisions to treat such disorders are predicated exclusively on symptoms or related complications. Prostate size is generally of secondary importance to nature and severity of symptoms.

5. What operative approach is appropriate for the majority of patients with BPH?

BPH—Operative Options

Transurethral prostatectomy	Prostatic urethral stent
Suprapubic prostatectomy	Balloon dilatation, prostatic urethra
Retropubic prostatectomy	Laser prostatectomy
Perineal prostatectomy	Transurethral incision of prostate

Perineal prostatectomy is rarely performed for benign disease and is generally limited to the patient who is vulnerable to pulmonary or other complications associated with alternative surgical approaches. Suprapubic and retropubic approaches are similar open procedures and are often used for larger glands; blood loss and fluid absorption are considerably less than what may occur with lengthy transurethral resection. Transurethral resection is appropriate for the majority of patients, however, because it limits hospitalization and convalescence. "Prostatectomy" for BPH is in reality adenomectomy that involves removal only of the obstructing hypertrophied periurethral adenoma and leaves the prostate largely undisturbed.

Treatment alternatives currently under investigation include incision rather than resection of smaller obstructive prostates, balloon distention of the prostatic urethra, permanent dilating prostatic urethral stents, and application of laser and hyperthermic tissue destruction.

6. Discuss the three hormonal therapies available to reduce prostate size in patients with symptomatic BPH.

1. **Agonists of luteinizing hormone-releasing hormone** (LH-RH), which include leuprolide and nafarelin acetate, produce significant benefits but require permanent uninterrupted therapy. Side effects include decreased libido, impotence, gynecomastia, hot flushes, and decreased levels of serum prostate-specific antigen (PSA). Therapy therefore is ideally restricted to impotent patients. An additional disadvantage is the requirement for intramuscular administration.

2. **Antiandrogen medication** is presently limited to flutamide, which has similar advantages and fewer side effects than LH-RH agonists but also alters PSA levels. Side effects include gastrointestinal upset and gynecomastia or nipple tenderness. Sustained serum testosterone levels produce the advantage of undiminished libido, potency, and ejaculation. Flutamide is administered orally but may require up to 6 months to achieve maximal benefit. Uninterrupted maintenance therapy is necessary.

3. **Inhibitors of 5-alpha reductase** (finasteride/Proscar) is a once-daily medication that has no significant side effects and may reduce prostatic volume and modestly improve symptoms in 30–50% of patients. Six months may be required for maximal benefit, and permanent maintenance therapy is required. PSA levels may fall by as much as 50%. An added advantage is the potential for halting disease progression owing to suppressed androgen stimulation of the prostate.

All three agents appear equally effective in reducing prostatic volume by approximately 25% and improving obstructive symptoms and urinary flow rate.

7. What other type of medical therapy is available to treat outlet obstruction in patients with BPH?

Selective alpha$_1$ antagonists relax smooth muscle fibers at the vesicle outlet, thus reducing outlet resistance and improving urinary flow. Nonselective alpha antagonists (phenoxybenzamine/Dibenzyline) may reduce voiding symptoms but also have adverse side effects. Selective alpha$_1$ antagonists include prazosin (Minipress), terazosin (Hytrin), and doxazosin. Lightheadedness, dizziness, and tiredness may occur early in the administration period but improve thereafter; it is advisable to administer the first several doses under conditions that minimize the risk of complications. Dosage options are 1, 2, 5, and 10 mg; the greatest benefit is associated with the 5- and 10-mg doses.

The potential role of estrogens in the pathogenesis of BPH has prompted assessment of a potential therapeutic role for aromatase inhibitors, which interrupt the final step of estrogen synthesis in men. Preliminary clinical investigations have generated enthusiasm for atamestane, which appears capable of decreasing urinary frequency and nocturia, improving urinary flow rates, and perhaps decreasing prostatic volume. Atamestane may prove effective alone or in combination with the other agents listed.

8. What is the preferred management of acute urinary retention?

The obvious answer is catheter decompression of the bladder. Decisions regarding removal or maintenance of catheter drainage relate to the level of bladder overdistention: retained volumes exceeding 700 cc are probably best treated by a few days of catheter drainage to permit recovery of detrusor tonus. Smaller volumes are usually amenable to stat drainage, restoring pre-retention voiding dynamics. Patients in whom urethral catheterization is unsuccessful should be referred to a urologist for alternative methods of achieving decompression.

9. When urethral catheterization cannot be performed and consultation with a urologist is unavailable, what can be done emergently to relieve urethral obstruction?
When urologic consultation is unavailable, temporary relief is obtainable by suprapubic trocar cystostomy or by suprapubic insertion of a large needle into the bladder through which a polyethylene drainage tube is passed. Suprapubic maneuvers require a distended bladder and the absence of previous surgical procedures that may jeopardize bowel and colon because of adhesions.

10. What is the recommended practice for improving early diagnosis of prostate cancer?

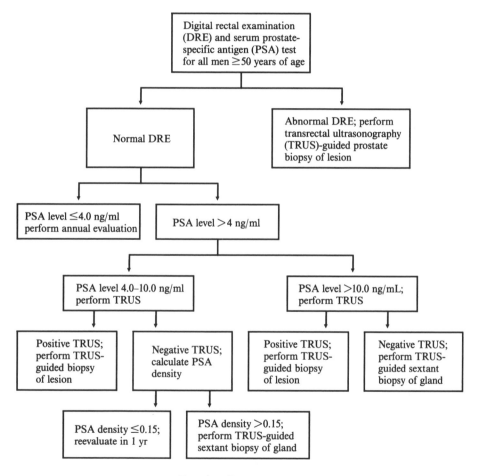

Detection of prostate cancer.

The above approach is directed at men 50 years of age or older. PSA elevation without abnormalities at DRE or TRUS warrants referral for needle biopsy of all major areas of the prostate. PSA levels not exceeding 20 ng/ml are statistically unassociated with identifiable metastatic dissemination; dissemination is more likely as levels progressively exceed 20 ng/ml. Elevation of the serum prostatic acid phosphatase is associated in most cases with cancer escaping the confines of the prostate gland.

11. What conditions other than prostatic carcinoma may elevate the PSA to intermediate levels?
Prostatitis, prostate infarction, large BPH, and trauma, including biopsy or surgery.

12. Describe the staging of prostatic cancer.

Staging Systems for Prostate Cancer

WHITMORE-JEWETT	DEFINITION
A1–A2	No palpable tumor, incidental finding in operative specimen; positive random biopsy
B1–B3	Palpable tumor confined to the gland, or small nodule, confined to one lobe
C1–C2	Extension beyond prostatic capsule with/without involvement of lateral sulci and/or seminal vesicles
D1–D2	Metastases to any site, including a persistently elevated prostatic acid phosphatase

13. What is the recommended contemporary management of prostatic cancer?
Management differs according to staging. **Stages A and B disease** (localized within the prostatic capsule) are actively treated by hormonal suppression, radiotherapy, or radical prostatectomy. External beam radiotherapy recently has shown improved results. Radical prostatectomy is preceded by pelvic lymphadenectomy (open or laparoscopic) to ensure the absence of latent disseminated disease. Prospective, randomized controlled clinical trials in early prostatic carcinoma are needed to ascertain the efficacy of treatment modalities in improving survival.

Stage C prostatic carcinoma (invasion of prostatic capsule or seminal vesicle) increases the likelihood of local and disseminated recurrence after surgery or radiotherapy. Some patients may respond to hormonal suppression by cytoreduction to a volume amenable to radical extirpation.

Disseminated prostatic cancer **(stage D)** into bone or regional lymph nodes may derive palliation and survival benefit from hormonal suppression by castration, estrogen therapy (diethylstilbestrol, 3 mg/day), or LH-RH stimulation (leuprolide, 7.5 mg/month intramuscularly) with or without antiandrogen therapy (flutamide, 250 mg every 8 hr).

14. List the potential complications or side effects seen with the various forms of therapy for prostatic carcinoma.

Surgery
  Impotence
  Incontinence
  Anastomotic stricture
  Rectal injury
External radiotherapy
  Cystitis
  Bladder contracture
  Urethral stricture
  Enteritis or proctitis
  Incontinence
  Impotence

Estrogen therapy
  Breast enlargement and tenderness
  Increased incidence of cardiovascular events
Isolated leuprolide therapy
  Testosterone flare (temporary increase in bone pain and other symptoms, suppressible with antiandrogen therapy)
  Testicular atrophy
  Loss of libido
  Impotence
Flutamide therapy
  Gynecomastia
  Nausea and vomiting
  Diarrhea
  Hepatic dysfunction

15. What is meant by prostatitis?
A misdiagnosis of prostatitis is often applied to nonspecific complaints of low back pain, perineal pain or discomfort, constipation, premature ejaculation, or vague voiding discomfort or dysfunction. Prostatitis or prostatic inflammation, which is subcategorized into acute bacterial prostatitis, chronic bacterial prostatitis, nonbacterial prostatitis, prostadynia, or granulomatous prostatitis (rare), requires specific diagnosis and treatment.

16. Describe the presentation and management of a patient with acute prostatitis.
Acute bacterial prostatitis presents as a florid clinical disorder characterized by toxic systemic symptoms: extreme dysuria with increased frequency, urgency, and strangury; severely tender prostate; and rusty urine containing red blood cells, white blood cells, and bacteria. The prostatic barrier to antibiotic penetration is destroyed by the acute inflammatory process; therefore, any effective antibiotic suffices. Potentially severe local and systemic symptoms often necessitate hospitalization for parenteral administration of antibiotics, fluid repletion, pain control, and urethral catheter drainage. Recovery is typically prompt with appropriate therapy.

17. Why should chronic bacterial prostatitis be distinguished from acute prostatitis?
Accurate diagnosis is important because several weeks or months of uninterrupted antibacterial therapy are required to produce symptomatic relief and cure in patients with chronic bacterial prostatitis. Diagnosis depends on culture positivity of prostatic secretions (after prostatic massage) or semen, in the presence of sterile urine. Clinical manifestations are dominated by recurrent episodes of bacterial cystitis. Effective therapy is usually provided by trimethoprim sulfamethoxazole or quinolone agents.

18. How is nonbacterial prostatitis managed?
Nonbacterial prostatitis is manifested as vague, nonspecific symptoms (see question 15) in the absence of culture positivity. By definition antibiotic therapy is inappropriate. Symptoms are nonetheless dominant, and therapy is designed for symptomatic alleviation. Prostatic congestion may benefit from massage to express accumulated secretions. Other modalities include pharmacologic relaxation of the pelvic floor, warm sitz baths, pyridium for urethral discomfort, and occasionally dilation of the anal sphincter.

19. Define prostadynia.
Prostadynia is a term intended to incorporate the nonspecific symptoms often misinterpreted as prostatitis. Management is the same as for chronic nonbacterial prostatitis.

20. What is the significance of a diagnosis of prostatic abscess?
Prostatic abscess is uncommon and possible contributing factors should be considered, including diabetes, AIDS, and other immunosuppressive states, and specific bacterial diagnosis is warranted to identify atypical opportunistic infections. A prostatic abscess may present as either an acute systemically toxic disorder or as a chronic low-grade, nonspecific state. Urethral obstruction may contribute and should be evaluated. Digital rectal examination reveals asymmetry and nonhomogeneity; the involved lobe is open, bulging, fluctuant, and variably sensitive. Prostatic abscess frequently ruptures spontaneously into the rectum or urethra, with resolution of the acute clinical status. Interventional drainage may be accomplished by transurethral resection or by transrectal needle aspiration.

BIBLIOGRAPHY

1. Cooner WH: Early diagnosis of prostate cancer. In Walsh PC, Retik AB, Stamey TA, Vaughn ED (eds): Campbell's Urology. Philadelphia, W.B. Saunders, 1992, pp 1–10.
2. Graham SD Jr: Localized adenocarcinoma of the prostate. Mediguide Urol 5:1–7, 1993.
3. Lee ET, Kuzel TM: Medical oncology in urology. Mediguide Urol 6:1–7, 1993.

4. Littrup PJ, Lee F, Mettlin C: Prostate cancer screening. Cancer 42:198, 1992.
5. Meares EM: Prostatitis and related disorders. In Walsh PC, Gittes RF, Perlmutter AD, Stamey TA (eds): Campbell's Urology. Philadelphia, W.B. Saunders, 1986, pp 868–887.
6. Oesterling JE: PSA leads the way for detecting and following prostate cancer. Contemp Urol Feb:68–81, 1993.
7. Peterson NE: Emergency management of common urologic problems in men. Part 2: Urethritis and prostatitis. Emerg Med Rep 7:9–15, 1986.
8. Peterson NE: Peer review editor: Acute urinary retention, by Fontanarosa PB. Emerg Med Rep 14:57–66, 1993.
9. Peterson NE: Urinary retention. In Wolfson AB, Harwood-Nuss A (eds): Renal and Urologic Emergencies. New York, Churchill Livingstone, 1986, pp 179–200.
10. Peterson NE: Urinary obstruction and retention. In Callaham ML (ed): Current Therapy in Emergency Medicine. Philadelphia, B.C. Decker, 1987, pp 522–525.
11. Peterson NE: Urinary incontinence and retention. In Callaham MC, Barron CW, Schumaker HM (eds): Decision Making in Emergency Medicine. Ontario, B.C. Decker, 1990, pp 225–229.
12. Peterson NE: Urinary incontinence and retention. In Harwood-Nuss A, Linden CH, Luten RC, Sternbach G, Wolfson AB (eds): The Clinical Practice of Emergency Medicine. Philadelphia, J.B. Lippincott, 1990, pp 225–229.

50. SCROTAL MASSES

Norman Peterson, M.D.

1. List the benign, inflammatory, and malignant masses that may involve intrascrotal contents, and specify the presence or absence of pain in each.

Scrotal Masses

Benign	PAIN +/–	Inflammatory	PAIN +/–
Hydrocele	–	Epididymitis	+
Varicocele	–	Orchitis	+
Spermatocele	±	Abscess	+
Inclusion cyst	–	Tuberculosis	–
Lipoma	–	**Malignant**	
Adenomatoid tumor	–	Seminoma	–
Hematocele	+	Embryonal carcinoma	–
Spermatic cord torsion	+	Teratocarcinoma	–
Torsion, testis	+	Yolk sac carcinoma	–
appendage		Choriocarcinoma	–

Hydrocele and varicocele are often described as painful, but actual discomfort is uncommon. Spermatocele is more painful in its earliest and smallest manifestations, and pain at the globus major (upper pole of testis) may indicate the presence of a subclinical spermatocele when no cyst or mass is palpable. As the spermatocele enlarges, the fibers of its capsule separate, thereby relieving the pain of distension, and explaining why the smallest lesions are most symptomatic.

Malignant testicular lesions are typically painless, but acute pain occasionally is associated with intralesional hemorrhage, and chronic discomfort may result from the weight and mass of larger lesions.

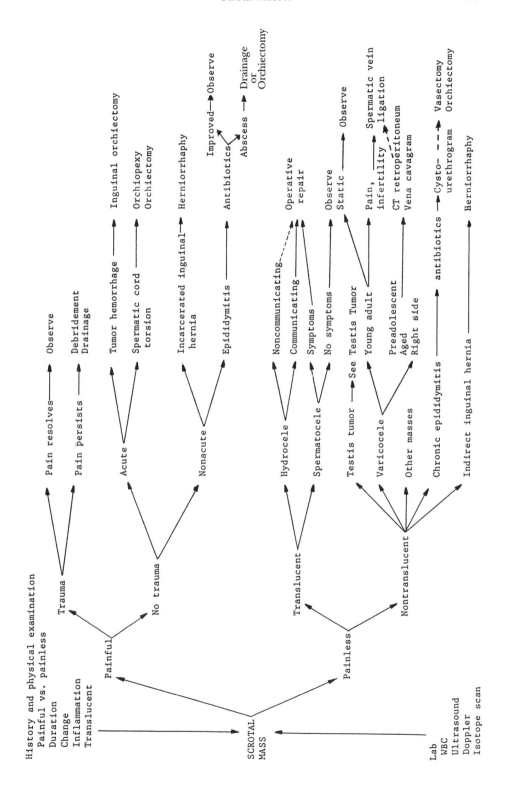

2. What is the significance of acute versus chronic scrotal pain?
Scrotal pain of acute onset characterizes torsion of the spermatic cord or testicular appendages, and acute epididymitis. Acute pain also may result from hemorrhage into a tumor, or from traumatic rupture of the testicular capsule (tunica albuginea).

Chronic scrotal pain may occur with any subacute inflammatory disorder, including epididymitis or orchitis. It also may result from the weight and mass of larger testis tumors. Chronic testicular pain is a frequent complaint with hydrocele, varicocele, and spermatocele, but the validity of such claims is questionable.

3. Why is orchiectomy not indicated for chronic orchidynia?
Occasionally a patient describes debilitating chronic testicular discomfort resistant to every form of analgesic and mood-altering therapy (termed "orchalgia" or "orchidynia"). Both psychotherapy and orchiectomy are often unsuccessful. Spermatic cord stump pain or transference of symptoms to the opposite testis may follow therapeutic orchiectomy.

4. What diagnostic adjuncts are available for evaluation of the scrotum?
Urinalysis (to exclude infection)   Ultrasound scanning
Color Doppler ultrasound (for blood flow)   Serum tumor marker evaluation
Isotope scintigraphy   Drainage cultures
Plain radiographs (for evidence of calcification)   Surgical exploration

5. How may physical examination be implemented in the patient with severe pain?
Pain resulting from epididymitis, spermatic cord torsion, or posttraumatic hematocele inhibits palpation. Injection of local anesthetic (1% lidocaine) into the spermatic cord above the testis provides instant relief, and examination may then proceed.

6. What is the most helpful clinical feature for distinguishing spermatic cord torsion from epididymitis?

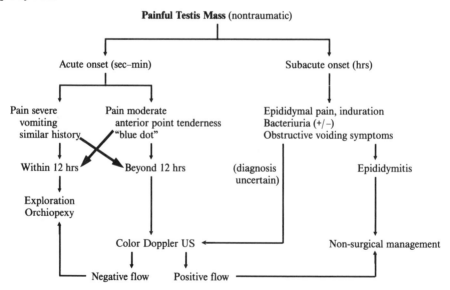

Despite published references to clinical distinctions between torsion and epididymitis (e.g., transverse epididymal position, Prehn's sign, testicular elevation, cutaneous erythema), the most differentiating feature is the rate of onset of testicular pain. Pain of spermatic cord torsion evolves almost instantaneously to maximal intensity; emesis frequently occurs in pediatric patients. Pain of epididymitis escalates gradually over many hours or 1–3 days to maximal intensity. Diagnosis may be confirmed by localization of induration and tenderness to the posterior aspect of the testis, and perhaps even to the upper or lower epididymal pole.

7. Is spermatic cord torsion restricted to young patients?
Classically spermatic cord torsion is restricted to boys under age 16 years and epididymitis to adults. Neither statement is accurate. Acute severe testis pain is spermatic cord torsion until proved otherwise, regardless of age or other clinical features.

8. What is the recommended management of possible spermatic cord torsion?
The recommended management is prompt detorsion, usually surgical. Occasionally manual derotation permits elective (nonemergency) scheduling for bilateral orchiopexy. Manual or spontaneous derotation occurs more frequently in adults, perhaps related to less fixation by fibrin exudate in adults than in pediatric patients. When manual derotation is not attempted or unsuccessful, emergency operative scrotal exploration is required for derotation, appraisal of viability, orchiectomy or orchipexy, and prophylactic fixation of the opposite uninvolved testis. When the diagnosis is uncertain or when excessive time has elapsed between onset and presentation (thereby questioning testicular viability), color Doppler ultrasound, or isotope scintigraphy is recommended. Orchiectomy for definitive infarction may be deferred or omitted.

9. Describe the management of acute epididymitis.
Symptoms of acute epididymitis range from nominal polar tenderness to extreme indurated painful mass with systemic toxicity. Management therefore ranges from outpatient antibiotics and pain medication to hospitalization for fluid repletion, intravenous antibiotics, and perhaps therapeutic orchiectomy.

10. What is the anticipated response to therapy for acute epididymitis?
Epididymitis that does not respond to therapy within 24–48 hours implies inappropriate antibiotic treatment, inaccurate diagnosis, or abscess formation.

11. What is the potential significance of an episode of epididymitis in a pediatric patient?
Epididymitis is uncommon in pediatric patients and therefore suggests the possibility of obstructive or fistulous urinary defects, usually identified by voiding cystourethrogram.

12. What is the potential significance of recurrent epididymitis in an adult?
Recurrent epididymitis suggests lower urinary tract obstruction. An alternative possibility in patients engaged in vigorous work or exercise is retrograde reflux of urine into the vas deferens with straining, producing a chemical epididymitis that tends to be recurrent.

13. What is the potential significance of a varicocele to a child? To an adult?
Varicoceles usually become manifest in early or mid-adolescence, and often spontaneously regress during the fourth decade. Thus the published incidence of varicocele among military inductees is 12–15% compared with an insignificant incidence of varicocele or history of varicocelectomy among older men. Pathologic etiologies such as intraabdominal or retroperitoneal masses that produce venous obstruction and collateral venous drainage should be considered in preadolescent or presenile patients.

Nonpathologic varicoceles in preadolescent boys are significant owing to possible deleterious influences on testicular growth and maturation. Therefore varicocelectomy is recommended to reverse suppressive influences in a testis that is noticeably smaller than its mate.

Fertility dysfunction and abnormal seminalysis may improve after varicocelectomy in adults. Semen defects associated with varicocele include reduced sperm motility and increased numbers of immature and abnormal forms. Although both defects may improve after varicocelectomy, the greatest benefit is increased sperm motility; absolute sperm count is often not significantly improved.

14. What is the usual presentation of a testicular tumor?
Testicular tumors present as a painless mass. Lack of symptoms is reflected in the frequent delay of presentation until the size of the mass is several times normal.

15. Should needle aspiration of a painless testicular mass be undertaken for diagnosis?
No. The mainstay of diagnosis is inguinal orchiectomy for establishment of tumor histology. Needle aspiration is contraindicated, because tumor seeding and inaccurate histologic subtyping may result. Also needed are a chest radiograph and assessment of serum tumor markers (alpha fetoprotein and beta human chorionic gonadotropin) as an index of tumor volume, aggressiveness, and histology and later as a measure of response to therapy. Additional diagnostic maneuvers include computerized abdominal scanning and excretory urography (See figure on following page).

16. Is testicular carcinoma curable?
Yes. Therapy is determined by histology, volume, and staging (degree of dissemination) of the tumor as well as response to previous therapy. Seminoma is traditionally curable with small doses of radiotherapy; large-volume seminoma or extranodal disease warrants chemotherapy. Nonseminomatous germ-cell carcinoma (embryonal carcinoma, teratocarcinoma, choriocarcinoma) requires platinum-based chemotherapy with or without retroperitoneal lymph node dissection.

17. How does management of pediatric tumors differ?
Pediatric yolk sac tumor is best managed by routine retroperitoneal lymph node resection; chemotherapy is reserved for supradiaphragmatic, incompletely resected, or recurrent malignancy. Pediatric testicular teratoma is a benign lesion that requires no management after orchiectomy. In contrast, benign teratoma in adults is capable of malignant dissemination and is therefore routinely managed as a malignant lesion.

18. What should be considered in the management of indurated testicular enlargement in a neonate?
Intrauterine testicular torsion presents as an apparently painless, smooth, homogeneously enlarged testis that may appear blue through the scrotal integument, and may be distinguished from hydrocele or other lesions by testicular ultrasound. Orchiectomy is usually not necessary.

19. What is the presentation and significance of torsion of a testicular appendage?
Torsion of a testicular appendage presents with symptoms of spermatic cord torsion, but much less intense. Vomiting is unlikely. Less extreme pain and swelling contribute to delayed presentation, which is provoked more often by chronicity than intensity of symptoms. Therefore, emergency operative intervention is avoided in favor of adjunctive diagnostic maneuvers (color Doppler ultrasound, isotope scanning). The natural history of a twisted appendage is symptomatic resolution and regression of the tender mass (which may appear blue through the skin, producing the "blue dot" sign). Such lesions may calcify and become separated, accounting for the floating lesion occasionally discovered at routine physical examination.

20. What is the significance of acute pain and testicular enlargement after scrotal trauma?
Acutely painful post-traumatic testicular enlargement reflects rupture of the testicular capsule (tunica albuginea) with parenchymal extrusion and hematoma formation (hematocele). Pain may be extreme, with pallor, sweating, and nausea. Diagnosis may be confirmed in equivocal circumstances by scrotal ultrasound. Patients managed conservatively usually recover

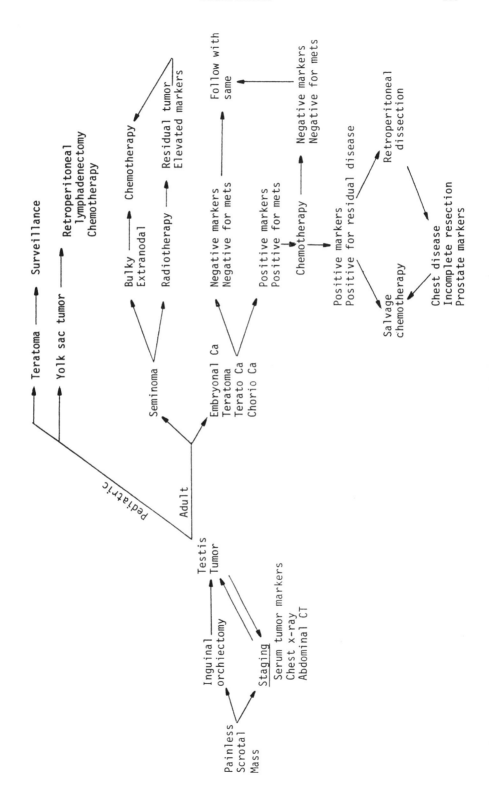

spontaneously after an extended symptomatic convalescence, whereas scrotal exploration, evacuation of hematoma and infarcted tissue, and surgical repair of the testicular capsule contribute to a brief and relatively benign convalescence.

BIBLIOGRAPHY

1. Peterson NE: Scrotal mass. In Norton LW, Steele G Jr, Eiseman B (eds): Surgical Decision Making. Philadelphia, W.B. Saunders. 1992, pp 266–267.
2. Peterson NE (consulting editor), Schwab R: Acute scrotal pain requires quick thinking and plan of action. Emerg Med Rep 13:11–18, 1992.
3. Peterson NE: Emergency management of common urologic problems in men. Part I: Physical examination and differential diagnosis of scrotal masses. Emerg Med Rep 7:1–7, 1986.
4. Peterson NE: Painless scrotal mass. In Norton L, Eiseman B (eds): Surgical Decision Making. Philadelphia, W.B. Saunders, 1985, pp 276–277.
5. Peterson NE: Painful scrotal mass. In Norton L, Eiseman B (eds): Surgical Decision Making. Philadelphia, W.B. Saunders, 1985, pp 278–279.
6. Peterson NE: Testis tumors. In Norton L, Eiseman B (eds): Surgical Decision Making. Philadelphia, W.B. Saunders, 1985, pp 280–281.
7. Wettlaufer J, Peterson NE: Germinal testis tumor. In Eiseman B (ed): Prognosis of Surgical Disease. Philadelphia, W.B. Saunders, 1980, pp 464–466.

51. IMPOTENCE

Norm Peterson, M.D.

1. What is impotence?
Impotence is a diagnostic term that should be supplanted by *erectile dysfunction*, which refers to the inability to obtain or maintain penile erection satisfactory for intercourse. Erectile dysfunction is distinct from infertility and also must be distinguished from the patients' unrealized ambitions of sexual potency.

2. How common is impotence in the United States?
The number of men with erectile dysfunction is estimated at 10–20 million. Figures for the year 1985 included 525,000 office visits and 30,000 hospital admissions for erectile dysfunction. Erectile dysfunction is thought to be grossly underdiagnosed because of embarrassment, and reluctance to acknowledge symptoms and to pursue remedies.

3. What are the potential etiologies of erectile dysfunction?
In the broadest terms, erectile dysfunction is categorized as organic or nonorganic:

Organic Causes
Trauma
Inflammatory disorder (prostatitis)
Neurogenic disorders: Spinal cord injury
    Multiple sclerosis
    Temporal lobe epilepsy
    Cerebrovascular accident
    Autonomic neuropathy
    Peripheral neuropathy
Vasogenic disorders: Arterial
    Venous
    Mixed

Endocrine (hormonal):	Hypogonadism
	Decreased testosterone
	Increased prolactin
Systemic disorders:	Diabetes
	Hypertension
	Hypercholesterolemia
	Hyperthyroidism
Pharmacologic impotence	
Miscellaneous factors:	Cigarettes
	Priapism
	Peyronie's disease
	Dialysis
	Alcoholism
	Zinc deficiency
	Angina
	Arthritis
	Chronic obstructive pulmonary disease
	Postoperative dysfunction
	Abdominoperineal resection
	Prostatectomy
	Renal transplantation

4. What are clues to psychogenic impotence?

Clues to psychogenic impotence include complaints of erectile dysfunction despite the presence of periodic erections or coitus, spontaneous nocturnal or early morning erections, or the ability to attain satisfactory potency only in certain circumstances, such as illicit romance or under the influence of drugs or alcohol. Psychogenic impotence typically involves patients in younger age groups in the absence of other potential pathologic influences.

5. Can psychogenic erectile dysfunction be treated?

Therapeutic remedies for psychogenic erectile dysfunction include psychiatric counseling, which may be prolonged and of variable benefit, and initiation of therapy to artificially induce erection.

6. List the indications for psychiatric counseling.

Sex therapy	Personality disorder
Ambiguous impotence	Hypochondriasis
Psychiatric fitness for prosthesis	History of psychiatric disorder
Preexisting functional impotence	Situational impotence
Ethanol or drug abuse	Emotional problems

7. Are objective means available for identifying or verifying nocturnal erections?

Yes. Erectile response to intracavernous injection of erection-inducing agents is satisfactory evidence of intact erectile physiology. Thus, referral to the urologist for this test may eliminate greater expense and help direct therapy.

8. What drugs or medications may deleteriously influence penile erection?

Diuretics	Antihypertensive agents
Hydrochlorothiazide	Hydralazine
Chlorthalidone	Minoxidil
Spironolactone	Clonidine
Hydroflumethizide	Guanethidine
	Methyldopa
	Reserpine

Tranquilizers
  Phenothiazines
  Butyrophenones
  Thioxanthines
Antiandrogens—flutamide
Addictive and abused substances
  Alcohol
  Opiates
  Barbiturates
  Nicotine
  Cannabis
Alpha-adrenergic blockers
  Phenoxybenzamine
  Phentolamine
  Prazosin
  Terazosin
Beta-adrenergic blocker
  Propranolol
  Metoprolol
Anticholinergic agents
  Atropine
  Clinidium
  Dicyclamine
  Isopropamide
Antidepressants
  Tricyclics
  Monoamine oxidase (MAO)
    inhibitors
Antianxiety agents
  Benzodiazepines
  Meprobamate

Antispasmodic agents
  Propantheline
Antiparkinsonian agents
  Benztropine
  Biperiden
  Procyclidine
  Trihexyphenidyl
Antihistamines
Muscle relaxants
  Cyclobenzaprine
  Orphenadrine
Miscellaneous drugs
  Cimetidine
  Clofibrate
  Digoxin
  Estrogens
  Indomethacin
  Lithium carbonate
  Methysergide
  Metoclopramide
  Metronidazole
  Phenytoin
  Antineoplastic agents
  Thiabendazole
  Tolazoline
  Ethionamide
  Phentolamine
  Dicyclomine
  Diethylpropion
  Phentermine

When it is suspected that such an agent may be responsible for erectile dysfunction, discontinuation of the drug, and rechallenge, if necessary, should be undertaken. A supportive history connects erectile dysfunction with initiation of drug therapy.

9. What is the most important systemic cause of erectile dysfunction?
Diabetes may be the single most frequent etiology of erectile dysfunction. Impotence occurs in 35–75% of diabetic men. Whereas many studies claim no correlation between impotence and the duration and severity of diabetes, other reports assert that impotence affects 50% of male diabetics after 10 years. Impotence is often associated with peripheral and/or autonomic diabetic neuropathy. Patients with erectile dysfunction and poorly controlled hyperglycemia may improve with careful medical management.

10. Which hormone tests are important in evaluating patients with erectile dysfunction?
A serum testosterone value within the normal range obviates the need for additional endocrine testing or exogenous testosterone therapy. The rare patient with hypogonadism has a serum testosterone level 200 mg/dl or less, a small prostate, and small soft testes. (< 3.5 cm).
  Impotence occasionally results from hyperprolactinemia (> 15–20 mg/dl), which is typically associated with reduced serum testosterone and diminished libido. Bromocriptine is a specific antagonist, but therapy depends on the specific etiology:

Idiopathic etiology
Postoperative factors
Posttraumatic factors
Primary hypothyroidism
Renal disease
Hypothalamic-pituitary disease
Craniopharyngioma
Sarcoid
Pituitary tumors

Drugs
  Phenothiazines
  Trycyclic antidepressants
  Meprobamate
  Haloperidol
  Methyldopa
  Reserpine
  Amphetamines

11. What medical therapy is available for erectile dysfunction?

Medical Therapy for Impotence

Oral agents		Intracavernous	
Yohimbine	6 mg 3 times/day	Papavarine HCl	30–90 mg
Intramuscular agents		Phentolamine	5 mg
Testosterone propionate	400 mg every 3 wk	Prostaglandin E-1	5–25 ng

Oral therapy is limited to yohimbine, 2–6 mg 3 times/day. This therapy is expensive and of no objective benefit, although some patients claim improvement; placebo effect may explain their claim.

Intramuscular testosterone (either proprionate or ethionate, 400 mg every 3 weeks) is directed to patients with documented subnormal levels of serum testosterone. Some patients with normal serum testosterone claim benefit from such therapy, but placebo effect is likely. For men with normal testosterone levels, endocrine treatment is inappropriate.

Intracavernous therapy of any combination of papaverine (30–90 mg), regitine (5 mg), and/or prostaglandin E-1 (PGE-1; 5–25 ng) injected directly into one cavernous compartment usually induces erection within 10 minutes and maintains erection for 30–90 minutes. Smaller doses are required for neurogenic erectile dysfunction and for agents given in combination. Responsible patients can be educated to perform self-injection so that urologic evaluation and prescription refills are necessary only 3–4 times/year. Potential problems include cavernous scarring (papaverine), which requires discontinuance; local pain (PGE-1); priapism, which often is associated with injection of excessive volumes; and drop-out due to patient dissatisfaction with the procedure itself.

12. What is a vacuum erection device?

The vacuum erection device is a plastic tube that fits over the penis. Air is evacuated from the tube by an attached hand pump, resulting in attraction of blood into the cavernosal tissues by negative pressure. An elastic constriction applied to the penile base maintains an erection satisfactory for coitus. Such devices are effective for many patients and have a low incidence of side effects. Cost ranges between $250–400 and may be partially covered by insurance.

13. What role does penile and pelvic vascular surgery play in therapy for erectile dysfunction?

Penile vascular surgery is of uncertain value and may be best limited to investigational centers. Such therapy is traditionally indicated for younger patients with posttraumatic vascular obstructions amenable to repair. Surgery has a high failure rate: many early successes deteriorate later.

14. What are penile prostheses?

Penile prostheses are intracavernosal implants available to patients who fail or refuse other forms of treatment. Several models are available, including semirigid devices with malleability features for convenience, and inflatable–deflatable hydraulic models. Semirigid devices are reliable and have a low failure rate. Improvements in materials and bioengineering have reduced the mechanical dysfunction of inflatable models, although cost remains significant.

BIBLIOGRAPHY

1. Kabalin JN, Kessler R: Five year followup of the Scott inflatable penile prosthesis and comparison with semirigid penile prosthesis. J Urol 140:1428–1430, 1988.
2. Klavans MS, Padma-Nathan H, Goldstein I: A pharmacologic treatment for impotence. Contemp Urol Feb/Mar:17–21, 1989.
3. Lipman AG: Drugs associated with impotence. Mod Med May:31–82, 1977.
4. Lue T, Tanagho E: Physiology of erection and pharmacological management of impotence. J Urol 137:829–836, 1987.
5. Michie DD: Causes of impotence in elderly men and considerations for treatment. Gen Med Today 7:38–44, 1988.
6. Morley JE: Impotence in older men. Hosp Pract 139:158, 1988.
7. Van Arsdalen KN, Malloy TR, Wein AJ: Erectile physiology, dysfunction, and evolution. Manage Urol 1983, pp 165–185.
8. Van Arsdalen KN, Wein AJ: Drug-induced sexual dysfunction in older men. Geriatrics 39:63–70, 1984.

VIII. Common Disorders of the Renal and Urinary Systems

52. URINARY TRACT INFECTIONS

Randall R. Reves, M.D.

1. Are urinalysis and urine culture always necessary to confirm the diagnosis of a urinary tract infection?

No. By age 65 years up to one-third of women experience one or more episodes of cystitis, the great majority of which are uncomplicated. Such infections are usually due to *Escherichia coli* (80%) or *Staphylococcus saprophyticus* (5–15%), follow predictable susceptibility patterns, and respond to a short course of antimicrobial agents. Thus a young woman with typical symptoms and signs of uncomplicated cystitis and with pyuria documented with a positive urine dipstick test for leukocyte esterase may be treated without urine microscopy or culture. If the leukocyte esterase test is negative in such patients, microscopic examination of urine or a urine culture should be done.

2. How can one be certain that genitourinary symptoms in young women are due to cystitis?

Dysuria may be due to cystitis, urethritis, vulvovaginitis with or without urethritis, or noninfectious inflammatory processes such as chemical irritation. Urinary tract infection is the cause of dysuria in about one-half of female patients. Among young women cystitis is characterized by the abrupt onset of rather severe symptoms of urgency, dysuria, and urinary frequency, often with suprapubic or low back pain. Women with urethritis or vaginitis are more likely to report gradual onset of symptoms, vaginal discharge, and a recent new sexual contact; examination often reveals cervicitis or vulvovaginitis. Significant pyuria is strongly associated with urinary tract infection.

3. Define "significant pyuria."

Most recent studies indicate that 8–10 leukocytes/mm^3 (as determined by cytometer) correlate with urinary tract infection. This level is probably similar to 10 cells per high power field on examinations of centrifuged urinary sediment.

4. What is the role for single-dose treatment of urinary tract infections?

Uncomplicated cystitis in young women may be treated with a single dose of trimethoprim, trimethoprim/sulfamethoxazole, or a fluoroquinolone (which is far more expensive), but treatment failures are slightly higher than with 3-day courses of therapy. Beta lactam drugs are less effective. Treatment for 7 days should be considered for women who are diabetic or pregnant, who have recently experienced a urinary tract infection or have had symptoms for over a week before treatment, or who use a diaphram for contraception.

5. Should young women with repeated episodes of cystitis be evaluated differently?

Repeated episodes of cystitis usually are due to recurrent episodes of infection rather than relapses of chronic infection. At least one culture should be done for confirmation, but cultures during recurrent infections are not necessary. Frequent recurrences can be managed by daily or thrice-weekly prophylaxis or postcoital prophylaxis. Self-diagnosis with prompt single-dose or 3-day treatment is an effective alternative.

6. Why is a colony count of $> 10^5$/ml of urine no longer the single standard for defining urinary tract infection?

Colony counts of $> 10^5$/ml of a single species of bacteria are found in about 80% of individuals with pyelonephritis; this concentration also reliably distinguishes between true (significant) asymptomatic bacteriuria and low-level contamination that occurs during specimen collection (frequently with several species). The value of $> 10^5$ is not useful in defining significant bacteriuria among several other populations (see Table below). Only about 50% of young women with documented cystitis are correctly identified with such a definition.

Colony-forming Units (CFU)/ml of Urine Used to Define Significant Bacteriuria among Different Populations

POPULATION	CFU/ml	COMMENTS
Patients with pyelonephritis	$> 10^5$	80% have $> 10^5$; most $> 10^6$
Asymptomatic individuals	$> 10^5$	Repeat to confirm
Young women with cystitis	$> 10^2$	Pyuria/dysuria syndrome
Men with urinary tract infection	$> 10^3$	Contamination uncommon
Recently catheterized inpatients	$> 10^2$	CFUs usually rise; symptoms develop

7. How important is it to discriminate between upper and lower urinary tract infections before considering a 3-day course of therapy?

Up to one-third of women with symptoms of cystitis have been shown to have occult pyelonephritis. Nonetheless, single-dose antibiotic therapy is 85–95% effective, and 3-day treatment is even less likely to fail. When symptoms and signs of upper tract involvement are present, however, urine culture should be obtained, and treatment for pyelonephritis should be given.

8. Should all patients with symptoms of pyelonephritis be admitted to the hospital?

Young women who have relatively mild symptoms without nausea and emesis that preclude oral therapy and for whom follow-up can be ensured may be treated as outpatients. Pyelonephritis during pregnancy generally should be treated in the hospital. Resistance to amoxicillin and first-generation cephalosporins is noted in 20–30% of bacteria causing community-acquired pyelonephritis. Treatment may be initiated with trimethoprim/sulfamethoxazole; if trimethoprim resistance is common in the community, a fluoroquinolone should be used. Two weeks of therapy appears adequate in most cases. Amoxicillin is less effective than trimethoprim/sulfamethoxazole, even for susceptible strains.

Blood cultures should be obtained from patients requiring hospitalization; up to 20% are positive. Options for initial empirical intravenous therapy include a third-generation cephalosporin such as ceftriaxone (1 gm/day), a fluoroquinolone, or gentamicin (often with ampicillin if enterococci are suspected). After several days of intravenous therapy, treatment often can be completed with an oral agent.

9. What is the value of a Gram stain of uncentrifuged urine?

The detection of one or more bacteria per oil-immersion field correlates well with a colony count of $> 10^5$/ml and identifies the organism in about 80% of cases of pyelonephritis. In addition, the detection of gram-positive cocci provides rapid indication of an enterococcal etiology.

10. Should imaging procedures or urologic evaluations be used in all cases of pyelonephritis?
When fever and other symptoms fail to resolve after 72 hours of appropriate therapy, ultra-sonography or computed tomography should be considered to look for obstruction, urologic abnormalities, or complications such as perinephric abscess.

11. When should a complicated urinary tract infection be suspected?
Complicated urinary tract infections are defined as those due to organisms resistant to antibiotics or occurring among patients with urinary tract abnormalities. Complicated infections should be considered in patients who recently received antibiotics or acquired infections following urinary tract instrumentation, during urinary tract catheterization, or nosocomially. Urinary tract infections are more likely to be complicated among men, diabetics, pregnant women, and immunosuppressed individuals.

12. What is the recommended therapy for complicated urinary tract infections?
Recommendations vary depending on the severity of the illness and the known or anticipated drug-susceptibility patterns of the infecting organism. A greater frequency of *Proteus* sp., enterococci, and nosocomial pathogens such as *Pseudomonas aeruginosa* can be anticipated. Empiric therapy of the seriously ill patient should include coverage for *P. aeruginosa* and *Enterococcus* sp. pending culture results.

13. Should all men with a single urinary tract infection receive a urologic evaluation?
Urinary tract infections in men have traditionally been considered to be complicated by definition, but it is clear that a small number of men experience uncomplicated cystitis. Sexual partners of women with vaginal colonization with *E. coli* or homosexual men engaging in insertive anal intercourse appear to be at greater risk. A 7-day course of therapy with pre- and posttreatment cultures is recommended. If the infection responds promptly to treatment, urologic evaluation may be deferred. Recurrent infections, pyelonephritis, or other complicating factors warrant urologic evaluation.

14. What are the indications for repeat cultures after treatment of a urinary tract infection?
Routine posttreatment cultures of asymptomatic patients are not recommended except for individuals with pyelonephritis, complicated urinary tract infections, urinary tract infections associated with pregnancy, and infections in men. Follow-up cultures should be obtained 2 weeks after treatment.

15. Who should be screened and treated for bacteriuria?
Only two patient groups are known to benefit from treatment of asymptomatic bacteriuria and to warrant screening with two separate urine cultures. Bacteriuria during pregnancy should be treated to prevent pyelonephritis and the risks of premature delivery. Patients with bacteriuria before urologic surgery should be treated to prevent infectious complications of surgery.

16. When should one consider treatment of urinary tract infection for longer than 2 weeks?
Women with positive posttreatment cultures following pyelonephritis may have subclinical pyelonephritis and may require 4–6 weeks of antibiotics for a cure. Men with positive post-treatment cultures may have either an upper tract or prostatic source of infection and benefit from a 4–6 week course of therapy.

17. Should one treat patients with indwelling urinary catheters and positive urine cultures?
Bacteriuria in patients with indwelling urinary catheters should not be treated unless patients become symptomatic. Removal or replacement of catheters that have been in place for more than 2 weeks may be helpful.

18. What is the significance of staphylococcal isolates from urine cultures?
S. saprophyticus is a recognized cause of cystitis in young women. *Staphylococcus aureus* is an unusual cause of community-acquired urinary tract infection, and the diagnosis of

staphylococcal bacteremia with or without a renal cortical abscess should be considered. Diabetes mellitus, hemodialysis, and intravenous drug use are predisposing factors for staphylococcal sepsis. Complications of pyelonephritis may lead to a perinephric abscess, usually due to *E. coli* or other enteric bacilli. Ultrasonography or computerized tomography is usually required to diagnose either type of renal abscess.

19. What factors may alter the vaginal flora and increase the risk of urinary tract infection?
The use of spermicides with or without a diaphram for contraception increases the frequency of both vaginal colonization with uropathogens and urinary tract infections. Estrogen deficiency in postmenopausal women leads to a decrease in the frequency of vaginal colonization with *Lactobacillus* sp., a higher vaginal pH, and increased frequency of colonization with *E. coli*. Topical application of estriol has been shown to decrease the frequency of recurrent urinary tract infections in postmenopausal women.

BIBLIOGRAPHY

1. Hooton TM, Stamm WE: Management of acute uncomplicated urinary tract infection in adults. Med Clin North Am 75:339–357, 1991.
2. Johnson CC: Definitions, classification, and clinical presentation of urinary tract infections. Med Clin North Am 75:241–252, 1991.
3. Kamaroff AL: Urinalysis and urine culture in women with dysuria. Ann Intern Med 104:212–218, 1986.
4. Kunin CA, White LVA, Hua TH: A reassessment of the importance of "low-count" bacteriuria in young women with acute urinary symptoms. Ann Intern Med 119:454–460, 1993.
5. Lipsky BA: Urinary tract infections in men. Ann Intern Med 110:138–150, 1989.
6. Neu HC: Urinary tract infections. Am J Med 92(Suppl 4A):63S–70S, 1992.
7. Raz R, Stamm WE: A controlled trial of intravaginal estriol in postmenopausal women with recurrent urinary tract infections. N Engl J Med 329:753–756, 1993.
8. Stamm WE, Hooton TM: Management of urinary tract infections in adults. N Engl J Med 329:1328–1334, 1993.

53. SEXUALLY TRANSMITTED DISEASES

Mary Ann De Groote, M.D.

1. Why should women be especially targeted for control of gonorrhea?
An estimated one million new cases of gonorrhea develop each year in the United States. While screening and treatment of all patients with gonorrhea is important, most men with new infection develop symptoms and seek care. Many women are asymptomatic until complications such as pelvic inflammatory disease (PID), tubal scarring, or ectopic pregnancy occur. Undiagnosed chronic pelvic infections are considered the major cause of infertility.

2. What nongenital infections and complications can occur due to *Neisseria gonorrhoeae*?
    1. **Pharyngeal infection** may be asymptomatic. A pharyngeal culture should be obtained in patients with a history of orogenital contact. Occasionally, overt pharyngitis with cervical lymphadenitis may occur.
    2. **Anorectal infection** occurs in women and homosexual men.
    3. **Disseminated gonococcal infection** (DGI) occurs in up to 1% of patients. Patients present with fever, tenosynovitis, petechial or pustular skin lesions, and occasionally septic arthritis.
    4. **Perihepatitis**, also known as Fitz-Hugh-Curtis syndrome, is most often caused by *Chlamydia trachomatis* but may be a rare complication of gonococcal infection.

5. **Tubo-ovarian abscess and pelvic peritonitis** may be serious complications of *N. gonorrhoeae* infection that requires hospitalization.

6. **Long-term complications** of gonorrhea include tubal scarring, which leads to ectopic pregnancy, infertility, and chronic pelvic pain.

3. What anatomic sites may be involved in women with *C. trachomatis* infection of the genital tract?

1. The **endocervix** is the most frequent site of infection. Most patients present with a vaginal discharge. On examination of the cervix, a yellow or green mucus is often visible. Although not specific for *Chlamydia*, a swab obtained of the discharge reveals polymorphonuclear cells (PMNs) without gram-negative intracellular diplococci.

2. The **urethra** is also a common site of infection. In up to 65% of women with dysuria or urgency and a negative urine culture for bacteria, *C. trachomatis* is the etiologic agent.

3. Numerous studies have shown that chlamydial infection of the **endometrium** may be the most common cause of endometritis and PID.

4. Damage to the **fallopian tubes** leading to obstructive infertility and ectopic pregnancy has been linked to *C. trachomatis*.

4. How is chlamydial infection diagnosed?

The diagnosis begins with a careful history. Chlamydial infection is most common in younger women ($\leq$ 24 years old), women with a new sexual partner, and women who do not use barrier contraceptives. The patient may present with no symptoms, abdominal or pelvic pain, or vaginal or urethral symptoms. In most women, the cervix is the initial site of infection. Vaginal discharge, vaginal bleeding, and postcoital spotting may occur. On examination the cervical discharge may be clear or purulent, and cervical bleeding after using a culture swab is common. Culture for *C. trachomatis*, the gold standard, is not always available. Culture is performed using a Dacron swab (after mucus has been removed from the endocervix) and must be sent on ice within 24 hours. Other diagnostic modalities include direct fluorescent antibody, enzyme linked immunosorbent assay, DNA probe, and polymerase chain reaction (PCR). These techniques are more widely used than culture because of ease of collection, transport, and performance. They carry a sensitivity rate of 75–90% and a specificity rate of 95%. Empirical therapy while the patient is still in the clinic is often begun before the results are confirmed. The treatment of choice is doxycycline or tetracycline. If the patient is pregnant, erythromycin is the drug of choice.

5. Which organisms are thought to cause PID?

PID may be caused by one or more organisms. The most common is *C. trachomatis*, but *N. gonorrhoeae* is also important. Polymicrobic infection, including facultative aerobic and anaerobic bacteria, also occurs. Laparoscopic cultures of fallopian tubes and culdocentesis from patients with PID often reveal a combination of aerobic and anaerobic organisms, such as *Bacteroides, Escherichia coli*, group B streptococci, *Gardnerella vaginalis*, and other anaerobic cocci. These organisms are frequently isolated in the presence of *N. gonorrhoeae* or *C. trachomatis* from endocervical cultures.

6. Discuss the evaluation of a man who presents with urethritis.

Although some men may be asymptomatic, a history of urethral discharge, dysuria, itching, and a recent history of a sexually transmitted disease (STD) in a partner should be ascertained. In homosexual men, a history of rectal and/or pharyngeal contact should be looked for. A Gram stain of the urethral discharge typically reveals increased PMN cells. A first-void urine sediment also may be used. The presence of intracellular gram-negative diplococci is diagnostic of gonorrhea. Because the Gram stain may miss some cases, a urethral swab culture for *N. gonorrhoeae* also should be done. When no bacteria are detected in the presence of PMNs, the diagnosis of nongonoccocal urethritis (NGU) is made. NGU is most frequently caused by *C. trachomatis* but *Ureaplasma urealyticum, Trichomonas vaginalis*, and other organisms also may be responsible.

Treatment of NGU consists of doxycycline. Because the coisolation of *N. gonorrhoeae* and *C. trachomatis* is common, patients with evidence of gonorrhea should be treated for both. For treatment of gonorrhea, options include ceftriaxone (given intramuscularly) or ciprofloxacin, cefixime, or ofloxacin; (all given once orally).

7. Name the three most common causes of genital ulcers.

1. **Herpes simplex virus** (HSV). Although the incidence varies geographically, in the U.S., HSV is the most common cause of genital ulcers and appears to be increasing.

2. **Syphilis**. The classic syphilitic ulcer is a painless indurated chancre. Syphilis is a frequent cause of genital ulceration both in the United States and in developing nations.

3. **Chancroid**. This common cause of genital ulcers in the developing world is also gaining a foothold in the U.S. *Haemophilus ducreyi*, the etiologic agent, needs to be cultured on special media.

More than one pathogen may exist in a small number of lesions (3–10%). Less common causes are lymphogranuloma venereum and donovanosis (granuloma inguinale). The presence of a genital ulcer is a risk factor for transmission of the human immunodeficiency virus (HIV). All patients should be evaluated with syphilis serology. Other miscellaneous noninfectious causes include trauma, allergic reactions, Behçet syndrome, malignancy, and Stevens-Johnson syndrome.

8. Describe the clinical stages and the consequences of untreated syphilis.

There are no pathognomonic presentations for each stage, and a high index of suspicion is needed to make the diagnosis. Syphilis is a systemic disease caused by the spirochete *Treponema pallidum*. Primary syphilis is manifested by a chancre that begins as a macule at the site of inoculation (usually on the genitals) and then becomes an indurated ulcer. Secondary syphilis, which usually appears 3–6 weeks after the initial chancre, includes a wide variety of signs and symptoms that reflect the systemic nature of the infection. The skin rash is a hallmark and characteristically appears on the palms and soles but may be highly variable. Lymphadenopathy, mucous membrane lesions, arthritis, hepatitis, nephrotic syndrome, meningitis, and cranial nerve abnormalities may be seen with secondary syphilis. Syphilis is called the great masquerader because of the plethora of findings; most patients, however, display only one or a few of these findings.

If untreated, the disease progresses to a latent stage with no evidence of disease, although serologic tests are positive. Early latent infection refers to a duration of less than 1 year. Patients who have been infected more than 1 year or for an unknown duration are considered to have late latent infection. In the preantibiotic era, approximately 25% of untreated patients with latent syphilis progressed to the tertiary stage, which includes gummas, granulomas of bones and soft tissues, cardiovascular symptoms, and neurosyphilis. Currently rates of complications of unrecognized latent syphilis are probably lower because of the likelihood of receiving antibiotics with antisyphilitic activity for unrelated reasons.

9. How can the laboratory assist the clinician in making the diagnosis of syphilis?

The definitive diagnosis of syphilis is made by demonstrating the presence of characteristic spirochetes on a darkfield examination of infected tissue. However, two types of serologic tests assist in diagnosis: nontreponemal and treponemal. The first consists of the rapid plasma reagin (RPR) and venereal disease research laboratories (VDRL) tests. The two specific treponemal tests include the fluorescent treponemal antibody-absorbed assay (FTA) and the microhemagglutination assay for antibody to *Treponema pallidum* (MHATP). The nontreponemal serologic tests may be quantitated and followed to assess response to therapy and to diagnose reinfection. The RPR and VDRL are associated with occasional false-positive results and must be confirmed with a specific treponemal test. Both abnormally high and low syphilis titers have been described in patients infected with HIV, but serologic tests remain reliable for the vast majority of patients. The diagnosis of neurosyphilis relies on serology of the cerebrospinal fluid (CSF). A positive CSF VDRL is considered diagnostic, but the test may be falsely negative.

10. Does the treatment of syphilis depend on the stage of infection?

Yes. Although the drug of choice for all stages is penicillin, late latent, tertiary, and neurosyphilis require a longer duration of therapy. Careful follow-up includes history, physical examination, and serologic tests. Failure of the nontreponemal test to decline fourfold or more by 3 months for primary or 6 months for secondary syphilis warrants close follow-up and consideration for retreatment.

STAGE	THERAPY*
Primary	Benzathine PCN G, 2.4 million units IM once
Secondary	Benzathine PCN G, 2.4 million units IM once
Latent (early)	Benzathine PCN G, 2.4 million units IM once
Latent (late or unknown)	Benzathine PCN G, 2.4 million units IM weekly for 3 weeks
Neurosyphilis	12–24 million units aqueous crystalline PCN G daily for 10–14 days or 2.4 million units procaine PCN, intramuscularly + probenecid, 500 mg 4 times/day for 10–14 days

*For HIV infection, PCN allergy and treatment of pregnant patients, see Centers for Disease Control: 1993 Sexually Transmitted Diseases Treatment Guidelines. MMWR 42(RR-14), 1993.

11. Genital warts are caused by the human papilloma virus (HPV). Which malignant lesions are also linked to the virus?

HPV has been linked to cervical and vulvar cancer in women and squamous cell cancer of the penis and anus in men. Genital warts are commonly caused by HPV types 6 or 11. Other types, including 16, 18, 31, 33, and 35, have been associated with dysplasia and cancer. External warts can be removed in a number of ways, including cryotherapy with liquid nitrogen, podophyllin, and trichloroacetic acid, but recurrences are common. Laser treatment and surgery are reserved for extensive warts. Patients should be counseled regarding recurrences, use of condoms, and the importance of annual Papanicolaou smears.

12. What is the most common parasitic STD?

The most common parasitic STD is infection with *Trichomonas vaginalis*, a flagellated protozoan. Signs and symptoms include vaginal inflammation and malodorous discharge. Some women and most men are asymptomatic. Occasionally men have mild urethritis. Organisms can be demonstrated in 30–40% of sexual partners. Diagnosis can be made in the office by performing a microscopic evaluation of vaginal secretions and demonstrating typical motile organisms. The microscopic examination is only 60–70% sensitive compared with culture. Treatment consists of a single 2-gm dose of metronidazole. Patients should be warned about a disulfiramlike reaction. Metronidazole is relatively contraindicated in the first trimester of pregnancy because of teratogenic effects observed in laboratory animals. Male sexual partners also should be treated.

13. Differentiate between the clinical manifestations of primary and recurrent genital herpes infections.

The two serotypes of herpes simplex virus are HSV-1 and HSV-2. Most cases of genital herpes are caused by HSV-2. Although the course may vary, primary disease is usually more severe. The patient lacks specific antibodies at the time of the lesions. Mucosal lesions may be multiple. Urethritis, cervicitis, lymphadenopathy, fevers, headaches, and occasionally aseptic meningitis or sacral nerve symptoms (urinary retention or laxness of the anal sphincter) may complicate primary genital herpes infection. Primary disease is often treated with acyclovir to reduce the duration of symptoms, although therapy does not cure or prevent latent infection.

Recurrent disease tends to be milder. The small clusters of lesions usually crust over in a few days. Some patients have a prodromal tingling sensation, numbness, or paresthesias before the development of vesicles. Experimental evidence demonstrates that in patients with frequent recurrences prophylactic acyclovir may decrease the recurrence of lesions by 40–50%. Recurrent and mild disease usually does not require therapy. Of importance, many persons with a history of symptomatic genital HSV experience asymptomatic recurrences. During such generally brief periods they have infectious HSV in genital secretions but no symptoms of a herpes outbreak.

14. Why are the diagnoses and treatment of genital herpes important? Describe each.
In addition to the morbidity associated with genital ulcers, the major serious sequela of genital HSV infection is transmission to the newborn infant at the time of delivery. The greatest risk occurs when the mother acquires a primary infection near the time of delivery. Viral cultures of the birth canal at delivery are helpful in guiding management of the neonate.

In nonpregnant patients with HSV, clinicians should suspect the diagnosis and perform a careful examination with culture of suspicious lesions. Transmission of virus is most efficient in the presence of overt lesions. However, virus can be shed in the absence of obvious lesions, and many cases are thought to be transmitted during asymptomatic periods. Patients should be advised to refrain from sexual activity in the presence of overt lesions. Condoms are not foolproof but should be encouraged during all sexual exposures. Sexual partners benefit from evaluation and counseling, even if they are asymptomatic.

15. How can the clinician help to decrease the spread of STDs?
The mnemonic **STEPS** summarizes a common sense approach to STDs:

S = Signs and symptoms. Be familiar with the common and not-so-common STDS to facilitate accurate diagnosis.

T = Treatment. Know the treatment and appropriate follow-up.

E = Education. It is crucial to disseminate information about STDs by verbal communication with the patient during the office visit and the written materials available from most health departments.

P = Partner notification. It is crucial (and required by law in some diseases) to notify the partner so that he or she can be evaluated. It is not sufficient to give the patient medications for his or her partner(s) without direct evaluation.

S = Serious counseling in a nonconfrontational manner. The patient needs to understand how to protect himself or herself in the future. Because of the sensitive nature of a diagnosis with an STD and implications for sexual behavior in the future, emotional support is needed.

Counseling should include frank and nonjudgmental discussions about all options, including abstinence, mutually monogamous relationships, careful choice of partners, and use of condoms for all sexual encounters. When used correctly, condoms are effective in preventing STDs as well as unwanted pregnancy. Latex offers better protection, and the quality is regulated by the Food and Drug Administration (FDA). The link between substance abuse (alcohol and drugs) and STDs should be looked for. Counseling should include education about the risks of needle sharing. At the very least, needles should be cleaned with bleach and water.

16. Do STDs pose special risks to travelers?
All general guidelines apply to STDs during travel, but a few points deserve special mention:
1. Frequently the incidence of STDs is much higher in developing countries than in most areas of the U.S. In addition to gonorrhea, chlamydia, and syphilis, two other important STDs—hepatitis B and HIV—are often more common. Hepatitis B antibody prevalence is well over 50% in some countries of Africa and Asia, and carriage of the surface antigen (HBsAg) may be as high as 25%.
2. HIV-1 and HIV-2 seroprevalence rates are high in certain areas of the world. The major route of transmission is heterosexual intercourse. Solid evidence suggests that the presence of an STD increases the risk of transmisssion of HIV.

3. Avoidance of high-risk sexual behavior is clearly the best course, but barrier contraception is also effective at decreasing the transmission of STDs.

BIBLIOGRAPHY

1. Ault KA, Faro S: Pelvic inflammatory disease: Current diagnostic criteria and treatment guidelines. Postgrad Med 93(2):85–91, 1993.
2. Centers for Disease Control: 1993 Sexually Transmitted Diseases Treatment Guidelines. MMWR 42(RR-14): 1993.
3. Freund KM: Chlamydial disease in women. Hosp Pract 27(2):175–186, 1992.
4. Hansfield HH: Recent developments in STDs: I. Bacterial diseases. Hosp Pract 26(7):47–56, 1991.
5. Hansfield HH: Recent developments in STDs: II. Viral and other syndromes. Hosp Pract 27(1):175–200, 1991.
6. Holmes KK, Mardh PA, Sparling PF, Wiesner PJ (eds): Sexually Transmitted Diseases, 2nd ed. New York, McGraw-Hill, 1990.
7. Mandell GL, Douglas RG, Bennett JE (eds): Principles and Practice of Infectious Diseases, 3rd ed. New York, Churchill Livingstone, pp 931–975, 1990.
8. Mogabgab WJ: Recent developments in the treatment of sexually transmitted diseases. Am J Med 91(Suppl 6A): 140-143S, 1991.
9. Parenti DM: Sexually transmitted diseases and travelers. Med Clin North Am 76:1449–1461, 1992.
10. Vinson RP, Epperly TD: Counseling patients on proper use of condoms. Am Fam Physician 43:2081–2085, 1991.
11. Wooldridge WE: Syphilis: A new visit from an old enemy. Postgrad Med 89(1):193–202, 1991.

54. PROTEINURIA AND HEMATURIA

Arlene B. Chapman, M.D.

1. How should one prepare a urine specimen for analysis?

A fresh urine specimen voided at the beginning of the day gives the most concentrated and acidic urine, which preserves formed elements. Urine specimens should be reviewed within 30 minutes of collection to avoid disintegration of red cells and red cell casts. All samples should be collected in midstream; therefore, a moderately full bladder is required. At least 200 ml of urine should be voided before the specimen is collected. Contamination is avoided by foreskin retraction in men and good labial separation in women. Proper preparation includes gentle cleansing with cotton wool swabs moistened with saline. Even midstream urine collections in the majority of women demonstrate contamination unless cleaning instructions are clear. If it is impossible to obtain a good midstream urine specimen, as in patients with physical handicaps, a catheter specimen may be required.

2. What are the two main components of urinalysis?

1. **Dipstick or chemical analysis.** Commercially available dipsticks measure a number of different components including pH, glucose, ketones, hemoglobin, protein, leukocyte esterase, and bilirubin. Dipsticks screen most accurately for the presence of proteinuria, whereas microscopic analysis is a more informative method for the evaluation of hematuria. Dipstick evaluation of protein involves a pad that contains tetrabromophenol, which changes from yellow to green to blue as increasing amounts of protein are available for binding. Dipstick evaluation of hematuria involves hemoglobin or myoglobin to catalyse a reaction between hydrogen peroxide and the chromogen O-toluidine. When hemoglobin or myoglobin is present in the urine, the test pad turns blue.

2. **Microscopic analysis.** Fixed volumes of fresh urine samples are aliquoted into a 10-ml test tube and centrifuged at 2500–3000 rpm for 5 minutes. The supernatant is poured off,

and after resuspension the sediment is poured onto a slide and placed under a coverslip. A bright-field microscope is commonly used for analysis of urinary sediment, although phase-contrast microscopy provides better vision of all elements. Microscopic analysis is commonly viewed without staining. This approach allows rapid preparation. Two magnifications are required, with the lower (100×) for a general overview and the higher (400×) for details and cell evaluation. The complete slide should be evaluated, which can take 10–15 minutes; most formed elements, however, adhere to the edges of the coverslip.

3. What is considered normal proteinuria?
Under physiologic conditions, urinary excretion of protein does not exceed 150–180 mg/day. The main proteins normally excreted are albumin, immunoglobulins, immunoglobulin light chains, and Tamm-Horsfall protein. In some conditions excessive proteinuria is benign, including functional proteinuria in patients with fever or after exercise; idiopathic transient proteinuria, as in patients with congestive heart failure; and orthostatic proteinuria.

4. What conditions produce false-negative and false-positive results for proteinuria?
False-negative results for proteinuria occur when urine is extremely dilute or when Bence Jones albumin (immunoglobulin light chains) is the predominant source of protein. Dipsticks are more sensitive to albumin, and sulfosalicylic acid should be added to determine if immunoglobulin light chains are present.

False-positive results occur when urine is highly concentrated, when urine pH is greater than 8, when the dipstick has been immersed too long (> 30 seconds), and in the setting of gross hematuria when plasma proteins accompany blood.

5. What is proteinuria?
The three types of proteinuria are glomerular, tubular, or overproduction proteinuria. Proteinuria is most commonly of glomerular origin, and albumin is the major component of protein that leaks through an abnormal glomerular basement membrane. Tubular proteinuria is due to decreased tubular reabsorption of proteins contained in the glomerular filtrate, as in tubulointerstitial disorders. Overload proteinuria is secondary to increased production of immunoglobulin light chains, as in monoclonal gammopathies, or lysozyme, as in some forms of leukemias.

6. How does one evaluate a patient with proteinuria?
The first approach is to quantify the amount of protein in the urine by collecting a 24-hour urine specimen and determining rates of creatinine and protein excretion. Creatinine excretion rates are determined to assess the accuracy (total time) of urine collection. Men should excrete 15–25 mg/kg/day and women 12–20 mg/kg/day of urinary creatinine. Nephrotic range proteinuria is more than 3.5 gm/day. Protein/creatinine ratios have been found to be extremely useful in patients with established creatinine excretion rates, noncompliant patients, or in patients for whom rapid diagnoses are sought. Ratios greater than 3.5 in a single voided sample represent more than 3.5 gm of proteinuria in 24 hours, and ratios less than 0.2 represent less than 0.2 gms of proteinuria in 24 hours.

After quantitation, qualitative analysis of proteinuria should be performed. Qualitative analysis of proteinuria is typically carried out by using electrophoresis on cellulose acetate or agarose after concentrating the urine specimen. This procedure reveals dense bands in β and γ regions. Immunoelectrophoresis is used to identify a monoclonal component.

7. What is considered normal hematuria?
Normal hematuria is defined simply as no red blood cells (RBCs). The dipstick method is extremely sensitive for detecting RBCs in the urine and is positive with as little as 3–5 RBC/hpf. Normal individuals excrete as many as 1×10^6 RBCs every 24 hours. Therefore, occasional RBCs seen microscopically in urine sediment are normal. Approximately 10% of normal people excrete up to 10 RBC/hpf of centrifuged urine sediment. However, less than 3% of normal people excrete more than 3 RBC/hpf. When repeat urinalyses demonstrate 1–3 RBC/hpf, further investigation for a cause of hematuria is warranted.

8. Are the characteristics of hematuria clinically useful?

Yes. Increased excretion of erythrocytes is a nonspecific finding and may be associated with bleeding at any site in the urinary tract. Patterns of hematuria usually are determined by four parameters:

1. Color and appearance of urine (gross or macroscopic vs. covert or microscopic hematuria)
2. Timing of the hematuria (persistent or constant, intermittent or recurrent)
3. Presence or absence of symptoms
4. Isolated hematuria or evidence of proteinuria, leukocyturia, or bacteriuria

9. What may cause false-positive hematuria?

A color of red or dark brown may be seen in conjunction with dyes in foods, including beets, paprika, and senna. Drugs such as rifampin, phenothiazines, and dilantin also may have this effect. Myoglobin also gives a red-brown color to the urine. After intravascular hemolysis, free hemoglobin may be excreted, giving a distinct red color to the urine. Both myoglobin and hemoglobin pigments cause the standard urinary dipstick to give a positive reaction in patients with microscopic hematuria, but the correct diagnosis of urinary RBCs is based on microscopic analysis of the same urine specimen. In female patients, menstrual blood occasionally finds its way into an improperly collected urine specimen. Such patients need to return when they are not having menstrual bleeding. Microscopically, candidal spherules, calcium oxalate crystals, starch granules, and air bubbles have been mistaken for hematuria.

10. What are the causes of isolated hematuria?

Isolated hematuria is almost always due to an extrarenal source. The major causes of both gross and microscopic hematuria include acute and chronic prostatitis or urethritis, hemorrhagic cystitis, renal stones, and tumors of the kidney, renal pelvis, ureter, bladder, prostate, and urethra.

11. How does one approach a patient with isolated hematuria?

Patients need repeat urinalyses to demonstrate persistent hematuria. Examination of the prostate and external urethra in conjunction with a urine culture is the basic first step in evaluation. A three-glass urine test is helpful in diagnosing lower urinary tract hematuria. The patient voids into three different containers. Hematuria only in the initial void suggests urethral bleeding, whereas hematuria in the terminal void suggests a prostatic or bladder origin. Intravenous pyelography and renal ultrasonography are the next tests to be performed if the above studies are uninformative. Renal stones, cysts, or urinary tract tumors can be identified in this fashion. Cystoscopy or retrograde pyelography then should be undertaken in an attempt to identify the source of bleeding. If these studies are uninformative, renal biopsy should be considered.

12. What suggests that hematuria may be renal in origin?

Associated proteinuria almost always suggests a renal origin of hematuria. However, in renal diseases in which proteinuria alone predominates (e.g., diabetes mellitus), evaluation for extrarenal sources of hematuria should be done, such as cystoscopy to screen for transitional cell carcinoma of the bladder. When red cell casts (RBCs enmeshed in Tamm-Horsfall protein) are found, the hematuria is almost always glomerular in origin.

Glomerular hematuria also is suspected when abnormalities in size, shape, and membrane appearance of the RBCs are present (dysmorphic erthyrocytes). Phase-contrast microscopy is necessary to identify such abnormalities. RBCs from a nonglomerular source have normal and regular morphology (isomorphic erythrocytes). More recently, automated blood-cell volume analysers have been proposed to distinguish glomerular from nonglomerular hematuria. Decreased cell volumes are more commonly found in glomerular bleeding.

13. What is the most common cause of hematuria?
Extrarenal sites are the most common source of isolated hematuria. Of a consecutive series of 1000 patients with gross hematuria, 67% demonstrated a lesion in the bladder or lower urinary tract. The most common causes of gross hematuria originating in the kidney are nephropathy and polycystic kidney disease. In 10–15% of patients, no cause for hematuria can be found.

BIBLIOGRAPHY

1. Abuelo JC: Proteinuria: Diagnostic principles and procedures. Ann Intern Med 98:186–191, 1983.
2. Ginsberg JM, Chung BS, Materese RA, Garella S: Use of single voided urine samples to estimate quantitative proteinuria. N Engl J Med 309:1543–1546, 1983.
3. Glassock RJ: Hematuria and pigmenturia. In Massry S, Glassock R (eds): Textbook of Nephrology, vol. 1. Baltimore, Williams & Wilkins, 1989, pp 4.14–4.22.
4. Kubota M, et al: Mechanism of urinary erythrocyte deformity in patients with glomerular disease. Nephrol 48:338–339, 1988.
5. Raman VG, Peud L, Leu HA, Haskell R: A blind controlled trial of phase-contrast microscopy by two observers for evaluating the source of hematuria. Nephrology 44:304–308, 1986.

55. NEPHROLITHIASIS

Jonathan Slater, M.D., and Arlene B. Chapman, M.D.

1. What is the chemical composition of kidney stones?
Kidney stones consist of solutes that are normally dissolved in the urine; however, under the appropriate circumstances they can precipitate out of solution to form crystals that can grow to varying sizes. In general, most kidney stones can be classified into one of the following five categories:

	FREQUENCY IN U.S. (%)
Calcium oxalate	65
Calcium phosphate	7.5
Magnesium ammonium phosphate (struvate)	20
Uric acid	5
Crystine	1

2. Which kidney stone is lucent on radiograph?
Uric acid stones are lucent; all others are opaque.

3. Why do kidney stones form?
In the appropriate urinary environment, precipitation of solute(s) results in formation of a kidney stone. Concentration of the solute is a major factor in determining whether stone formation occurs in urine. Hence, the volume of excreted urine is of utmost importance. For example, the urinary concentration of cystine is normally so low that precipitation is impossible. However, a defect in the normal tubular reabsorption of cystine increases the concentration significantly, and precipitation of this relatively uncommon stone may occur.

4. Does stone formation depend only on urinary solute concentration?
No. The factors listed below have varying importance in promoting or inhibiting stone formation:

1. Urinary pH

Low pH ($<$ 5.5)	Promotes	uric acid stones + + +
		cystine stones + +
	Inhibits	phosphate-containing stones –
		struvite stones – – –
High pH ($>$ 7.0)	Promotes	struvite stones + + +
		phosphate-containing stones +
	Inhibits	Uric acid stones – – –
		Cystine stones – –
2. Hypocitraturia	Promotes	calcium stones + + +
3. Hypomagnesiuria	Promotes	calcium stones + + +
4. Increased sodium in the urine	Promotes	calcium stones +

5. What factors contribute to the formation of calcium-containing stones?
Hypercalciuria. Generally defined as $>$ 4 mg calcium/kg body weight in the urine over 24 hours, hypercalcium is present in approximately 60% of all patients with stones. Hypercalciuria may result from absorptive hypercalciuria (most common cause; inherited); renal hypercalciuria; or primary hyperparathyroidism.
Hypocitraturia. Since urinary citrate inhibits stone formation, low urine citrate (as in distal renal tubular acidosis) promotes stone formation.
Hyperuricosuria. Stone formation is promoted by urinary uric acid and may be found in up to 30% of patients with calcium stones.
Hyperoxaluria. Increased excretion of oxalate, as in terminal ileal disease, also increases the propensity to form calcium (not only oxalate) stones.

6. When should the clinician anticipate an increased risk of oxalate stones?
Enteric hyperoxaluria occurs when a disturbance of normal ileal function (Crohn's disease, ileal resection) results in increased intestinal absorption of oxalate. The fatty acids and bile salts normally reabsorbed by the ileum now are increased in concentration in the intestinal lumen and compete with oxalate for binding to divalent ions (calcium). Thus, more free oxalate is available to be absorbed in the colon and excreted into the urine. Primary oxaluria is a rare inherited disorder; high-oxalate foods (dark green vegetables, chocolate, tea, nuts) occasionally cause hyperoxaluria.

7. When are struvite stones seen?
The major predisposing factor for struvite stones is recurrent urinary tract infections with urease-splitting bacteria (*Proteus* sp., *Pseudomonas* sp., *Escherichia coli*).

8. What causes hyperuricosuria?
Increased excretion of uric acid ($>$ 800 mg/24 hours) may be associated with hyperuricemia (resulting from conditions of increased cellular turnover or breakdown) or uricosuric agents (such as probenecid, sulfinpyrazone, salicylates, thiazides). Dietary purines may exaggerate hyperuricosuria (organ meats, sardines). Otherwise, hyperuricosuria, which is found in 30% of patients with calcium and urate stones, is idiopathic.

9. Is there a correlation between symptoms and anatomic location of stone?
Stone formation occurs most often in the proximal portion of the urinary collecting system, then passes down through the calyces, pelvis, ureter, and bladder, and finally exits the body through the urethra. When the stone obstructs the ureter, either completely or partially, it causes renal colic (writhing and excruciating pain of acute onset, often fluctuating in intensity). The location and radiation of the pain depends on the anatomic location of the stone in the ureter. In general, as the stone makes its journey, it is prone to obstruct the ureter in the following five locations where the collecting system narrows:

1. Calyx/pelvis: abdominal distension, colicky pain localized to flank or costovertebral angle or occasionally radiating into the groin and testicle
2. Ureteropelvic junction: similar pain pattern as in 1
3. Pelvic brim: pain in the lateral flank and lower abdomen
4. Posterior pelvis: (especially in women) bladder irritation and/or genital pain
5. Ureterovesical junction: similar pain pattern as in 4

10. What tests should be performed to diagnose kidney stones?
When the patient presents acutely with renal colic, the following steps should be taken: history, physical examination, serum chemistries, urinalysis, kidneys, ureter, and bladder (KUB) radiographs, and intravenous pyelogram (IVP). Typically the combination of a suggestive history and hematuria (almost always present) helps to make the diagnosis. The abdominal radiograph (KUB) reveals the stone in approximately 90% of cases. The IVP clearly demonstrates the location of the stone and whether hydronephrosis (complete obstruction) is present. To avoid contrast-induced acute renal failure, all patients should be well hydrated; if azotemia, diabetes mellitus, or multiple myeloma is present, further precautionary prophylactic measures (e.g., mannitol, furosemide) may be warranted.

Drug-seeking patients also know that renal colic causes excruciating pain and often requires narcotic analgesia. Hence one must exercise caution in the evaulation and treatment of patients presenting with symptoms of renal colic.

11. What percentage of first-time stone formers develop a subsequent stone?
In the United States there are approximately 250,000–350,000 new cases of nephrolithiasis each year. It was previously thought that the majority of patients who presented with their first kidney stone would not develop another stone in their lifetime; hence a complete medical evaluation was not indicated and not cost-effective. It is now known that the chance of recurrence of kidney stones within 10 years is 70%; thus all patients should have a complete medical evaluation. Furthermore, in 85–90% of patients, evaluation yields a positive test result.

12. What tests should be performed in evaluating a patient with a kidney stone(s)?
Stone analysis plays a key role in the medical evaluation of the patient with kidney stones. Patients should be instructed to pass all urine through a strainer until they spontaneously pass the stone, which then can be analyzed. This point cannot be overemphasized.

Other important tests may diagnose medical conditions that identify patients at risk for recurrent kidney stones (see quesion 5); then treatment can be targeted to decrease risk for subsequent stone formation. In approximately 10–15% of patients, no underlying metabolic disturbance is discovered; low urine volume may be the only problem.

The following tests should be performed: two separate 24-hour urine collections for assessment of total volume and excretion of calcium, uric acid, creatinine, oxalate, citrate, cystine, magnesium, and sodium; a random urine sample for culture and metered pH; and assessment of serum calcium, creatinine, phosphorus, and uric acid.

13. Does it matter in what setting the 24-hour urine collection is done?
Yes. Collection should be performed on an outpatient basis while the patient follows normal dietary habits, because urinary excretion depends in large degree on food and liquid intake. Measurement of urine creatinine (normal values for men and women are 15–25 and 12–20 mg/kg/24 hr, respectively) allows one to determine whether an adequate urine collection was performed.

14. What treatment should be instituted in patients with first-time kidney stones?
In many cases before subjecting patients with first stone to lifelong pharmacologic intervention, it is prudent to initiate so-called general treatment programs. All patients should be encouraged to ingest enough fluids to ensure at least 2 liters of urine output/day. Depending on the type of stone and 24-hour urine results, further dietary restriction and limitations may

be initiated (for example, decreasing calcium, oxalate, and purines in the diet). In patients with hypercalciuria, sodium restriction is also advantageous, because it further decreases urinary calcium excretion.

15. What recommendations should be made for recurrent stone formers who fail general treatment?

If the general treatment programs are not effective, the following specific treatments may be added, depending on the results of stone analysis and urine and serum tests:

Hypercalciuria can be treated with thiazide diuretics which increase tubular reabsorption of calcium, thus directly counteracting the hypercalciuria in patients with renal calcium leak. It also is often effective in patients with absorptive hypercalciuria in combination with dietary calcium restrictions.

Hyperoxaluria in the majority of cases is due to dietary intake and thus can be effectively treated by dietary restrictions. However, if the levels are markedly elevated or refractory to dietary alterations, one should consider further tests to diagnose primary or enteric hyperoxaluria; and if either is present, treatment should be directed at the specific problem. In either situation it is often helpful to add potassium citrate to the diet to help to inhibit stone formation. If renal insufficiency is present serum potassium must be monitored when potassium citrate is prescribed.

Hypocitraturia can be treated effectively by either sodium or potassium citrate, both of which have a dramatic preventive effect. Potassium citrate, if tolerated, is preferred because the sodium tends to increase calciuria.

Hyperuricosuria, which promotes both calcium-containing and uric acid stones, usually can be decreased by changes in dietary habits. However, if the patient cannot comply or if urinary uric acid levels remain high, allopurinol is very effective.

Uric acid stones can be effectively prevented by alkalinizing the urine with potassium citrate or other alkalinizing agents. In some patients, alkalizing of the urine promotes formation of calcium-containing stones.

16. How often do patients spontaneously pass kidney stones?

Most patients with kidney stones can be managed as outpatients with analgesics and large fluid intake (8 oz of fluid/hr while awake). Approximately 80% of patients pass stones spontaneously; the other 20% of patients ultimately require some form of intervention. The probability of spontaneously passing the stone depends in large part on the size of the stone:

　< 4 mm　　75% probability
　> 8 mm　　10% probability

17. What techniques are available to remove kidney stones?

1. **Ureteroscopy.** A wire is placed with a cystoscope past the stone, if possible; the distal ureter is dilated with a balloon; and the ureteroscope is advanced to the stone. Using either a basket or forceps, the stone is pulled downward through the ureter. The success rate for stones in the lower third of the ureter is 90%, whereas the success rate of stone removal from the upper ureter is only 30%.

2. **Percutaneous nephrolithotomy.** Under either fluoroscopy or ultrasound, first a needle and then a wire and tube are placed into the renal pelvis percutaneously. Next the nephroscope is advanced into the collecting system to allow direct visualization of the stone. Depending on the size of the stone, different methods are available for its removal. Stones less than 10 mm can be directly withdrawn from the nephroscope, whereas stones that are greater than 10 mm must be fragmented either by ultrasonic or electrohydraulic lithotripsy. This procedure is successful in removing approximately 98% of renal and 88% of ureter stones.

3. **Extracorporeal shock wave lithotripsy (ESWL).** Shock waves are used to fragment stones into sandlike particles that can pass through the urinary system and be excreted over the next 2–3 weeks. ESWL can be used for kidney stones in the renal pelvis that are < 3 cm in diameter or stones in the middle or upper portion of the ureter. Overall success depends on

stone location: 97% vs. 67% success rate in renal pelvis vs. middle portion of the ureter respectively. In general contraindications to ESWL include staghorn calculi, solitary kidney, and current infection.

4. **Open surgery.** General surgery with actual visualization of the ureter and direct physical removal of the stone is required only in highly unusual circumstances.

18. How should one approach the treatment of an infected stone?
By far the majority of infected stones are composed of struvite (staghorn calculi) and result from ongoing infection with urease-splitting bacteria. Management requires initial evaluation, as described previously; however, infected stones always require invasive intervention for removal. Furthermore, patients should be treated with antibiotics before and after stone removal to prevent sepsis and recurrence of stone formation. Interventions to prevent recurrence are still controversial; however, frequent follow-up and urine cultures to allow for early detection of recurrent infections are important.

BIBLIOGRAPHY

1. Coe FL, Favus MJ: In Brenner BM, Rector FC (eds): The Kidney, 4th ed. Philadelphia, W.B. Saunders, 1991.
2. Crowley AR, Smith AD: Percutaneous ultrasonic lithotripsy: A simplified treatment of renal stones. Postgrad Med 79:57–64, 1986.
3. O'Brien WM, Rotolo JE: New approaches in the treatment of renal calculi. Am Fam Physician 36:181–194, 1987.
4. Pak CYC: Citrate and renal calculi. Miner Electrolyte Metab 13:257–266, 1987.
5. Pak CYC: In Resnick MI, Pak CYC (eds): Nephrolithiasis. Philadelphia, W.B. Saunders, 1990.
6. Pak CYC: Etiology and treatment of urolithiasis: In-depth review. Am J Kid Dis 18:624–637, 1991.
7. Pak CYC: In Wyngaarden JB, Smith LH, Bennett JC (eds): Cecil Textbook of Medicine, 19th ed. Philadelphia, W.B. Saunders, 1992.
8. Streem SB: Kidney stones: How new technology has improved management. Postgrad Med 84:77–89, 1988.

56. INCONTINENCE

Evelyn Hutt, M.D.

1. What percentage of community-dwelling elders are incontinent?
Prevalence of urinary incontinence varies by age and gender. Among the population aged 65–74 years, approximately 5–7% are incontinent. Over age 75 years, at least 10% of men and 15–20% of women living in the community are incontinent. About 10 million Americans suffer from urinary incontinence; annual costs are estimated at $10.3 billion.

2. What is the differential diagnosis of acute incontinence?
About 50% of incontinence is acute and therefore readily treatable. It may be the only presenting sign of a serious underlying disorder, such as delirium or spinal cord compression. A simple mnemonic, **DRIP**, helps to remember the differential diagnosis:

D = Delirium and Drugs. Any patient with new-onset incontinence should have formal mental status testing (e.g., Mini-Mental Status Exam) and a review of medications, including over-the-counter (OTC) preparations. Drugs that precipitate incontinence can be divided into three main groups: diuretics, sedatives, and anticholinergics. Alcohol is both a sedative and a diuretic. It is easy to miss the diagnosis of excessive alcohol intake in older women. Anticholinergics may precipitate acute urinary retention by direct action on bladder innervation and by central sedative effect; they are common in OTC cold preparations.

R = Restricted mobility and **R**etention. Many older people have impaired mobility, which limits their ability to get to the bathroom quickly. Retention of urine may be caused by drugs, as mentioned above; an enlarged, obstructing prostate; or neurologic damage from an acute spinal cord compression. New-onset incontinence in the setting of back pain is a medical emergency and should prompt an immediate work-up for spinal cord lesions.

I = Infection, Inflammation, and Impaction. Every patient with new-onset incontinence should have a urinalysis and rectal examination.

P = Polyuria, which serves as a reminder that diabetes and hypercalcemia may present in the elderly as incontinence.

3. What simple clinical test distinguishes between inability to retain urine and inability to empty the bladder?

Bladder catheterization to measure postvoid residual volume (PVR) determines whether or not the patient is retaining urine. A volume greater than 60 cc immediately after the patient voids freely is abnormal and suggests retention.

4. Is it useful in women to distinguish between stress and urge incontinence?

In reality, most incontinent women have a mixture of stress and urge syptoms and pathophysiology. Predominance of one type of symptom may suggest what treatment modality to start with.

5. What is detrusor instability? How is it treated?

Detrusor instability is defined as uninhibited bladder contraction sufficient to overcome urethral resistance. It is the most common cause of incontinence. Because bladder contraction is cholinergically mediated and urethral contraction is sympathetically mediated, one can either give an anticholinergic to block bladder contraction or an alpha-adrenergic agonist to increase urethral resistance. Alpha agonists are generally better tolerated than anticholinergics.

6. Define bedside cystometrics. When is it useful?

Bedside cystometrics is a series of maneuvers, described by Ouslander, Leach, and Staskin, that assesses stress incontinence, detrusor instability, and bladder capacity. The patient is asked to come to the exam with a full bladder and to cough 3 times in the standing position, with a small pad held over the urethral area. Then the patient voids privately. A 14-French straight catheter is inserted into the bladder with the patient supine to measure PVR. A 50-ml catheter tip syringe is attached to the catheter, and the bladder is filled with room-temperature sterile water at 50-ml increments until the patient feels the urge to void and then at 25-ml increments until bladder capacity is reached. The catheter is removed, and the stress maneuvers are repeated. The patient voids again privately. Involuntary contractions visible as a rise in the meniscus of the syringe or urgency at relatively low volume (< 300 cc) suggests detrusor instability.

The tests are useful in women for whom a drug trial is contraindicated (e.g., dementia) and in men with benign prostatic hypertrophy (BPH) who are contemplating transurethral pros-tatectomy to detect the presence of detrusor instability and to plan for the possible onset or worsening of incontinence postoperatively.

7. How effective are nonpharmacologic treatments for incontinence?

Nonpharmocologic treatment consists either of timed toileting techniques or pelvic floor muscle-strengthening techniques. In timed toileting the patient is taught to void on a schedule determined by the frequency of incontinent episodes as revealed by a diary. With or without biofeedback in several small trials, this technique achieved a 60–80% reduction in incontinent episodes. The technique is also effective in demented patients with conscientious caregivers.

Pelvic muscle (Kegel's) exercises have been shown to be effective in stress incontinence. One study found them to be as effective as alpha agonist therapy. Their utility is limited, however, by the need for strong motivation and a clear sensorium.

8. What is the role of estrogen in the treatment of stress incontinence?
Estrogen has not been shown to affect pure stress incontinence, but it improves dysuria and urgency caused by atrophic vaginitis. Because most incontinent women have both stress and urge symptoms as well as atrophic vaginitis, a trial of estrogen is often beneficial. It is contraindicated, however, in women with breast cancer. For women reluctant to try hormone therapy, a 3-week trial of vaginal estrogen cream may help to assess its utility.

9. How effective are alpha agonists in the treatment of stress and urge incontinence?
Alpha agonists have been shown to be 60–80% effective in reducing episodes of wetness, but placebo-controlled trials are lacking. The side-effect profile of alpha agonists compares favorably with that of anticholinergics; therefore, alpha agonists should be tried first.

10. When should an incontinent woman with cystocele be referred for surgery?
Only a grade 3 cystocele, with extension to the back of the vaginal vault or through the introitus, is likely to cause incontinence. Such patients are unlikely to benefit from drug or behavioral therapy and should seek surgical attention. All other patients deserve a trial of conservative management.

11. How useful are alpha antagonists in the treatment of urinary retention from BPH?
Alpha antagonists may be of some benefit in the treatment of retention from BPH. They are particularly useful in patients who are too frail for surgery or who have concomitant hypertension. Caution must be exercised to prevent syncope with the first dose, and the patient should be checked for orthostatic hypotension after initiation of therapy.

12. What is the role of finasteride in the treatment of retention due to BPH?
Finasteride is a 5-alpha-reductase inhibitor that may reduce prostate volume by approximately 25% and improve urine flow rates in 30% of patients. Side effects include decreased libido and a confounding of the prostate-specific antigen (PSA) values used to screen for prostate cancer. It is at least twice as expensive as an alpha antagonist. Whether finasteride can be combined with alpha antagonists to increase benefit is currently under investigation.

13. When is an indwelling Foley catheter indicated in the management of chronic incontinence?
The clearest indication for long-term use of a Foley catheter is protection of skin in a patient who has or is at risk for pressure ulcers and who has failed condom catheterization. Patients with urinary retention who are difficult to catheterize intermittently or who are too frail for surgery also may benefit from an indwelling Foley catheter.

BIBLIOGRAPHY

1. Fanti JA, Wyman JF, McClish DK, et al: Efficacy of bladder training in older women with urinary incontinence. JAMA 265:609–613, 1991.
2. Kane RL, Ouslander JG, Abrass IB: Incontinence. In Essentials of Clinical Geriatrics, 2nd ed. New York, McGraw-Hill, 1989, pp 139–191.
3. Monda JM, Osterling JE: Medical treatment of benign prostatic hypertension: 5 Alpha-reductase inhibitors and alpha-adrenergic antagonists. Mayo Clin Proc 68:670–679, 1993.
4. Ouslander JG, Leach GE, Staskin DR: Simplified tests of lower urinary tract function in the evaluation of geriatric urinary incontinence. J Am Geriatr Soc 37:706–714, 1989.
5. Resnick NM, Ouslander JG: NIH Conference on Urinary Incontinence. Urinary incontinence—Where do we stand and where do we go from here? J Am Geriatr Soc 38:263–368, 1990.
6. Wells TJ, Brink CA, Diokno AC, et al: Pelvic muscle exercise for stress urinary incontinence in elderly women. J Am Geriatr Soc 39:785–791, 1991.

57. RENAL FAILURE

Alan B. Cooper, M.D., and Arlene B. Chapman, M.D.

1. What is renal failure?
Renal failure is an *irreversible* loss of nephrons and is usually asymptomatic until 70–80% of the nephron population is destroyed. Renal disease progresses through various stages:

Decreased renal reserve: nephron loss without the loss of measured renal function.

Renal insufficiency: a measurable decline in renal function (azotemia), usually associated with an impaired ability to concentrate the urine or a decreased maximal urinary osmolality that causes nocturia or polyuria and is often accompanied by hypertension.

Renal failure: a progressive decline in renal function to the point that homeostasis cannot be maintained; associated with worsening azotemia, anemia, hyperphosphatemia, hypocalcemia, and metabolic acidosis.

Uremia: a clinical syndrome with severe decline in renal function, associated with dysfunction of multiple organ systems potentially manifested as anorexia, taste change, nausea, epigastric pain, pruritus, chest pain (pericarditis), shortness of breath, fatigue, weakness, and depression.

2. How does one differentiate acute from chronic renal failure?
History, supported by medical records, is the most important way to differentiate acute from chronic renal failure. Often records are not available. Classically, hypocalcemia, hyperphosphatemia, and anemia have been associated more often with chronic than acute renal failure. However, calcium, phosphorus, and acid-base derangements are often seen in patients with acute renal failure as early as 48 to 72 hours after the onset of illness. Anemia is also a nonspecific indicator. A more reliable indicator of chronic renal failure is the finding of small kidneys with a decrease or absence of renal cortex, as assessed by ultrasonography. Ultrasound is noninvasive with image resolutions of 0.5 cm and is highly effective in determining renal size and ruling out obstructive disease. A kidney length of less than 9 cm is abnormal and indicates chronic and significant renal disease. A difference of greater than 1.5 cm in renal length indicates unilateral or asymmetric renal disease. The echogenicity of the renal cortex is increased in chronic renal disease.

Another reliable indication of chronic renal failure is the presence of renal osteodystrophy; osteitis fibrosa cystica, osteomalacia, and osteoporosis are present to varying degrees in all patients with chronic renal disease.

3. What conditions causing chronic renal failure are associated with normal to increased renal size?

Diabetic nephropathy   Polycystic kidneys
Hydronephrosis   Nephropathy associated with the
Amyloidosis   human immunodeficiency virus
Congenital malformations   Myeloma kidney

4. What evaluation should be done in patients with renal insufficiency?
In the evaluation of patients with renal disease, it is important to establish the degree of renal impairment and to identify reversible factors causing a decrease in renal function, such as infection, obstruction, volume depletion, nephrotoxic drugs, less than optimal cardiac output with or without hypotension, uncontrolled hypertension, hypercalcemia, and hyperuricemia. A thorough history and physical examination should be performed, including orthostatic blood pressure and pulse measurements. Besides the history and physical, the database should include urinalysis by dipstick and microscope; assessment of serum electrolytes, blood urea

nitrogen (BUN), and creatinine; complete blood count; evaluation of postvoid residual; and ultrasonography.

5. How does urinalysis aid in the evaluation of renal failure?

The simplest, most cost-effective element of the evaluation of a patient with chronic renal failure is routine urinalysis. In chronic renal disease, one may see unconcentrated or isosthenuric urine, as indicated by a specific gravity of 1.010 or less. Dipstick glucose may be seen in diabetes mellitus or in chronic renal failure as the ability of the proximal tubule to reabsorb glucose decreases with progression of disease. The urine pH in chronic renal failure is usually less than 7.0; if it is greater than 8.0, the question of infection with urease-splitting organisms should be raised. Proteinuria is the hallmark of intrinsic renal disease; nephrotic-range proteinuria is seen in glomerular lesions and 1–2 gm of protein excretion in interstitial diseases. If the dipstick is positive for blood but no red blood cells are seen microscopically, the question of myoglobulinuria and rhabdomyolsis should be raised. Cellular or red blood cell casts indicate active renal disease of a glomerular or vascular etiology. White blood cells are usually seen in infections but may be present in allergic interstitial nephritis, renal tuberculosis, glomerulonephritis, or chlamydial infection. Hansel's stain for eosinophils helps to differentiate allergic interstitial nephritis from other conditions.

6. Aside from correcting reversible factors, what can be done to change the chronic progression of renal disease?

Relatively few renal diseases are responsive to therapy, and once the serum creatinine concentration is greater than 2.0 mg/dl, progression often occurs even if the initial insult completely resolves. However, control of blood pressure is paramount in slowing the progression of renal disease. Some antihypertensive agents also show promise of slowing the progression of renal disease independent of blood pressure control, particularly in diabetic nephropathy, including angiotensin-converting enzyme (ACE) inhibitors such as enalopril or captopril and the non-dihydropyridine calcium channel blockers, such as diltiazem or verapamil. The beneficial effects of the ACE inhibitors are secondary to their predominant actions on the postglomerular efferent arteriole. Both groups of drugs demonstrate antiproteinuric effects, which are important because proteinuria is an independent risk factor for progressive loss of renal function.

Dietary modification may slow the progression of renal disease. Protein restriction (with attendant phosphorus restriction) has been demonstrated to decrease loss of renal function in animal studies and has been used for decades to prevent loss of renal function in humans. However, clinical trials demonstrate no clear benefit. Because of the risk of malnutrition, patients should not be placed on long-term severe protein restriction without careful monitoring. According to conservative recommendations, patients should ingest no more than 0.8–1 gm of protein/kg/day with dietetic counseling to ensure adequate nutritional intake. Three-day dietary recall and diet diaries are reliable ways to determine the level of protein intake.

7. Which antihypertensive agents are contraindicated in patients with chronic renal failure?

Contraindicated antihypertensives in patients with renal disease include the potassium-sparing diuretics, such as triamterene, spironolactone, and amiloride. Medications that cause large changes in systemic blood pressure or in potassium handling by the kidney (such as ACE inhibitors) require close monitoring in patients with chronic renal failure.

8. When do patients with renal failure have problems maintaining potassium balance?

Without renal tubular acidosis, patients with renal failure are able to maintain potassium balance on a regular diet until the glomerular filtration rate (GFR) is reduced to 5–10 ml/min/ 1.73 m^2. In chronic renal failure, total body stores of potassium are either normal or low; shifts of potassium from the intracellular to extracellular compartment predominate. The colon secretes potassium, but its contribution to potassium balance is negligible until chronic renal failure occurs, at which point stool potassium excretion increases to 35% of intake.

9. How should acute hyperkalemia be managed? When should hyperkalemia be treated in renal failure?

Patients with chronic renal failure may have chronically elevated concentrations of serum potassium; chronic hyperkalemia is often better tolerated by the cardiovascular system than acute hyperkalemia. The predominant effects of hyperkalemia are cardiac and require treatment when EKG changes are present. Peaked T waves (isosceles triangle) or widening of the PR interval, which may be followed by widening of the QRS complex and a sine wave complex and asystole, require emergent therapy. Intravenous calcium should be given to stabilize the cardiac membrane; the effect of this treatment lasts for approximately 20 minutes. An insulin drip with glucose should be infused (10 units in 250 cc D10W at 75 to 100 cc/hr) to increase cellular uptake of potassium. If volume overload is not a problem, 1 ampule of sodium bicarbonate should be added to the insulin infusion. Beta agonists such as albuterol have been shown to potentiate the potassium-lowering effects of insulin and should be used as a prolonged nebulizer treatment. The effects of this regimen last as long as the treatment continues, but some method of potassium removal must be provided—either Kayexelate (sodium polystyrene exonate) (30–50 gm with 20% sorbitol) or dialysis. Intracellular shifts of potassium should be avoided during hemodialysis, because they prevent effective removal of potassium. Continued monitoring of serum potassium is required to avoid severe hypokalemia during dialysis.

10. What indications are used for the treatment of chronic metabolic acidosis in renal failure?

Exogenous alkali treatment should be used in symptomatic patients with renal failure. Symptoms include dyspnea (from respiratory compensation) and persistent hyperkalemia. Treatment of milder asymptomatic metabolic acidosis minimizes the loss of skeletal calcium with resultant osteodystrophy. In addition, acidemia interferes with protein metabolism and may lead to muscle wasting and cardiac dysfunction. Treatment of metabolic acidosis secondary to uremia is recommended when serum bicarbonate levels reach 15 mg/dl.

11. Which agents are available to provide exogenous alkali in chronic renal failure?

The most commonly used agents are sodium bicarbonate or citrate. The sodium content may worsen blood pressure control or contribute to volume overload; citrate should be used with caution when patients are also taking aluminum as a phosphate binder (e.g., Amphojel, Basogel). Citrate increases aluminum absorption and may lead to toxic aluminum levels, which are associated with dementia in patients with renal failure. Calcium carbonate has been advocated as a buffering agent, but it is not as effective as the others in restoring neutral pH, because large doses (more than 1500 mg/day) are required. This dosage may increase the calcium-phosphorus product, resulting in metastatic calcium deposition, and predispose patients to calcium oxalate stone formation.

12. Are patients with renal failure at increased risk for depression?

Many believe that depression is the most common psychiatric disorder in patients with renal disease. However, the true incidence is unknown, because the data are scarce. Presenting symptoms of depression in renal failure may mimic a primary depressive illness (e.g., anhedonia, sense of helplessness, depressed mood) or may involve more subtle findings. Such findings include increased irritability, bad dreams, or somatic complaints that cannot be explained after careful diagnostic evaluation. Treatment of depression should be strongly considered in patients with chronic renal failure. Because tricyclic antidepressants are predominantly metabolized by the liver and are not dialyzable, no dosage adjustments need be made. Some investigators have found that patients with renal failure respond better to certain antidepressants, such as imipramine or sertraline.

13. What bleeding diathesis is associated with renal failure?

A qualitative platelet defect is present and manifested only by an increased bleeding time. The platelet count is normal, whereas platelet aggregation and adhesion are abnormal. Treatment, directed at increasing release of von Willebrand's factor, consists of administration of 1-

deamino-8-D-arginine vasopressin (DDAVP) at 3 $\mu l/kg$. This treatment, which is effective for 4–6 hours after administration, is accompanied by tachyphylaxis. Cryoprecipitate rapidly corrects the diathesis and is effective for 24–36 hours but carries the risk of blood-borne viruses. Estrogens (25 mg orally or 3 mg/kg divided over 5 days intravenously) have been shown to be effective for as long as 3–10 days. Maintaining the patient's hematocrit at greater than 30% is also beneficial. Dialysis improves platelet function without normalizing the bleeding time and should be considered as an adjunctive therapy for life-threatening hemorrhage that is attributed to uremia.

14. How common is upper gastrointestinal (GI) bleeding in patients with renal failure?
Upper GI bleeding is a major complication in patients with renal failure and accounts for 3–7% of deaths. Superficial mucosal abnormalities are more common than ulcerative disease. Duodenitis and gastritis have been reported in 10–60% of patients with moderate-to-severe renal failure. The incidence of angiodysplasia is also increased in renal failure and is believed to be the source of bleeding in 23% of patients. Therapy for upper GI bleeding in renal failure is the same as for patients without renal disease, except that H_2 receptor antagonists, such as cimetidine, should be given at reduced dosages because they are cleared by the kidney.

15. List the five indications for acute hemodialysis.
  1. Medically unresponsive hyperkalemia with EKG changes
  2. Profound metabolic acidosis causing cardiovascular compromise and hypotension
  3. Medically unresponsive pulmonary edema with hypoxemia
  4. Drug ingestions (lithium, theophylline, salicylates, methanol, or glycols)
  5. Uremic encephalopathy

16. When is hemodialysis contraindicated?
Most contraindications to hemodialysis are relative and depend on the individual patient. However, in acute hemorrhage involving the central nervous system, hemodialysis should be deferred, because rapid fluid shifts between the arachnoid and subarachnoid space may worsen the injury. Peritoneal dialysis is the modality of choice.

17. What therapeutic options are available for patients with endstage renal disease?
The three forms of renal replacement are hemodialysis, peritoneal dialysis, and transplantation. Chronic hemodialysis is performed for 2.5–4 hours 3 times/week based on patient characteristics and may be provided at home or in a dialysis center. Peritoneal dialysis, which allows patients more freedom and control of therapy, is either continuous over a 24-hour period or performed at night for approximately 8 hours on a cycler machine. The cycler machine allows the patient to hang the dialysate before going to bed; the cycler performs the exchanges throughout the night. Renal transplantation can be performed using either a living or cadaveric donor; good outcomes are expected with either source. The life expectancy for patients on dialysis is 4–5 years for those less than age 60 years and 2–3 years for those older than 60 years. Survival after renal transplantation is 90% at 3 years with cadaveric transplantation and approximately 95% with living related donations.

BIBLIOGRAPHY

1. Giovannetti S, Cupisti A, Barsotti G: The metabolic acidosis of chronic renal failure: Pathophysiology and treatment. Contrib Nephrol 100:48–57, 1992.
2. Kupin WL, Narins RG: The hyperkalemia of renal failure: Pathophysiology, diagnosis and therapy. Contrib Nephrol 102:1–22, 1993.
3. Malluche HH, Monier-Faugere MC: Uremic bone disease: Current knowledge, controversial issues, and new horizons. Miner Electrolyte Metab 17:281–296, 1991.
4. Murphey MD, Sartoris DJ, Quale JL, et al: Musculoskeletal manifestations of chronic renal insufficiency. Radiographics 13:357–379, 1993.

5. Oldrizzi L, Rugiu C, De Biase V, Maschio G: The place of hypertension among the risk factors for renal function in chronic renal failure. Am J Kidney Dis 5(Suppl 2):119–123, 1993.
6. Peterson JC, Tisher CC, Wilcox CS (eds): Nephrology for the House Officer. Baltimore, Williams & Wilkins, 1989.
7. Procci WR, Massry SG, Glassock RJ (eds): Textbook of Nephrology. Baltimore, Williams & Wilkins, chapter 66(Pt 1), 1989.
8. Remuzzi G: Bleeding in renal failure. Lancet i:1205–1208, 1988.
9. Sevy N, Snape WJ, Massry SG, Glassock RJ (eds): Textbook of Nephrology. Baltimore, Williams & Wilkins, chapter 70(Pt 1), 1989.

IX. Common Problems of the Blood and Lymph System

58. ANEMIA

Lori Jensen, M.D., and Jeanette Mladenovic, M.D.

1. Define anemia.

Normal hemoglobin levels are influenced by age, sex, ethnic group, and altitude. Normal values were calculated to a 95% reference range for a large population, thus providing the laboratory reference. Values for men are higher than for women, a finding attributed to testosterone. For children, the lower hemoglobin level at age 2 years (10.7 g/dl) rises gradually until normal limits are reached by age 15 and 18 for girls and boys, respectively. Values for Afro-Americans are approximately 0.5–0.6 gm lower than for Caucasian Americans. In men older than 65 years, hemoglobin tends to decline; if the value of 12 g/dl is used as the norm, 25% of patients may be abnormal, but the anemia has no pathologic etiology. It is also important to compare the patient's hemoglobin values over time, thus determining when deviation from the norm occurs. Mild anemia may be important primarily as a barometer of the patient's overall health and as an early clue to disease.

2. What are the most common causes of anemia?

Iron deficiency	25%
Blood loss	25%
Anemia of chronic disease	25%
Megaloblastic anemias	10%
Hemolysis	10%
Other bone marrow failure	5%

3. Can anemia be diagnosed by the physical exam?

Often physical examination is diagnostic only indirectly when anemia is severe: by resting tachycardia, wide pulse pressure, hyperdynamic precordium, or evidence of high-output heart failure. Pallor is highly subjective and influenced by vascular tone and intrinsic skin hue. Even absence of palmar creases in severe anemia is currently in question. When a patient appears pale in the face, conjunctiva, and mucous membranes, the physician is likely to order a complete blood count (CBC) to evaluate systemic illness. In most other instances, anemia is diagnosed asymptomatically or during the evaluation of other complaints.

4. How does the mean corpuscular volume (MCV) help in the differential diagnosis of anemia?

Classification of anemia has traditionally relied on the size of the red blood cell (RBCs), as determined by the RBC volume. The normal MCV is 80–95 fl; values above and below this range define macrocytic and microcytic anemias, respectively. However, because the value represents the arithmetic mean of all RBCs, a mixed population of cells may contribute to the overall value. Furthermore, in several instances a single deficiency may be masked by a combined deficiency. Thus, low or high values of the MCV are useful in directing the diagnosis, but a normal MCV does not exclude any of the causes that may contribute to the etiology of the anemia. The table below outlines the classification of anemia based on the MCV in conjunction with the reticulocyte count.

Practical Evaluation of Anemia

RETICULOCYTE	HALLMARK ON SMEAR	LABORATORY TESTS
RETICULOCYTE < 2%		
MCV low	**MICROCYTOSIS**	
Iron deficiency	—	Ferritin < 12 μg/L or $\downarrow$Fe/$\uparrow$TBC = Sat $< 16\%$
		$\downarrow$Fe/$\uparrow$TIBC = Sat $< 16\%$
Chronic disease	—	$\downarrow$Fe/$\uparrow$TIBC = Sat $< 20\%$
		Ferritin low or may be > 100 μg/L
Thalassemia	—	Hemoglobin electrophoresis normal,
($\alpha\alpha^-$, β-minor, or HbE)		$\uparrow$A$_2$ or E
MCV high	**MACROCYTOSIS**	
B$_{12}$ deficiency	Multilobed neutrophils	B$_{12}$ level
Folate deficiency	Multilobed neutrophils	Serum/RBC folate
Myelodysplasia, or other stem cell defect	—	Bone marrow aspiration and biopsy
MCV normal		
Early iron deficiency or chronic disease	Normal	As above
Renal or endocrine disease	Normal	As indicated
Marrow replacement or stem-cell diseases	Abnormal cells from the marrow; teardrops, or nucleated red cells	Bone marrow biopsy
Mixed defects	Large and small cells, or normal	As needed from clinical suspicion
CORRECTED RETICULOCYTES > 2%		**TESTS FOR RBC BREAKDOWN**
Extravascular hemolysis	Spherocytes	Direct Coombs' test
Intravascular hemolysis	Abnormal RBC shapes and sizes	Tests for free hemoglobin, DIC evaluation
Intrinsic RBC defects	Clues: shapes, Heinz bodies	Evaluation for defect in RBC membrane, hemoglobinopathy, enzyme

5. When is a reticulocyte count helpful?

The reticulocyte count is the only available measure of daily marrow production. As such, it is the most important test for determining whether anemia is due to increased RBC destruction or inadequate marrow production. Normal production of RBCs is 1–2% per day. Thus, any number less than 2% in the patient with anemia is considered inadequate production, which may be due to hematinic deficiencies (iron, vitamin B12, folate); chronic inflammatory, endocrine, or renal disease; or infiltrating marrow diseases, such as tumor or primary stem-cell failure.

However, when the reticulocyte count is greater than 2%, further analysis is required to determine whether chronic stimulated marrow production due to increased destruction of RBCs is truly present. Because the reticulocyte count is expressed as a percentage of RBCs, measurement of daily production of RBCs requires correction of this percentage when the absolute RBC count is decreased (as in anemia). The following equation may be used for the correction:

Corrected reticulocyte = observed hematocrit/45 (used as the normal hematocrit)
× measured reticulocyte count

Alternatively, an absolute reticulocyte count $> 90 \times 10^9$ is considered increased. In reality, the severity of the increased destruction (hemolysis) tends to be reflected in the measured reticulocytosis. More importantly, correction of the reticulocytosis is a helpful reminder of underlying pathophysiology in the following circumstances: mild reticulocytosis with intra-medullary hemolysis in B12 or folate deficiency when the underlying problem is hypoprolifer-ative; after a single episode of acute hemorrhage with an appropriate marrow response; and in the instance of hemolytic disease, when it is necessary to determine whether the marrow is adequately responding (i.e., is the amount of iron or folate sufficient to maintain the marrow production needed for the increased destruction, or is the patient entering an aplastic crisis?).

6. When may the red blood cell volume distribution width (RDW) be useful?

The RDW reflects the degree of homogeneity or heterogeneity in size among the RBCs. This measurement is meant to detect the degree of anisocytosis on a peripheral blood smear. A wide RDW may be the first clue to iron deficiency; a manifestation of dual populations of cells; or a sign of anisocytosis due to RBC fragments. The RDW may be highly sensitive for early iron deficiency, but it is not specific. A normal value is helpful in distinguishing thalassemia minor from iron deficiency as a cause of microcytosis.

7. When should the clinician evaluate the peripheral blood smear?

Ideally the smear should be evaluated in all patients with anemia or even leukocytosis, but this often becomes practically unfeasible and does not change the primary care provider's evaluation. Thus, it is important to determine when the smear should be further evaluated— a heretical but realistic approach. Often the smear needs to be viewed to confirm abnormalities detected by automated procedures before further work-up is pursued. Automated values require review of the smear in the following circumstances:

- Abnormal types of circulating cells; for example, blasts or lymphocytes
- Confirmation and evaluation of extremely high or low values of blood counts (especially platelets and neutrophils)
- RBC fragments of any type (teardrops, schistocytes, sickle cells)
- Perplexing hypoproliferative anemia to look for clues of rouleaux (paraprotein) or mixed populations of cells (large and small)
- Anemia with reticulocytosis to search for spherocytes or other clues, such as shape abnormalities in hereditary membrane disease

8. What are the indications for a bone marrow aspirate and/or biopsy?

The provider should obtain consultation for the purpose of a bone marrow analysis under the following circumstances:

1. Pancytopenia or bicytopenias
2. A peripheral blood smear that shows abnormal early cells (i.e., blast, myelocytes) or evidence of myelophthisis (teardrops)
3. For rare causes of anemia, such as sideroblastic anemia and pure RBC aplasia, which must be suspected because of unique clinical situations or in patients in whom the anemia is unexplained
4. Severe thrombocytopenia
5. Severe leukopenia
6. Monoclonal serum protein
7. Culture for granulomatous diseases in unique situations

A biopsy is not always indicated; however, when evaluation of cellularity or a search for tumor cells or other infiltrating disease is required, a biopsy is necessary along with the aspirate. Although bone marrow examination has traditionally been advocated for the evaluation of iron stores, the diagnosis of iron deficiency usually is made by other means.

9. Which single test most frequently yields a diagnosis of iron deficiency anemia?

Two laboratory tests are in common use to detect iron deficiency: the ferritin level, a measure of iron stores, and the serum iron saturation (serum iron/total iron binding capacity [TIBC] = iron saturation; a value less than 16% in the presence of a normal-to-high TIBC reflects iron deficiency). In uncomplicated cases of iron deficiency, the ferritin level most often leads to the diagnosis (level less than 12 μg/L). However, this test lacks sensitivity. A normal value does not exclude iron deficiency, but a value greater than 100 μg/L is inconsistent with iron deficiency. Both tests are not necessary in the initial evaluation; on occasion, however, both may prove helpful.

10. When is the ferritin level likely to be falsely elevated?

Ferritin reflects true iron overload at values greater than 1000 μg/ml (hemochromatosis; hemosiderosis from blood cell dyscrasias). However, both inflammation and liver disease with destruction of hepatocytes increase ferritin to values ranging from 100 to > 1000 μg/ml.

11. What are the hallmarks of the anemia of chronic disease?

1. Nonprogressive anemia that usually does not fall below a hematocrit of 25% and parallels the severity of the underlying inflammatory disease. In this instance, inflammation is a broad term that includes systemic diseases accompanied by a major cellular response. An elevated sedimentation rate often correlates with the presence of chronic disease.

2. MCV that is not increased and usually is mildly decreased

3. Low reticulocyte count (less than 2%)

4. Low serum iron. The pathophysiologic problem appears to be tissue avidity for iron and failure to release iron to the serum; thus, although ferritin may be above normal, serum iron is characteristically low. This defect may be seen immediately in infectious processes, even before the 1–2 months required for the development of anemia with chronic inflammation. Thus, low serum iron, often with a low TIBC, results in low iron saturation, which characterizes the anemia of chronic disease.

12. What further evaluation is required for the diagnosis of iron deficiency?

The etiology of the iron deficiency must be evaluated. A chronic loss of 3–4 cc blood per day (1–2 mg of iron) leads to iron deficiency. Although gastrointestinal (GI) blood loss may occur with common entities, including use of nonsteroidal anti-inflammatory drugs, aspirin, and anticoagulants, hemorrhoids, and various acid peptic entities (ulcers, esophagitis), they should not be assumed to be the etiology. Chronic loss of iron from the lower GI tract as an initial manifestation of malignancy must always be considered.

Another common cause of iron deficiency is menses. The history may provide clues to excessive menstrual loss: menses greater than 7 days in duration; passage of clots greater than 2 cm in size; and inability to control flow with tampons. In the absence of such manifestations, excessive menstrual flow is poorly assessed by the history alone.

Urinary blood loss is not a cause of iron deficiency, unless excessive gross hematuria is chronically present or unless intravascular hemolysis is persistent (as in the presence of a cardiac valve that causes hemolysis or in rare blood disorders, such as paroxysmal nocturnal hemoglobinuria).

The above observations have led to the practical clinical recommendations that men with GI blood loss and women over the age of 35–40 years require evaluation of iron deficiency anemia to exclude sources of occult GI blood loss due to malignant or premalignant lesions.

13. What is runner's anemia?

Iron deficiency has been seen in up to one-half of long-distance competitive runners. The cause of the iron loss appears to be chronic and multifactorial: low-grade intravascular hemolysis; low-grade hematuria; and low-grade GI loss. However, this diagnosis remains one of exclusion in populations at risk.

14. Can a patient have both iron deficiency and chronic disease?

Yes. Iron deficiency is particularly common in patients with rheumatoid arthritis, although it may be seen in other conditions. Clues to iron deficiency include a fall in the usually low hematocrit of chronic disease; ferritin < 100 $\mu g/l$; and iron saturation $< 5\%$. Oral iron supplementation may be given on a trial basis, with an anticipated increase in the hematocrit or hemoglobin to low plateau levels consistent with the inflammatory state.

Iron deficiency also may occur with a defect in folate or vitamin B12 and initially high iron studies. Thus normal iron studies in the presence of or at the initiation of treatment for folate or B12 deficiencies are not helpful in excluding iron deficiency. A more accurate reflection of iron stores is obtained when normal marrow maturation has resumed after replacement of B12 or folate.

15. How should iron deficiency be treated?

Multiple preparations are available to treat iron deficiency, with variable amounts of iron available for absorption. Overall, lower amounts of iron are better tolerated. Thus, ferrous gluconate or slow-release preparations may be better tolerated than traditional ferrous sulfate, 300 mg 3 times/day. However, the required rate of correction determines the choice of preparation. In any case, iron supplementation must be continued for 3–6 months beyond correction of the anemia.

Failure to correct iron deficiency is due to poor compliance, inadequate absorption, continued blood loss that exceeds supplementation, or incorrect diagnosis. Absorption may be enhanced by changing preparations or mode of administration. Systemic iron should be reserved for patients at extreme risk of malabsorption (inflammatory bowel disease).

16. When is evaluation of the folate level useful?

Evaluation of folate level is rarely useful in the usual patients at risk, such as nutritionally deficient patients who consume alcohol or the nutritionally replete patient who consumes alcohol but has a mildly elevated MCV. It is much more important to eliminate B12 deficiency as the cause of the macrocytosis than to evaluate the serum folate level, which is easily and rapidly corrected by alcohol cessation or food intake. If the B12 level is normal, folate deficiency may likely be treated with multivitamin and folate supplements. If the B12 level is low, further evaluation is necessary, because spuriously low levels may be seen in folate deficiency. Although the evaluation of multiple levels, including folate, B12, red blood cell folate, and iron, is common in the shotgun evaluation of anemia, the cost-effectiveness of this approach is suspect. As a marker of malabsorption in high-risk patients or in the evaluation of a difficult-to-diagnose anemia with megaloblastosis, evaluation of levels of serum and erythrocyte folate is clearly useful.

17. When should levels of vitamin B12 be measured?

In addition to the evaluation of megaloblastic anemia, certain conditions lead predictably to B12 deficiency or result from B12 deficiency in the absence of hematologic defects:

1. Gastrectomy, ileal resection, or malabsorption. Because stores of B12 are large, deficiency is not suspected until years later. The average time to deficiency after gastrectomy is 5 years (2–12-year range).

2. Dementia or manifestations consistent with posterior column disease. The initial evaluation should determine whether B12 deficiency contributes to the neurologic defect.

18. What regulates the red blood cell mass?

RBC mass is maintained within well-defined limits through a feedback mechanism regulated by the hormone erythropoietin. Tissue oxygenation, as sensed within the kidney, governs the amount of hormone released from renal peritubular cells. Erythropoietin stimulates early marrow cells to undergo differentiation, proliferation, and maturation. Production and destruction of RBCs in the spleen are carefully matched to tissue oxygen demands. Thus, maintenance of hemoglobin also depends on bone marrow that can respond adequately to external demands.

19. When is measurement of the erythropoietin level helpful?

In the presence of anemia, erythropoietin should be appropriately elevated for the level of hematocrit and is especially high with bone marrow failure. Measurement of erythropoietin is most useful for distinguishing high from normal values. The hormone level also is useful in distinguishing causes of erythrocytosis: high levels indicate secondary causes of erythropoietin secretion, whereas low levels indicate primary marrow-induced polycythemia. Measurement is helpful in considering therapy for patients with infection by the human immunodeficiency virus (HIV) and zidovudine (AZT)-induced anemia; an extraordinarily high level ($>$ 500 IU/ml) suggests that erythropoietin will not be effective.

20. Which patients are candidates for therapy with erythropoietin?

1. Patients with debilitating anemia of chronic renal failure. Hormone therapy, although costly, decreases transfusions and enhances the quality of life.

2. HIV-positive patients with AZT-induced anemia that requires drug modification or transfusion and erythropoietin levels less than 500 IU/ml.

3. In rare instances, patients with anemia of chronic disease may have inappropriately low erythropoietin levels and may respond to therapy. However, the cost-effectiveness of this approach currently requires careful individual assessment.

21. When may anemia be attributable to chronic renal failure?

The anemia of chronic renal failure, which is due to deficient production of erythropoietin, is not likely to become manifest clinically until the creatinine clearance is $<$ 40 ml/min 1.73 m^2. There is a rough correlation between creatinine and anemia, although this correlation cannot be extrapolated to the individual patient. With polycystic kidney disease, the erythropoietin level appears to be maintained; patients become anemic much later (if at all) in the natural course of the disease. With progressive renal failure, additional causes of anemia must be considered, especially iron deficiency and volume expansion.

22. What laboratory tests support the diagnosis of hemolysis or increased RBC destruction?

Measures of cellular breakdown of RBCs

• Bilirubin: A slightly elevated bilirubin may be a clue to underlying RBC destruction in the absence of a hepatic explanation. However, the liver can compensate tremendously for increased bilirubin production. Thus, values over 4 mg/dl are likely to reflect liver disease as well as excessive RBC breakdown.

• Lactate dehydrogenase (LDH): Although nonspecific for red cells or hemolysis, the presence of an elevated LDH is consistent with the diagnosis of hemolysis.

Evidence of free hemoglobin

• Low haptoglobin: This protein, one of the measurable carriers of free hemoglobin falls to undetectable levels as it is catabolized when it is bound to free hemoglobin. Thus haptoglobin may not be low in patients who have decreased RBC survival that is localized to the spleen (extravascular). Because haptoglobin may be elevated in inflammatory disease, the absolute value is not helpful clinically. However, an undetectable or very low level is consistent with hemolysis.

• Free serum hemoglobin: When overwhelming hemolysis is present, as in a mismatched transfusion reaction, free hemoglobin results in pink serum. Otherwise, hemoglobin is cleared and degraded quite rapidly.

• Urine hemoglobin: When haptoglobin is saturated, free hemoglobin dissociates into molecules that pass freely through the glomerulus and thus are detected in the urine when the tubular reabsorption threshold is exceeded. Therefore, urine hemoglobin is also a measure of hemolysis due to excessive RBC breakdown, if other mechanisms cannot clear serum hemoglobin.

• Urine hemosiderin: With excessive free serum hemoglobin, free heme pigment may precipitate in the distal tubular cells. Hemoglobin iron in the renal epithelial cell is rapidly stored as hemosiderin or ferritin. As the tubular cell sloughs, hemosiderin and iron can be measured in the urine. Thus, urine hemosiderin is a good measure of chronic intravascular hemolysis. After a single episode of hemolysis, measurement of urine hemosiderin may not be positive for 2–3 days, but it may persist for up to 14 days. Thus it is a useful clue for an earlier event.

23. What classic disease results in extravascular hemolysis?
Autoimmune hemolytic anemia results in shortened RBC survival due to complement and/or antibody detection on the RBC membrane by the splenic macrophage. Hallmarks of the disease are the spherocyte and the direct Coombs' positive antibody test in the presence of reticulocytosis. A spleen tip is palpable in one-half of patients. The majority of all other hemolysis is due to intravascular causes, including RBC mechanical or fibrinous breakdown in the vascular space or intrinsic RBC defects.

BIBLIOGRAPHY

1. Denton TA, Diamond GA, Matloff JM, Gray RJ: Semin Oncol 21(Suppl 2):29–34, 1994.
2. Eichner ER: Runner's macrocytosis: Runner's anemia as a benefit versus runner's hemolysis as a detriment. Am J Med 78:321–325, 1985.
3. Eschbach J, Adamson JW: Guidelines for recombinant human erythropoietin therapy. Am J Kidney Dis 14(Suppl 2):2–8, 1989.
4. Guyatt GH, Oxman AD, Willan M, et al: Laboratory diagnosis of iron deficiency anemia: An overview. J Gen Intern Med 7:145–153, 1992.
5. Hillman RS, Finch CA: The Red Cell Manual, 5th ed. Philadelphia, F.A. Davis, 1985.
6. Krause JR: Blood smear evaluation. Hematol Oncol Clin North Am 8:631, 650, 1994.
7. Lee EGR, Bittell TC, Forester J, et al (eds): Wintrobe's Clinical Hematology. Philadelphia, Lea & Febiger, 1993, pp 715–745.
8. Mladenovic J, Roodman D: Normocytic anemia. In Spivak J (ed): Textbook of Hematology. Baltimore, Johns Hopkins Press, 1993, pp 91–100.
9. Nardone DA, Roth KM, Mazur DJ, McAfee JH: Usefulness of physical examination in detecting the presence of absence of anemia. Arch Intern Med 150:201–204, 1990.
10. Pinevich AJ, Peterson J: Erythropoietin therapy in patients with chronic renal failure. West J Med 157:154–157, 1992.
11. Sears DA: Anemia of chronic disease. Med Clin North Am 76:567–579, 1992.

59. LYMPHADENOPATHY AND SPLENOMEGALY

Jeanette Mladenovic, M.D.

1. Why is it important to know the common drainage patterns of lymph nodes amenable to palpation?
Recognizing common drainage patterns of lymph nodes facilitates assessment of the anatomic location of infectious etiologies and potential serious pathology.

Cervical nodes:	Head, ears, eyes, nose, and throat (HEENT) area
	Submental and submandibular area: salivary glands and mouth
	Pre- and postauricular area: eyes, scalp, ears
Supraclavicular nodes:	Intrathoracic and intra-abdominal area, in addition to ears, nose, and throat
Axillary nodes:	Breast and thorax
Epitrochlear nodes:	Hand and forearm
Inguinal nodes:	Lower extremities and genitalia
	Femoral and pelvic area

2. Which palpable lymph nodes suggest a malignancy?
1. Supraclavicular nodes are generally not palpable. When they are enlarged, they suggest thoracic malignancy on the right and thoracic or upper gastrointestinal (GI) malignancy on the left (called a Virchow's node).
2. Enlarged femoral nodes complicating usual inguinal adenopathy should raise suspicion.
3. Enlarged periumbilical nodes (Sister Mary Joseph nodes) signify advanced GI malignancy.

3. Which palpable lymph nodes are likely benign?
1. Palpable nodes (1–2 cm) in anterior cervical area are common under age 12 years and persist with diminishing frequency to age 30 years. In addition, almost all children have palpable axillary and inguinal adenopathy.
2. Mild insignificant bilateral inguinal adenopathy is common throughout life.
3. Isolated posterior cervical lymphadenopathy is usually benign.

4. List the most common causes of generalized diffuse lymphadenopathy in the United States.
Infectious, inflammatory, and malignant diseases account for the majority of lymphadenopathy in clinical practice. Rare storage or lymph node diseases and occasionally hyperthyroidism also may present as generalized lymphadenopathy. If a patient has recently traveled to or is from an area with endemic parasitic infections, other causes must be considered.

Infectious diseases	Infectious mononucleosis, cytomegalovirus (CMV), hepatitis A
	Human immunodeficiency virus (HIV), syphilis, toxoplasmosis
	Coccidiomycosis, histoplasmosis
Inflammatory diseases	Sarcoidosis
	Rheumatoid arthritis, systemic lupus erythematosus, dermatomyositis
	Serum sickness
	Drug reaction (phenytoin)
Malignant diseases	Non-Hodgkin's lymphoma
	Acute or chronic lymphoid or myeloid leukemias
Nonhematologic malignancies	Germ cell tumors, melanoma, breast cancer

5. What is the classic difference between the presentation of Hodgkin's disease and non-Hodgkin's lymphoma?
Non-Hodgkin's lymphoma spreads and often presents with diffuse lymphadenopathy. Classic Hodgkin's disease has a predictable pattern of spread in contiguous groups; thus, isolated lymphadenopathy in contiguously draining areas is more characteristic of Hodgkin's disease.

6. What finding on peripheral blood smear almost always accompanies the diagnosis of infectious mononucleosis?
Mononucleosis is the most common infectious cause of lymphadenopathy in young people. It is often accompanied by pharyngitis and constitutional symptoms. The peripheral blood smear almost always (in > 95% of patients) shows atypical lymphocytes. Atypical lymphocytes and/ or lymphocytosis also may be seen in other conditions, such as CMV, hepatitis, lymphoid malignancy (especially chronic lymphocytic leukemia), toxoplasmosis, serum sickness, and phenytoin lymphadenopathy.

7. For what complications of infectious mononucleosis should corticosteroid therapy be considered?
After a confirmed diagnosis of infectious mononucleosis (monospot or Epstein-Barr virus testing), corticosteroids may be indicated for obstructing tonsillar enlargement, autoimmune thrombocytopenia, severe granulocytopenia, and/or hemolytic anemia. Patients with splenomegaly should limit sports involvement to avoid rupture.

8. When should a lymph node be biopsied?
Biopsy of a lymph node, in most instances, is a minor procedure. The timing of biopsy depends on the clinical presentation, age of the patient, and suspicion of the diagnosis. Certainly, systemic symptoms suggesting malignancy should prompt earlier diagnosis. Careful follow-up is essential, because infectious lymphadenopathy usually improves or recedes in 14 days. Thus, sampling of the lymph node should be performed:
    1. When the node is very large or has associated skin changes with matting;
    2. When the lymph node has increased in size in an area associated with a high incidence of malignancy; and
    3. When an isolated lymph node with no clear site of local infection has not receded in 2–3 weeks or when diffuse lymphadenopathy with no clear etiology has not improved in 2–3 weeks.

9. When is lymph node fine-needle aspiration (FNA) not the initial procedure of choice?
FNA is helpful to confirm a suspected diagnosis of infection or metastatic malignancy. It does not provide adequate tissue to distinguish architecture or type of lymphoma or to perform cellular or molecular studies that differentiate tumor origin. Because lymphoma is usually an important diagnostic consideration in many patients undergoing lymph node biopsy, time to diagnosis and treatment should be minimized; thus biopsy is the preferred initial procedure.

10. What is the significance of a nondiagnostic lymph node biopsy?
Lymph node biopsy provides a diagnosis in more than 50% of adults. Up to one-fourth of the patients with nondiagnostic biopsies develop lymphoma in the following year. Thus, careful follow-up of a patient with a nondiagnostic biopsy is mandatory.

11. Does bilateral hilar adenopathy always require a tissue diagnosis?
Isolated bilateral hilar adenopathy in a patient with characteristics and systemic manifestations of sarcoidosis may be followed. (The classic patient is an Afro-American woman with erythema nodosum). However, asymmetry and additional symptoms should prompt aggressive diagnosis, because the differential includes lymphoma, lung carcinoma, tuberculosis, and histoplasmosis.

12. How are retroperitoneal nodes evaluated?
Computed tomography (CT) delineates the size of all retroperitoneal nodes, including para-aortic nodal areas. The lymphangiogram is now rarely utilized. Although it may provide more distinct morphology, it does not easily visualize the upper para-aortic areas and is inconvenient and difficult to perform.

13. What is the significance of massive splenomegaly?
Massive splenomegaly is most consistent with diseases of hematologic origin:
    Myeloproliferative diseases
        Myelofibrosis
        Chronic myelogenous leukemia
        End-stage polycythemia vera or essential thrombocythemia
    Neoplastic diseases
        Hairy cell leukemia
        Hodgkin's or non-Hodgkin's lymphoma
        Chronic lymphocytic leukemia
        Malignant reticuloendotheliosis
    Other less common diseases are usually apparent by other symptoms and signs. Rarely, infiltrative disease (Gaucher's disease), infectious causes (malaria), or inflammatory diseases (sarcoidosis, Felty's syndrome) may present as isolated massive splenomegaly. Massive splenomegaly is seen with thalassemia major, but the majority of other hemoglobinopathies result in lesser splenomegaly.

14. What is the significance of a palpable spleen tip?

A palpable spleen tip usually suggests mild to moderate splenic enlargement (except in children) and may be due to any of the diseases that cause diffuse lymphadenopathy, because the spleen is yet another organ of the lymph system. Thus, systemic acute or chronic infection is the most common cause of palpable splenomegaly. Systemic inflammatory diseases that cause lymphadenopathy also may cause splenomegaly, with or without lymph node enlargement (e.g., rheumatoid arthritis, SLE). However, two other categories of diseases should be considered when a spleen tip is palpable:

Congestive diseases: Vascular congestion may be due to portal vein hypertension, hepatic vein thrombosis, or portal or splenic vein thrombosis.

Hematologic diseases: Hemolytic diseases due to immune, enzyme, or membrane etiologies. Sickle cell disease of the SS variety is not accompanied by splenomegaly.

15. How can one evaluate the size and function of the spleen?

Besides physical exam, splenic size and consistency (cysts, tumors) may be evaluated by technetium scan, CT, or ultrasound, depending on the level of suspicion. Splenic function may be evaluated by viewing the peripheral blood smear. The finding of Howell-Jolly bodies suggests a nonfunctional spleen. A splenic scan with labelled red cells also may determine size and function.

16. Which patients manifest hypersplenism?

Hypersplenism consists of mild-to-moderate pancytopenia; various cell types are affected to varying detectable degrees. Cells are sequestered in the spleen, as an exaggeration of the spleen's normal function. Thus, anemia with short survival, thrombocytopenia, and leukopenia constitute hypersplenism, which usually complicates diseases that cause splenomegaly by congestion or hypertrophy of the phagocytic elements. Infiltrative diseases (lymphoma, chronic lymphocytic leukemia) usually do not manifest hypersplenism.

BIBLIOGRAPHY

1. Fijlen GH, et al: Unexplained adenopathy in family practice: An evaluation of the probability of malignant causes and the effectiveness of the physician's work-up. J Fam Pract 27:373, 1988.
2. Kunitz G: An approach to peripheral lymphadenopathy in adult patients. West J Med 143:393, 1985.
3. Libman H: Generalized adenopathy: Clinical reviews. J Gen Intern Med 2:48, 1987.
4. Pierson FG: Staging of the mediastinum: Role of mediastinoscopy and computed tomography. Chest 103(Suppl 4):3465–3485, 1993.

60. BLEEDING AND THROMBOCYTOPENIA

Jeanette Mladenovic, M.D.

1. What history is important in diagnosing a congenital bleeding disorder?

Careful inquiry into prolonged bleeding with minor common surgeries or insignificant trauma is the most helpful element of the history. Specifically, unusual or prolonged bleeding with circumcision, tonsillectomy, or tooth extraction provides strong clues. A history of hemarthrosis also is suggestive. The common congenital bleeding abnormalities of varying severity that present early or late in life include hemophila A or B, von Willebrand's disease, and congenital platelet disorders. Of equal importance is the family history in patients who may be suspected of a congenital abnormality. Even mild symptoms may be compatible with inherited defects.

2. What are the major components of the hemostatic system?

The major components of the hemostatic system are platelets, blood coagulation proteins, and structural support of the vasculature. All components should be investigated in a bleeding patient or a patient with evidence of even a mild bleeding abnormality on physical exam. In acute bleeding, a structural lesion (e.g., a postoperative bleeder) is likely when platelets and coagulation parameters are corrected. In a patient complaining of recurrent bruisability, failure to consider problems in vascular support may lead to a missed diagnosis (e.g., amyloidosis, vasculitis).

3. What abnormalities on physical examination suggest a bleeding disorder?

Major findings include petechiae and ecchymoses. Isolated thrombocytopenia usually results in petechiae. However, petechiae are seen at lower levels of thrombocytopenia when the platelets are young and highly functional than when the defect is due to poor production and/or dysfunctional platelets, as in myeloproliferative diseases. Ecchymoses, especially in areas not usually subjected to trauma, suggest abnormalities of the coagulation proteins, platelet dysfunction, or vascular fragility. Mucosal bleeding from gingiva or as epistaxis in the absence of other explanations also may suggest a bleeding abnormality. Active oozing from puncture sites is consistent with severe defects in any component of the hemostatic system and also suggests activation of the fibrinolytic system, as in disseminated intravascular coagulation (DIC).

4. What tests measure function of the coagulation system?

The prothrombin time (PT) and the activated partial thromboplastin time (aPTT) measure separate components of the coagulation system in vitro. A normal PT suggests that factor VII and other vitamin K-dependent factors contributing to the common pathway are functionally adequate. A normal aPTT suggests adequate function of factors VIII, IX, and XI. Prolongation of the PT and or aPTT may be due to inadequate levels of factors or to specific or nonspecific inhibitors.

5. In what instances should PT and PTT be used as screening tools?

Hematologic malignancies	History of bleeding
Hepatobiliary disease	Anticoagulant use
Malnutrition or malabsorption	Systemic lupus erythematosus

6. Are abnormalities of the coagulation system possible in patients with normal PT and PTT?

PT and PTT may be normal in rare patients with mild acquired von Willebrand's disease or abnormalities in factor XIII, alpha-2 plasmin inhibitor, or platelet coagulant. If a strong history of bleeding (recurrent mucosal bleeding, large muscle hematoma with minimal trauma) is suspected, such disorders are still possible; referral to a hematologist is helpful.

7. List the critical levels of platelets that should direct assessment of bleeding risk.

20,000/mm³: Spontaneous bleeding in the absence of trauma is unusual until platelet counts fall below this level. Spontaneous bleeding is routinely seen with platelet counts of 5000/mm³.

50,000/mm³: This level is recommended to prevent bleeding after surgery and to maintain hemostastis postoperatively or with trauma.

100,000/mm³: This level, which is compatible with a normal bleeding time, may be required for patients who must undergo major surgery in which hemostasis is paramount (neurosurgery, cardiac surgery) or who have severe defects in the coagulation system or their endogenous platelets before surgery.

8. How are platelets evaluated?

Platelets are evaluated by number and function. A low number should be confirmed by viewing the peripheral blood smear and estimating a count of 15,000/mm³ per single platelet viewed on high-power field. The presence of large platelets may help to diagnose immune destruction. Function is evaluated by bleeding time, which also is related to platelet number (100,000 platelets/mm^3 are needed for a normal bleeding time). Evaluation of bleeding time, however, is subject to variability in performance and in correlation with bleeding diathesis (especially preoperative or preprocedure evaluation). It may be most helpful in the positive diagnosis of a platelet defect, such as in von Willebrand's disease, or a myeloproliferative disease with thrombocytosis. In addition, the diagnosis of immune thrombocytopenia is corroborated by a short bleeding time with thrombocytopenia.

9. What common acquired systemic diseases are associated with bleeding?
Liver and renal failure.

10. List the causes of bleeding in liver diseases.
Abnormalities that lead to bleeding in liver disease may be due to structural, hemostatic, or therapeutic causes.

Structural causes
　　Portal hypertension with varices
　　Increased incidence of peptic ulceration and gastritis
Hemostatic causes
　　Decreased hepatic synthesis of procoagulant proteins (fibrinogen, prothrombin, factors V, VII, IX, X, and XI)
　　Decreased absorption and metabolism of vitamin K
　　Decreased clearance of activated coagulation proteins
Therapeutic causes
　　Dilution of proteins and platelets from massive transfusions
　　Increase in bleeding with therapeutic endoscopy

11. Why are patients with renal failure at risk for increased bleeding?
Chronic uremia is associated with abnormalities in platelet function, which may be improved with dialysis (although the bleeding time does not correct). The bleeding diathesis may be corrected by desmopressin, cryoprecipitate, estrogen, or erythropoietin therapy, depending on which is most appropriate for the patient's clinical needs.

12. What contributes to thrombocytopenia in patients who chronically abuse alcohol?
Direct toxicity of alcohol: once alcohol is discontinued, the platelet count should rise and return to normal within 1 week in most patients.

Hypersplenism due to portal hypertension: Hypersplenism alone should not lead to a platelet count significantly lower than 50–60,000/mm^3.

Folate deficiency: Folate is required for hematopoiesis; thus folate deficiency may contribute to thrombocytopenia, usually when megaloblastosis and leukopenia are also evident.

13. What diagnosis is likely in a young child with petechiae?
If the complete blood count demonstrates isolated thrombocytopenia, the likely diagnosis is immune thrombocytopenic purpura. This syndrome follows a viral exanthum or upper respiratory illness, and the majority of patients recover spontaneously, usually in 4–6 weeks. Diagnosis is made by the history; by evaluation of the peripheral blood smear, which shows isolated decreased numbers of large platelets; and by bone marrow aspiration, which eliminates an atypical presentation of a more severe hematologic disease as the cause. Transfused platelets are short-lived and sensitize the patient; thus, transfusion should be reserved for severe bleeding. An increased incidence of central nervous system bleeding is seen with severe thrombocytopenia (< 5–10,000 platelets/mm^3). If needed, prednisone is the drug of choice for initial therapy.

14. What drugs are the most common offenders in drug-induced thrombocytopenia?
Besides alcohol, the best-documented drugs in common practice that cause thrombocytopenia include thiazide diuretics; quinidine and quinine (from tonic water); sulfathiazole; heparin;

estrogens; and myelosuppressive chemotherapy. Many other drugs are suspect; the exact cause is documented in only 10% of patients with drug-induced thrombocytopenia. Thus, the best confirmation of drug-induced thrombocytopenia is a prompt rise in platelet count after removal of the drug (in most patients, within 7–10 days). This reaction to a drug should be clearly documented in the patient's chart so that rechallenge does not occur.

15. How is DIC diagnosed?

Clinical setting: DIC should be considered in obstetric catastrophes or in severely ill patients with sepsis, hypoperfusion, nonviable tissue, massive cell breakdown, or malignancy.

Laboratory confirmation: Ongoing activation of the clotting system is evidenced by consumption of coagulation factors, platelets, and secondary fibrinolysis (as demonstrated by circulating dimers, a specific manifestation of plasmin cleavage). Thus, thrombocytopenia or prolongation of the PT and aPPT in the presence of a low fibrinogen level confirms DIC in the appropriate setting. Clinical bleeding correlates best with the fibrinogen level; levels less than 100 $\mu g/ml$ are likely to require therapy. The presence of nonspecific fibrin degradation products and schistocytes on peripheral blood smear is confirmatory, but their absence does not rule out the diagnosis.

16. When are patients who have used aspirin no longer at risk for bleeding?

Patients who discontinue aspirin for 3 days are likely to have enough newly produced, unaffected platelets to prevent bleeding. The platelets of such patients also may be used in a donor pool. Total replacement of the platelet pool does not occur until 8–16 days.

BIBLIOGRAPHY

1. Eberst ME, Berkowitz LR: Hemostasis in renal diseases: Pathophysiology and management. Am J Med 96:168–179.
2. Hassouna HI: Laboratory evaluation of hemostatic abnormalities. Hematol Oncol Clin North Am 7:1161–1249, 1993.
3. Kirchner JT: Acute and chronic immune thrombocytopenic purpura. Postgrad Med 92(6):112–118, 125–126, 1992.
4. Kitchens CS: Approach to the bleeding patient. Hematol Oncol Clin North Am 6:983–989, 1992.
5. Mammen EF: Coagulated defects in liver disease. Med Clin North Am 78:545–554, 1994.
6. Messmore HL, Godwin J: Medical assessment of bleeding in the surgical patient. Med Clin North Am 78:625–634, 1994.
7. Rutherford CJ, Frenkel EP: Thrombocytopenia: Issues in diagnosis and therapy. Med Clin North Am 78:555–575, 1994.

61. THROMBOSIS AND ANTICOAGULATION

Jeanette Mladenovic, M.D.

1. When is chronic anticoagulation indicated to prevent thrombosis?

Chronic anticoagulation may be indicated on a short-term (3–6 months) or long-term (lifelong) basis.

Short-term use
    Pulmonary emboli
    Proximal deep venous thrombosis
    New bioprosthetic mitral valves with sinus rhythm
    Anterior wall transmural infarction with congestive heart failure

Long-term use (1 year or lifelong)
  Cardiac disease
    Prosthetic mechanical valves
    Recurrent (not lone) or persistent atrial fibrillation
    Cardiomyopathy with chronic congestive heart failure
    Rheumatic valve disease with embolism, atrial fibrillation, or atrium > 5.5 cm
  Malignancy with recurrent emboli
  Inherited disorders of proteins C or S or antithrombin III with multiple thromboses
  Systemic emboli from unknown source

2. When should heparin be given?

Heparin should be administered in the acute management of thromboses, for the prevention of thromboses in operative or hospitalized patients, and in patients in whom sodium warfarin (Coumadin) is contraindicated.

  Acute management
    Venous thromboembolism
    Acute arterial thromboembolism (if not fibrinolysed)
    Unstable angina (3–5 days only)
  Prophylaxis
    General surgery
    Patients with congestive heart failure, infarction, or cardiomyopathy
  Coumadin contraindicated
    Maintenance of anticoagulation during invasive surgical procedure
    Pregnancy, acutely or as prophylaxis
    Coumadin necrosis
    Coumadin failure in malignancy

3. How is heparin administered and monitored?

Heparin interacts with antithrombin III to potentiate the rate of inhibition of the serine proteases (most of the coagulation proteins). Heparin is usually given by continuous infusion to provide a rapid, consistent level of anticoagulation; this approach has a decreased incidence of bleeding compared with intermittent dosing. Recent data have demonstrated the importance of obtaining therapeutic levels within 24 hours of initiation of treatment to prevent recurrent thromboses.

The standard regimen is a loading dose of 5000–10,000 U (higher in patients with pulmonary embolus), followed by continuous infusion of 1000 U/kg/hr. More recent evidence, however, demonstrates that efficacy is improved by higher doses, based on body weight. One such protocol is a loading dose of up to 80 U/kg/body weight, followed by 18 U/kg/hr, with adjustment based on activated partial thromboplastin time (aPTT). Heparin therapy is followed by the aPTT, a test with significant laboratory variability. Values of 1.5–2.0 times the pretherapy value have been used; alternatively, an aPTT of 55–85 seconds may be a more appropriate guideline to follow. This test requires frequent follow-up in the first 48 hours, i.e., 6 hours after initiation and every 6 hours thereafter.

4. When is sodium warfarin (Coumadin) therapy effective?

There is a time lag between the peak level of Coumadin, the prothrombin time (PT), and therapeutic functional anticoagulation. This lag is due to the time required for normal anticoagulation factors to disappear from plasma after their synthesis has ceased. Thus, the PT is maximally prolonged at 72 hours after Coumadin administration, when levels of factor VII and protein C fall, but the antithrombotic action does not peak until 7 days, when factors IX and X are significantly depressed. For this reason, heparin administration must continue for 3–5 days while Coumadin is instituted. Large loading doses of Coumadin are not indicated, because they cannot hasten the initial action.

5. What is the international normalized ratio (INR)?

Coumadin impairs the synthesis of vitamin K-dependent coagulation factors in the liver. Because the PT reflects 3 of the 4 vitamin K-dependent coagulation factors, this test historically has been used to monitor the anticoagulant effect of Coumadin. However, standardizing optimal therapeutic regimens has been difficult, because the laboratory reagent used in the test (the thromboplastin) varies widely and thus produces significant variation in results. The INR compares the patient's PT to a population control adjusted for thromboplastin. Thus, the INR allows physicians to follow published recommendations for anticoagulation. Most indications require an INR of 2–3; the exceptions are patients with mechanical valves, arterial emboli, or recurrent emboli, in whom the INR should be maintained at 3–4.5.

6. When should fibrinolytic agents be considered?

Fibrinolytic agents activate plasminogen and are directed to the site of fibrin thrombi to cause dissolution. Currently streptokinase (in some instances, the more expensive tissue plasminogen activator [TPA]) is indicated in the following circumstances: acute coronary occlusion, acute peripheral artery occlusion, and massive pulmonary embolus resulting in hemodynamic compromise. Streptokinase also should be considered in the therapy of axillary vein thromboses and massive iliofemoral vein thromboses. Likewise, thrombolysis with fibrinolytic agents is useful locally in thrombosed arteriovenous shunts and arterial or venous cannulas.

7. When is anticoagulation contraindicated?

In general	Active bleeding
	Recent cerebrovascular hemorrhage
	Severe congenital or acquired defects in hemostasis
	Recent major surgery, especially of the central nervous system or eye
	Malignant hypertension
Heparin	Thrombocytopenia with thrombosis
Coumadin	Skin necrosis
	Pregnancy
Fibrinolytic agents	Immediately after external cardiac massage
	Patients with a predisposition to intracranial bleeding: untreated hypertension, head trauma, intracranial neoplasms
Relative contra-indications	Severe hepatic or renal disease
	History of falling or unstable gait
	History of GI, genitourinary, or intracranial hemorrhage
	Requirement for high-dose salicylate or nonsteroidal therapy
	Poor compliance

8. How do other drugs affect the PT?

Numerous drugs affect Coumadin therapy by various mechanisms. Recall of all specific drug effects is impractical; thus, the *Physicians' Desk Reference* (PDR) should be consulted. In addition, the results of drug interactions in individual patients require regular monitoring (every 4–6 weeks when stabilized). However, some general classes of drugs and their effects should be commonly recognized as complicating warfarin therapy.

Increased PT or INR through enhanced potency

Reduced Coumadin clearance or binding	Disulfiram
	Metronidazole
	Trimethoprim-sulfamethoxazole
	Phenylbutazone
Increased vitamin K turnover	Clofibrate

Decreased PT or INR through decreased potency

Increased hepatic metabolism	Barbiturates
	Rifampin
Reduced drug absorption	Cholestyramine

9. Which clinical situations are likely to yield increased sensitivity to Coumadin or bleeding while on Coumadin?

Systemic diseases	Liver disease
	Renal disease
	Hyperthyroidism
Additive to other anti-coagulant states	Vitamin K deficiency
	Thrombocytopenia
	Therapy with heparin
	Therapy with aspirin

10. What is the risk of bleeding from Coumadin?
Up to 10% of patients taking Coumadin for 1 year have bleeding complications that require medical intervention. Fatal complications occur as frequently as 1/100 patient years of therapy, despite careful medical management. The highest risk for bleeding is at the initiation of therapy, when patients should be seen frequently. Factors that increase the risk for bleeding are underlying GI, urologic, or neurologic lesions and hypertension. Bleeding usually can be controlled by administration of vitamin K and infusion of fresh frozen plasma.

11. Who is at risk of bleeding from heparin?
Bleeding has not been prevented by frequent monitoring and does not correlate with any clinical assay. Bleeding after surgery or trauma may be severe. Certain patients are at particular risk:
    Patients on drugs that inhibit platelet function
    Patients with renal failure
    Patients with thrombocytopenia
    Postmenopausal women
    Patients with underlying anatomic lesions
Bleeding usually can be managed by discontinuation of heparin therapy, because the half-life of the drug is so short. If necessary, rapid reversal can be accomplished by the slow administration of protamine sulfate (50 mg), a specific antidote.

12. Should guaiac positivity and hematuria be attributed to vascular mucosal leak from anticoagulant therapy?
No—not until a structural lesion has been ruled out. Several studies have demonstrated the high incidence of demonstrable anatomic lesions in patients who bleed even on therapeutic doses of anticoagulant agents. Thus, the source of bleeding should be carefully evaluated.

13. How should heparin-induced thrombocytopenia be managed?
Heparin therapy is associated with two types of thrombocytopenia. A mild thrombocytopenia in as many as 10% of patients predictably occurs at approximately 7 days of therapy. Thus, the platelet count should be measured before and after initiation of heparin. By 7 days, patients usually are taking Coumadin, and thrombocytopenia rapidly resolves once the heparin is discontinued; in some instances, however, it may resolve even if continued heparin therapy is indicated. Alternatively, low-molecular-weight heparin does not appear to cause thrombocytopenia and may be substituted. The more severe form of thrombocytopenia is associated with multiple thromboemboli (white clot syndrome), and may be heralded by initial heparin resistance. This reaction may result in severe thrombocytopenia accompanied by paradoxical clotting. Clinical recognition is paramount. The mortality rate is as high as 25%; heparin must be discontinued.

14. List ten critical elements of education for all patients on Coumadin therapy.
    1. Take Coumadin at the same time each day; never take extra doses to compensate for missed doses.
    2. Report excessive bleeding or ecchymoses immediately.
    3. Regularly check for blood in the stool and urine.
    4. Notify your provider of all changes in medication.

   5. Do not take aspirin or aspirin-containing drugs; use acetaminophen instead.
   6. Avoid circumstances that lead to injury in normal daily activities.
   7. Limit alcohol to a single beer or 1–2 ounces of liquor daily.
   8. Minimize dietary changes and erratic eating.
   9. Women of child-bearing age should notify the provider of any delay in menses
(3–4 days), when pregnancy may be possible.
   10. Prevent epistaxis and learn techniques for its control.

15. List the indications for antiplatelet treatment.

Cardiovascular disease	Unstable angina
	Primary and secondary prevention of myocardial infarction
	Postoperatively for coronary bypass grafting or insertion of certain prosthetic valves
Cerebrovascular disease	Transient ischemic attacks
	Secondary prevention of stroke
Renal disease	Prevention of clotting in arteriovenous fistulas

16. Which systemic diseases are associated with an increased incidence of thrombosis?
Chronic congestive heart failure
Carcinoma, especially mucin-producing types
Hyperviscosity from plasma proteins, red blood cells, or white blood cells
Nephrotic syndrome
Hematologic diseases
   Myeloproliferative diseases
   Paroxysmal nocturnal hemoglobinuria
   Hemoglobinopathies (sickle cell disease)
Homocystinuria
Systemic lupus erythematosus (SLE) with lupus anticoagulant

17. What physiologic, environmental, or iatrogenic conditions contribute to a hypercoagulable state?

Physiologic conditions	Stasis
	Pregnancy
	Postpartum
	Increasing age
Environmental conditions	Smoking
Iatrogenic conditions	Surgery
	Oral contraceptive drugs

18. Who should be screened for an inherited or acquired disorder of hypercoagulability?
The most common inherited disorders that predispose to hypercoagulability are deficiencies of antithrombin III, protein C, and protein S. Proteins C and S are readily assessed either functionally or immunologically. Of patients with recurrent thromboses and a family history of thromboses, about 35% have an identifiable inherited defect in coagulation that appears causative. No known test predicts patients who will thrombose, but the following clinical clues should trigger screening for antithrombin III, protein C, protein S, and lupus anticoagulant:

Thromboses at age less than 40 years	Thromboses during pregnancy
Thromboses in unusual sites	Coumadin necrosis (protein C)
Recurrent thromboses	Resistance to heparin therapy
Recurrent spontaneous abortions	(antithrombin III)

19. When should levels of antithrombin III, protein C, and protein S be measured?
Acute thromboses and therapy with heparin or Coumadin may alter levels of proteins C and S. Optimally, levels should be measured when the individual is off therapy and asymptomatic.

If the patient is on therapy, only a tentative diagnosis may be established if the level is decreased. In addition, because all defects are inherited autosomal dominant traits, confirmation of deficient levels in family members should be pursued.

20. Should patients with hypercoagulable states be treated with lifelong anticoagulation after the first thrombosis?
No. Common practice is to place patients on chronic Coumadin therapy after a second documented episode of thromboses. Patients with low levels of functional proteins and no episodes of thromboses require no treatment.

21. Why is the term lupus anticoagulant a misnomer?
The term is a misnomer because it refers to a group of antiphospholipid antibodies that prolong the aPTT but lead to thromboses in up to 30% of individuals. Thus, it is a true hypercoagulable state associated with SLE but also found in other settings, such as increased age, drug use (phenothiazines), and postinfectious states. In women it may present as recurrent spontaneous abortions. However, it also may be found in men, in whom the specificity of the antiphospholipid antibody may differ. Asymptomatic individuals do not routinely require treatment. If thrombosis occurs, heparin therapy and monitoring by heparin assay are indicated.

BIBLIOGRAPHY

1. Alving B: The hypercoagulable states. Hosp Pract 28:109–114, 119–121, 1993.
2. Antiplatelet Trialists' Collaboration: Collaborative overview of randomized trials of antiplatelet therapy: I. Prevention of death, myocardial infarction, and stroke by prolonged antiplatelet therapy in various categories of patients. BMJ 308:81–106, 1994.
3. Bithell TC: Thrombosis and antithrombotic therapy. In Lee GR, Bithell TC, Foerster J, et al (eds): Wintrobe's Clinical Hematology. Philadelphia, Lea & Febiger, 1993, pp 1515–1551.
4. Cook DJ, Guyatt GH, Laupacis A, Sackett DL: Rules of evidence and clinical recommendations on the use of antithrombotic agents. Chest 102(Suppl):305–311, 1992.
5. Ezekowitz MD, Bridgers SL, James KE, et al for the Veterans Affairs Stroke Prevention in Nonrheumatic Atrial Fibrillation Investigators: Warfarin in the prevention of stroke associated with nonrheumatic atrial fibrillation. N Engl J Med 327:1406–1414, 1992.
6. Fihn S, McDonnell M, Martin D, et al for the Warfarin Optimized Outpatient Follow-up Study Group: Risk factors for complications of chronic anticoagulation. Ann Intern Med 118:511–520, 1993.
7. Hirsh J, Poller L: The internationalized normalized ratio: A guide to understanding and correcting its problems. Arch Intern Med 154:282–288, 1994.
8. Hull RD, Raskob GE, Ginsberg JS, et al: A noninvasive strategy for the treatment of patients with suspected pulmonary embolism. Arch Intern Med 154:289–297, 1994.
9. Hull RD, Raskob GE, Rosenbloom DR, et al: Optimal therapeutic levels of heparin therapy in patients with venous thrombosis. Arch Intern Med 152:1589–1595, 1992.
10. Laupacis A, Albers G, Dunn M, Feinberg W: Antithrombotic therapy in atrial fibrillation. Chest 102(Suppl):426–433, 1992.
11. Meijer A, Verheugt F, Werter C, et al: Aspirin versus Coumadin in the prevention of reocclusion and recurrent ischemia after successful thrombolysis: A prospective placebo-controlled angiographic study. Results of the APRICOT Study. Circulation 87:1524–1530, 1993.
12. Meyer BJ, Chesebro JH: Treatment of arterial thromboembolic disease. Curr Opin Hematol 1:336–340, 1994.
13. Nachman R: The hypercoagulable states. Ann Intern Med 119:819–827, 1993.
14. Raschke RA, Reilly BM, Guidry JR, et al: The weight-based heparin dosing nomogram compared with a "standard care" nomogram: A randomized controlled trial. Ann Intern Med 119:874–881, 1993.
15. Raskob GE, Durica SS: Treatment of venous thromboembolism. Curr Opin Hematol 1:329–335, 1994.
16. Stroke Prevention in Atrial Fibrillation Investigators: Warfarin versus aspirin for prevention of thromboembolism in atrial fibrillation: Stroke Prevention in Atrial Fibrillation II Study. Lancet 343:687–691, 1994.
17. Turpie A, Gent M, Laupacis A, et al: A comparison of aspirin with placebo in patients treated with warfarin after heart-valve replacement. N Engl J Med 329:524–529, 1993.

62. SICKLE CELL DISEASE AND OTHER HEMOGLOBINOPATHIES

Jeanette Mladenovic, M.D.

1. How do globin abnormalities result in clinical hemoglobinopathies?

Hemoglobin, the major component of red cells, is a tetramer of four globin chains covalently linked to heme and arranged in two polypeptide chains. Each globin subunit is determined by inherited genes: two alpha genes on chromosome 16 and one nonalpha gene (normally beta) on chromosome 11. Thus, the hemoglobin in each cell may be composed of various globin types, depending on quantitative or qualitative defects in genes inherited from each parent. Remembering the genetic possibilities facilitates an understanding of the common clinical diseases. Alpha globin is inherited on four genes (two from each parent on chromosome 11), and the severity of quantitative defects (alpha thalassemias) increases with each missing gene. Because chromosome 16 contains a single gene not only for beta hemoglobin but also for other normal hemoglobins that are present in varying amounts during fetal and adult life, quantitative and qualitative defects commonly involve the beta gene. In addition, combined abnormalities may arise from quantitative and/or qualitative defects of genes on both chromosomes. The common abnormalities are as follows:

Qualitative defects in the beta gene are structural:

Hemoglobin S, C, E (usually due to specific mutations)

Quantitative defects in both alpha and beta genes are seen with progressive defects in hemoglobin formation as demonstrated by microcytosis and varying clinical severity:

Alpha thalassemias: usually deletions of one or more genes

Beta thalassemias: quantitative defects in the beta gene

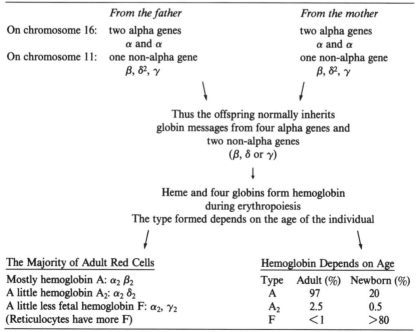

Hemoglobin Production

	From the father	From the mother
On chromosome 16:	two alpha genes α and α	two alpha genes α and α
On chromosome 11:	one non-alpha gene β, δ^2, γ	one non-alpha gene β, δ^2, γ

Thus the offspring normally inherits
globin messages from four alpha genes and
two non-alpha genes
(β, δ or γ)

Heme and four globins form hemoglobin
during erythropoiesis
The type formed depends on the age of the individual

The Majority of Adult Red Cells	Hemoglobin Depends on Age		
	Type	Adult (%)	Newborn (%)
Mostly hemoglobin A: $\alpha_2 \beta_2$	A	97	20
A little hemoglobin A_2: $\alpha_2 \delta_2$	A_2	2.5	0.5
A little less fetal hemoglobin F: α_2, γ_2	F	<1	>80
(Reticulocytes have more F)			

2. What groups in the United States are at risk for carrying a gene related to one of the common hemoglobinopathies?

S gene	1 in 12 Afro-Americans
	Combined with beta thalassemia in people from the Mediterranean countries and Africa.
C gene	1 in 50 Afro-Americans
E gene	Southeast Asians, especially from Laos, Thailand, and Cambodia (almost one-fifth of Laotian and Cambodian refugee children in the U.S.)
Beta thalassemia	Americans of African, Italian, and Greek descent
Alpha thalassemia	Americans of African (1/9), Southeast Asian, Chinese, Italian, and Greek descent

3. Why is it important to recognize the populations with high gene frequencies, even though the diseases may be clinically insignificant to patients who are heterozygous or carriers?
Affected individuals may require genetic counseling. Because the genes follow Mendelian inheritance patterns, prevention or early knowledge of the homozygous state (especially sickle cell disease and beta thalassemia major) is possible with prenatal screening.

4. Which defects are lethal in utero or early in life?
Three major defects are severe and require serious genetic counseling or early recognition:
   Alpha thalassemia with four deleted genes leads to hydrops fetalis.
   Beta thalassemia major (Cooley's anemia), a homozygous variant, leads to severe hemolysis, growth retardation, iron overload, and shortened survival.
   Heterozygotes of beta thalassemia and hemoglobin E disease are similar to beta thalassemia major.

5. What abnormality causes sickle hemoglobin?
Because of a structural abnormality in the beta gene, a single amino acid substitution (valine for glutamic acid) creates an unstable hemoglobin instead of the normal beta hemoglobin. When the unstable hemoglobin deoxygenates, the normal biconcave red blood cell (RBC) becomes sickled, stiff, and sticky.

6. How does the primary care provider screen for hemoglobin?
The usual screen is a solubility test (deoxyhemoglobin S is poorly soluble). If the result is positive, a confirmatory test of hemoglobin electrophoresis should be performed. Sickle cell trait or disease is detected by the amounts of hemoglobins S, A, and F. The usual percentage of hemoglobin F and S should be known for patients with homozygous sickle cell disease, because it may be helpful in therapy.

7. Should persons with heterozygous sickle cell disease be considered high risk for insurance or employment purposes?
No. Affected individuals have normal life expectancy and no clinical illness related to hemoglobin. However, they may be unable to concentrate their urine and occasionally (at low oxygen tension) have asymptomatic splenic or renal infarcts; the latter may result in painless hematuria. They are not required to restrict athletic activity.

8. Describe the four major manifestations of sickle cell disease.
   1. **Anemia.** Because of markedly shortened RBC survival, each patient has a characteristically low hematocrit (usually between 18 and 30%) with a compensatory reticulocytosis. If the reticulocytosis is depressed by infection (especially with parvovirus) or folate deficiency, aplastic crises or critical anemia may develop emergently.
   2. **Constitutional symptoms.** Growth and development are delayed because the illness presents in early childhood. In addition, patients soon become functionally asplenic; thus overwhelming sepsis from encapsulated organisms poses a life-threatening risk.

3. **Acute pain crises.** Vaso-occlusive phenomena lead to recurrent and unpredictable pain, which presents most frequently in the abdomen, joints, back, and chest. Patients usually are familiar with their own patterns of precipitating events and periodicity. A prior infection is known to precipitate crises. The chest syndrome is treated as both infection and infarction, because the differentiation is not possible. Abdominal pain is particularly difficult, because it may mimic an acute abdomen. Joint crises may be accompanied by noninflammatory effusions.

4. **End-organ damage.** As patients with sickle cell disease reach adulthood, they experience end-organ damage in essentially all systems because of repeated microvascular occlusions. Most prominently affected are the lungs, heart, kidneys, bones, skin, and eyes. Macrovascular events are particularly apparent in the incidence of cerebral thromboses.

9. How should painful crises be managed?
Acute painful crises should be managed supportively with analgesia and hydration. Oxygen should be administered when low oxygen saturation is present. Infection should be ruled out or treated. Transfusion to decrease the percentage of hemoglobin S or to improve oxygen-carrying capacity should be reserved for severe illness or surgery; it usually is given with consultation of a hematologist.

10. What preventive measures should the primary care provider institute in the care of patients with sickle cell disease?
1. Folate supplementation
2. Immunization: Pneumococcal vaccine
3. Prophylaxis: Penicillin in children to prevent sepsis
                  Malaria prophylaxis for travel to endemic areas
4. Regular ophthalmologic follow-up
5. Consideration of supply of narcotics for early prevention of crises, with recognition of the risk of abuse

11. What therapies are available to diminish the effect of sickle hemoglobin on the clinical course of the disease?
Therapies are usually aimed at diminishing the percentage of hemoglobin S, often through monitored hypertransfusion programs for unique indications. In addition, experimental therapies are aimed at enhancing hemoglobin F, which prevents sickling. Thus, in many instances, the care of a patient with sickle cell disease should be undertaken in conjunction with a hematologist, especially when the patient becomes pregnant or requires surgery.

12. Why is hypertransfusion not routinely used in patients with sickle cell disease?
Although hypertransfusion may appear to be an easy answer to decreasing the percentage of sickle hemoglobin, it is not routinely practiced because of its complications. Iron overload, isoimmunization, and infection may be anticipated with repeated transfusions.

13. Can sickle cell disease present late in life?
Yes. In some populations, disease severity varies considerably. Thus, hemolytic anemia should raise the possibility of sickle cell disease in a patient who belongs to a susceptible group and has not previously been screened.

14. What are the four major causes of death in patients with sickle cell disease?
Cardiopulmonary failure, renal failure, cerebrovascular events, and infection.

15. Is hemoglobin SS the only genotype associated with the phenotype of sickle cell disease?
No. Two additional disorders may mimic sickle cell disease. Sickle beta thalassemia (one gene for S and one for beta thalassemia) and sickle C (one S and one C gene on each of the two 16 chromosomes) present similarly to sickle cell disease. Sickle beta thalassemia may be seen in Caucasians of Mediterranean descent. If no beta chains are made, this condition may be difficult to distinguish from hemoglobin SS disease on electrophoresis.

16. What inherited hemoglobin abnormalities commonly result in microcytosis?
Prominent microcytosis is seen in three settings: alpha thalassemia trait, beta thalassemia trait, or hemoglobin E (hetero- or homozygous). All may demonstrate a low mean cell volume in routine complete blood counts with no detectable anemia. Alpha thalassemia trait, a common asymptomatic finding in Afro-Americans, may have a normal electrophoresis. If so, no further evaluation is usually necessary. A silent carrier of alpha thalassemia with one alpha gene missing has no detectable abnormalities. Electrophoresis in patients with beta thalassemia trait usually shows an increase in A_2 hemoglobin. Patients with hemoglobin E, both homo- and heterozygotes, may have microcytosis without anemia or only mild anemia. This condition may be diagnosed by electrophoresis.

17. What happens to the patient with alpha thalassemia in whom three genes are missing?
This defect produces a compensated hemolytic disease, with anemia, reticulocytosis, many target cells, and precipitated beta chains in the RBCs, called Heinz bodies.

18. What other hemoglobin abnormalities may cause a congenital hemolytic anemia?
The major defects to consider in children or young adults who present with a relatively compensated hemolytic anemia are of three types: RBC enzyme defects (G6PD deficiency); RBC membrane defects; or other mutant hemoglobins. Many other mutants of the beta genes lead to hemolytic anemia and often demonstrate precipitated hemoglobin as Heinz bodies. Whereas these mutants may result in a relatively compensated hemolytic anemia, their structural abnormalities may give rise to hemoglobins that have varying oxygen affinities or that are susceptible to precipitation with oxidant stress by drugs.

19. Which patients are at risk for gallstones?
All patients with congenital hemolytic anemia have an increased incidence of gallstones. In patients with sickle cell disease, the diagnosis is complicated by abdominal pain associated with sickle crisis and liver abnormalities that may result from repeated hepatic infarcts. Generally, cholecystectomy is recommended in symptomatic patients.

BIBLIOGRAPHY

1. Bunn HF: Disorders of hemoglobin. In Isselbacher KJ, Braunwald E, Wilson JD, et al (eds): Harrison's Principles and Practices of Medicine. New York, McGraw-Hill, 1994, pp 1734–1743.
2. Dabrow MB, Wilkins JC: Hematologic emergencies. Management of transfusion reactions and crises in sickle cell disease. Postgrad Med 93:183, 1993.
3. Embury SH: The clinical pathophysiology of sickle cell disease. Ann Rev Med 37:361–376, 1986.
4. Kazazian HH: The thalassemia syndromes: Molecular basis and prenatal diagnosis. Semin Hematol 27:209, 1990.
5. Pollack CV: Emergencies in sickle cell disease. Emerg Med Clin North Am 11:365–378, 1993.
6. Steingart R: Management of patients with sickle cell disease. Med Clin North Am 76:669–682, 1992.
7. Weinberger M: Approach to the management of fever and infection in patients with primary bone marrow failure and hemoglobinopathies. Hematol Oncol North Am 7:865–885, 1993.

X. Disorders of the Musculoskeletal System

63. PRINCIPLES OF MUSCULOSKELETAL INJURY AND SPORTS MEDICINE

Richard Fisher, M.D.

1. In taking a history from a trauma patient, why is it important to inquire about the mechanism of injury?

Knowing the mechanism of injury in the severely traumatized patient often aids in identifying high-risk areas and in determining treatment. High-energy injuries, such as occur in automobile or motorcycle accidents, have profound effects on multiple systems in addition to the musculoskeletal system. Low-energy injuries, such as simple falls, have different implications for patient survival and complications.

2. During the initial evaluation of a severely traumatized patient, what are the important priorities to consider?

As with all patients seen on an emergency basis, the ABCs (airway, breathing, and circulation) should take precedence over other exams. The patient also should be evaluated for chest injuries, abdominal trauma, and head trauma before beginning definitive therapy for musculoskeletal injuries.

3. During the evaluation of other sites of injury, how should the musculoskeletal system be protected?

If the extremities or spine appear to be injured, they should be protected with splinting or simple immobilization to prevent further damage.

4. In evaluating a traumatized extremity, what are the principal tissue priorities to consider?

In order of importance, the six tissues to be considered are the vascular system, neurologic system, skin and underlying soft tissue, muscle-tendon units, joint and ligament complexes, and bone.

5. How may the vascular integrity of the extremity be evaluated?

Major arteries should be palpated, and the temperature and color of the extremity should be evaluated and compared with noninjured extremities, recognizing that extremities often feel cool in the patient with shock. The capillary refill can be evaluated in the nailbeds. If pulses are difficult to palpate, the Doppler may be used. In cases of suspected major vascular injury, arteriography is indicated.

6. Describe the neurologic evaluation of an injured extremity.

Extremities should be checked for sensation and motor function with an attempt to cover all major peripheral nerves as well as dermatomes. Testing of the deep tendon reflexes also is helpful. Interruption of the tendon or muscle units at times may be mistaken for neurologic injury. Serial exams always should be performed. A change in status is a good indicator of developing problems.

7. What are the potential stages of injury of a nonfunctioning peripheral nerve? Describe the prognosis for each.

1. A **contusion or neurapraxia** injures the nerve, but the nerve cell processes remain in continuity. Function usually returns within 6 weeks.

2. A **crush injury or axonotmesis** interrupts the nerve cell, and the axon must be regrown distally from the point of injury before recovery occurs. Regrowth takes place at about 1 mm/day.

3. **Neurotmesis or complete division** of the nerve is associated with a laceration or injury from the sharp ends of a fractured bone. The nerve will not regain function without surgical repair.

8. What is the importance of the skin exam?

In addition to cosmetic change and disfigurement associated with injuries to the skin, the clinical courses of open and closed fractures are entirely different. The same is true for open injuries of a joint or tendon sheath. The skin should be checked on all sides of the body.

9. Why does an open fracture require emergent management?

Open fractures should be treated with tetanus prophylaxis and antibiotics as soon as possible. The patient should be transported to the operating room for thorough debridement and irrigation of the fracture to remove all possible contamination. In addition, the fracture should be properly stabilized. The incidence of complications, including infection and nonunion, increases in proportion to delay in treatment. The goal is definitive debridement in less than 6 hours from the time of injury.

10. Describe the severity rating for muscle strains.

Muscle strains are graded into three stages, depending on the severity of the injury. **First-degree strains** consist of a mild pulled muscle. The muscle-tendon unit remains intact. The muscle should be protected from use until painless function returns. **Second-degree strains** from a moderate pull to the muscle results in some tearing of the muscle fibers but continuity of the muscle-tendon unit is maintained. Signs and symptoms include impaired muscle function, moderate amounts of pain with muscle use or stretching, swelling, and ecchymosis. **Third-degree strains** are severely pulled muscles that disrupt the continuity of the muscle-tendon unit. Treatment depends on the site of the injury.

11. Any muscle-tendon unit may be injured by direct laceration. List the six most common sites of indirect third-degree muscle tendon injuries.

1. The long head of the biceps tendon at the shoulder
2. The quadriceps tendon at its insertion into the patella
3. The patella tendon, which ruptures either from the surface of the patella or in mid-substance
4. The Achilles tendon
5. The extensor tendon at the distal interphalangeal (DIP) finger joints
6. The flexor digitorum profundus tendon at the DIP joint

12. Describe the typical signs and symptoms of joint injuries.

A dislocated joint is held in an abnormal position, and because of pain the patient will not allow the joint to be moved. Injured joints usually show a detectable amount of fluid that is either effusion or hemarthrosis; the distinction is made by aspiration. In the presence of ligament injury, careful testing may reveal the associated instability. Testing at times is difficult because of the acute pain and swelling in the joint. The joint should be examined under anesthesia or several days later when the pain subsides.

13. What are the stages of ligament injury?

Stage I injuries involve tearing of some of the ligament fibers without disruption of individual or collective fibers. **Stage II injuries** involve tearing of multiple ligament fibers without disruption of individual or collective fibers. In both stage I and stage II injuries the joint remains stable to testing. In more severe stage II injuries, however, tearing of the ligament fibers may involve partial disruption of the ligament complex. The joint may show mild instability but not complete laxity, and the exam is usually painful. **Stage III injuries** involve complete disruption of the integrity of the ligament, usually with demonstrable instability. Treatment depends on the joint involved but generally is nonsurgical for stages I and II. Stage III injuries may require surgical repair or reconstruction.

14. Why does clipping in football invoke a 15-yard penalty?

Clipping is a block from the posterolateral side at the level of the knee. The foot is usually planted on the ground, and a valgus force is produced across the knee. Clipping often results in a tear of the medial collateral ligament, the anterior cruciate ligament, and the medial meniscus. The treatment is surgical, and rehabilitation is often prolonged. Full functional recovery is not guaranteed.

15. Describe the signs and symptoms of a fractured bone.

Although signs and symptoms vary, the cardinal findings are swelling, point tenderness, visible or palpable deformity, and crepitus at the fracture site. Stress fractures and torus (greenstick) fractures in children may show minimal signs on physical exam. Radiographs are indicated once the area of injury is determined.

16. What principles should be followed when ordering radiographs for the traumatized patient?

Generally plain roentgenograms are indicated after examination of the patient and determination of the site to be examined; 90-90 radiographs are almost always indicated, because deformities may be missed when only one view is taken. In addition, the joint above and the joint below the involved bone should always be included in the exam. Special studies, such as computed tomography (CT) or magnetic resonance imaging (MRI), are indicated to evaluate certain fractures. Injuries most likely to require special imaging studies involve the calcaneus, tibia plateau region, pelvis, and spine. Occult fractures or stress fractures are often diagnosed earliest with bone-scanning techniques.

17. What are the most commonly missed fractures in the polytrauma patient?

The most commonly missed fractures involve the odontoid process, C7 vertebral body, scaphoid, radial head, pelvis, femoral neck, tibial plateau, and talus. The incidence of missed fractures is about 10%.

18. Under what special circumstances does musculoskeletal trauma lead to extreme blood loss that may be missed by the clinician?

Although blood loss needs to be monitored in all trauma patients, musculoskeletal injuries involving the femur, hip, and pelvis and all open fractures are especially prone to large amounts of blood loss. In closed fractures of the femur or pelvis, the loss may not be apparent, and many units of blood may be sequestered before external signs become obvious.

19. Occasionally a patient presenting with a history of trauma may in fact have a preexisting underlying condition responsible for the acute signs and symptoms. Name the more common conditions that may cause confusion.

Underlying problems, such as infection and tumor, are often unmasked by simple and seemingly insignificant injury, including pathologic fractures through the lesion and simple contusions that exacerbate symptoms. Gouty arthritis often occurs after trauma and presents as a painful joint at the site or remote from the area of injury.

20. Name the three most common delayed complications in patients following musculoskeletal injury.

The three most common delayed complications are compartment syndrome, fat embolism syndrome, and Sudeck's atrophy. Compartment syndromes usually occur in the region of a long bone fracture but may occur in remote areas with muscle or crush injuries. Symptoms are usually present within the first 24 hours after injury. Fat embolism syndrome usually presents within 12–72 hours of multiple trauma, long bone fractures, or burns. Symptoms include confusion, shortness of breath, tachycardia and petechiae. The partial pressure of oxygen (PO_2) is usually low. Sudeck's atrophy is usually seen later in the course of injury and presents as swelling, redness, and pain out of proportion to the underlying injury.

21. How do the presenting symptoms of a stress fracture differ from those of acute traumatic fractures?
The stress fracture is usually produced by overuse of the extremity and is of gradual onset. The history usually includes an increase in activity levels about 3 weeks before the onset of symptoms, which are exaggerated by repetition of the activity. This pattern of injury occurs commonly in runners when they suddenly increase their distance or time. Some recent data suggest that patients prone to stress fractures have a decrease in bone density. In elite female athletes, decreased production of estrogen may lead to an increased incidence of stress injuries.

22. What are the most common locations for stress fractures?
The location depends to some extent on the activity producing the injury. The stress fracture was first described in the second metatarsal in association with prolonged walking. Fractures of the proximal tibia and mid- and proximal femur are common in runners. Fractures in the area of the femoral neck are especially dangerous and should be stabilized surgically. Fractures of the upper extremities are seen in gymnasts and others involved with prolonged upper extremity activities. Stress fractures associated with osteomalacia also may be seen in the pelvis, scapula, and ribs.

23. Describe the common signs and symptoms of spinal column injury.
The mechanism of injury is important in assessing the potential severity of spinal column and associated injuries. Falls from heights, diving injuries, and motor vehicle accidents are common mechanisms. Pain is usually reported at and below the level of the injury, and a careful history should be taken with regard to neurologic symptoms, such as ascending numbness and loss of motor control. The physical exam should include evaluation of cutaneous reflexes, muscle power, muscle tone, deep tendon reflexes, sensation, and anal sphincter tone. The spine should be palpated carefully for areas of tenderness and possible deformity. A multiply injured patient should be treated as if a spinal column injury were present until history, physical exam, and radiographic studies prove otherwise.

24. What are the two most common areas of injury in the spinal column?
The two most common areas are the mobile parts of the column—the cervical spine and the thoracolumbar junction.

25. What is the proper management of patients with suspected cervical spine injuries?
Such patients should be immobilized, and anteroposterior and cross-table lateral radiographs should be taken. A careful neurologic examination should be performed, and the patient should not be moved until it is proved that the spinal column is intact. An unconscious patient should be assumed to have a cervical spine injury until the above studies are shown to be normal.

26. Which two injuries most commonly occur in combination with spinal column injuries?
Fractures of the calcaneus associated with lumbar spine fractures and head injuries associated with cervical spine injuries.

27. Describe the common medically important systemic conditions that often interface with musculoskeletal injuries.
The most significant medical illnesses that seem to be found in patients with musculoskeletal illnesses include diabetes, seizure disorders, high-dose steroid use, and various central nervous system disorders, such as stroke or Parkinson's disease.

BIBLIOGRAPHY

1. Browner BD, Jupiter JB, Levine AM, Trafton PG: Skeletal Trauma. Philadelphia, W.B. Saunders, 1992.
2. D'Ambrosia RD: Musculoskeletal Disorders: Regional Examination and Differential Diagnosis. Philadelphia, J.B. Lippincott, 1986.
3. Fabian TC: Unraveling the fat embolism syndrome. N Engl J Med 329:961–963, 1993.
4. Frymoyer JW (ed): Orthopaedic Knowledge Update 4. Rosemont, IL, American Academy of Orthopaedic Surgeons, 1993.
5. Iverson LED, Clawson DK: Manual of Acute Orthopaedic Therapeutics. Boston, Little, Brown, 1987.

64. MONARTICULAR ARTHRITIS

David H. Collier, M.D.

1. What diseases may present as a swollen, painful, warm and frequently also erythematous joint?

Such symptoms, which may present as monarticular or polyarticular disease, are typical of an inflammatory response to an immune reaction, crystals, or infection.

Immune-induced disease	Rheumatoid arthritis and other autoimmune diseases (systemic lupus erythematosus, mixed connective tissue disease, vasculitides) Spondyloarthropathies
Crystalline-induced disease	Gout and pseudogout
Infection	Bacteria, fungi, viruses

2. What is the differential diagnosis of an acutely warm, painful joint (monarticular inflammatory arthritis)?

The examiner must first ascertain that inflammation is in the joint space and not in the surrounding supportive tissue (such as tenosynovitis). The typical patient with a truly inflamed joint guards the area from movement and will not allow any range-of-motion testing by the examiner. A patient with periarticular inflammation may allow careful movement of the joint and often localizes pain and tenderness to the area around the joint. An effusion may be present in either case.

Once it is determined that a joint is involved, the differential diagnosis commonly centers on determining whether the joint is inflamed from infection (bacterial or fungal) or in response to crystals (monosodium urate, as in gout, or calcium pyrophosphate dihydrate (CPPD) as in pseudogout). Bleeding into the joint also may induce inflammation, and the spondyloarthropathies may present initially as isolated monarticular arthritis or rarely as atypical rheumatoid arthritis.

A single joint that is chronically swollen with limited evidence of synovitis is more likely to be due to an isolated posttraumatic degenerative arthritis or indolent or granulomatous inflammation.

3. What characteristic radiographic findings are helpful in the differential diagnosis of arthritis?

Soft-tissue swelling, periarticular osteopenia, and joint space loss followed by erosions at the site of the capsular insertion into the bone are characteristic of inflammatory arthritides. Crystal-induced arthritis may show dramatic erosions or calcified cartilage (pseudogout) with intact cartilage space. In contrast, degenerative joint disease (osteoarthritis) demonstrates cartilage loss in stress areas, with sclerosis along the joint line and osteophyte formation.

4. What test helps to determine the etiology of a monarticular arthritis?

A sample of the synovial fluid should be aspirated from the inflamed joint. Several joints, such as the knee, are easily amenable to aspiration; other joints are better approached with the aid of an experienced rheumatologist or orthopedic surgeon.

5. What helpful information is obtained from evaluation of the joint fluid?

Although several tests are available to analyze joint fluid, examination of the fluid for white and red blood cell counts with differentials, assessment of crystals, and microbiologic cultures for infectious organisms are the most useful. White blood cell counts > 2000 cells/mm^3 are consistent with inflammation; the highest counts are seen with septic joints. A Gram stain, even in the presence of crystals, should be done; even if the results are negative, however, a negative culture is required to exclude suspected diagnosis of septic arthritis. A noninflammatory arthritis is suggested by the finding of < 2000 white cells/mm^3.

Examination of the fluid for crystals requires a rose-quartz filter and a polarizing microscope. Gout is confirmed by the presence of negatively birefringent crystals, seen as yellow crystals with the slow wave of the polarizer parallel to the crystals. Pseudogout is suggested by small positively birefringent crystals, seen as blue crystals with the slow wave of the polarizer parallel to the crystals.

6. Does an overlying cellulitis preclude aspiration through the apparently infected area?

No. A diagnosis of septic arthritis must be pursued, if suspected. However, before the aspiration, systemic antibiotics should be given for the cellulitis. The only contraindication to arthrocentesis is suspected hemarthrosis due to coagulopathy, either congenital or acquired.

7. Does crystalline deposition occur only in joints?

No. Deposition of both uric acid and CPPD in periarticular tissue may present as acute attacks of tenosynovitis or bursitis. Tenosynovitis is also a characteristic presentation of the initial arthritis of disseminated gonoccocemia.

8. Should a fluid-filled bursa be aspirated?

When monarticular swelling occurs in the prepatellar area or over the extensor surface of the elbow, the likely diagnosis is bursitis, which often is caused by repeated trauma or crystalline or other arthritic disease. Surface temperature change (compared to the opposite side) or other signs of inflammation over the swelling suggest the possibility of infection, caused by the typical pathogens of *Staphylococcus aureus* or *S. epidermidis*, or streptococci. Thus, aspiration of fluid for Gram stain, culture, and crystal analysis is indicated in the first episode of bursitis. The white blood cell count of the fluid may be similar in infection and inflammation. Therefore, in the absence of a positive Gram stain, therapy with a cephalosporin or antistaphyloccocal penicillin should be given on the basis of clinical suspicion. Complications of systemic infections or overlying cellulitis require intravenous therapy. If sterility of the synovial fluid is assured, bursitis may be treated with aspiration, compression dressing and extensor pads, nonsteroidal anti-inflammatory drugs (NSAIDs), or steroid injection, which shortens the course of the disease.

9. What may precipitate a gouty attack?

1. Medication that causes a change in the uric acid level
2. Hospitalization for medical or surgical causes (Patients with a history of gout have a high incidence of recurrence during hospitalization.)
3. Stress, trauma, infection
4. Weight reduction, hyperalimentation, and fluid shifts

10. How should gout be treated acutely?

Therapy of gout is effective if begun early in the attack. Gout responds well to NSAIDs. Indomethacin is commonly used but should be avoided in patients with congestive heart failure, cirrhosis, renal disease, or a history of gastrointestinal (GI) bleeding. Colchicine, the traditional specific therapeutic intervention, is helpful when the diagnosis is uncertain; however, the frequency of GI side effects usually makes it a less popular alternative. Intravenous colchicine, used in the past, is now unavailable in the United States. Intra-articular steroids are also effective but should not be the first line of therapy. Oral adrenocorticosteroids are used when NSAIDs and colchicine are contraindicated or in cases resistant to those therapies.

11. Why should the level of uric acid not be treated during an acute attack?

An acute attack may be prolonged or precipitated when the level of uric acid is treated. Thus, it is wise to wait 4 weeks or more before instituting therapy to lower the level of uric acid. Treatment is begun once it is determined whether the patient is an overproducer or underexcreter of uric acid. Underexcreters are the most common type. Probenecid is a cost-effective drug to treat underexcreters (in the absence of renal disease or tophi); allopurinol treats both underproduction and overproduction but may cause exfoliative dermatitis.

12. What is the spectrum of pseudogout?

Acute synovitis caused by deposition of CPPD crystals mimics gout and thus has been called pseudogout. However, CPPD crystalline deposition results in a spectrum of disease that includes subacute or chronic forms as well as complicating osteoarthritis, and may mimic rheumatoid arthritis, even producing calcification of intervertebral disks with no symptoms. Although the knee is the most common presenting joint, radiographic evidence of polyarticular disease is common. CPPD deposition increases in incidence with age and is precipitated by the same factors that precipitate gouty attacks.

13. Can therapy prevent crystalline deposition in pseudogout?

No. Therefore deposition frequently results in chronic arthritis. Therapy of pseudogout is symptomatic with NSAIDs. Colchicine also leads to improvement and may be given prophylactically for frequent recurrence. Joint aspiration may provide symptomatic relief, and glucocorticoid injection is an option, although it should be used with care.

14. Which joints are most likely to become bacterially infected?

Usually bacteria are hematogeneously spread from a remote focus. Organisms resist serum and reticuloendothelial defenses and colonize synovial tissue. This resistance accounts for the increased likelihood of infection in a damaged joint or impaired host and in joints with the greatest amount of synovium. Therefore, the most commonly affected joints are the knee, hip, shoulder, ankle, wrist, and elbow. Intravenous drug abusers usually have staphylococcal infections, but atypical infections are also possible. The most common joints affected in intravenous drug abusers include the vertebral column, sacroiliac joint, sternoclavicular joint, and lower extremities, often on the side used for drug injection.

15. What organisms are commonly responsible for acute pyogenic arthritis in adults?

Organism	Incidence (%)
Neisseria gonorrhoeae	50%
Staphylococcus aureus	35%
Streptococcus pyogens	10%
Gram-negative bacilli	5%
Mycobacteria, other fungi	< 1%

Suspicion or diagnosis of septic arthritis requires intravenous antibiotic therapy.

BIBLIOGRAPHY

1. Espinoza L, Goldenberg DL, Arnett FC, Alarcon GS (eds): Infections in the Rheumatic Diseases: A Comprehensive Review of Microbial Relations to Rheumatic Disorders. Orlando, FL, Grune & Stratton, 1988.
2. Kelly WN, Harris ED, Ruddy S, Sledge CB (eds): Textbook of Rhematology, 4th ed. Philadelphia, W.B. Saunders, 1993.

3. Klippel JH, Dieppe PA (eds): Rheumatology. St. Louis, Mosby, 1994.
4. McCarty DJ, Koopman W (eds): Arthritis and Allied Conditions, 12th ed. Philadelphia, Lea & Febiger, 1993.

65. POLYARTICULAR ARTHRITIS

David H. Collier, M.D.

1. What is the "gel" phenomenon?

The gel phenomenon refers to the complaint of stiffening with inactivity and is characteristic of systemic arthritides. Typically, it is manifest as morning stiffness that requires loosening with a hot shower or activity. The stiffening returns when patients are inactive (e.g., prolonged sitting) but improves with activity. Quantitating the morning stiffness can be helpful in gauging the severity of the disease and its response to therapy.

2. How do the history and physical examination help to determine whether complaints of polyarticular arthritis are more likely due to rheumatoid arthritis or degenerative joint disease (osteoarthritis)?

	Rheumatoid arthritis	Degenerative joint disease
History		
Morning stiffness	Long ($>$ 1 hr)	Short ($<$ 0.5 hr)
Movement	Improves stiffness	Increases pain
Systemic symptoms	Common	Uncommon
Physical examination		
Inflammation	Red, warm synovitis	Not evident
Swelling	Invariable	Variable
Symmetry	Characteristic	Variable
Joints	Distal small joints	Variable
Hands and feet	Proximal interphalangeal (PIP) joint, metacarpophalangeal (MCP) joint	Distal interphalangeal (DIP) joint, first carpometacarpal (CMC) joint, first metatarsophalangeal (MTP) joint

3. What are risk factors for generalized osteoarthritis (more than 3 joints)?

Risk factors include obesity, trauma, congenital hip abnormalities, and familial history of hand arthritis. Osteoarthritis also may occur after an inflammatory process or secondary to metabolic defects (such as hemochromatosis).

4. How is rheumatoid arthritis diagnosed?

Rheumatoid arthritis is diagnosed by a constellation of clinical and laboratory abnormalities, often appearing over 1–2-year period. Criteria developed by the American College of Rheumatology have a high sensitivity (90–95%) and specificity (89%) in establishing the diagnosis but cannot be used to exclude early disease. Four of the seven following criteria should be observed by a physician for 6 weeks:

1. Morning stiffness of more than 1 hour's duration
2. Polyarticular arthritis: simultaneous involvement of 3 or more joint areas
3. Arthritis of the hands or wrist
4. Simultaneous symmetric arthritis
5. Rheumatoid nodules
6. Positive rheumatoid factor
7. Typical radiographic changes of rheumatoid arthritis in the hands adjacent to affected joints

5. Is rheumatoid arthritis a disease only of joints?

No. The spectrum of rheumatoid arthritis ranges from mild, seronegative disease to high titers of rheumatoid factor accompanied by vasculitis. High-titer rheumatoid factor is associated with rheumatoid nodules, small vessel vasculitis involving skin and peripheral nerves, pleuropericardial or pleuropulmonary disease, eye disease (episcleritis, scleritis), and Felty's syndrome.

6. What is the standard therapeutic approach to a patient with rheumatoid arthritis?

1. Education by trained individuals (often physical therapists).
2. Occupational and physical therapy, even for prevention of complications.
3. Pharmacologic therapy for inflammatory control. The first approach is to control pain and function with nonsteroidal anti-inflammatory drugs (NSAIDs), prescribed at optimal doses. Control of inflammation may be adequate for patients with mild disease.
4. Remittive therapy. Patients who are young or have high titers of rheumatoid factor, evidence of joint destruction, or systemic vasculitis should be referred to a rheumatologist for management and consideration of remittive therapy (e.g., gold, penicillamine, methotrexate, prednisone).

7. What is the characteristic difference between rheumatoid arthritis and systemic lupus erythematosus (SLE) arthritis?

Both are a polyarticular symmetric inflammatory arthritis that most commonly affects the hands (PIP, MCP) and feet. SLE, however, is nonerosive. Alignment abnormalities, swelling, pain and even subcutaneous nodules may be seen in both diseases.

8. What constellation of findings suggests systemic vasculitis?

Multiorgan involvement	**Systemic manifestations**
Renal disease, including glomerulitis	Fever
Diffuse arthritis or arthralgias	Fatigue
Skin lesions such as purpura, necrosis,	Weight loss
ulcerations, or Raynaud's	Hypertension
phenomenon	**Laboratory findings**
Possible pulmonary disease	Mild anemia
	Elevated sedimentation rate

9. Describe the approach to effective treatment of systemic vasculitis.

Effective treatment depends on classification of the vasculitis according to specific vessels involved and known syndromes.

10. Describe the four major characteristics of the spondyloarthropathies.

1. Seronegative arthritis (absence of rheumatoid factor and nodules)
2. Asymmetric involvement of peripheral joints (often in the lower extremity), accompanied usually by sacroiliitis (whether symptomatic or evident only on radiographs) and often by spondylitis involving the posterior intervertebral apophyseal joints
3. Involvement of synchondroses (cartilaginous junction between bones), specifically in the vertebral bodies and discs, pubic symphysis, and manubriosternal joints
4. Enthesopathies or inflammation at insertions of ligaments, tendons, and fibrous structures into the bone.

11. What diseases constitute the spondyloarthropathies?

Spondyloarthropathies are characterized by the level of involvement of the sacroiliac joint:

Bilateral sacroiliitis	**Unilateral sacroiliitis**	**Variable sacroiliac involvement**
Ankylosing spondylitis	Reiter's disease	
Enteropathic arthropathies	Psoriatic	Whipple's disease
due to ulcerative colitis or	arthropathy	Behçet's syndrome
inflammatory bowel disease		

12. What five organ systems may be involved in patients with spondyloarthropathies?
1. Eyes: iritis, uveitis, or conjunctivitis
2. Skin: psoriasis, keratoderma blenorrhagicum (similar to psoriasis)
3. Cardiovascular system: aortitis, conduction defects
4. Pulmonary system: apical pulmonary fibrosis
5. Gastrointestinal tract: diarrhea, ulcerations of the small and large intestines

13. What five questions about back pain may distinguish an inflammatory cause, as seen with the spondyloarthropathies, from a mechanical cause?
1. Did the back pain begin before the age of 40 years? Most mechanical back problems start after 40, whereas most spondyloarthropathies are symptomatic before 40.
2. Was the onset of pain insidious? The pain of ankylosing spondylitis typically has a slow, vague onset, whereas most mechanical back problems start suddenly.
3. Is the duration of the pain over 3 months? The vast majority of acute back injuries improve after 2 months, whereas pain of the spondyloarthropathies is slowly progressive.
4. Is the pain worse in the morning and associated with morning stiffness? A major complaint of most patients with inflammatory problems is severe back stiffness and pain in the morning which last over 1 hour. Mechanical back problems typically improve after a night's rest.
5. Does the pain improve with exercise? Moving the back exacerbates pain due to a mechanical problem, whereas a patient with ankylosing spondylitis may exercise each morning to feel more comfortable and to carry out daily activities.

14. Which physical maneuvers may point to a diagnosis of spondyloarthropathies?
1. **Measurement of spinal range of motion.** Two points—10 cm above and 5 cm below L5–S1—are marked on the patient's back, and the patient is asked to bend over in an attempt to touch the toes. A normal change between the two marks is 5 cm, or a total range of motion of 20 cm. A smaller change suggests restricted range of motion of the lower spine.
2. **Palpation of the sacroiliac joints.** The effects of direct palpation may be exaggerated by having the patient lie on one side and flex the ipsilateral hip (knee to chest) while the examiner hyperextends the contralateral hip.

15. What constitutes Reiter's syndrome?
Reiter's syndrome refers to a spectrum of reactive arthritis (ReA) that is not consistent with other spondyloarthropathies. The syndrome characteristically is an acute, asymmetric arthritis of the lower extremities that may involve the subtalus or present a dactylitis (sausage digit). It may be isolated to joints or include systemic illness characterized by fatigue, fever, and weight loss. Classic accompanying or intercurrent manifestations involve the following three systems:
1. Urethritis or cervicitis (including prostatitis and salpingitis)
2. Ocular manifestations ranging from sporadic conjunctivitis to debilitating uveitis
3. Mucutaneous disease ranging from painless oral or genital ulceration to a keratoderma blenorrhagicum, a psoriaticlike skin lesion typically on the palms and soles.

16. What organisms have been cultured from patients with reactive arthritis?
The following organisms have been cultured from stool or genitourinary discharge: *Shigella flexneri, Chlamydia trachomatis, Yersinia enterocolitica, Campylobacter jejuni,* and *Salmonella* species. Other organisms also have been implicated.

17. Are antibiotics of benefit in the therapy of ReA?
Treatment of ReA has classically centered on NSAIDs; refractory cases are treated with sulfasalazine or immunosuppressive drugs. In the past antibiotics were thought to play no role. Recently, however, chlamydia-induced disease was shown to respond to a prolonged course of long-acting tetracycline. However, effectiveness of other antibiotics remains to be determined.

18. When should the human leukocyte antigen B27 (HLA-B27) be assessed in a patient suspected of having a spondyloarthropathy?

Seronegative spondyloarthropathy probably arises from interaction of a susceptible genetic background and an environmental factor that induces the disease. HLA-B27 is strongly associated with the spondyloarthropathies, especially in Caucasians (over 80% of Caucasians with ankylosing spondylitis are HLA-B27–positive). Although its presence or absence does not confirm or deny the diagnosis, HLA-B27 may be helpful in family counseling or in particularly enigmatic cases in which every piece of evidence may help to determine a probable diagnosis.

BIBLIOGRAPHY

1. Arnett FC: Seronegative spondyloarthropathies. Bull Rheum Dis 37:1–12, 1987.
2. Calin A, Elswood J, Rigg S, Skevington SM: Ankylosing spondylitis—an analytical review of 1500 patients: The changing pattern of disease. J Rheumatol 15:1234–1238, 1988.
3. Calin A, Porta J, Fries JF, Schurman DJ: Clinical history as a screening test for ankylosing spondylitis. JAMA 237:2613–2614, 1977.
4. Danzi JT: Extraintestinal manifestations of idiopathic inflammatory bowel disease. Arch Intern Med 148:297–302, 1988.
5. Harris ED: Rheumatoid arthritis: Pathophysiology and implications for therapy. N Engl J Med 322:1277–1289, 1990.
6. Hurd ER: Extraarticular manifestations of rheumatoid arthritis. Semin Arthritis Rheum 8:151–176, 1979.
7. Khan MA (ed): Spondyloarthropathies. Rheumatic Disease Clinics of North America, Philadelphia, W.B. Saunders, 1992.
8. Reveille JD, Conant MA, Duvic M: Human immunodeficiency virus associated psoriasis, psoriatic arthritis, and Reiter's syndrome: A disease continuum. Arthritis Rheum 33:1574–1578, 1990.
9. Utsinger PD, Zvifler NJ, Ehrlich GE (eds): Rheumatoid Arthritis Etiology, Diagnosis, Management. Philadelphia, J.B. Lippincott, 1985.

66. LOW BACK PAIN

Joseph Anderson, M.D.

1. Why should the primary care provider develop expertise in the management of low back pain?

Low back pain is one of the most common presenting symptoms in a doctor's office. Approximately three-quarters of all adults experience back pain during their life. In addition, disability from chronic low back pain is growing at an alarming rate. Practitioners should be prepared to help patients with low back pain maintain functional status and be vigilant about spotting diseases that may present as low back pain, such as an aortic aneurysm.

2. Which structures in the body can be the source of low back pain?

Musculoskeletal structures	Visceral structures
Vertebral periosteum	Renal disease
Outer layer of the annulus fibrosus	Gastrointestinal disease
Nerve roots	Pelvic disorders (e.g., prostate,
Muscles	ovary, uterus)
Apophyses	Aorta
Posterior longitudinal ligaments	Endocrine system

3. Which potentially serious diagnoses should be considered in the evaluation of back pain?

Osteomyelitis, malignancy, aortic aneurysm, and unstable spine fractures.

4. What are the relative frequencies of diseases that cause low back pain?
Unfortunately, a large percentage (up to 85%) of patients cannot be given a definite diagnosis. Less than 5% of all patients with low back pain present with sciatic complaints. Another small fraction, also less than 5%, have malignancy, infection, fracture, or visceral disease as a cause of pain.

5. In addition to a careful history aimed at determining the organic etiology of the pain, what additional elements of the history should be elicited from the patient with low back pain?
The practitioner should extract a thorough and careful history from the patient, because the differential diagnosis of low back pain encompasses many organ systems. However, it is also important to question the patient about motor vehicle accidents, sports injuries, and previous back surgery. In addition, a full employment history as well as date of eligibility for disability should be obtained. The practitioner also should ask about lifestyle behavior such as weight, exercise, and smoking.

6. Most mechanical back pain is relieved by bed rest. What diagnoses may be considered when low back pain persists in the presence of bed rest?
Malignancy and spondyloarthropathy are two diagnoses in which pain may persist even during bed rest. Malignancy also may be suspected in the presence of weight loss and/or a previous history of malignant disease. Spondyloarthropathies tend to present with insidious onset of pain and morning stiffness.

7. What are good predictors of compression fractures?
Steroid use and age greater than 70 years are good predictors for the presence of compression fractures. Although trauma may be a cause, most patients have no history of trauma.

8. What is sciatica? What does it indicate?
Sciatica is a sharp, burning pain radiating posteriorly or laterally down the leg past the knee, often in association with numbness. Such pain is usually increased with coughing and sneezing. The complaint of sciatica is a clue to nerve root irritation and may herald neurologic compromise. The presence of sciatica usually signifies disc herniation, which most commonly occurs at the level of L4–L5 or L5–S1; however, sciatica also may be seen in spinal stenosis.

9. What characteristic history suggests the diagnosis of spinal stenosis?
Spinal stenosis is a degenerative disease of the spine and thus usually begins after the age of 50 years. Patients complain of pseudoclaudication or back pain accompanied by lower extremity pain with paresthesias or dysesthesias that worsen with standing but are not present in the sitting position.

10. What maneuvers should be performed during the physical examination of patients who present with low back pain?
  1. Inspection of the back, looking for leg-length discrepancies and spinal curvature abnormalities.
  2. Palpation of the vertebral column and the sacroiliac joints. Point tenderness may be found in malignancy or infection, whereas sacroiliac (SI) joint tenderness suggests spondyloarthropathies.
  3. Range of motion of the spine. Two lines are drawn (at L5–S1 and 10 cm above), and the distance between the two lines is measured during spinal flexion. A distance of less than 15 cm during flexion suggests decreased range of motion and may be one of the earliest manifestations of spondyloarthropathy. This test is called the Schober test.
  4. Straight leg-raising. With the patient supine, the examiner raises the affected leg in the extended position. Pain at less than 60° signifies nerve root irritation.
  5. Motor exam. See the table below for correlation of nerve with muscle innervation. Foot dorsiflexion testing is particularly useful.

6. Sensory exam. Careful attention must be paid to the dermatomal or lack of dermatomal distribution of numbness. The saddle area must be included.

7. Reflexes, especially ankle reflexes, which are diminished when the S1 nerve root is affected.

NERVE	MOTOR	SENSORY	REFLEX
L1	Hip flexion	Back/groin	Cremasteric
L2	Hip adduction Hip flexion	Back Anterior thigh	Cremasteric
L3	Same as L2 and Knee extension	Back Upper buttock Anterior thigh	Patellar
L4	Knee extension	Medial foot/calf	Patellar
L5	Toe extension Ankle dorsiflexion	Lateral lower leg Medial dorsum of foot	Tibialis posterior
S1	Ankle plantar flexion Knee flexion	Sole/heel Lateral foot	Achilles
S2	Ankle plantar flexion Toe flexion	Posterior upper and lower leg	None
S3	No text	Medial buttocks	Bulbocavernosus
S4	No test	Perirectal	Bulbocavernosus
S5	No test	Perirectal	Anal

11. What is the utility of plain radiographs of the spine?
Plain radiographs, although inexpensive, are often not helpful or misleading. Since by the age of 50 years, two-thirds of individuals have narrowing between vertebrae and 20% have osteophytes, radiographs are of greatest use after trauma or when systemic disease is suspected from the history or physical exam.

12. What routine laboratory studies may be helpful clues in the diagnosis of a patient with low back pain?
An elevated erythrocyte sedimentation rate (ESR) is highly specific for malignancy and infection. A complete blood count, urinalysis, and assessment of calcium, and alkaline phosphatase levels may be considered in patients who are older than 50 years, have failed conservative management, or have signs or symptoms suggestive of systemic disease.

13. When should an HLA-B27 test be ordered?
The HLA-B27 test should be considered only when the radiographs are normal, but the clinical history, setting, and physical exam are perplexing and highly suggestive of a spondyloarthropathy.

14. When are other imaging tests indicated?
A bone scan may detect malignancy or infection before radiograph. However, it is not specific and does not detect lytic lesions. Computed tomography (CT) or magnetic resonance imaging (MRI) should be ordered only in patients for whom surgery is contemplated. Both are sensitive for disc pathology. However, a significant percentage of asymptomatic patients will have evidence of disc herniation.

15. What is the cauda equina syndrome?
The cauda equina syndrome is the constellation of bowel dysfunction and/or urinary retention, saddle anesthesia, and bilateral leg weakness or numbness. This syndrome constitutes a true surgical emergency.

16. When should back pain result in surgical referral?

Cauda equina syndrome (emergency)

Progressive or severe neurologic deficit at presentation (the presence of fever should suggest epidural abscess as an emergency)

Persistent neurologic deficit and sciatica after 4–6 weeks of conservative management

17. How should patients with acute back pain be managed?

1. Education

    Explanation of symptoms

    Advise to return for worsening neurologic deficits

    Strong reassurance about the natural history (resolution expected)

    Counseling: weight loss, smoking cessation (if applicable)

2. Activity

    Limit activity only as desired (2–3 days) in patients without neurologic deficits.

    Bed rest should be described for longer periods (up to 1 week) for patients with neurologic deficits.

3. Pain control

    NSAIDs may control inflammation and pain but should be used with caution in elderly patients or patients with renal disease.

    Narcotics and muscle relaxants should be used only for short, well-defined periods (1 week).

    Heat may be used as desired after the acute injury.

4. Follow-up

    One month–6 weeks if the patient does not improve

18. What is the role of exercise in the treatment of low back pain?

An exercise program, in the absence of neurologic deficit, should be encouraged. Stretching exercises for the lower back and extremities and general anaerobic fitness may improve back mobility, increase energy levels, and decrease recurrent acute episodes of back pain. Such a program may begin within 2 weeks of the acute episode, assuming that it has resolved.

19. What are the indications for hospitalization?

The patient should be hospitalized only if surgery is contemplated. Traction has not been shown to be beneficial in the treatment of low back pain.

20. What methods may be used to determine whether the patient is a malingerer?

Waddell[11] reported five ways to elicit nonorganic signs in a patient who amplifies symptoms:

1. Spinal loading or rotation. Lightly press down on the head of the patient and rotate the patient's hips and pelvis. These maneuvers should not cause back pain.

2. Nonorganic tenderness. If lightly touching the paraspinal muscles causes pain, the patient may be amplifying the symptoms.

3. Distraction straight leg-raising. When the patient is seated, straighten the leg while asking about the knee. This maneuver should produce pain in the back, causing the patient to lean backward, especially if the straight leg-raising test is positive.

4. Inappropriate sensory findings. Check for reproducibility of sensory abnormalities as well as dermatomal distribution.

5. Overreaction during examination.

21. List five basic principles in treating patients with chronic back pain.

Only 10% of all patients with back pain will develop chronic symptoms. The patient must understand that complete resolution of chronic pain is an unrealistic goal. The mnemonic **TREAT** summarizes the appoach to preventing chronic back pain:

T = Transfer some responsibility to the patient. The patient must adhere to lifestyle changes such as weight loss and smoking cessation.

R = Reassurance. The patient should understand that the back pain is not life-threatening and should not interfere with most activities of daily living.

E = Early mobilization. The patient should understand that activity will not be detrimental for his back and might be beneficial.

A = Avoid drug dependency. It is unrealistic for the patient to expect total relief from medication.

T = Titrate medications upward only for short, preset periods during occasional flare-ups.

CONTROVERSY

22. Should strict bed rest always be prescribed for acute low back pain, even if sciatica is present?

Strict bed rest has been the cornerstone of conservative treatment. The rationale is to limit disc pressure so that the disc may resume its previous form. However, most low back pain does not originate with the disc. Furthermore, little evidence supports bed rest as a therapeutic modality. Deconditioning, loss of muscle, and demineralization of bone are among the deleterious effects of just a few days of bed rest. On the other hand, the back must be given sufficient recovery time to prevent chronic injury. Thus it appears unwise to prescribe bed rest for a patient without a neurologic deficit or sciatic complaints. Individualized treatment plans should be the rule with an emphasis on early mobilization. Patients with a neurologic deficit should stand periodically to decrease the negative effect of bed rest. Standing causes only a slight increase in disc pressure over the supine position.

BIBLIOGRAPHY

1. Borenstein D: Epidemiology, etiology, diagnostic evaluation, and treatment of low back pain. Curr Opin Rheumatol 4:226–232, 1992.
2. Borenstein D, Wiesel S: Low Back Pain: Medical Diagnosis and Comprehensive Management. Philadelphia, W.B. Saunders, 1989.
3. Deyo R, Roinville J, Kent D: What can the history and physical exam tell us about low back pain? JAMA 268:760–765, 1992.
4. Deyo R, Loeser J, Bigos S: Herniated lumbar intervertebral disk. Ann Intern Med 112:598–603, 1990.
5. Deyo R: Early diagnostic evaluation of low back pain. J Gen Intern Med 3:230–238, 1986.
6. Deyo R, Mayer T, Pedinoff S, et al: An attack on low back pain. Patient Care 21:106–143, 1987.
7. Gran J: An epidemiological survey of the signs and symptoms of ankylosing spondylitis. Clin Rheumatol 4:161–169, 1985.
8. Hall S, Bartleson J, Onotrio B: Lumbarspinal stenosis. Ann Intern Med 103:271–275, 1985.
9. Mazanec D: Low back pain syndromes. In Panzer R, Black E, Grinzer P (eds): Diagnostic Strategies for Common Medical Problems. Philadelphia, American College of Physicians, 1991.
10. McConin P, Borenstein D, Wiesel S: The current approach to the medical diagnosis of low back pain. Orthop Clin North Am 22:315–325, 1991.
11. Waddell G, McCulloch J, Kummel E, Vernner R: Nonorganic physical signs in low back pain. Spine 5:117–125, 1980.
12. Waldvogel F, Vassey H: Osteomyelitis: The past decade. N Engl J Med 303:360–370, 1980.

67. HIP AND KNEE PAIN

Richard C. Fisher, M.D.

1. What are the most important questions to characterize pain in the hip or knee regions?
The purpose of the history is to focus attention on possible etiologies of the pain. The following areas are the most important.

1. **Localization of the pain.** Pain originating in the pelvis is often felt throughout the low back, gluteal muscles, and thighs. Pain from bursae or tendons is sharply localized. Hip joint pain is often felt in the anterior groin area or medial thigh and knee in the distribution of the obturator nerve.

2. **Onset and duration of pain.** Onset is slow in inflammatory conditions but rapid with trauma or infections.

3. **Relation of the pain to activities.** It is important to know whether the pain occurs at rest, whether it has changed the lifestyle of the patient, and whether it requires the use of walking support such as a cane or walker.

4. **Associated systemic symptoms.** Of specific importance are back pain, abdominal complaints, other joint involvement, and associated fever, chills, and malaise.

2. What is the first change seen in the physical examination of a patient with a disorder of the hip joint?
The first change in the physical examination usually is loss of joint motion, specifically internal rotation. Motion should be measured with the patient supine, including flexion, extension, abduction, adduction, and internal-external rotation. Loss of motion and pain should be noted. Other findings include a limp thigh of decreased circumference due to secondary disuse atrophy. At times, pain with deep palpation is noted over the anterior aspect of the hip joint.

3. List the most common etiologies of hip joint pain.

Degenerative, inflammatory and occasionally infectious arthritides	Stress fractures
	Paget's disease
Avascular necrosis of the femoral head	Tumors, especially pigmented
Acute fractures	villonodular synovitis

4. What is the differential diagnosis of traumatic hip pain in elderly patients?
The most obvious consequence of trauma to the hip region in elderly patients is a fracture of the proximal femur. Occasionally the initial films appear normal, but the patient continues to have varying degrees of pain with activity. In such situations establishing the correct diagnosis is important. The most common diagnoses include simple contusion to the soft tissue, fractures of the greater trochanter, occult fractures of the pelvis, and occult fractures of the femoral neck or intertrochanteric region. The latter are the most significant, because an initial occult fracture may become a displaced fracture without appropriate treatment. Focused routine radiographs may show a fracture line; if no fracture line is seen, the diagnosis may be confirmed with a radionucleotide bone scan. This test, however, may not be diagnostic for as long as 3 days after the onset of trauma. Magnetic resonance imaging (MRI) scans recently have been reported to be useful in assessing occult femoral neck fractures immediately after injury.

5. What common problems may masquerade as hip and thigh pain?
Spinal problems
Atraumatic pelvic fractures (pelvic insufficiency fractures)
Lower abdominal abnormalities, including tumors and infection
Meralgia paresthetica
Claudication of the internal iliac artery

6. Name the common causes of avascular necrosis of the femoral head.

Among the many etiologies of avascular necrosis, the most common are trauma (e.g., femoral neck fracture or hip dislocation); use of corticosteroid medication; alcohol overuse; rapid decompression (caisson disease); sickle cell disease; and radiation.

7. How is avascular necrosis diagnosed?

MRI evaluation may show the earliest changes. The technetium 99-m bone scan is abnormal before plain radiographs. The scan is usually cold for a very short time initially and then shows increased uptake as revascularization begins. Plain radiographs show changes at a much later time when an increase in bone density and subchondral fractures become apparent.

8. Describe the treatment options for avascular necrosis.

The value of surgical decompression of the femoral head remains controversial. Decompression in the stage prior to radiographic changes but subsequent to changes on the MRI scan may improve the prognosis for revascularization without collapse, but this remains unproved. Once the femoral head has begun to deform, decompression is not indicated. Osteotomy or total joint replacement is indicated at this stage.

9. What are the manifestations of overuse syndromes in the region of the hip and knee?

1. **Stress fractures.** The most commonly seen overuse problem is stress fractures in the proximal or mid-femur or proximal aspect of the tibia. Of greatest concern is a stress fracture of the femoral neck and intertrochanteric region, which often results in displaced fractures. Patients who may have this diagnosis should be removed from weight bearing immediately and considered for referral to an orthopedic surgeon for surgical stabilization.

2. **Soft-tissue injury.** Soft-tissue injuries develop from repetitive motion of the fascia lata over the greater trochanter (greater trochanteric bursitis) and latertal femoral condyle (iliotibial tract friction syndrome) of the femur.

3. **Tendinitis.** Quadriceps and patella tendinitis are more frequent in young patients at the tendon insertion sites.

10. Which bursae about the hip or knee are more commonly involved in clinical symptoms?

Greater trochanteric bursa, prepatellar bursa, infrapatellar bursa, and pes anserinus bursa seem to be the most commonly involved. Others include the iliopsoas bursa and occasionally the ischiogluteal bursa (with prolonged wheelchair use).

11. Describe the treatment for bursitis and tendinitis.

Initial treatment consists of rest from aggravating activities. Rest may be supplemented with application of ice and use of nonsteroidal anti-inflammatory agents (NSAIDs). Various physical therapy modalities are also effective, including ultrasound treatments. When such conservative therapy is not effective, injection of corticosteroids into the bursa or tendon sheath may be indicated. The use of steroids about ligaments and tendons should be carefully considered, because the steroids may lead to tendon or ligament rupture because of changes in collagen synthesis. The same is not necessarily true of bursitis. Surgical excision of the bursa or release of the tendon sheath is occasionally indicated for unremitting and disabling cases.

12. Enlargement about the knee may be associated with bursitis, knee effusion, or generalized swelling. How are the three differentiated?

Prepatellar bursitis causes fluid accumulation between the skin and the patella. A fluctuant area superficial to the bony patella is palpable.

A **knee effusion** elevates the patella, which is readily palpated beneath the skin with no intervening fluid. In addition, the suprapatellar pouch, which extends approximately 3 fingerbreadths above the superior pole of the patella, feels full superiorly, medially, and laterally.

Generalized swelling in the knee, such as occurs from acute injuries, is not localizable to either the bony patella or the suprapatellar pouch. Swelling is diffuse, usually extends to the proximal tibia and distal femur, and is often circumferential in nature. It is frequently associated with ecchymosis.

13. What are the most common causes of true knee effusions?

1. **Traumatic effusions** usually contain blood or a mixture of blood and synovial fluid. The fluid may contain fat droplets in the presence of an associated fracture.

2. **Posttraumatic effusions** occur after meniscal tears, ligamentous injuries, or other destabilizing injuries of the knee. Posttraumatic effusions show an increased amount of normal synovial fluid.

3. **Inflammation**, such as seen in rheumatoid arthritis or gout, often causes an effusion with an abnormal synovial analysis.

4. **Purulent fluid** is seen in both acute and chronic types of infection.

14. What are the indications for joint aspiration?

The predominant indication is diagnosis. After trauma the knee occasionally swells to the extent that it becomes tense and painful, at which time removal of some of the blood and synovial fluid relieves the patient's pain.

15. Describe the classic signs and symptoms associated with early degenerative arthritis of the knee.

The history usually includes pain with weight-bearing activities. Often patients report removal of a meniscus or a ligamentous injury some years before. A mild effusion may be present, and crepitus is felt with joint motion. The early radiographic changes include flattening of the femoral condyles, osteophyte formation beginning at the joint margins, and narrowing of the cartilage space. Weight-bearing films provide the best evaluation.

16. Describe the history and physical findings associated with patellofemoral disease.

The major finding in the history is pain with walking up or down stairs or inclines, rising from a chair, and kneeling. The pain is felt directly beneath the patella and associated with crepitus or a rough feeling as the patella glides over the femoral condyle. On physical examination the patella may track laterally as the knee reaches full extension. Patellar instability, detectable by palpation, is not uncommon, and the patient often becomes apprehensive as the patella is pushed to the lateral side.

17. What treatment is available for patellar pain?

The treatment depends to some extent on the cause of the pain. In general, treatment is symptomatic, as in other inflammatory conditions, and consists of rest, ice or heat, and NSAIDs. Protection of the patella femoral joint is sometimes possible with a patellar orthosis or a special type of taping to correct malalignment. Physical therapy consists primarily of short arc quadriceps-strengthening exercises. In patients with severe malalignment and recurrent subluxation or dislocation, surgical correction protects the underlying articular cartilage. The value of arthroscopic or open patella debridement and shaving remains controversial.

18. When are imaging techniques useful in the evaluation of knee problems?

Imaging techniques are useful for bony lesions such as osteochondritis dessicans, fractures, tumors, and early degenerative changes. Routine radiographs are indicated for the initial evaluation. The MRI scan has become increasingly useful for diagnosing soft-tissue problems such as meniscal and anterior and posterior cruciate injuries and for evaluating possible bony or soft-tissue tumors about the knee. The arthrogram has been largely supplanted by the MRI scan for the evaluation of meniscal injuries, although it may be of value in diagnosing the size and extent of popliteal cysts. Ultrasound is also useful for evaluating popliteal cysts and distinguishing fluid-filled from solid lesions. Computerized or plain tomography is of value in evaluation of certain fractures, particularly in the proximal area of the tibia and distal femur.

19. When is total hip or total knee arthroplasty indicated?

Replacement arthroplasty is a serious undertaking and should be used only in patients with no other alternatives for treatment. Failure of arthroplasties may result in either a flail or a fused joint. Arthroplasty should be recommended only as an endstage procedure when the joint is destroyed by an arthritic or traumatic process beyond the point at which conservative measures are effective. The failure rate in young patients is high, and surgery is usually discouraged before the age of 60 years. However, in young patients who have incapacitating joint destruction and are not candidates for either osteotomy or arthrodesis, arthroplasty may be an appropriate procedure.

20. What are the expected outcomes from total hip or total knee arthroplasty?

The expected outcome is return to a painfree functional status. Rarely does the involved joint regain full motion or become totally painfree. The goal is return of enough function to allow activities of daily living and low-impact recreational activities. The major short-term complications are infection (reported incidence of 0.5–4%) and mechanical failure (reported incidence of 5% at 2 years). Both complications usually require revision surgery. The major long-term complication is mechanical failure or loosening, which at 10-year follow-up is reported in the range of 10–40%.

21. Discuss the treatment options for pyogenic infections of the hip and knee joint.

The choice of open drainage, arthroscopic drainage, or needle drainage of pyogenic infections remains controversial, although authorities agree that some type of drainage is needed. Antibiotics also are mandatory in the treatment of these potentially destructive infections. In general, the two most important considerations are the type of organism involved in the infection and ease of access to the joint. The most destructive organisms include the gram-negative bacilli, and staphylococci, whereas streptococci and gonococci are known to be particularly benign. Joint accessibility is important for adequacy of drainage and monitoring of clinical response.

Pyogenic hip joint infections in children should be treated with open drainage. Treatment of other joints remains controversial. No clear evidence indicates an advantage of one treatment over another for adult hips and knees. If clinical response is not adequate within 3–4 days of aspiration, open or arthroscopic drainage is indicated. Failure of needle drainage is probably related to the virulence of the organism and inability to evacuate loculated areas within the joint. Acute infections following total joint arthroplasty should be treated by open drainage.

BIBLIOGRAPHY

1. D'Ambrosia RD: Musculoskeletal Disorders: Regional Examination and Differential Diagnosis. Philadelphia, J.B. Lippincott, 1986.
2. Frymoyer JW (ed): Orthopaedic Knowledge Update 4. Rosemont, IL, American Academy of Orthopaedic Surgeons, 1993.
3. Fulkerson JP, Shea KP: Disorders of patellofemoral alignment. J Bone Joint Surg 72A:1424–1429, 1990.
4. Holder LE, Schwarz C, Wernicke PG, et al: Radionuclide bone imaging in the early detection of fractures of the proximal femur (hip): Multifactorial analysis. Radiology 174:509–515, 1990.
5. McCarty DJ, Koopman WJ (eds): Arthritis and Allied Conditions. Philadelphia, Lea & Febiger, 1993.
6. Turek SL: Orthopaedics: Principles and Their Application. Philadelphia, J.B. Lippincott, 1984.

68. SHOULDER AND ELBOW PAIN

Richard C. Fisher, M.D.

1. What questions are important in taking a history from a patient presenting with shoulder or elbow pain?

1. Time of onset and patient's perception of the cause of pain, such as a fall or other trauma, overuse, or systemic illnesses
2. Duration of the pain and its change over time
3. Anatomic location of maximal discomfort
4. Activities that increase or decrease the pain
5. Functional limitations caused by the pain, specifically decreased range of motion, inability to use the arm for certain activities of daily living, and difficulty in sleeping.
6. Treatment modalities that have been tried

2. Describe the measurement of range of motion for the shoulder and elbow.

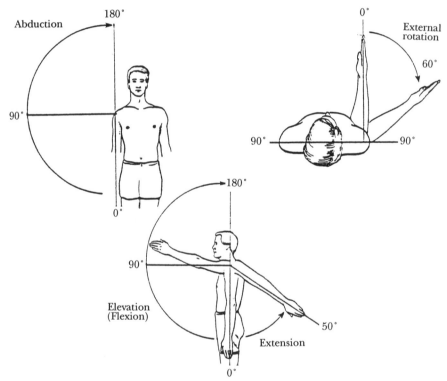

Measurement of the range of motion of the shoulder joint. (From Greene WB, Heckman JD: The Clinical Measurement of Joint Motion. Rosemont, IL, American Academy of Orthopaedic Surgeons, 1994.)

3. Describe the visible deformities that may suggest the cause of the patient's pain.

After trauma deformity may be seen with acromioclavicular (AC) separations, shoulder or elbow dislocations, and fractures of the clavicle and humerus. AC separations show a prominence and/or swelling at the AC joint and may be accompanied by an abrasion over the tip of the shoulder. Patients with shoulder dislocations have a hollow area inferior to the acromion with a palpable humeral head more distally. Elbow dislocations show a prominence of the distal humerus or the olecranon with loss of motion. Fractures of the clavicle are usually in the mid-portion and present with swelling and/or bony angulation. Some fractures of the mid-humerus have visible angular deformity; the arm is held in abduction and cannot be adducted to the side. Pain of neurogenic origin may be associated with muscle atropy about the shoulder and arm region. The most common abnormality is atrophy of the deltoid muscle following axillary nerve injury or of the supraspinatous and infraspinatous muscles following compression injuries to the suprascapular nerve. Patients with spastic neuropathies often have an internal rotation contracture at the shoulder.

4. Can palpation help to delineate the cause of pain?
Yes. Patients with olecranon and subacromial bursitis have point tenderness over the tip of the elbow or shoulder. Traumatic deformity, even if not visible, often can be delineated by palpation about the clavicle, acromioclavicular joint, shoulder joint, and elbow joint. In patients sustaining acute AC separations, instability of the joint may be palpable with gentle downward stress on the arm. Patients with referred pain often have a diffuse area of discomfort that does not correspond to any specific anatomic abnormality and may have no tenderness at the site at which they perceive the pain.

5. What common sites refer pain to the shoulder and upper arm region?
1. Cervical spine
2. Brachial plexus
3. Thoracoabdominal region, including tumors of the lung, ischemic heart disease, subphrenic abscesses, stomach problems, and gallbladder disease

6. How are the causes of referred pain differentiated?
Referred pain due to cervical spine and brachial plexus abnormalities usually is accompanied by local discomfort that is aggravated by motion of the neck and palpation over the brachial plexus. Neurologic deficits may be present. In thoracic and abdominal problems symptoms are referrable to those areas and usually accompanied by physical findings or radiographic abnormalities.

7. Name the common locations of compression neuropathies of the shoulder, upper arm, and elbow regions.
Suprascapular nerve entrapment occurs as the nerve transverses the suprascapular notch on the superior border of the scapula. The presenting complaint is weakness of shoulder abduction and external rotation as well as diffuse, nonspecific shoulder pain. Atrophy of the scapular fossa muscles is usually present. Suprascapular nerve entrapment is often seen in throwing athletes and in patients performing other repetitive motions.
Thoracic outlet syndrome is commonly associated with pain after using the upper extremity in the elevated or abducted position and with symptoms of ulnar nerve dysfunction.
Congenital lesions such as those of the syrinx also cause neurologic change leading to a neuropathic (Charcot) shoulder joint. **Ulnar nerve compression** at the olecranon groove at the elbow is one of the most common compression neuropathies of the upper extremity. **Median nerve compression** at the pronator muscle in the proximal forearm is seen less frequently.

8. Describe the diagnostic features of thoracic outlet syndrome.
Usually the patient complains of pain in the shoulder region with radiation into the arm. If the arm is held in the abducted position, the palpable pulse at the wrist decreases, and a bruit may be audible over the subclavian artery. This test also may produce pain and dysesthesias in the upper extremity. The ulnar nerve is most commonly involved, but median and radial nerves also may be affected. Adson's test is performed with the arm at the side and the head turned from one side to the other while the patient inhales. A positive test reproduces the patient's symptoms, and a decreased radial pulse is noted.

9. What are the diagnostic features and treatment options for ulnar nerve entrapment at the elbow?

Diagnostic signs include (1) a postitive Tinel's sign (tingling sensation with percussion of the nerve) at the olecranon groove on the medial aspect of the humerus and (2) motor and sensory changes in the ulnar nerve distribution distal to the elbow. Electromyography and nerve conduction tests are confirmatory in most cases, if the diagnosis is unclear. Treatment initially consists of rest with a splint or sling and often a trial of anti-inflammatory medications. Corticosteroid injections may be used but are somewhat hazardous because of the tight compartment in which the nerve travels at the medial epicondyle. Surgical decompression is indicated for persistent symptoms or progressive neuropathy.

10. Name the most common sites of bursitis in the shoulder and elbow region.

The subacromial bursa and the olecranon bursa are the most frequently involved. The **subacromial bursa** can be palpated directly distal to the tip of the acromion process on the lateral aspect of the shoulder. If inflamed, it is tender to palpation and painful with shoulder abduction approaching 90°. **Olecranon bursitis** produces swelling directly over the tip of the olecranon process, which is tender to palpation. In acute cases, surrounding skin appears red and indurated. Olecranon bursitis is differentiated from an infected bursa by the lack of systemic signs of infection and by the results of aspiration.

11. How does the cause of bursitis in the subacromial and olecranon bursae differ?

The principles of overuse and compression apply to both bursae. The subacromial bursa is injured indirectly by impingement of the greater tuberosity of the inferior aspect of the acromion when the arm is used in the abducted position. Olecranon bursitis is secondary to direct pressure on the tip of the elbow over the bursa. It may be initiated by an acute traumatic event but most often results from chronic irritation. If an abrasion is present over the bursa, the chances of infection are increased.

12. Discuss the common lesions in the elbow region that are secondary to repetitive trauma.

The most common problem is **lateral epicondylitis** (tennis elbow), which is caused by repetitive use of the upper extremity for a variety of activities, such as tennis or gripping a hammer or saw. **Medial epicondylitis**, although less frequent, results from similar activities. In both conditions the area directly over the epicondyle at the insertion of the extensor or flexor muscle mass is usually tender. On the lateral side other causes of pain include **entrapment of the radial nerve** just distal to the elbow and **inflammation of the annular ligament** about the radial head.

13. Explain the treatment protocol for tennis elbow.

Initial treatment includes avoidance of aggravating activity, ice before and after use, and anti-inflammatory medication. Physical therapy modalities and a graded biceps- and triceps-strengthening program are useful. A tennis elbow band, which fits just below the elbow, acts as a damper for the extensor muscle mass and may be beneficial during activity. If noninvasive therapy has not helped, an injection with corticosteroid may be tried. Surgical release and reimplantation of the extensor muscle mass into the lateral epicondyle may be indicated in resistant cases.

14. List the pathologic stages of shoulder impingement syndrome.

Inflammation, fibrosis, tendon rupture, and degeneration are the four pathologic stages of shoulder impingement syndrome. During the inflammatory stage, which includes acute bursitis, the lesion is reversible with rest, steroid injection (in select patients), or surgical decompression. Once the degeneration has become advanced or the lesion has progressed to overt rupture of the tendon, surgical correction is usually necessary for symptomatic and functional improvement.

15. Describe the treatment for shoulder impingement syndrome.

Treatment depends in part on the stage of the impingement syndrome. For acute inflammation and early fibrosis, initial treatment consists of decreased activity or rest followed by physical therapy for gentle extension of range of motion and muscle strengthening. Active use of the extremity may be resumed if the acute symptoms are controlled. If the impingement syndrome involves rotator cuff rupture and degenerative changes about the joint, conservative treatment often fails, and operative intervention is indicated.

16. What are the diagnostic features of rotator cuff tear?

A history of decreasing function and increased pain about the shoulder is fairly typical. Often the pain is worse at night or when the patient lies in the supine position. Degenerative tears occur over a long period of time after repetitive use. Traumatic tears usually are associated with an injury that the patient can identify as the onset of symptoms. The physical examination typically demonstrates the patient's inability to abduct the arm beyond 30–40°. If the arm is passively abducted above 90°, the patient can maintain the arm in this position. On lowering the arm, the patient loses control at about 90°, and the arm causes discomfort as it falls. Often patients learn to maneuver the arm into abduction by circumducting the shoulder. Imaging techniques that have become useful in recent years include routine shoulder arthrography, computed tomographic arthrography, and magnetic resonance imaging.

17. Describe the common mechanisms of injury in the shoulder region.

Falls onto the outstretched arm and hand commonly result in injuries at many levels, including the radial head, the supracondylar area of the humerus, the humeral shaft, and the midclavicle area. If the arm remains tucked close to the side in a position of adduction, a fracture of the proximal humerus is likely. Such a fall is typical among older people, who may slip while holding a grocery bag. Falls onto the tip of the shoulder, often accompanied by an abrasion, are the classic cause of acromioclavicular separations. This mechanism is common with forward falls from bicycles and horses. Injuries with the arm abducted are associated with shoulder joint dislocations.

18. Explain the functional classification of acromioclavicular (AC) joint injuries.

Grade I injuries are mild and may affect both the coraclavicular and AC joints. The ligaments are stretched and become painful but remain intact; no separation or deformity is present. Grade II separations involve a partial ligament injury with instability at the AC joint but without gross upward displacement of the clavicle. The coracoclavicular ligaments remain intact. Grade III separations occur secondary to disruption of the coracoclavicular ligaments, and the clavicle is displaced upward. With severe grade III separations, which often are classified as grade IV injuries, the tip of the clavicle penetrates the deltoid and trapezius muscle sling and occupies a subcutaneous position. Treatment of grades I, II, and III injuries is usually a sling followed by physical therapy for rotation and strengthening. Grades III and IV injuries may require surgical stabilization.

19. Why should an axillary radiographic view be obtained of all shoulder dislocations?

Dislocations caused by trauma to the abducted arm usually result in an anterior dislocation of the shoulder; the humeral head is anterior and usually inferior to the glenoid cavity. The incidence of posterior dislocations due to trauma is about 10%. Seizures, however, result in a much higher incidence of posterior dislocations. Care should be taken in diagnosis, because the joint often appears normal in the anteroposterior radiograph. Thus it is important to obtain an axillary view in all suspected cases of shoulder dislocation. Recurrent dislocations require much less trauma and at times occur with simple reaching activities.

20. Describe the treatment for acute and recurrent dislocations of the shoulder.

The recurrence rate for a first-time shoulder dislocation depends on the age of the patient. Patients in the second and third decades of life at the time of the initial dislocation have a recurrence rate as high as 70%; the rate decreases with age. Although the efficacy of treatment is controversial, the initial step consists of immobilization with the arm in a position of abduction and internal rotation; limited range-of-motion exercises should begin at 2–3 weeks. Abduction and external rotation of the shoulder should be limted for 6–8 weeks, and sporting and other high-risk activities should be avoided. The decision to perform surgical stabilization of the shoulder is based on the number and ease of recurrent dislocations and the inconvenience or risk caused by dislocation.

21. What are the indications for total shoulder and elbow arthroplasty?
As with the knee and hip, total joint arthroplasty in the upper extremity is indicated when the joint is destroyed to a sufficient degree that conservative measures fail to relieve pain and to provide adequate function for daily activities.

22. What are the expected results of total shoulder and elbow arthroplasties?
Total shoulder arthroplasty has shown results comparable to those of knee and hip procedures. A 90% relief of pain can be expected, along with a failure or revision rate at 10 years of 10–20%. The cause of the joint destruction makes some difference in the outcome. Patients with osteonecrosis or degenerative arthritis have better results than patients with rheumatoid arthritis. The worst results are seen in traumatic arthritis following fractures about the shoulder with scarring and interruption of the rotator cuff tendons. Total elbow arthroplasty is less reliable than arthroplasty of the shoulder, but with newer techniques it is becoming a more efficacious procedure. Its primary indication is joint destruction due to inflammatory arthritis.

BIBLIOGRAPHY

1. Crenshaw AH (ed): Campbell's Operative Orthopaedics. St. Louis, Mosby, 1992.
2. D'Ambrosia RD: Musculoskeletal Disorders: Regional Examination and Differential Diagnosis. Philadelphia, J.B. Lippincott, 1986.
3. Dawson DM: Entrapment neuropathies of the upper extremities. New Engl J Med 329:2013–2018, 1993.
4. Frymoyer JW (ed): Orthopaedic Knowledge Update 4. Rosemont, IL, American Academy of Orthopaedic Surgeons, 1993.
5. Greene WB, Heckman JD: The Clinical Measurement of Joint Motion. Rosemont, IL, American Academy of Orthopaedic Surgeons, 1994.
6. Lord JW: Critical reappraisal of diagnostic and therapeutic modalities for thoracic outlet syndromes. Surg Gynecol Obstet 168:337–340, 1989.
7. Peterson GW, Will AD: Newer electrodiagnostic techniques in peripheral nerve injuries. Orthop Clin North Am 19:13–25, 1988.

69. HAND PAIN

Richard C. Fisher, M.D.

1. What are the most common causes of atraumatic hand pain?

Referred pain from the shoulder or cervical spine	Inflammatory conditions
Overuse syndrome	Compression neuropathies
	Arthritis

2. List the common compression neuropathies involving the forearm and hand.
Median nerve compression at the wrist (carpal tunnel syndrome)
Anterior interosseous syndrome (pain in the proximal forearm associated with weakness of flexion of the index fingertip)

Pronator syndrome (median nerve compression in the region of the pronator teres muscle)
Ulnar nerve compression at Guyon's canal at the wrist joint
Radial nerve compression at the waist (Wartenberg's sydrome)

3. How is carpal tunnel syndrome diagnosed?

The classic history includes pain at night, sufficient to wake the patient from sleep. Pain may be referred to the elbow and shoulder. In addition, the patient may have pain with repetitive hand use, a feeling of clumsiness, and numbness and tingling in the median nerve distribution on the radial side of the hand. Physical findings include decreased sensation in the thumb, index and long fingers, and half of the ring finger; weakness of thumb opposition; dysesthesias with percussion of the median nerve at the wrist (Tinel's sign); and reproduction of the carpal tunnel symptoms with acute flexion of the wrist (Phalen's sign). Radiographs may show changes due to an old fracture or lesion in the bone, but these are rare causes of carpal tunnel syndrome. Electrodiagnostic studies help to confirm the diagnoses by showing prolonged conduction latency across the wrist.

4. List the general medical conditions that may be associated with carpal tunnel syndrome.

Hypothyroidism	Hemophilia
Rheumatoid arthritis	Pregnancy
Multiple myeloma and amyloidosis	Gout
Diabetes mellitus	

5. What is the best approach for treating carpal tunnel syndrome?

The primary treatment is to decrease repetitive activities and to use night splints. Nonsteroidal anti-inflammatory drugs (NSAIDs) also may be used. Injection of corticosteroids into the carpal canal is controversial but at times it may be helpful. Surgical release of the transverse carpal ligament is usually the definitive procedure.

6. What is reflex sympathetic dystrophy?

Reflex sympathetic dystrophy is characterized by pain, swelling, discoloration, and stiffness in the hand and distal forearm after trauma. However, the symptoms are out of proportion to those expected from the instigating trauma.

1. Pain may be of a cutting or searing nature, usually worsens with range of motion, and usually is felt with light touch.

2. Swelling usually is extensive in and about the hand and often spreads from the point of initiation to encompass the whole distal aspect of the extremity.

3. Discoloration often begins as redness accompanying the swelling, changes to a dusky color in secondary stages, and may become pale in the chronic stages.

4. Stiffness initially is caused by pain with attempted range of motion but as the fibrosis progresses, the joints become markedly limited in range of motion. The final stages may actually be painless despite marked limitations of function.

5. Osteoporosis is seen initially as spotty areas of demineralization and later progresses to involve the entire extremity.

7. Explain the relationship of the shoulder-hand syndrome to reflex sympathetic dystrophy.

The physical findings in both conditions are similar, but the patient with shoulder-hand syndrome usually reports a history of proximal trauma to the neck or shoulder region, chest injury, cervical spine disc disease, myocardial infarction, stomach ulcer, or Pancoast's tumor. The physical findings in shoulder-hand syndrome include involvement and stiffness of the shoulder and elbow in addition to the hand symptoms in reflex sympathetic dystrophy.

8. What do de Quervain's disease and trigger finger syndrome have in common? Outline the treatment for both.

Both hand abnormalities result from stenosing tenosynovitis. The two most commonly involved areas are the tendon sheaths of the abductor pollicis longus and extensor pollicis brevis (de Quervain's disease) and the flexor tendon sheaths in the palm (trigger finger syndrome).

de Quervain's disease is caused by a repetitive use of the hand, especially the thumb, and characterized by mild swelling over the tendon sheath at the radial styloid as well as tenderness to palpation and pain with adduction of the thumb across the palm. Treatment may consist of splinting, NSAIDs, injection of corticosteroids into the tendon sheath, or surgical release of the tendon sheath on the radial side of the wrist.

Trigger deformities involve a tendon nodule at the opening of the flexor sheath at about the level of the distal palmar crease. The nodule becomes entrapped either within or outside the tendon sheath and makes a snapping sensation accompanied by discomfort in the area of the nodule when the fingers or thumb is flexed or extended. Treatment with injection into the sheath has been beneficial, but surgical release of the sheath opening is indicated for persistent problems.

9. Patterns of arthritic involvement of the joints of the hand are somewhat characteristic of the specific diagnosis. Name the regions commonly involved with osteoarthritis and rheumatoid arthritis.
Osteoarthritis involves the distal interphalangeal joints, predominantly with production of Heberden nodes or distal osteophytes. In addition, the first metaphalangeal (MP) joint and the first carpometacarpal joint (Bennett's joint) of the thumb are common sites of degenerative change. Rheumatoid arthritis involves predominantly the proximal interphalangeal and metacarpophalangeal joints of the hand as well as the intracarpal joints at the wrist. Synovial hypertrophy is common at the wrist and digital joints, and late changes typically include swan-neck deformity and ulnar deviation at the MP joints.

10. What are the common causes of posttraumatic midwrist discomfort?
Several entities may follow minimal trauma to the wrist that may be overlooked initially but manifest at a later time. The most common is fracture of the scaphoid bone that has progressed to nonunion, often with avascular necrosis of the proximal fragments. Untreated, it leads to late degenerative changes. Various syndromes of carpal instability that follow intercarpal ligament injury may cause diastasis of the carpal bones. The most common is scapholunate separation. Kienböck's disease (avascular necrosis of the lunate) follows trauma or a congenital discrepancy between the length of the radius and the ulna. Radiographic changes include irregular density of the lunate, often with collapse or change in shape of the bone. In addition, the most common location for ganglion cysts is the dorsal aspect of the wrist, and at times the cysts become painful because of impingement with the extensor tendons. A mass is usually palpable, and its size often changes in relation to activity.

11. Describe the clinical presentation of common types of hand infections.
Infection usually follows some type of puncture injury and involves several characteristic locations. Perionychia often develops around the nailbed on the dorsal aspect of the digit. Volar infections may involve the closed space of the palmar side of the tip of the digit (felon), which becomes red, swollen, and exquisitely tender. Because of the many spaces in the hands, swelling of the palmar surface with tenderness is the first sign of a deep space infection. If the tendon sheath is involved, the finger is held in a moderately flexed position and becomes painful with attempted passive extension or active flexion. In addition, fullness and tenderness may be palpated in the distribution of the tendon sheath into the palm. Because of the lymph drainage pattern, the swelling secondary to infection eventually involves the dorsal aspect of the hand, although the primary focus of the infection is usually on the palmar surface. Prompt treatment is imperative and usually involves both antibiotics and surgical drainage.

12. Discuss the common tumors that involve the hand.
The common benign lesions include ganglion cysts, giant-cell tumors of tendon sheaths, epidural inclusion cysts, and enchondromas. The first three are soft-tissue lesions that are

easily treatable with simple excision. Enchondromas occur most commonly within the bones of the phalanges, usually are not clinically symptomatic until the bone fractures through the cyst, and most often are diagnosed by incidental radiographs. Primary malignant musculoskeletal tumors or metastatic tumors to the hand, although not unknown, are extremely rare.

BIBLIOGRAPHY

1. D'Ambrosia RD: Musculoskeletal Disorders: Regional Examination and Differential Diagnosis. Philadelphia, J.B. Lippincott, 1986.
2. Green DP: Operative Hand Surgery. New York, Churchill Livingstone, 1988.
3. Idler RS (ed): The Hand: Examination and Diagnosis. New York, Churchill Livingstone, 1990.

70. LEG PAIN

Jeffrey M. Sippel, M.D.

1. Aside from obvious trauma, what are the most common causes of acute leg pain?
Bone and joint disorders and deep venous thrombosis.

2. List the common causes of chronic leg pain.

Intermittent claudication	Muscle cramps
Peripheral neuropathy	Reflex sympathetic dystrophy
Chronic venous insufficiency	Myofascial and rheumatologic illnesses

3. What are risk factors for the development of deep venous thrombosis (DVT)?
DVT is the formation of a blood clot within the deep venous plexus of the calf or within the popliteal, deep femoral, superficial femoral, or iliac veins. Any component of Virchow's triad— endothelial damage, stasis, or hypercoagulability—increase the risk for developing DVT. Endothelial damage usually results from trauma; stasis, from immobility (as after surgery or prolonged travel); and hypercoagulability, from various protein deficiency states such as protein C or S or antithrombin III, nephrotic syndrome, chronic liver disease, or certain malignancies.

4. What historical and physical findings support the diagnosis of DVT?
Patients who suffer from DVT complain of pain and swelling in the affected limb, usually acute or subacute in duration. Pain often is associated with use of the calf muscles, and frequently warm and erythematous skin is present. However, as many as one-half of patients may be completely asymptomatic. Physical exam focuses on at least four areas:
    1. The calf is often tender to compression, and pain sometimes is elicited with forced dorsiflexion of the foot (Homans' sign).
    2. Palpation along the superficial femoral vein (medial thigh) and into the popliteal fossa may reveal a palpable venous cord or clot.
    3. The affected limb may be swollen with pitting edema; circumferential measurements (traditionally made 10 cm below and 20 cm above the tibial plateau) may objectively verify asymmetry.
    4. The skin may be warm and red in the affected leg.

5. How reliable is the physical examination in diagnosing DVT?
Even in the face of abnormal findings, the clinician's ability to diagnose DVT accurately by examination alone is poor, probably not exceeding 50%. Numerous reliable tests are available to facilitate the diagnosis.

6. Discuss the different radiologic tests available for diagnosing DVT and their sensitivity and specificity.

1. **Contrast venography** is considered the gold standard of diagnostic tests for DVT. It is capable of visualizing clots in the deep calf veins as well as in the popliteal and femoral system. Contrast venography is an invasive test and in up to 25% of cases cannot be performed or interpreted for technical reasons. Risks include contrast dye allergy, nephrotoxicity, and induction of thrombosis. For these reasons, contrast venography is generally not the first choice when DVT is considered.

2. **Impedance plethysmography** (IPG) is a noninvasive test that measures changes in blood volume of the legs by using inflationary cuffs on the thighs. It is most sensitive for detecting clots in the iliac, femoral, and popliteal veins and much less sensitive for clots below the knee. False positives may occur in states of hypotension, congestive heart failure, pregnancy, and severe obstructive pulmonary disease.

3. **Doppler ultrasonography** (US) assesses the patency of veins, looking for alterations in blood flow with direct venous compression. Like IPG, it is most useful for DVTs at or above the knee. It is highly operator-dependent but has excellent sensitivity and specificity when performed by trained personnel. False positives occur with any condition that may cause external compression of the suspected vein, such as hematomas, edema, and popliteal (Baker's) cysts. False negatives may occur with total vein occlusion. Duplex US combines the modalities of Doppler with real-time imaging and has improved sensitivity for clots in the lower leg. In certain cases it also differentiates fresh intraluminal clot from chronic thickening of veins due to old clots.

4. **Radioactive fibrinogen uptake** is not frequently used except in research. It has excellent sensitivity and specificity for DVTs of the calf but is not as accurate for above-the-knee DVTs.

Diagnostic Tests for DVTs (Compared with Contrast Venography)

TEST	SENSITIVITY (%)	SPECIFICITY (%)	LOCATION OF CLOT
IPG	94	94	thigh
Doppler US	76–100	87–100	thigh
Duplex US	92–95	96–100	thigh
Fibrinogen uptake	95	90	calf

7. What complications may arise from an untreated DVT?

Of DVTs in the calf, 10–20% propagate to the popliteal system or higher; once the DVT reaches the level of the knee, the risk of subsequent **pulmonary embolus** (PE) is about 25%. If the DVT remains below the knee, the incidence of PE is less than 2%. Therefore, in patients with contraindications to anticoagulation and DVT limited to the calf, the clot may safely be followed by serial noninvasive testing. If on repeat examinations the DVT does not progress, anticoagulation can be deferred with a low risk for PE. The recurrence rate for inadequately treated DVTs is approximately 50%, regardless of the location. The incidence of **postphlebitic syndrome** is greatly increased with inadequately treated DVTs (see question 17). Within the 10 years following DVT, 85% of patients have some clinical evidence of postphlebitic syndrome.

8. Which hospitalized patients should receive prophylaxis for DVT?

The prevalence of hospital-acquired DVT is significant (see table below). Several studies have shown that incidence of DVT, subsequent pulmonary embolus, and even overall mortality can be successfully reduced. Prophylaxis includes low-dose subcutaneous heparin, adjusted-dose heparin, low-molecular-weight heparin, intermittent pneumatic compression, Coumadin, and elastic compression stockings.

Prophylaxis for DVT

POPULATION	PREVALENCE OF DVT (%)	RISK REDUCTION (%) WITH PROPHYLASIS
Myocardial infarction	24	72 (LDH)
Ischemic stroke	47	45–80 (LDH, LMWH)
General surgery	25	20–80 (LDH, LMWH, IPC, CS)
Knee surgery 50–80	50–80	60 (IPC)
Elective hip surgery	50–75	20–80 (LMWH, ADH, Coumadin)
Hip fractures	50–75	43 (LMWH, Coumadin)

LDH = low-dose subcutaneous heparin; LMWH = low-molecular-weight heparin; ADH = adjusted-dose heparin; IPC = intermittent pneumatic compression; CS = elastic compression stocking.

9. Discuss the use of low-molecular-weight heparin (LMWH) in treating DVT.

Hull et al.[10,11] randomized 432 patients with documented DVT to receive either conventional intravenous infusion of heparin, followed by oral anticoagulation, or once daily subcutaneous LMWH, followed by oral anticoagulation. The investigators found a reduced rate of DVT recurrence (2.8% vs. 6.9%), fewer major bleeding complications (0.5% vs. 5%), and an overall lower mortality rate (4.7% vs. 9.6%) with LMWH. LMWH should be available for clinical use in the United States in the near future; it is expected to simplify and reduce the cost of care for patients with DVT.

10. What are risk factors for intermittent claudication or peripheral arterial disease (PAD)?

Intermittent claudication occurs when oxygen delivery fails to meet the oxygen requirements of a specific muscle group, usually during exertion. Inadequate delivery most commonly results from significant arteriosclerosis in the affected limb. The risks for PAD closely parallel those for coronary artery disease:

    1. **Diabetes** carries a relative risk of three; in fact, 13–30% of adult-onset diabetics have laboratory evidence of PAD.

    2. **Hypertension** is associated with a two- to threefold increase in disease and is seen in one-third of patients with PAD.

    3. **Cigarette smoking** increases the risk of disease by two- to sevenfold.

    4. **Hypertriglyceridemia** or **low levels of high-density lipoprotein** (HDL) carry a relative risk of two. The prevalence of PAD is approximately 20% in the general population over 70 years of age; PAD reduces life expectancy by 10 years.

11. Describe the typical complaints of patients with intermittent claudication.

Intermittent claudication typically causes a cramping or aching pain in the calf, thigh, or buttock, reproducibly triggered by mild to moderate walking. Calf pain is the most common. The pain persists throughout walking, often causing the person to reduce or stop activity. Symptoms typically resolve within 10 minutes of rest. Disease of the iliac arteries is generally manifested as thigh, buttock, and calf pain; impotence also may be present. Isolated calf or foot claudication reflects disease of the femoral, popliteal, or tibial arteries. Symptoms are often severe enough to affect normal daily activities and force a change in lifestyle.

12. Explain the significance of ischemic rest pain.

Ischemic rest pain is caused by tissue hypoxia when the patient is in a resting state; that is, exercise and increased oxygen demand are not necessary to cause hypoxia and subsequent painful ischemia. With sudden arterial occlusion, as in embolic disease, the pain is acute and severe. In most patients, however, ischemic rest pain results from progressive arteriosclerosis; pain may be subacute in onset, with numbness, paresthesias, and muscle weakness. The presence of ischemic rest pain indicates that a significant number of vessels have become occluded and that collateral flow is inadequate to meet the basal metabolic demands. Patients with this marker of more severe disease are at greater risk to develop complications of PAD, including infection, focal necrosis, and amputation.

13. What physical findings are present with intermittent claudication?
The initial examination focuses on at least three components:

1. Begin by palpating the arterial pulses of the leg, including femoral, popliteal, dorsalis pedis, and posterior tibial arteries. Check for asymmetry in pulse amplitude and duration. Pulses in legs affected by PAD often are diminished or absent. If pulses are not palpable, a hand-held Doppler device may be used to auscult the arterial pulse. This technique is also used for calculating ankle-brachial indices (see question 14).

2. Check for asymmetry in leg size that may be due to muscle atrophy in the affected leg. If the patient has bilateral disease, however, this finding may be absent.

3. Cutaneous changes are numerous and include thinning of skin, loss of hair on the digits, and predisposition to developing ulcers. Elevation of the foot produces dependent rubor and blanching. After the leg is lowered, venous filling in the foot may be delayed by 15 or more seconds (delayed capillary refill).

14. What tests help to establish a diagnosis of PAD?
The most commonly used noninvasive screening test is comparison of the ankle systolic pressure with the arm systolic pressure, referred to as the ankle-brachial index (ABI). Doppler ultrasound is used to detect the ankle pressure, over either the posterior tibial or dorsalis pedis arteries. In a normal person, the ratio is near 1.0 and does not decrease after exertion. A resting ratio < 0.94 or a postexertion ratio < 0.73 is suggestive of PAD in the appropriate clinical setting. If available, segmental limb pressures may be used to help in defining a level of blockage; pulse volume recording is helpful in defining sites at which focal calcifications may be present. Lower extremity angiography also may be used in the diagnosis of PAD, but it is not a screening test and generally is not performed unless surgical intervention is considered.

15. Discuss surgical vs. medical management of PAD.
Surgical measures for the treatment of intermittent claudication include percutaneous transluminal angioplasty (PTA) and surgical bypass. The goal of both therapies is to improve symptoms and function and possibly to slow progression of disease, thereby reducing the need for limb amputation. Both modalities have been shown in trials to improve symptoms, walking ability, and hemodynamics. Direct comparisons have shown the two modalities have similar rates of success, complication, and disease progression at 3-year follow-up. However, a population-based study by Tunis et al.[17] showed that the large increase in the number of PTA and bypass procedures over a 10-year period did not decrease the rate of limb amputation, indicating that such invasive procedures may not be effective in limb salvage.

Medical management traditionally includes risk modification, and scheduled walking programs. Smoking cessation has been shown in some studies to improve maximal walking times and to reduce disease progression; although this finding may be inconsistent, smoking cessation is generally recommended. Lipid-modifying regimens have been shown to reduce progression of disease by 66%. Hiatt et al.[8] showed that a supervised progressive treadmill walking program over a 12-week period was associated with improved peak walking time (123%), pain-free walking time (165%), and peak oxygen consumption (30%). In contrast, the control group increased peak walking time by 20%, but other parameters showed no improvement. Other investigators have shown similar benefits from increased walking distance with daily exercise programs. At least one study[3] directly compared PTA and exercise. The 20 patients who underwent PTA showed a significant improvement in ABIs at 9-month follow-up but no increase in walking distances, whereas 16 patients enrolled in an exercise program showed significant increases in walking distances at 18 months without concomitant increases in ABIs.

16. Are any drugs available to treat claudication?

Several drugs have been studied with limited success. In some clinical trials pentoxifylline has been shown to increase pain-free and maximal walking distances by 66%. Other studies show favorable results only in patients with ABIs less than 0.8, and with symptoms for over 1 year. Pentoxifylline is the only agent approved for clinical use in the United States.

17. What causes chronic venous insufficiency? What physical findings are characteristic of this condition?

Chronic venous insufficiency of the legs is characterized by dependent edema and venous engorgement and frequently associated with local pain. Valvular incompetence within the thigh and/or deep venous system of the calf causes venous hypertension, which is responsible for the subsequent skin changes and swelling. Superficial varicosities also may develop, either from valvular incompetence or from inability of the thin wall to support high venous pressure. Skin changes include subcutaneous fibrosis, brawny edema, hyperpigmentation (typically on the medial and lateral aspects of the ankle), and predisposition to developing ulcers. Chronic venous insufficiency caused by DVTs is referred to as the postphlebitic syndrome. In many cases, however, other risk factors are implicated, such as obesity, advanced age, pregnancy, or occupational hazards (e.g., heavy lifting and prolonged standing). Diagnostic tests include ambulatory venous pressure monitors, Doppler venous surveys, and contrast venography.

18. How and why is chronic venous insufficiency treated?

Therapy includes leg elevation to a level above the heart and knee-high compression stockings, both directed at improving venous drainage. In fitting stockings it is important to ensure that a torniquet effect is not created at the knee by an improperly fitted stocking. In addition, the patient should avoid prolonged periods of standing and elevate the legs several times a day. Because patients are prone to develop skin complications such as ulcers, stasis dermatitis, and bacterial or fungal suprainfections, local skin hygeine is important. Specific therapy for treatment of skin conditions may be found in chapter 99. When conservative treatment of secondary varicosities fails, surgery should be considered, including ligation and removal of the incompetent valves and varicosities. Sclerotherapy is sometimes used as an adjunct to surgery.

19. Which peripheral neuropathies can cause leg pain?

The most common type of painful neuropathy encountered by the primary care provider is diabetic neuropathy, which typically is a symmetric distal sensory neuropathy but may have mixed sensory and motor findings. Burning pain, numbness, and paresthesias are common in the stocking-glove distribution. Other conditions that may cause painful neuropathy are listed below:

Medical illnesses	Toxins
Chronic liver disease	Cis-platinum
Hypothyroidism	Vincristine
Paraproteinemias	Isoniazid
Multiple myeloma	Lead
Waldenstrom's macroglobulinemia	Nitrofurantoin
Cryoglobulinemia	Pesticides
Uremia	Phenytoin
Vitamin B12 deficiency	

20. What physical findings are present in patients with diabetic neuropathy?

Decreases in vibratory sensation and pinprick vs. light touch as well as impaired two-point discrimination may be demonstrated in patients with diabetic neuropathy. Such sensory findings occur most commonly in a stocking-glove distribution and do not follow dermatomes. Autonomic neuropathy may manifest as orthostatic hypotension or abnormal heart rate/blood pressure responses to maneuvers such as Valsalva, deep inspiration, squatting, or sustained handgrip.

21. Describe muscle cramps.
A true muscle cramp is a palpable and visible muscle contraction caused by a hyperactive motor neuron unit with increased frequency of muscle action potentials. Cramps may occur in a muscle group that is already contracted and commonly involve the gastrocsoleus and plantar foot muscles. They often occur at night and are recurrent. Cramps may be triggered by voluntary isometric contractions of susceptible muscles. Isolated fasciculations are seen in 70% of patients. The prognosis of muscle cramps is good, given an otherwise normal neuromuscular examination. Therapy includes stretching, and trials have shown the efficacy of quinine, methocarbamol, and chloroquine.

22. Can cramps be associated with systemic illnesses?
Yes. Hypoglycemia and hyponatremia may cause true cramps. Thyroid disease may cause cramps, contractures, and myotonia, whereas hypocalcemia, hypomagnesemia, and hyper- or hypokalemia may cause tetany. Drugs such as beta agonists, calcium channel blockers, and ethanol also may be implicated.

23. What are heat cramps?
Heat cramps follow strenuous or repetitive muscle activity, often in supranormal heat with concomitant fluid loss (sweat) and hypotonic fluid replacement. Salt depletion with volume depletion rather than hyponatremia per se is believed to be the cause. Treatment is directed at replacement of salt and fluid.

24. What is relex sympathetic dystrophy (RSD)?
RSD is an uncommon pain syndrome of an extremity and almost always follows local trauma. In the leg, many types of blunt trauma may cause RSD, especially when nerves are crushed or stretched. Patellofemoral joint injury, including operative intervention, is also a common precipitating event.

25. Describe the historical and physical findings in patients with RSD.
The constellation of symptoms and signs includes burning pain, hyperesthesias, tenderness to palpation of the extremity, autonomic changes, and muscular atrophy. If untreated, the disease progresses through three stages. Stage I is characterized by the gradual onset of pain and burning with allodynia (pain caused by nonnoxious stimuli). The extremity initially is warm and dry, and patients guard against unnecessary movements. In stage II (2–3 months), the skin becomes cold and clammy; accompanying cutaneous changes include loss of hair and thinning of the skin. Osteopenia develops at a higher rate than expected from limb disuse. Stage III includes limb contracture and severely limited range of motion, due to disuse.

26. How is RSD treated?
Therapy centers on early diagnosis with physical therapy directed at improving and maintaining range of motion. Narcotic analgesics are not uniformly helpful, and their use may be complicated by side effects and addiction potential. Although nonsteroidal anti-inflammatory drugs are rarely helpful, a trial may be warranted, given the low risk.

BIBLIOGRAPHY

1. Clagett GP, et al: Prevention of venous thromboembolism. Chest 102:391S–407S, 1992.
2. Coffman JD: Intermittent claudication—be conservative. N Engl J Med 325:577–578, 1991.
3. Creasy TS, et al: Is percutaneous transluminal angioplasty better than exercise for claudication? Preliminary results from a prospective randomised trial. Eur J Vasc Surg 4(2):135–140, 1990.
4. D'Amico A: Imaging for deep venous thrombosis. Emerg Med Clin North Am 10:121–132, 1992.
5. DeFelice M, Gallo P, Masotti G: Current therapy of peripheral obstructive arterial disease: The nonsurgical approach. Angiology 41:1–11, 1990.
6. Goldberg RJ, et al: Occult malignant neoplasm in patients with deep venous thrombosis. Arch Intern Med 147:251–253, 1987.

7. Heijboer H, et al: A comparison of real-time compression ultrasonography with impedance plethysmography for the diagnosis of deep-vein thrombosis in symptomatic outpatients. New Engl J Med 329:1365–1369, 1993.
8. Hiatt WR, et al: Benefit of exercise conditioning for patients with peripheral arterial disease. Circulation 81:602–609, 1990.
9. Hiatt WR, et al: Diagnostic methods for peripheral arterial disease in the San Luis Valley Diabetes Study. J Clin Epidemiol 43:597–606, 1990.
10. Hull RD, et al: A comparison of subcutaneous low-molecular-weight heparin with warfarin sodium for prophylaxis against deep-vein thrombosis after hip or knee implantation. N Engl J Med 329:1370–1376, 1993.
11. Hull RD, et al: Subcutaneous low-molecular-weight heparin compared with continuous intravenous heparin in the treatment of proximal-vein thrombosis. N Engl J Med 326:975–982, 1992.
12. Lindgarde F, et al: Conservative drug treatment in patients with moderately severe chronic occlusive peripheral arterial disease. Scandinavian Study Group. Circulation 80:1549–1556, 1989.
13. McGee SR: Muscle cramps. Arch Intern Med 150:511–518, 1990.
14. Radlack K, Wyderski RJ: Conservative management of intermittent claudication. Ann Intern Med 113:135–146, 1990.
15. Regensteiner JG, et al: Functional benefits of peripheral vascular bypass surgery for patients with intermittent claudication. Angiology 44:1–10, 1993.
16. Sinatra RS, et al (eds): Acute Pain: Mechanisms and Management. St. Louis, Mosby, 1992, pp 440–442.
17. Tunis SR, Bass EP, Steinberg EP: The use of angioplasty, bypass surgery, and amputation in the management of peripheral vascular disease. N Engl J Med 325:556–562, 1991.

71. FOOT CARE IN PATIENTS WITH DIABETES OR PERIPHERAL VASCULAR DISEASE

Stephen F. Albert, D.P.M.

1. What are the three most common foot problems in the United States?

Based on the 1990 National Health Interview Survey,[7] ingrown nails and other toenail problems, foot infections, and corns or calluses were the three most common foot problems. Each of these problems troubled over 11 million civilian noninstitutionalized Americans.

Incidence of Foot Problems in the United States, 1990

PROBLEM	NUMBER IN MILLIONS
Ingrown nails or other toenail problem	11.3
Foot infection, including tinea and warts	11.3
Corns and calluses	11.2
Foot injury	5.6
Flat feet	4.6
Bunions	4.4
Arthritis of toes	3.9
Toes and joint problems	2.5
Bone spurs	0.95
Nerve damage to foot	0.23
Clubfoot	0.16
Others	2.7

2. What are the chances of success when one treats an ingrown nail by avulsion only?

At 1-year follow-up the success rate is poor. Ingrown toenails most commonly affect the great toes, but any digit may be involved. Although the condition may occur in either sex or at any age, it is seen most frequently in boys and young men. A prospective British study randomized 163 patients with ingrown nails into three groups: total nail avulsion, nail edge excision, and nail edge excision with chemical cautery (phenolization) of the germinal nail matrix. The recurrence rates at 1 year were 73%, 73%, and 9%, respectively.[10]

Phenolization of the germinal nail matrix can be performed by primary care practitioners, but the technique requires attention to procedural details. Under application of phenol may result in a greater than expected rate of recurrence, whereas overapplication may result in a persistently draining periungual wound that is prone to infection.

3. Why is foot care important to patients with diabetes mellitus?
Twenty-five percent of patients with diabetes develop related foot problems. Foot ulcers and amputation rank high among the many disabling complications of diabetes. Multiple foot problems may quickly progress to a critical point; without immediate and definitive measures, amputation may soon follow. Of all nontraumatic amputations, 50–70% occur in patients with diabetes. Although the precise location and number of amputations are unknown, it is estimated that 56,000 per year involve the foot and leg.[3]

4. Which factors contribute to amputations in diabetics?
Infection and gangrene are common causes for diabetic amputations. Contributing causes include minor trauma, cutaneous ulceration, and failure of wound healing. All of these factors are exacerbated by the nearly universal occurrence in diabetics of peripheral neuropathy (motor, sensory, and autonomic), peripheral arterial disease, and mechanical dysfunction in the lower extremities.

5. What is the most frequent cause of hospitalization of diabetic patients?
Serious foot or lower extremity problems[4] (1 of 5 admissions of diabetics to hospitals in the United Kingdom[22]).

6. Plantar calluses and plantar warts are often confused. How does the clinician differentiate the two?
Warts (verruca plantaris) result from viral infection, whereas a plantar callus (also called tyloma or plantar keratoma) is a dermal response to the vertical and shear forces of standing and walking on a foot with mechanical dysfunction, osseous plantar prominences, or a thinned plantar fat pad. Both are painful, visible skin lesions that are exacerbated by weightbearing.

Warts may be solitary with a clearly circumscribed border or mosaic with a patchy and irregular border. They have a rough surface with hypertrophic papillae and are tender with side-to-side squeezing. Individual papillae may become darkly colored from capillary hemorrhage secondary to standing and walking. Plantar warts are surrounded and covered by keratotic tissue. They may or may not be associated with an osseous plantar prominence. After paring, a "cauliflower" center is visible, the patient experiences pain, and pinpoint capillary hemorrhages readily appear.

Initial management of discrete plantar warts most commonly involves patient application of 40% salicylic acid plasters every 2–3 days after removal of overlying hyperkeratosis. Removal of macerated hyperkeratosis is best accomplished if the patient soaks the foot for 5 minutes in water and then uses an emory board or pumice stone only on the treated area, avoiding surrounding skin. Salicylic acid paint (10%) with lactic acid (10%) in flexible collodion, may be used for mosaic warts or warts that coalesce over larger areas. The paint is commonly applied once daily and again is most effective if the macerated hyperkeratotic tissue is removed.

Plantar callus presents as a hyperkeratotic mass at a site of friction or pressure. The lesion consists of raised, often clear, compressed layers of stratum corneum without a definite border. The more severe lesions may be pared below the level of the surrounding skin without pain or pinpoint capillary hemorrhage. Calluses are commonly managed by periodic paring of the hyperkeratosis and use of cushioning innersoles or foot orthoses to alleviate mechanical dysfunction and to accommodate osseous plantar prominences and thinned plantar fat pads.

7. What advice about foot care should be given to vascularly impaired or diabetic patients?
1. Wash and inspect the feet daily.
2. Use foot creams or lubricating oils, except in toe webs.
3. Cut toenails straight; do not bevel the sides.
4. Do not attempt to cut corns or calluses.
5. Avoid self-medication and extreme temperatures.
6. Do not walk barefooted.
7. Wear appropriate shoes and inspect the insides daily.
8. Seek early medical care for all skin lesions.
9. Do not delay medical care for abrupt foot swelling.

8. What guidelines assist a patient in attaining properly fitting shoes?
Properly fitted shoes are necessary to avoid aggravating or precipitating foot problems. A recent study of 356 women aged 20–60 years found that 88% wore improperly fitting shoes.[7]

Proper fit implies correct shape and size. The shape of the foot and shoe should match. Both feet should be measured. Size should be assessed while the patient stands in both shoes; there should be approximately 1 cm between the tip of the longest toe and the distal aspect of the shoe, the metatarsal heads should be in the widest part of the shoe (particularly the first metatarsal), and the heel should have a snug fit. In feet with high insteps (pes cavus) laces are preferred. For feet subject to edema, shoes should be purchased later in the day. It is important to be aware that shoe size tends to increase with age.

9. What medical diseases are commonly associated with foot deformity?
Rheumatoid arthritis and gout.

10. How often does rheumatoid arthritis affect the feet?
Rheumatoid arthritis involves the feet in over 50% of patients.[18] Patients commonly present with hallux valgus, hallux varus, hallux rigidus, hammertoes, fibular deviation at the metatarsophalangeal joints, and/or rheumatoid nodules. The distribution is symmetric, particularly at the distal metatarsals, with warmth, tenderness, and edema. The metatarsal heads often become plantarly prominent as the nonfunctional joints develop mechanical adaptations, including dislocation of the digits and displacement of the plantar fat pad. Radiographs show demineralization at the ends of the metatarsals, with joint space narrowing, articular erosions, soft-tissue edema, joint malalignment, and eventually subluxation. Women are affected more commonly than men.

11. Describe the acute and chronic presentations of hyperuricemia or gout.
The **acute presentation**, most commonly seen in men, is characterized by sudden onset of escalating pain that progresses to excruciating levels, accompanied by an edematous and inflamed first metatarsophalangeal joint. The patient is often apprehensive and quite uncomfortable. The condition is aggravated by weightbearing but may be less painful in the elderly and in patients with peripheral neuropathy. It also may occur at other sites. Often it is mistaken for a bacterial infection or septic joint.

The **chronic presentation** is characterized by deposition of monosodium urate crystals in tissues and joints. The crystals induce gouty arthritis characterized by cartilage destruction, bony erosions, radiolucent pockets with sclerotic overhanging bony margins, and "punched out" lytic lesions. In advanced stages, pathologic fractures, bony ankylosis, and draining sinuses from mechanically irritated and enlarging tophi may be found.

12. What condition should be suspected in a normal-appearing foot with lateral forefoot pain, a point of maximal tenderness at the third intermetatarsal space, normal radiographs, and negative laboratory tests?
Intermetatarsal neuroma, also known as Morton's neuroma, is often a diagnostic challenge. Foot radiographs, ultrasound, nerve conduction velocity, magnetic resonance imaging, clinical

laboratory tests, and visual appearance of the foot usually reveal nothing out of the ordinary. The diagnosis is made through history and examination of the foot. The patient commonly indicates a sharp lancinating, radiating pain in the lateral forefoot that is relieved by removal of the shoe and massage. Palpation or squeezing of the affected intermetatarsal interspace and numbness or burning in the associated toes are common features.

A neuroma of the foot is an irritative process of the common digital nerve that supplies the plantar aspect of adjacent toes. The term "neuroma" is a misnomer because the entity does not demonstrate neoplastic growth of nerve tissue or fibers; instead, histopathology reveals degenerative changes with perineural fibrosis. Repetitive trauma and/or constriction are the presumed underlying causes. Intermetatarsal neuroma occurs in all adult age groups and affects women 9 times more frequently than men. The third intermetatarsal interspace is most often involved. Neurectomy of the affected area is the treatment of choice; the rate of patient satisfaction is reported to be 93%.[12]

13. Why should cigarette smokers be counseled to stop smoking before undergoing amputation?
In a 1991 study of 88 nonsmokers and 77 smokers undergoing amputation,[14] smokers had a 2–5 times higher risk for infection and re-amputation. Thus, amputees should avoid smoking at least 1 week before surgery and during wound healing.

14. What patients should be referred to podiatrists routinely and acutely?
With the exception of congenital foot deformities and severe acute trauma presenting to emergency departments, most podiatrists treat the foot problems listed in question 1. Podiatrists excel in treating the chronic recurring foot problems that tend to increase as people age, particularly when periodic care is required, when prior interventions by the primary care provider have not been successful, or when the diagnosis is unclear. Of the acute presenting foot conditions, by far the most potentially devastating are infections in a diabetic, immuno-compromised, or vascularly compromised patient.

The primary care provider should be aware that podiatrists' educational credentials, interests, and expertise vary. In general, podiatrists that are hospital-affiliated, residency-trained, and board-certified are better prepared to deal adeptly with acute conditions.

15. What is the role of homologous platelet-derived wound-healing factors (PDWHFs) in the treatment of recalcitrant dermal ulcers of the lower extremity?
Several investigators[2,6,20] have reported improved healing of recalcitrant foot and leg dermal ulcers and higher rates of salvaging presumably lost limbs with the use of PDWHFs. Their report included 315 diabetic wounds that had not healed after an average of 32 weeks of treatment. Use of PDWHFs achieved the following outcomes: 88% of 127 wounds healed in an average of 9.5 weeks; 85% of 103 wounds healed in an average of 10.3 weeks; and 88% of 85 wounds healed in an average of 13.3 weeks. They also have reported a 90% salvage rate for diabetic limbs considered for below-the-knee or transmetatarsal amputation.

Krupski,[13] among others, has questioned the conclusion that the outcomes are a direct result of PDWHF. His findings in 18 patients with 26 lower extremity wounds refractory to conventional treatments contradicted prior studies. He found the rate of healing to be no better in PDWHF-treated wounds than in placebo-treated wounds and concluded that PDWHF treatments provided no additional benefit over traditional therapies. Several explanations were offered to explain the divergent results, including investigator/institutional bias (4 of 5 early studies were performed at the same facilities by the same team), failure to design most of the trials with placebos, failure to determine the mitogenic activity of each batch of PDWHF, confounding variables such as use of topical antibiotics, and differing patient populations.

16. What is the likelihood that osteomyelitis underlies a diabetic foot ulcer when the ulcer does not appear inflamed?
Newman et al.[16] at the 1993 Annual Meeting of the American Diabetes Association reported that approximately two-thirds of 12 patients had clinically unsuspected osteomyelitis. Leukocyte

scans appear to be more sensitive than bone scans and radiographs. Schauwecker[21] concurred, reporting a sensitivity of 88% and a specificity of 85% for osteomyelitis.

Many practitioners believe that the radionuclide spatial resolution among the numerous bones and joints of the foot is inadequate and that none of the imaging modalities are entirely specific for osteomyelititis. In addition, [111]indium scanning is time-consuming and costly and requires considerable experience, including knowledge of factors leading to both false-negative and false-positive results:

Scanning for Osteomyelitis with [111]Indium-labeled Leukocytes

Reported reasons for false-positive results
Noninfected acute closed fractures
Diabetic neurotrophic osteopathy
Noninfected prostheses
Rheumatoid arthritis
Stress fractures
Synovitis
Neuromas
Tumors

Reported reasons for false-negative results
Avascular bone marrow
Poor blood supply
Tissue necrosis

No matter what imaging modality is used, it is quite difficult to differentiate foot osteomyelitis in diabetics from diabetic osteopathy or osteoarthropathy (Charcot foot).

BIBLIOGRAPHY

1. American College of Foot Surgeons: Ingrown Toenail—Preferred Practice Guidelines. Park Ridge, IL, American College of Foot Surgeons, 1991, p 3.
2. Atri SC, Misra J, Bisht D, et al: Use of homologous platelet factors in achieving total healing of recalcitrant skin ulcers. Surgery 108:508, 1990.
3. Bild DE, Selby JV, Sinnock P, et al: Lower extremity amputation in people with diabetes: Epidemiology and prevention. Diabetes Care 12:24–31, 1989.
4. Boulton AJM: The diabetic foot. Med Clin North Am 72:1513–1530, 1988.
5. Cicchinelli LD, Corey SV: Imaging of the infected foot: Fact or fancy? J Am Podiatr Med Assoc 83:10, 1993.
6. Dosick SM, Hobson RW, Krosnick A: Mangement of ulcers on the ischemic limb. In Treatment of Chronic Wounds 2. City Curative Technologies, 1991.
7. Frey C, Thompson F, Smith, et al: American Orthopedic Foot and Ankle Society Women's Shoe Survey. Foot Ankle 14:2, 1993.
8. Fylling P, Knighton DR: Amputation in the diabetic population: Incidence, causes, cost treatment and prevention. J Enterostom Ther 16:247–255, 1989.
9. Greenberg L, Davis H: Foot problems in the US: The 1990 National Health Interview Survey. J Am Podiatr Med Assoc 83:8, 1993.
10. Grieg JD, Anderson JH, Ireland AJ, Anderson JR: The surgical treatment of ingrowing toenails. J Bone Joint Surg 73B:1, 1991.
11. Janisse DJ: The art and science of fitting shoes. Foot Ankle 13:5, 1992.
12. Keh RA, et al: Long-term follow-up of Morton's neuroma. J Foot Surg 31:1, 1992.
13. Krupski WC: Growth factors and wound healing. Semin Vasc Surg 5:249, 1992.
14. Lind J, Kramhoft M, Bodtker S: The influence of smoking on complications after primary amputations of the lower extremity. Clin Orthop 267:211, 1991.
15. Macauley KE, Sartoris DJ, Resnick D: Diseases of the foot: Test of radiographic interpretation. J Foot Surg 30:4, 1991.
16. Newman LG, Waller J, Palestro CJ, et al: Leukocyte scanning with ^{111}In is superior to magnetic resonance imaging in diagnosis of clinically unsuspected osteomyelitis in diabetic foot ulcers. Diabetes Care 15:11, 1992.

BIBLIOGRAPHY

17. Oyen WJ, Netten PM, Lemmens JA, et al: Evaluation of infectious diabetic foot complications with indium-111–labeled human nonspecific immunoglobulin G. J Nucl Med 33:7, 1992.
18. Patton JP, Murdoch DP, Lindsey J, Young G: Rheumatoid arthritic foot. J Am Podiatr Med Assoc 83:5, 1993.
19. Pecoraro RE, Reiber GE, Burgess EM: Pathways to diabetic limb amputation. Basis for prevention. Diabetes Care 13:5, 1990.
20. Poucher RL, Leahy JD, Howells G: Active healing of diabetic wounds utilizing growth factor therapy. Wounds 3:xx, 1991.
21. Schauwecker DS: The scintigraphic diagnosis of osteomyelitis. Am J Roentgenol 158:9, 1992.
22. Sussman KE, Reiber G, Albert SF: The diabetic foot problem—a failed system of health care? Diabetes Res Clin Pract 17:1–8, 1992.
23. Yale JF (ed): Yales's Podiatric Medicine, 3rd ed. Baltimore, Williams & Wilkins, 1987.

72. FIBROMYALGIA AND RELATED SYNDROMES

Danny C. Williams, M.D.

1. Define soft-tissue rheumatism.

The term "soft-tissue rheumatism" (i.e., nonarticular rheumatism) defines a heterogeneous group of common ailments involving musculoskeletal structures other than the bones and joints. Soft-tissue disorders are categorized according to their distribution: focal (e.g., bursitis, tendinitis), regional (e.g., myofascial pain syndromes), or generalized (e.g., fibromyalgia).

2. What is fibromyalgia?

Fibromyalgia is a chronic, generalized muscle pain syndrome of unknown etiology. Fibromyalgia is characterized subjectively by multiple, diverse somatic symptoms and objectively by the physical presence of widespread muscle tenderness.

3. Who develops fibromyalgia?

Although predominantly a disorder of young women (aged 20–45 years), fibromyalgia may occur in anyone, including children (usually adolescents) and the elderly.

4. In what settings may fibromyalgia be seen?

Fibromyalgia may develop at any time, either spontaneously or in relation to a stressful life event, such as severe, flulike illness, whiplash injury, or divorce. Fibromyalgia also may occur as a secondary disorder in patients with preexisting chronic illnesses, such as rheumatoid arthritis, alcoholism, and acquired immunodeficiency syndrome (AIDS).

5. Describe the clinical features of fibromyalgia.

The cardinal features of fibromyalgia are diffuse subjective pain and physically demonstrable areas of muscle tenderness (i.e., tender points). Despite extensive muscle pain, there is no objective muscle weakness. Protracted fatigue coupled with a nonrestorative sleep pattern is also a major manifestation. Other somatic symptoms may include headaches (tension or migraine), arthralgias with subjective swelling, atypical chest pain, diffuse stiffness, irritable bowel syndrome, paresthesias, and depression. Raynaud's phenomenon and mitral valve prolapse are also common. Fibromyalgic symptoms may be exacerbated by various factors, including physical and mental stress, weather changes, inactivity, exercise, and poor quality of sleep.

6. What are tender points?

Aside from an abnormal stage 4 sleep pattern, tender points are the only objective clinical finding in patients with fibromyalgia. Tender points are discrete areas (2–3 cm in diameter) of normal-appearing skin at which application of pressure elicits focal pain. Adequate pressure is the pressure required to blanche the thumbnail. Palpation of a tender point frequently causes a sudden withdrawal response—the "jump sign." Control points (e.g., forehead, anterior thigh, and thumbnail) are used to differentiate fibromyalgia from functional disorders.

7. How does myofascial pain differ from fibromyalgia?

Myofascial pain differs from the diffuse pain of fibromyalgia by being localized to a specific region, usually a single muscle or closely related muscle group.

Trigger points, which are typical of myofascial pain syndromes, consist of palpable abnormalities (taut band or thickened nodule) usually found in the bellies of traumatized muscles. Palpation of a trigger point produces local tenderness and generates referred pain throughout the involved muscle and/or muscle group.

8. How is fibromyalgia diagnosed?

Fibromyalgia is a diagnosis of exclusion, particularly in elderly patients. The American College of Rheumatology developed the following classification criteria in 1990:
1. Generalized pain > 3 months affecting all four body quadrants and the axial skeleton
2. Palpable, subjective pain in 11 of the following 9 pairs of tender points:

Occipital	Lateral epicondyle (2 cm distally)
Lower cervical (posterolateral C5–C7)	Gluteal (upper, lateral quadrant)
Midtrapezius (upper fold)	Greater trochanter (2 cm posteriorly)
Suprasupraspinatus (origin)	Knee (medial fat pad)
Second rib (costochondral junction)	

A patient is classified as having fibromyalgia if both criteria are present.

From Wolfe F, Smythe HA, Yunus MB, et al: The American College of Rheumatology 1990 criteria for the classification of fibromyalgia: Report of the multicenter criteria committee. Arthritis Rheum 33:160, 1990.

9. Is fibromyalgia a systemic disease?

Many systemic illnesses may present with the clinical features of fibromyalgia. However, fibromyalgia per se is not a systemic disorder, either by physical or laboratory findings. Therefore, evidence of inflammation or other systemic disease suggests diagnoses other than fibromyalgia. The following disorders may manifest features consistent with fibromyalgia:

Rheumatoid arthritis (early)	Chronic fatigue syndromes
Spondyloarthropathy (early)	Paraneoplastic disorders
Systemic lupus erythematosus	Hyper- or hypothyroidism
Polymyositis	Hyper- or hypoparathyroidism
Polymyalgia rheumatica	Viral infections
Giant cell arteritis	Metastatic cancer
Generalized osteoarthritis	Somatiform disorders or depression

Fibromyalgia may occur secondarily to any of the above disorders.

10. What laboratory screening tests are useful in establishing fibromyalgia as a diagnosis of exclusion?

Complete blood count and differential	Rheumatoid factor
Erythrocyte sedimentation rate and/or C-reactive protein	Radiographs (may be required to convince the patient that the pain is not of articular origin)
Creatine phosphokinase	Bone scan (may be required to convince the physician that there is no synovitis)
Serum calcium	
Thyroid-stimulating hormone	
Antinuclear antibody	

11. Describe the nonpharmacologic management of patients with fibromyalgia.

Reassurance is a major therapeutic tool for patients with fibromyalgia. Many patients suspect that their symptoms are the result of occult malignancy, crippling arthritis, or an aberrant psyche. Simply providing a diagnosis may be therapeutic. Local measures such as heat packs, gentle massage, gentle stretching exercises, and avoidance of cold may provide temporary relief. The best therapeutic intervention at present is the adoption of a graduated (progressing over 4–6 months) aerobic exercise program. Aquatic aerobics or stationary bicycle riding seem to be most effective. Older patients may warrant an initial treadmill test to determine exercise tolerance.

12. Is pharmacologic management of patients with fibromyalgia effective?

Simple analgesics and muscle relaxants usually provide little relief from the symptoms of fibromyalgia. Narcotics and benzodiazepine derivatives may exacerbate symptoms and are not recommended for patients exhibiting the potential for chronic pain syndrome. Systemic steroids have no role in the treatment of fibromyalgia. A trial of nonsteroidal anti-inflammatory drugs is warranted in most patients with fibromyalgia, but the response is variable. Improvement in the duration of morning stiffness is typical.

Pharmacologic therapy for fibromyalgia is directed primarily at improving the quality of restorative sleep with low doses of cyclobenzaprine (10–30 mg) or amitriptyline (12.5–50 mg) 2 or 3 hours before bedtime. Tender point injection with local anesthetics and/or corticosteroids is effective in select patients. The difficulty lies in knowing which tender points to inject.

BIBLIOGRAPHY

1. Bennet RM: Fibromyalgia and the facts: Sense or nonsense. Rheum Dis Clin North Am 19:45, 1993.
2. Campbell SM: Regional myofascial pain syndromes. Rheum Dis Clin North Am 15:31, 1989.
3. Kelley WN, Harris ED, Ruddy S, et al (eds): Textbook of Rheumatology, 4th ed. Philadelphia, W.B. Saunders, 1993.
4. McCarty DJ (ed): Arthritis and Allied Conditions, 12th ed. Philadelphia, Lea & Febiger, 1993.
5. Moldofsky H: Sleep and fibrositis syndrome. Rheum Dis Clin North Am 15:91, 1989.
6. Simons DG: Fibrositis/fibromyalgia: A form of myofascial trigger points? Am J Med 81(Suppl 3A):93, 1986.
7. Wolfe F, Smythe HA, Yunus MB, et al: The American College of Rheumatology 1990 criteria for the classification of fibromyalgia: Report of the multicenter criteria committee. Arthritis Rheum 33:160, 1990.
8. Yunus MB, Holt GS, Masi AT, et al: Fibromyalgia syndrome among the elderly: Comparison with younger patients. J Am Geriatr Soc 36:987, 1988.
9. Yunus MB, Masi AT: Juvenile primary fibromyalgia syndrome. Arthritis Rheum 28:138, 1985.

XI. Common Disorders of the Nervous System

73. DEMENTIA

Lawrence A. Meredith, M.D.

1. Define dementia.

Dementia is the persistent loss of previously acquired cognitive skills in 3 of the 5 following categories: memory, language, spatial concepts, personality, and executive function (ability to perform tasks). In general, memory is affected first and foremost by dementing processes. However, as dementia progresses, other brain systems may be affected.

2. How does dementia differ from delirium?

It is important to differentiate dementia from the acute confusional state of delirium. Acute confusional states are characterized primarily by disordered attention. When attention mechanisms are impaired, detailed testing of mental status is difficult and often fruitless. For example, testing of memory is impossible with a patient who cannot attend to the task long enough to encode the information properly.

In acute confusional states arousal mechanisms may be normal, suppressed, or exaggerated and so may give rise to a normally alert, lethargic, or hypervigilant, agitated patient. Patients in various degrees of stupor or coma (i.e., with disorders of arousal) cannot be evaluated accurately for underlying dementia. Demented patients, on the other hand, typically do not exhibit disorders of attention or arousal until late in the course of illness.

3. What is the goal of evaluating dementia?

Finding a potentially reversible cause or component of dementia is the single most important goal.

4. What laboratory evaluation should be included in the initial evaluation of dementia?

All evaluations of dementia should include a brain image (computed tomography [CT] or magnetic resonance imaging [MRI]), assessment of thyroid-stimulating hormone and serum levels of vitamin B12, sedimentation rate, complete blood count, chemistry profile, and syphilis serology. Unfortunately, the yield is low. An electroencephalogram (EEG) is helpful with a history of seizures or blackouts and in patients suspected of cognitive impairment related to depression (so-called pseudodementia).

5. When should a lumbar puncture be performed in the evaluation of dementia?

Lumbar puncture should be strongly considered for patients under age 60 years or patients suspected of infection, meningeal irritation, rapid progression, compromised immunity, or positive syphilis serology. Dementia may occur relatively early in the course of infection with the human immunodeficiency virus (HIV) and is an increasingly important consideration, especially in at-risk patients.

6. How do patients with Alzheimer's disease frequently come to the attention of a physician?

Often the family brings the patient because of disorientation in familiar surroundings, problems with the checkbook, or failure at work. Some families clearly observe the loss of memory, whereas others notice only behavioral changes (anger, disinhibition, or social withdrawal). The patient may deny the accusations, but simple testing usually confirms a major impairment in short-term memory despite retention of long-term memory.

7. What is the usual diagnosis for a patient with "idiopathic dementia"?

Alzheimer's disease is the most common nontraumatic cause of dementia, affecting approximately 10% of people over 65 years old and 50% of those over 85 years. At present, absolute confirmation of the diagnosis depends on pathognomonic brain findings in autopsy specimens. The term "dementia of the Alzheimer type" is sometimes used when the diagnosis is suspected on clinical grounds but not proved pathologically. Experimental work has shown genetic markers for both familial and sporadic cases of Alzheimer's disease. Such research eventually may enable early diagnosis and effective treatments.

8. Why does dementia present acutely?

Although dementia may result from a sudden, severe brain injury, the typical cause is a previously undiagnosed condition unmasked by a stressful event such as moving to a new home, loss of a spouse, hospitalization, illness, or argument. Such dementia initially may be difficult to distinguish from an acute confusional state, to which the elderly are particularly susceptible. Family members or friends often provide the necessary historical clues of prior loss of intellect to reveal an underlying dementia that presents as an acute event.

9. When is tacrine useful in patients with dementia?

Tacrine (THA) is a centrally active anticholinesterase inhibitor that modestly improves cognition in early to moderate Alzheimer's disease. Because hepatic intolerance is common, slow titration to therapeutic doses is required, along with weekly transaminase testing. Transaminase elevations are dose-related rather than idiosyncratic; thus they are reversible and often avoidable with slower rechallenge. Most healthy patients with mild-to-moderate Alzheimer's disease deserve a trial of tacrine. If no real benefit is apparent after a few months, the drug may be discontinued.

10. What is MID?

MID is the acronym for multi-infarct dementia, the second leading cause of nontraumatic dementia. In contrast to the gradual, relentless deterioration of cognitive function and general lack of localizing neurologic signs in patients with Alzheimer's disease, patients with MID often exhibit a stepwise progression of mental deficits associated with focal neurologic signs (e.g., clumsiness of one hand, dysarthria, Babinski signs). The physician should be cautious about overuse of this diagnosis without both an appropriate clinical history and supporting radiologic evidence (i.e., focal lesions on CT or MRI scan of the brain).

The main goal of therapy is prevention of future strokes through reduction of risk factors, antiplatelet medications (aspirin or ticlopidine) and anticoagulation (if an embolic source is clearly identified). The majority of patients with MID have multiple bilateral, deep lacunar strokes. Multiple large cortical infarcts are a rare cause of MID. At autopsy, many patients with MID have concomitant Alzheimer's disease.

11. How does alcohol lead to dementia?

Alcoholic dementia continues to be a major cause of cognitive dysfunction. Alcoholic cognitive impairment results from two sources: nutritional deficiencies (most notably thiamine deficiency) and the direct toxic effects of alcohol. Acute alcohol-related thiamine deficiency results in irreversible damage to brain structures and chronic inability to encode new information (Korsakoff's psychosis). Patients with acute alcoholic dementia have ophthalmoplegia, gait ataxia, and confusion (Wernicke's syndrome). They require adequate thiamine replacement (100 mg intravenously immediately and 3 times/day) to prevent progression to a severe, permanent deficit in memory.

12. What other structural brain lesions should be considered in the differential diagnosis of a patient with dementia?

Structural brain lesions other than strokes may cause apparent dementia. Only a small percentage of the demented population has a treatable brain lesion. Both CT and MRI can identify such conditions, which are reversible with timely treatment. If stroke coexists with incurable dementia, it is still helpful to treat the vascular disorder.

13. How may the primary care provider unknowingly contribute to worsening dementia in an otherwise stable patient?

The brain of elderly patients is highly sensitive to pharmacologic effects. Thus, simple prescription of a new medication may cause an apparent decline in otherwise stable function. Normally innocuous medications, including nonprescription pills, may cause delirium that looks like dementia. The family of the patient must bring in every pill container to which the patient has access so that the physician can evaluate the role of medications in causing apparent dementia. All drugs that act on the central nervous system should be discontinued, if possible.

14. What advice should be given to the family of a demented patient?

Supportive care is necessary, including supervision of activities of daily living, thoughtful management of psychosocial issues, prevention of injury, and judicious use of low-dose medications (haloperidol, thioridazine) to manage aggressive behavior. Support from the family caregiver(s) is also necessary. Memory aids, companionship, and attention to grooming and cleanliness are particularly important.

The family caregiver also needs constant support, including (1) education about anticipated impairments, safety considerations, and the natural history of dementia and (2) encouragement to use respite care as needed (if the demented patient remains in the home) or alternative care settings as appropriate.

BIBLIOGRAPHY

1. Adams RD, Victor M: Delirium and other confusional states; Dementia and the amnesic (Korsakoff) syndrome. In Principles of Neurology, 5th ed. New York, McGraw-Hill, 1994.
2. Cummings J, Benson DF: Dementia—A Clinical Approach. Boston, Butterworth, 1992.
3. Katzman R: Delirium and dementia. In Rowland LP (ed): Merritt's Textbook of Neurology, 8th ed. Philadelphia, Lea & Febiger, 1989, pp 3–8.
4. Whitehouse P (ed): Dementia. Philadelphia, F.A. Davis, 1993.

74. TREMOR

C. Alan Anderson, M.D., and Richard Hughes, M.D.

1. Define tremor.

Tremor is an involuntary, unwanted movement characterized by a rhythmic oscillation ranging in frequency between 1 and 12 or more Hz.

2. What four questions help to classify a tremor?

1. Where in the body does it occur? Is it restricted to the hands?
2. Is it unilateral or asymmetrical?
3. Does it occur at rest or with movement?
4. Is it affected by sustained posture (postural or static tremor), movement (kinetic, action, or intention tremor), or a specific activity (task-specific tremor)?

3. If the tremor occurs at rest, what are the possible diagnoses?

Nearly all resting tremors are related to parkinsonian states. Possible diagnoses include idiopathic Parkinson's disease, drug-induced parkinsonism, other degenerative disorders, and, rarely, focal brain injury from stroke, tumor, trauma, or infections.

The tremor of Parkinson's disease is typically 4–6 Hz, asymmetric, and "pill-rolling" in appearance. The diagnosis of Parkinson's disease is supported by the presence of bradykinesia, rigidity, stooped posture, and festinating gait. Treatment includes anticholinergic agents (trihexyphenidyl, benztropine), dopamine precursors (levodopa), dopamine agonists (bromocriptine, pergolide), and monoamine oxidase inhibitors (selegiline).

4. Which drugs are most commonly responsible for drug-induced parkinsonism?

Drug-induced parkinsonism most commonly results from neuroleptic or antiemetic agents (e.g., metoclopramide). Occasionally the antidepressant amoxapine is responsible. Treatment of drug-induced parkinsonism is removal of the offending drug.

5. Describe the characteristics of postural tremor and the possible causes.

Postural tremors are of high amplitude and usually more proximal (i.e., the whole arm moves rather than just the finger and hand); the amplitude peaks with movements away from the body. Patients minimize postural tremors by holding their arms close to the trunk (e.g., folding the arms, holding the elbow against the chest wall, using both hands for stability) and by keeping the arms at rest.

The most common causes are familial tremor and essential tremor. Essential tremor, which occurs sporadically, and familial tremor, which follows an autosomal dominant pattern of inheritance, have identical characteristics. The head and distal upper extremities are most often affected. The tremor may begin at any time from childhood to late in life and is slowly progressive. It rarely persists at rest but worsens with use of the limb. Parkinson's disease occasionally involves a coexisting postural tremor along with the resting tremor. Wilson's disease, although rare, may present with postural tremor; other common clues include psychiatric problems, liver disease, or other abnormal movement. The tremor of Wilson's disease varies in amplitude and frequency and is more prominent proximally.

6. How does the response of a tremor to alcohol intake help with the differential diagnosis?

Many patients describe temporary improvement of essential or familial tremor with alcohol. This response is so specific that it is helpful diagnostically. Conventional therapy includes beta blockers, primidone, or injections of botulinum toxin.

7. Why do excitement and caffeine produce tremor?

All people experience a low-amplitude tremor with a frequency of 6–12 Hz when they maintain a fixed posture. This normal physiologic tremor may be exaggerated with anxiety, excitement, fatigue, caffeine, thyrotoxicosis, hypoglycemia, alcohol withdrawal, hysteria, and drugs. The most commonly involved drugs are stimulants, lithium, beta-adrenergic agents, theophylline, and valproate. Exaggerated physiologic tremor may be suppressed by removing or minimizing the underlying cause; if necessary and tolerated, beta blockers or anxiolytics may be used.

8. Characterize a kinetic tremor.

Kinetic (or action) tremors are usually irregular, jerky, severe, and ataxic; they are caused by diseases of the cerebellum or its outflow tracts. They may affect the trunk and limbs and interfere with all activities. Specific causes include chronic toxicity from alcohol, phenytoin, or other drugs and structural brain lesions such as multiple sclerosis, tumors, infection, stroke, and trauma. Hysteria should be considered if no obvious cause is present. If the underlying cause cannot be removed or treated, the only other option is neurosurgical ablation, which has limited success.

9. What is a task-specific tremor?
A task-specific tremor occurs only with repetitive hand-arm activity, such as writing. It is similar to the focal dystonia known as writer's cramp. Psychological factors are common, but cause and effect remain uncertain. Treatment includes beta blockers, anxiolytics, or anticholinergics, but the best results are achieved with injections of botulinum toxin.

10. What principles should be followed in treating the patient with tremor?
Tremor alone is rarely a painful or life-threatening diagnosis. The classification of the tremor should direct treatment, and the clinical response to therapy may help diagnostically. Treatment should be started slowly to minimize side effects, with the response measured over weeks to months.

11. When should a patient be referred for injections of botulinum toxin? How do they work?
Botulism is a potentially fatal disease caused by a neuromuscular junction toxin produced by the anaerobic bacterium, *Clostridium botulinum*. The toxin can be purified and injected into muscles to reduce excessive contractions, including those that cause tremor. As experience grows, more tremors are being treated with botulinum toxin, but results are mixed at best. Botulinum toxin is best for dystonias, chronic focal tremor, or spasms.

BIBLIOGRAPHY

1. Calne D: Treatment of Parkinson's disease. N Engl J Med 329:1021–1027, 1993.
2. Hallett M: Classification and treatment of tremor. JAMA 266:1115–1117, 1991.
3. Jankovic J, Fahn S: Physiologic and pathologic tremor. Ann Intern Med 93:460–465, 1980.
4. Lou J, Jankovic J: Essential tremor. Neurology 41:234–238, 1991.

75. MUSCLE WEAKNESS

Paul A. Foley, M.D., and Richard Hughes, M.D.

1. Describe the three patterns of muscle weakness that aid in determining cause.
1. The **upper motor neuron** or **elective pattern** of weakness involves the extensor muscles of the upper extremity and the flexor muscles of the lower extremity. This pattern is seen in cerebral hemisphere lesions, subdural hematoma, stroke, and tumor. The patient assumes a posture of arm flexion and adduction with wrist drop and leg extension that causes a spastic gait and circumduction of the affected leg.
2. **Proximal muscle weakness** involving the muscles of the shoulder and pelvic girdle usually occurs in patients with myopathy, which may be inherited (muscular dystrophy) or acquired (polymyositis, hypothyroidism).
3. A **distal pattern** of weakness involving primarily the hands and feet is seen in peripheral nerve disease associated with diabetes, trauma, and amyotrophic lateral sclerosis (ALS).

2. What physical maneuvers permit the best functional assessment of weakness?
Weakness may be evaluated both functionally and formally. Functional testing is carried out by the observation of simple everyday tasks such as walking on heels or toes, arising from a chair without assistance or use of hands, stepping onto a stool or step, raising the arms above the head, buttoning a shirt or closing a zipper, or "burying" eyelashes. Such observation of everyday activities allows an assessment of functional impairment.

3. How is muscle strength graded?

Formal testing of muscle strength involves isolating individual muscles or muscle groups for evaluation. Strength is graded with a 6-point scale developed by the Medical Research Council:

> 5 = Normal power
> 4 = Active movement against gravity and resistance
> 3 = Active movement against gravity only
> 2 = Active movement with gravity removed
> 1 = A trace or flicker of muscle contraction
> 0 = No muscle contraction detectable

This scale has significant shortcomings because of the high degree of interobserver variability and subjectivity; 90% of patients tend to be evaluated at grade four.

4. What is the most common motor neuron disease in adults?

ALS is the most common motor neuron disease in adults. It affects men more commonly than women, typically presents between 40 and 60 years of age, and is primarily a clinical diagnosis. Patients usually complain of weakness, atrophy, fasciculations, and muscle cramps. Some patients also have dysarthria and dysphagia. Diagnosis is based on a combination of diffuse upper and lower motor neuron findings and a rapidly progressive course.

Electromyography (EMG) proves most useful by demonstrating diffuse denervation; studies of the cerebrospinal fluids (CSF) are characteristically normal. Because no therapy for ALS currently exists, the need for a rapid diagnosis is lessened; clinicians often delay the diagnosis until progression is clearly observed. Once the diagnosis is confirmed, supportive measures such as physical therapy and symptomatic treatment for aspiration or depression are helpful.

5. In which patients should the physician consider Guillain-Barré syndrome (GBS)?

The most frequent cause of acute muscle weakness from a peripheral neuropathy is GBS. The clinical picture is dominated by acute weakness (duration of hours to days), with only minor asymmetries, that usually begins in the legs and ascends but occasionally begins in the arms or face and descends. Maximal weakness may occur distally or proximally and may involve both bulbar and respiratory muscles, making intubation necessary. Reflexes range from diminished to absent; sensory aberrations and autonomic dysfunction are not uncommon. CSF protein levels may remain normal early in the course of the disease but usually rise after the first week and peak within 4–6 weeks. The protein peak often coincides with the maximal amount of weakness. The CSF may demonstrate a mild leukocytosis. EMG studies support the diagnosis by demonstrating delayed nerve conductions.

Because GBS has an immunopathogenic basis, plasmapheresis or intravenous immuno-globulins are used to limit the severity and duration of disease. Supportive care to maintain respiratory functions and to avoid infections has dramatically reduced the mortality of GBS.

6. Describe the course of botulism.

Botulism occurs 12–48 hours after the consumption of contaminated food. It progresses rapidly over a matter of hours, causing death if respiratory support is not available.

7. What are the first symptoms of botulism?

Symptoms of cranial nerve dysfunction appear first, including diplopia, ptosis, blurred vision, dysphagia, and dysarthria. Dilated fixed pupils are a classic sign of botulism but often are not present. The five cardinal features of botulism, as outlined by the Centers for Disease Control, include (1) absence of fever, (2) normal mental status, (3) normal or slow pulse, (4) no sensory dysfunction, and (5) symmetric neurologic dysfunction. Respiratory failure may precede the onset of significant limb weakness. Treatment strategies include the removal of unabsorbed toxin via cathartics and emetics, neutralization of circulating toxins with antitoxin, and compensation for neurologic deficits through vigorous support.

8. How is myasthenia gravis differentiated from botulism?

Myasthenia gravis rarely presents as fulminantly as botulism and typically begins with progressive fatigability accompanied by intermittent diplopia, ptosis, dysarthria, and dysphagia. Most patients report that symptoms worsen throughout the day and improve after periods of rest. Diagnostic tests for myasthenia gravis include the edrophonium chloride test, repetitive nerve stimulation, and measurement of serum antibodies to acetylcholine receptors.

Although both myasthenia gravis and botulism are disorders of neuromuscular transmission, the pathology is quite different. Whereas botulism results from impaired release of acetylcholine at peripheral synapses, myasthenia gravis involves impaired binding of acetylcholine to postsynaptic receptors.

9. What is the difference between weakness and fatigue?

Patients often complain of "weakness" when in fact they are fatigued. Fatigue is defined as a lessened capacity for work, whereas weakness is a state of reduced power. The diagnosis of weakness is often clarified by a history of decreased strength or decreased muscular contraction with normal force. Some patients have both weakness and fatigue.

Patients with fatigue often state that they are "tired all the time" or "exhausted." They often have decreased interest in otherwise routine activities and decreased initiative. Fatigue is to be expected with sleeplessness, prolonged exertion, and excessive work. Fatigue associated with a psychiatric disorder is often worse in the morning, increases with mild activity, and generally relates more specifically to some activities than to others. Fatigue is often the first symptom of psychosocial stress and interferes with mental activity.

10. Which medical disorders may present as fatigue?

Medical disorders that may produce fatigue include common viral infections, hepatitis, tuberculosis, Lyme disease, mononucleosis, metabolic or endocrine disorders (e.g., Addison's disease, hypothyroidism, diabetes, hyperparathyroidism, anemia), and occult malignancy. Nutritional deficiencies and other causes of poor health also may present as fatigue.

11. What are myopathies?

The myopathies are a heterogeneous group of primary muscle disorders. They are characterized by clinical and laboratory evidence of muscle destruction with or without inflammation.

Inflammatory myopathies include polymyositis, dermatomyositis, inclusion body myositis, and infectious myopathies. They typically present as a chronic proximal muscle weakness accompanied by pain. EMG studies, elevated serum creatine phosphokinase (CPK), and muscle biopsy are helpful in making the diagnosis.

Noninflammatory myopathies include both inherited and endocrine myopathies. Common inherited myopathies include Duchenne's muscular dystrophy and the adult form, Becker's muscular dystrophy, both of which are X-linked and accompanied by calf hypertrophy. Endocrine myopathies include hypothyroid and steroid-induced myopathy.

12. Which myopathies are not accompanied by an elevated level of CPK?

Classically the level of CPK is not elevated in steroid-induced myopathy. It may be elevated in hypothyroidism because of decreased renal clearance and is characteristically elevated in inflammatory myopathies. In common inherited myopathies, although muscles are not painful, the CPK level may be markedly elevated.

13. When may steroid use cause myopathy?

Steroids can induce dramatic proximal weakness. Despite reports of onset within a few weeks or with low doses (e.g., 15 mg of prednisone), myopathy typically occurs in chronic users of high-dose steroids. Many steroids have a discrete dose threshold above which weakness predictably occurs. Similar weakness occurs with excessive endogenous production of glucocorticoids, as in Cushing's disease or ectopic production of adrenocorticotropic hormone

(ACTH). Fortunately, such myopathies resolve with correction of the endocrine condition or withdrawal of the steroid.

BIBLIOGRAPHY

1. Adams R, Victor M (eds): Principles of Neurology, 5th ed. New York, McGraw-Hill, 1993.
2. Campbell W, Swift T: Differential diagnosis of acute weakness. South Med J 74:1371–1375, 1981.
3. Dalakas MC: Polymyositis, dermatomyositis, and inclusion-body myositis. N Engl J Med 325:1487–1498, 1991.
4. Riggs JE: Adult-onset muscle weakness. Postgrad Med 78:217–226, 1985.
5. Rowland LP (ed): Merritt's Textbook of Neurology, 8th ed. Philadelphia, Lea & Febiger, 1989.

76. NUMBNESS AND TINGLING

Doug Redosh, M.D., and Richard Hughes, M.D.

1. When should a complaint of numbness and tingling raise the concern of a primary care provider?

Numbness and tingling, also known as paresthesias (or, if painful, dysesthesias) can originate anywhere in the nervous system, either peripheral or central. If severe or clearly localized to a focal brain or spinal cord lesion, the complaint may herald a serious condition, especially if the symptoms are continuous and progressive.

Fortunately, paresthesias are usually of little significance, especially if fleeting. For example, everybody experiences a limb "falling asleep" from compression of the ulnar, sciatic, or peroneal nerves, and simple anxiety with hyperventilation commonly produces paresthesias of the face, hands, and legs.

2. Describe the pathway of sensory fibers.

Sensory information is first registered in various specialized nerve endings in the skin, subcutaneous tissue, and deep tissue. It is then conveyed via the peripheral nerves to the dorsal roots. Here the fibers enter the spinal cord and split into the dorsal columns (proprioception and vibratory sense) and the spinothalamic tracts (pain and temperature). These tracts ascend into the medulla where the proprioception/vibration fibers synapse and cross over to form the medial lemniscus, whereas the pain/temperature fibers ascend laterally. All sensory information converges in the thalamus. From here the final step is through the deep white-matter tracts of the internal capsule to the sensory cortex, located in the parietal lobe of the brain. A lesion at any point in these pathways may produce sensory symptoms, including paresthesia, hypoesthesia (lack of sensation), or hyperesthesia (increased sensation).

3. What clues suggest that a lesion in the sensory cortex produced the paresthesias?

Lesions in the sensory cortex also produce objective signs. Examples include astereognosis, the inability to identify simple objects (e.g., paper clips, keys) placed in the hand by texture and shape, and graphesthesia, the inability to identify letters or numbers scratched on the palm. Many patients also have mild hemiparesis. Because many processes may affect this area of the brain, neurologic consultation is needed if more than subjective paresthesias are present on examination.

4. When may a cerebrovascular event cause isolated sensory loss?

Lacunar or small strokes result from small-vessel occlusions in the internal capsule, thalamus, or brainstem. The major symptom of such purely sensory strokes is objective numbness to pain and temperature in the contralateral face, arm, and leg. Thalamic infarction may cause a longlasting, painful unilateral "numbness" that is refractory to treatment.

An unusual but important situation is the lateral medullary infarction, also known as Wallenberg syndrome. Symptoms include numbness of the ipsilateral face but contralateral body. This split sensory loss occurs as the fibers responsible for facial sensation travel to the cervical spinal cord before crossing and synapsing in the thalamus. Other signs and symptoms of lateral medullary syndrome include hoarseness, ipsilateral Horner's syndrome, hiccoughs, vertigo, and ipsilateral ataxia.

5. What signs and symptoms suggest a lesion in the spinal cord?

Spinal cord lesions produce symptoms and signs at or below their cervical, thoracic, or lumbar level. The face is spared. Other clues include back pain, Lhermitte's sign (electric shocks or tingling sensations down the back with forward flexion of the neck), bladder dysfunction, and a discrete level at a sensory dermatome.

6. How common is paresthesia as a presentation of multiple sclerosis (MS)?

Patients with MS commonly complain of unilateral or bilateral paresthesias from demyelinating plaques in the cerebral hemisphere or spinal cord. Paresthesias may be the first symptom, but typically they are associated with other signs, such as upper motor neuron weakness, incontinence, ataxia, or optic neuritis (blurred vision in one eye).

7. Do herniated discs cause numbness and tingling?

Yes. In addition to pain, herniated discs may produce paresthesias radiating to the shoulder, arm, and hand (cervical) or to the buttocks, thigh, and foot (lumbar). Less commonly, other serious lesions may produce sciatica, including epidural abscess, strategically placed tumors, and osteophytes impinging on the neural foramina. Serious causes are usually suspected by the presence of excruciating pain, severe tenderness, fever, or sepsis.

8. Where do the most common causes of numbness and tingling originate?

The most common causes of numbness and tingling originate in the peripheral nerves. Both polyneuropathies and mononeuropathies have paresthesias as prominent symptoms. The causes of polyneuropathy are numerous, but the most common are diabetes, infection with the human immunodeficiency virus (HIV), hypothyroidism, alcohol abuse, nutritional deficiencies (including vitamin B12), drugs (chemotherapeutic agents), and idiopathic factors.

9. Why do polyneuropathies typically follow a stocking-glove pattern?

The patient with polyneuropathy typically has paresthesias in a stocking distribution, because these branches of the nerves are farthest from the cell bodies in the dorsal root ganglion. As neuropathies progress, the patient may experience similar symptoms in a glove distribution in the hands.

10. Which classic polyneuropathy is life-threatening and treatable?

A life-threatening but treatable polyneuropathy is Guillain-Barré syndrome or acute idiopathic demyelinating polyneuropathy (AIDP). Patients experience mild-to-severe symmetric paresthesias in the feet, legs, or thigh in association with progressive paralysis and areflexia. The syndrome may progress to respiratory failure requiring mechanical ventilation. Effective treatments include plasmapheresis or intravenous immunoglobulin. The recurrent form of this process is called chronic idiopathic demyelinating polyneuropathy (CIPD).

11. How does a claw hand deformity develop?

Compressions of the ulnar nerve at the elbow or "funny bone" produce paresthesias down the ulnar aspect of the forearm to the fourth and fifth fingers. If the condition is longstanding, atrophy may be seen in the first dorsal interosseous muscle on the dorsum of the hand in the web space between the thumb and the index finger. In a complete palsy, the claw hand deformity develops.

12. What causes a peroneal palsy?

Compression of the peroneal nerve at the fibular head occurs in bedridden patients, habitual leg crossers, and diabetics; it also may be associated with surgery, overly tight compression stockings, and trauma. In the days before soft luggage, peroneal palsy was called palsy of the "suitcase nerve," because hard valises often repetitively traumatized the lateral knee. Patients experience paresthesias and hypoesthesias down the lateral leg to the dorsum of the foot; footdrop may result from weakness of the tibialis anterior muscle.

13. What neural lesions do *not* produce numbness and tingling in the nervous system?

Amyotrophic lateral sclerosis (ALS, motor neuron disease) is a disease of the anterior horn cells and long motor tracts; sensory symptoms effectively exclude ALS. **Neuromuscular junction disease** (e.g., myasthenia, botulism) and **myopathies** (polymyositis and muscular dystrophy) produce weakness without sensory symptoms or signs.

14. What clues suggest the hysterical patient?

Be wary of the patient who complains of paresthesias in nonanatomic distributions. On repeated examinations, the location of the symptoms often changes. Hysterical patients often note decreased hearing, vision, smell, or taste. Many have typical functional complaints in other organ systems and historically have suffered from depression, anxiety, or stress-related disorders.

15. When should electromyographic (EMG) studies be ordered?

EMG and nerve conduction studies may be helpful in the diagnosis and prognosis of patients with nerve, plexus, and root lesions. EMG is not helpful in patients with diseases of the central nervous system except to exclude concomitant peripheral disease. Its usefulness depends on the clinical setting. Neurologic consultation is advisable before requesting EMG testing.

16. Any closing thoughts?

Remember—try to localize the lesion by the pattern of numbness and sensory loss and by associated findings. Most confusion is due to imprecise descriptions of sensory symptoms. Patients often use "numb" or "dead" for either sensory changes or weakness. With a clear description, a good localization, and knowledge of the patient's medical history, the etiology of the numbness or tingling becomes apparent.

BIBLIOGRAPHY

1. Adams R, Victor M: Other somatic sensation. In Principles of Neurology, 5th ed. New York, McGraw-Hill, 1993.
2. Branzis P, et al: Localization. In Clinical Neurology, 2nd ed. Boston, Little, Brown, 1990.
3. Devor M: Neuropathic pain and injured nerve: Periphreal mechanisms. BMJ 47:619–630, 1991.
4. Kanchardani R, Howe JG: Lhermitte's sign in multiple sclerosis: A clinical survey and review of the literature. J Neurol Neurosurg Psychiatry 45:308–312, 1982.
5. Manusov EG: Late life migraines accompaniments: A case preventative and literature review. J Fam Pract 24:541–544, 1987.
6. Schmahmann JD, Leifen D: Parietal pseudo-thalamic pain syndrome: Clinical features and anatomic correlates. Arch Neurol 49:1032–1037, 1992.

77. CEREBROVASCULAR DISORDERS

Rafael Villalobos, M.D., and Richard Hughes, M.D.

1. What is the difference between a transient ischemic attack (TIA) and a cerebrovascular accident (CVA)?

The nomenclature for stroke is less than ideal. Both CVA and TIA refer to ischemia in the brain that results in neurologic deficits. If the *clinical* deficit resolves by 24 hours, the ischemia is termed a TIA. If the deficit is persistent at 24 hours, even if it resolves over a few days, the ischemia is called CVA or stroke. The nomenclature becomes more complicated because 30–50% of patients with *clinically* defined TIA actually have a permanent abnormality in the brain on computed tomography (CT) or magnetic resonance imaging (MRI) or at autopsy. Thus TIAs are the clinical expression of small areas of cell death in the brain, even though the neurologic deficit is not permanent.

2. What is the value of the history and physical examination in patients with obvious stroke?

In most instances the history and physical examination explain the pathophysiology of the event. For example, small-vessel thrombosis or lacunae are associated with a history of hypertension and risk factors for arteriosclerosis (advanced age, high cholesterol, smoking, diabetes). Patients often awaken with the deficit and commonly present with either pure motor or pure sensory findings with proportional involvement (equal impairment of face, arm, and leg).

Some patients with cerebral embolism have a history of cardiac arrhythmias, valvular disease, or myocardial infarction. Artery-to-artery embolism is also common, as suggested by the finding of carotid bruits. The onset of an embolic deficit is immediate and usually associated with activity or physical exertion. Because superficial vessels are usually affected, a combination of cortical problems (aphasia, neglect) and motor and sensory findings with nonproportional involvement (greater impairment of face and arm than leg) is common.

3. Can a migraine cause a stroke?

Yes. The rare migraine that causes a stroke, however, must be differentiated from the more common complicated migraine, which presents with a neurologic deficit that resolves within 20–30 minutes. Actual strokes cause persistent symptoms and objective deficit. A careful search for unusual causes of stroke, such as hypercoagulable states and inflammatory conditions, is indicated in migraine-induced stroke.

4. How frequently does a CVA or TIA present as a seizure?

A seizure is the first manifestation of ischemia in 5–10% of embolic strokes. A seizure rarely, if ever, complicates a small nerve or lacunar stroke.

5. What is Todd's paralysis?

Postictal paresis or Todd's paralysis may mimic a devastating stroke. Fortunately, such deficits resolve. The differentiation between an embolus with seizure and a seizure with Todd's paralysis is always difficult and likely to require the help of a neurologist.

6. Why should patients with ischemic events be rapidly evaluated?

The risk of a recurrent stroke is highest in the first few days and weeks after an initial stroke or TIA. Therefore, it is crucial that patients have an appropriate evaluation to prevent, if possible, a second ischemic event. Furthermore, about 20% of acute cerebral infarcts progressively worsen during the first 24 hours after onset. Rapid, thorough clinical evaluation and management can prevent progressive brain injury.

7. What mistakes during early management of a patient with a CVA may worsen injury?

Overtreatment of hypertension   Failure to prevent aspiration
Failure to treat dehydration   Failure to treat concomitant cardiac disease

8. Is contrast CT necessary to evaluate the patient with an acute CVA?

Generally not. An acute imaging study, such as a CT scan, is useful mainly to exclude the presence of hemorrhage. If the patient has a history of a malignancy that theoretically could metastasize to the brain, a contrast scan is probably worthwhile.

9. Is anticoagulation indicated in a patient with acute stroke?

Anticoagulation is indicated to prevent recurrent embolization in either cardiogenic emboli (i.e., atrial fibrillation) or noncardiogenic emboli (i.e., artery–artery). It is not clear whether anticoagulation should begin immediately or after a few days. The duration of anticoagulation varies with the risk of recurrence. For example, atrial fibrillation or valvular diseases usually require anticoagulation for life. Transient conditions, such as myocardial infarction or carotid artery injuries (e.g., dissection), may need only short-term anticoagulation.

10. Does every patient with a CVA or TIA need an echocardiogram?

No. However, the mechanism of the stroke should be defined in every patient. Cardiac ultrasound, either transthoracic or transesophageal, has demonstrated unsuspected cardiac sources for emboli in many patients, including the common sources, such as atrial fibrillation, prosthetic valves, endocarditis, and mural thrombi, as well as paradoxical emboli through patent foramen ovale (PFO). Young victims of stroke (< 45 years old) have a 2–3 times greater prevalence of PFO than age-matched controls, suggesting that PFO plays an important role in causing strokes.

11. How much aspirin is required to prevent stroke?

The initial recommendation was 4 aspirin/day, but recent evidence has demonstrated that 1 aspirin/day is as effective as higher doses. It may be possible to reduce the dose further; for example, 80 mg/day or 1 aspirin 3 days/week may eventually become the standard. Reducing the dose of aspirin reduces the risk of gastrointestinal and perhaps cerebral hemorrhages. Ticlopidine is a newer antiplatelet agent that works a bit better than aspirin, especially in the first year after a stroke or TIA. It is a good alternative when therapy with aspirin or Coumadin fails.

A small number of patients with hyperaggregable platelets need higher doses of aspirin to block platelet aggregation effectively. Currently no standard guidelines specify which patients need platelet aggregation testing. The standard of care is to reserve such testing for patients in whom aspirin therapy has failed, young patients, migraineurs, or patients without typical risk factors for stroke.

BIBLIOGRAPHY

1. Adams RD, Victor M: Approach to the patient with neurologic disease and the major categories of neurologic disease. In Principles of Neurology, 5th ed. New York, McGraw-Hill, 1993.
2. De Tullio M, Sacco RL, Aasha G, et al: Patent foramen ovale as a risk factor for cryptogenic stroke. Ann Intern Med 117:461–465, 1992
3. European Carotid Surgery Trialists Collaborative Group: MRC European Carotid Surgery Trial: Interim results for symptomatic patients with severe (70–90%) or mild (0–29%) carotid stenosis. Lancet 337:1235–1243, 1993.
4. Gent M, et al: The Canadian American Ticlopidine Study (CATS) in thromboembolic stroke. Lancet 1:1215–1220, 1989.
5. North American Symptomatic Carotid Endarterectomy Trial Collaborators: Beneficial effect of carotid endarterectomy in symptomatic patients with high grade carotid stenosis. N Engl J Med 325:445–453, 1991.

78. HEADACHE

Catherine Amlie-Lefond, M.D.

1. Characterize the four migraine syndromes.
  1. **Common:** Common migraine occurs in 5–10% of the population and accounts for about 80% of all migraines. Symptoms include throbbing headache, nausea and vomiting, pallor, and sensitivity to light and noise. The headache usually lasts for hours and often is relieved by sleep.
  2. **Classic:** Classic migraine, which occurs in about 1% of people, has features of a common migraine as well as preceding or associated neurologic symptoms, which often include visual phenomena, such as scotomata or fortification spectra (zig-zag lines).
  3. **Basilar:** Basilar artery migraine is rare but usually occurs in young women. It is associated with symptoms referable to the territory of the vertebral and basilar arteries, such as vertigo, dysarthria, ataxia, and quadriplegia.
  4. **Complicated:** In complicated migraine, focal neurologic symptoms and signs outlast the headache and occasionally are permanent. In rare cases migrainous neurologic symptoms may precede the headache or occur without a headache.

2. How should migraine headaches be treated?
Therapy for migraine is divided into two stages: (1) treatment of acute migraine and (2) chronic therapy to prevent and reduce severity of headaches. Standard therapy for a moderately severe headache consists of nonsteroidal anti-inflammatory agents (NSAIDs; e.g., ibuprofen, 600 mg every 4 hr), vasoconstrictors (Midrin or Cafergot), or analgesics (fiorinal, acetaminophen with codeine), often accompanied by a sedating antinausea drug (metoclopramide or hydroxyzine). More severe headaches are treated with dihydroergotamine (DHE-45; 0.5–1.0 mg intramuscularly, usually combined with a sedating antinausea supplement. Recently, sumatriptan (6 mg subcutaneously) has been reported to be highly effective in treatment of acute, severe migraine. It may be self-injected by the patient, thus avoiding emergency department visits. Preventive therapies for migraine include tricyclic antidepressants, beta-blocking agents, daily NSAIDs, or methysergide.

3. How does cluster headache differ from migraine?
Cluster and migraine headaches differ in epidemiology, presentation, and treatment. Migraine is more common in young women; cluster headache is more common in middle-aged men. Cluster headache is defined by multiple episodes of unilateral orbital pain that last 0.5–1.5 hours/day over a period of several weeks. The headache may be accompanied by unilateral conjunctival injection, lacrimation, sweating, or even Horner's syndrome. Individual headaches are sometimes relieved by inhaled oxygen (6–8 L/min; 100% oxygen by mask for 10–15 minutes); clusters of headaches may be abbreviated with prednisone (60 mg/day for 7 days, followed by a rapid taper).

4. Define tension headaches. How are they treated?
The classic dichotomy of vascular (i.e., migraine and cluster) and tension (muscle contraction) headaches is useful but not fully accurate. The typical "bandlike" fronto-occipital tension headaches are presumably caused by increased contraction of scalp muscles due to life stress.
  Treatment is usually with NSAIDs; rarely are more potent analgesics used. However, many patients have headaches with features of both vascular and tension types. Such headaches are best treated as common migraines.

5. What characteristics of a headache should raise the suspicion of intracranial disease?
No headache is pathognomonic for brain tumor, although the classic triad of headache, vomiting, and papilledema may be seen. Nonetheless, the physician must recognize the headache

that is a sign of intracranial disease. Such headaches may awaken the patient from sound sleep and be more severe in the early morning. The pain usually progressively worsens over days or weeks and is increased by changing posture, cough, or Valsalva effort. Changes in mental status or focal neurologic signs also may be present. New-onset seizures in combination with headache often herald serious brain lesions.

6. When should benign intracranial hypertension be considered as a cause of headache? Is it in fact benign?

Benign intracranial hypertension (BIH), also called pseudotumor cerebri, is elevated intracranial pressure of unknown etiology. It often is associated with obesity, pregnancy, and use of oral contraceptives, vitamin A, tetracycline, or steroids. It usually presents in young women as a headache that is worse on waking. The headaches often respond poorly to treatment. Papilledema is present, often along with visual symptoms such as blurring, enlarged blind spot, constricted visual fields, or even blindness.

BIH is not benign. Without proper therapy (weight loss, discontinuance of inciting medications, and treatment with acetazolamide, corticosteroids, lumboperiteonal shunt, or optic nerve sheath fenestration) visual loss may be permanent.

7. What medical emergency is suggested by a unilateral headache in an elderly patient?

Temporal arteritis, or giant-cell arteritis, is a disease of the elderly that presents with headache centered over the temporal artery or around the eye. It also may be associated with fever, anorexia, myalgias, malaise, weight loss, or leukocytosis. On palpation the temporal artery is prominent and tender. The diagnosis is suggested by a sedimentation rate over 50 mm/hr. Definitive diagnosis depends on temporal artery biopsy, which shows granulomatous inflammation. The diagnosis represents an emergency because the central artery of the retina, a branch of the ophthalmic artery, may become thrombosed, causing unilateral or bilateral blindness in over 25% of patients. Prednisone, 50–75 mg/day, may diminish headache and help to prevent blindness.

8. What should be done for the patient who complains of intense sharp, stabbing pains through the eye?

Lancinating or "icepick" pains are a common phenomenon. They are sudden, brief (< 10 sec), highly localized, piercing pains, often through or behind one eye, temple, occiput, or ear. They may hit first one spot, then another. They are common in migrainous and anxious patients but occur in many other settings. They are always benign, do not require brain imaging, and are too brief to be treated. The best therapy is to reassure the patient.

9. What condition is suggested by the patient with daily or constant headache who takes daily NSAIDs, Tylenol, vasoconstrictors, or analgesics?

The patient probably has drug-withdrawal, rebound headaches. He or she needs consultation and treatment by a specialist experienced in the management of severe headaches, chronic pain, and drug withdrawal. Hospitalization may be required.

BIBLIOGRAPHY

1. Raskin NH: Headache. In Appel SH (ed): Current Neurology, vol. 10. Chicago, Year Book, 1990, pp 195–219.
2. Saper JR, Silberstein SD, Gordon CD, Hamel RL: Handbook of Headache Management. Baltimore, Williams & Wilkins, 1992.
3. Silberstein SD: Intractable headache: Inpatient and outpatient treatment strategies. Neurology 42(Suppl 2), 1992.

79. DIZZINESS AND SYNCOPE

Richard Hughes, M.D., and Kamasamudram Ravilochan, M.D.

1. What is the first thing to do when a patient complains of dizziness?
Because dizziness is a vague term, it is critical to understand the patient's definition. The first task is to distinguish dizziness from complaints referable to weakness, visual disturbances, or seizures. The second task is to distinguish between vestibular and nonvestibular types of dizziness. Vestibular dizziness or vertigo is accompanied by a sensation of movement, whereas nonvestibular dizziness is often described as a sensation of lightheadedness or imbalance.

2. What are the most common causes of dizziness?
The key role of the primary care provider is to identify the common causes of dizziness: postural hypotension, positional vertigo, hyperventilation, and multiple sensory deficits. Thus unnecessary referrals and expensive testing are often avoided.

3. What historical data are important in suggesting the cause of dizziness?
Vestibular causes are suggested by episodic attacks that may be precipitated by positional changes and often are accompanied by nausea and vomiting, with or without hearing loss or tinnitus. Nonvestibular causes usually result in a prolonged sensation of lightheadedness brought on by stress, hyperventilation, or standing and perhaps accompanied by palpitations, perspiration, paresthesias, and pallor. Syncope may result. The patient should be questioned about a history of head injury, recent viral infections, diabetes, or psychiatric disturbance.

4. Which medications most notably cause dizziness?
Antibiotics (e.g., gentamicin, streptomycin), anticonvulsants, high-dose salicylates, antiparkinsonian agents, and antihypertensives may be responsible. Any sedative medication may cause fatigue and unsteadiness that some patients call "dizziness."

5. Describe the specific elements of the evaluation of the dizzy patient.
The cardiovascular examination pays special attention to pulse and blood pressure (standing and supine), murmurs, arrhythmia, and carotid bruits. The otoscopic examination should focus on evidence of impacted wax and ear infection as well as a brief assessment of hearing loss. Hyperventilation for 2–3 minutes may reproduce the symptoms and confirm the diagnosis of primary hyperventilation. A careful neurologic exam with special attention to cranial nerve and cerebellar function is critical to exclude signs of a focal process.

6. When are laboratory tests helpful in evaluating the patient with dizziness?
Laboratory tests are dictated by the history and examination. A complete blood count and electrolyte panel are needed when the patient equates dizziness with "feeling generally unwell." A routine electrocardiogram (EKG) should be performed to search for evidence of cardiac disease. An imaging study (computed tomography [CT] or magnetic resonance imaging [MRI]) is useful when focal brainstem abnormalities, such as acoustic neuromas or multiple sclerosis, are suspected. Audiometry is useful in patients with hearing loss and tinnitus. Other tests, such as electromyogram, electroencephalography (EEG), brainstem-evoked potentials, and cervical spine films, are usually not needed.

7. Once a diagnosis of dizziness of vestibular origin is made, is the patient treatable?
Yes. Most dizziness or tinnitus of vestibular origin is self-limited. Symptomatic treatment with transdermal scopolamine, meclizine (Antivert), or dimenhydrinate (Dramamine) is helpful for vertigo. Promethazine hydrochloride (Phenergan) or trimethobenzamide (Tigan) is usually

effective for controlling associated nausea. Vestibular exercise therapy may be useful in benign positional or posttraumatic vertigo.

8. What diagnosis is suggested when vertigo is accompanied by tinnitus?
The triad of vertigo, tinnitus, and aural fullness suggests Ménière's disease, which is treated empirically with vasodilators, diuretics, low-sodium diet, antihistamines, and tranquilizers. Response varies from great success to dismal failure. When symptoms are severe, a shunt procedure between the membranous labyrinth and subarachnoid space is sometimes recommended.

9. Which serious central nervous system diseases may cause new-onset vertigo?
　　1. **Posterior circulation cerebrovascular disease** typically is associated with brainstem or occipital lobe complaints.
　　2. **Acoustic neuroma,** when unilateral, typically is associated with hearing loss in the telephone range.
　　3. **Other posterior fossa tumors** are associated with slow onset and coordination difficulties.
　　4. **Multiple sclerosis** typically is associated with more than one neurologic abnormality as well as episodic symptoms.

10. Can seizures cause dizziness?
Yes. **Complex partial seizures** may present with an aura of dizziness, vertigo, or unsteadiness. Without clear evidence of epilepsy the diagnosis may require electroencephalographic monitoring. Complex partial seizures are easily treated with appropriate anticonvulsants. **Basilar migraine,** an odd variant of complicated migraine, may be accompanied by lightheadedness, vertigo, or ataxia.

11. What systemic disorders may cause dizziness or even brief alterations of consciousness?
Hypoglycemia, allergic reactions, drug or alcohol blackouts, and orthostasis due to loss of blood, volume, or electrolytes (adrenal insufficiency).

12. Describe syncope.
Syncope is a brief loss of consciousness that occurs while standing and causes the patient to collapse to the floor. Syncope is usually preceded by a warm or "floating" feeling and perhaps by changes in vision. Such premonitory symptoms typically last a fraction of a second but on occasion may be prolonged. When patients experience premonitory symptoms and sit or lie down to prevent syncope, the condition is termed "presyncope."

　　Once the patient hits the floor, unconsciousness lasts from a few seconds to a minute. Typically patients are not confused or disoriented. During the period of unconsciousness muscle twitches, called myoclonic jerks, may be observed. When prominent, they are mistaken for seizures. Only rarely, however, does syncope induce a truly generalized tonic-clonic seizure. When patients try to stand too quickly, syncope commonly recurs; the autonomic system may require a few minutes to recover sufficiently to allow maintenance of an erect posture.

13. Is it important to discover the cause of syncope?
Most causes of syncope in the United States are not serious. Episodes of simple fainting or vasovagal syncope account for approximately 50% of all events. For the neurologist or cardiologist who sees a small subset of high-risk patients with syncope, a serious diagnosis is more common, accounting for another 20% of cases. This bias explains the variation in response, which depends on which group of patients is seen. Approximately 20% of patients have no known diagnosis after evaluation.

14. How do I know who is safe?
Perhaps the most important role of the primary care physician is to recognize and treat appropriately (or leave alone) simple vasovagal syncope or fainting. A good history includes

the instigating event (if any), premonitory symptoms, and typical resolution of the syncopal episode. If the neurologic and cardiovascular examinations are normal, little more needs to be done.

Common triggering mechanisms include heat and dehydration combined with physical stress or startle. Examples include fainting at the sight of blood or instrumentation, micturation syncope, tussive syncope, Valsalva syncope (e.g., diving, weight lifting, trumpet playing), and the notorious tendency of people to faint at church services or weddings. Military recruits often faint during routine immunizations. If the patient cannot recall a triggering event, a witness may help.

15. Which cardiovascular abnormalities are associated with syncope?

Cardiac syncope requires a 50% fall in cardiac output and thus is a harbinger of serious cardiac disease. Mechanical, ischemic, and arrhythmic etiologies may lead to syncope. Mechanical lesions include aortic and pulmonary obstruction, including hypertension. Arrhythmias, including complete heart block, sick sinus syndrome, and brady- or tachycardias, may cause syncope. Ischemia due to myocardial infarction or aortic dissection also may present with syncope. Thus, any syncopal patient over the age of 50 years or with known cardiac abnormalities on EKG or physical examination requires further evaluation.

16. When should prolonged EKG monitoring be performed in the evaluation of syncope?

Certainly patients with a history, physical examination, or routine EKG suggestive of cardiac disease should have prolonged EKG monitoring. However, prolonged EKG monitoring provides diagnostic information in only 20% of syncopal patients older than 50 years with *no* clues pointing to cardiovascular disease. Further study is needed to determine the cost-benefit ratio of this practice.

17. What is the value of invasive testing in the diagnosis of syncope?

A thorough history and physical examination, an EKG, and 24-hour cardiac monitor should be performed in older patients. If no abnormalities or clues are found, additional invasive testing, such as electrophysiology or coronary angiography, head CT, or EEG, seldom adds significant information.

18. How useful is the tilt table?

Unfortunately, a tilt table can make anyone faint, regardless of what symptoms they may have had in church last week. Perhaps the most useful information results from inducing a faint in the patient with an unexplained loss of consciousness, which confirms that the episode was indeed a faint rather than another type of spell (such as hysteria). Many investigators have remarked on the negative electrophysiologic studies of patients who have simple faints on the tilt table. However, the tilt table is not a good screening device to determine who may need a more involved evaluation.

19. Define "drop" spells.

Drop spells are vaguely defined attacks that usually affect older patients, especially women. Patients experience a sudden "giving way" of the legs, fall, and may injure themselves but do not lose consciousness. The cause is not known. Once a thorough history, physical, and EKG are performed, no additional evaluation is needed.

20. Can strokes or neurologic problems cause syncope?

Yes. Patients with basilar artery ischemia may lose consciousness but usually also have vertigo, unsteadiness, dysesthesia, weakness, or blindness. Furthermore, basilar artery ischemia usually involves a longer period of unconsciousness than simple syncope. Epilepsy is always a concern in patients whose syncope was unwitnessed or who do not recall the event. Typical postictal clues, such as headache, confusion, fatigue, tongue biting, or incontinence, are found. Many neurologic disorders cause fainting by loss of normal blood pressure and pulse responses to standing. Both central degenerative disorders (e.g., Alzheimer's disease, Parkinson's disease, Shy-Drager syndrome) and peripheral nerve disorders induce autonomic impairment sufficient to cause syncope.

21. What is the natural history of syncope?
Because most syncope occurs in the older population, mortality may be high. For simple vasovagal syncope the 1-year mortality rate is less than 5%, whereas the 1-year mortality rate for cardiac syncope is 20–30%. Electrophysiologic testing has probably increased understanding of the disorder more than it has changed mortality rates.

BIBLIOGRAPHY

1. Adams RD, Victor M: Principles of Neurology, 5th ed. New York, McGraw-Hill, 1993.
2. Brandt TH, Daroff RB: Physical therapy for benign paroxysmal vertigo. Arch Otolaryngol 42:290–293, 1980.
3. Kapoor WN, Hammil SC, Gersch BJ: Diagnosis and natural history of syncope and role of invasive electrophysiologic testing. Medicine 69:160–175, 1990.
4. Manolis AJ, Linzer M, Salem D, Estes NAM: Syncope: Current diagnostic evaluation and management. Ann Intern Med 112:850–863, 1990.
5. Samuels MA: Manual of Neurology, 4th ed. Boston, Little, Brown, 1991.
6. Troost BT, Patton JM: Exercise therapy for positional vertigo. Neurology 42:1441–1444, 1992.

80. SEIZURE DISORDERS
John Towbin, M.D., and Richard Hughes, M.D.

1. Define epilepsy.
The International League of Epilepsy defines epilepsy as an ongoing propensity to have seizures in the absence of provoking circumstances. Thus withdrawal seizures, childhood febrile seizures, and seizures during cardiorespiratory arrest do not constitute epilepsy.

2. When does the onset of epilepsy most frequently occur?
Although the onset of seizure disorders may occur at any age, the incidence of first seizure has been found to be highest in patients below the age of 20 years.[2]

3. Describe the different forms of epilepsy.
Primary generalized epilepsies begin in a widespread fashion, involving the entire cortex (i.e., generalized rather than focal pathology). They often follow an autosomal dominant pattern of inheritance with incomplete penetrance. The onset is usually in childhood (for example, 5–7 years of age for absence seizures or puberty for juvenile myoclonic epilepsy). Patients typically have a normal neurologic examination and normal IQ. The possible types of seizure include absence (petit mal), generalized tonic-clonic (grand mal), atonic (often called "drop attacks"), and myoclonic (often desribed simply as "jerks").

Acquired epilepsies begin focally but often invade the entire brain (generalize), thus making the focal onset difficult to confirm. Genetic factors may create a predisposition, but the onset is highest under age 20 and over age 60 years. Although some patients with acquired epilepsy have clear evidence of a focal brain lesion by history, examination, or neuroimaging, most are normal. Common seizure types include complex partial seizures (which affect mentation without loss of consciousness), simple partial seizures (which do not alter mentation), and secondarily generalized seizures (grand mal seizures immediately preceded by a brief complex partial or simple partial seizure).

4. When do traumatic seizures usually occur?
When the cause of trauma to the cortex is known, the onset of seizure disorder is most likely to occur within 1 year of injury, although it may occur several years later.[5,13]

5. Should prophylactic anticonvulsants be given to patients with significant head trauma?
No. The prophylactic administration of currently available anticonvulsant medications following trauma or disease of the central nervous system (CNS) probably does not alter the risk of developing a seizure disorder.[9,14]

6. When is CNS imaging warranted in the evaluation of new-onset seizure?
When the clinical manifestations of seizure disorder fit one of the syndromes of primary generalized epilepsy, with an appropriate family history, response to medications, and electro-encephalographic (EEG) findings, imaging of the brain may be unnecessary, unless specific findings or elements of the history suggest coexisting focal neuropathology. In contrast, evaluation of acquired seizure disorders always includes an imaging study of the brain in an attempt to elucidate the cause of the presumed focal cortical injury. The differential diagnosis is voluminous and includes almost all illnesses and mechanisms known to cause injury to the cortex.

7. How is epilepsy treated?
Treatment depends on whether the patient has a primary generalized or acquired seizure disorder. All of the seizures associated with primary generalized epilepsies, including absence, generalized tonic-clonic, atonic, and myoclonic seizures, may be effectively treated with Depakote (divalproex sodium). Absence seizures are also successfully treated with Zarontin (ethosuximide), which has little value in treatment of other seizure types.

Treatment of acquired seizure disorders is equally successful with either Tegretol (carbamazepine) or Dilantin (phenytoin). Three new medications—felbamate, gabapentin, and lamotrigine—recently have been approved by the Food and Drug Administration and are likely to be available by mid 1994.

Although inexpensive and effective against most types of seizures, barbiturates such as phenobarbital, primidone, and mephobarbital are less favored because of sedation, cognitive impairment, and emotional depression.

8. Are two drugs better than one in the treatment of seizures?
No. In general, polypharmaceutical treatment of seizures is not necessary and may be disadvantageous. Although it is true that the beneficial effects of most of the antiepileptic medicines may be additive, the side effects are synergistic and typically accumulate faster than the benefits. Most patients have the best profile of benefit/side effects with the use of a single, appropriately chosen, optimally titrated medication.

9. Can generic drugs be used to treat seizures?
Not usually. Most classes of medications do not require the precise degree of titration that is necessary in antiepileptic drugs. Because most antiepileptic drugs have narrow therapeutic windows, the differences in bioavailability among various generic preparations often cause clinically important fluctuations in serum levels. For these reasons, generic antiepileptic medications should not be used.

10. How frequently should laboratory tests be used to monitor patients on therapy?
In general, a complete blood count, assessment of electrolytes and liver function tests should be obtained before initiating therapy with antiepileptic medications and repeated 1–2 months later. The value of routine repetition of these tests in patients who are doing well with antiepileptic therapy is debatable.[1] A single assessment of serum levels may be useful when titration appears to be successful to document the appropriate level for the patient. This level

then may be maintained. If seizure control decreases or side effects increase, serum levels of medication should be assessed. Remember the tried and true aphorism: "Treat the patient, not the laboratory." Patients occasionally do best (no seizures or side effects) at levels below or above the usual laboratory range.

11. What is status epilepticus?

Convulsive status epilepticus is a life-threatening emergency defined as a generalized tonic-clonic seizure or a series of generalized tonic-clonic seizures without return of consciousness over a period of 30 minutes. Nonconvulsive status epilepticus involving partial or absence seizures is not associated with the poor outcomes common to generalized status epilepticus.

12. Do women with epilepsy have increased obstetric risks?

Because of the many misunderstandings about pregnancy in patients with epilepsy, it is important to educate all women of childbearing age who have seizure disorders. Whereas approximately 2% of all births in the United States involve fetal malformation, the incidence in infants born to epileptic mothers is 4–6%. This increased risk may be attributed to three causes: the underlying illness, if any, that created the mother's seizure disorder; the seizures themselves; and the medications taken by the mother to control the seizures.

As long as the mother does not experience trauma secondary to a seizure, nonconvulsive seizures have little, if any, significance to the fetus. Generalized tonic-clonic seizures in the mother have been shown to be associated with decelerations in fetal heart rate and thus place the fetus at significant risk. Therefore, patients with generalized tonic-clonic seizures should continue with antiepileptic medications from conception through delivery. The risks and benefits must be assessed on a case-by-case basis.

13. Should antiseizure medications be changed during pregnancy?

Although the teratogenicity of the various anticonvulsant medications differs, the current recommendation is to continue the regimen that has been most effective (best control with least toxicity) in the past. Because of changes in hepatic function, it is usually necessary to make gradual incremental changes in dosages of medications metabolized in the liver. Serum levels during the mother's monthly prenatal visit should guide drug dosage. At the time of delivery, the dosage should be restored to prepregnancy levels.

Epileptic mothers taking ethosuximide or barbiturates should be advised that these medications appear in breast milk in significant concentrations; thus breast feeding is inadvisable.

14. May patients with epilepsy drive a car?

The laws regarding driving (not including commercial or interstate driving) vary from state to state. Epileptics should not drive until it is clear that medication completely controls their seizures. The usual standard is a seizure-free period of 6–12 months.

15. What advice should be given to patients with epilepsy?

Routine "seizure precautions" include the advice to abstain from all activities, situations, or circumstances in which the patient may be injured (or injure others) in the event of seizure. Although certain risky activities, such as using power tools, climbing ladders, or swimming, are likely to be self-evident, other less obvious activities, such as exposure to hot tap water, may pose significant risk to the patient with an active seizure disorder.[8]

16. Do epileptics need to quit their jobs?

No. Most patients with epilepsy are able to continue working. Like patients with other chronic health problems, they are well advised to understand the Americans with Disabilities Act. Because of old fears and ignorance, employers, teachers, and/or family also may benefit from education.

17. Where can patients with epilepsy get more information?
The Epilepsy Foundation of America, which can be reached at 1 (800) EFA-1000, may be of importance to patients, families, caregivers, and clinicians who provide medical care for patients with seizure disorders.

Disclaimer: All treatment guidelines are made with the understanding that the ultimate responsibility for all evaluation and treatment decisions rests exclusively with the treating physician. The author takes no responsibility for outcome or appropriateness of treatment guidelines.

BIBLIOGRAPHY

1. Dodson WE: Level off [editorial]. Neurology 39:1009–1010, 1989.
2. Hauser WA, Hesdorffer DC: Epilepsy: Frequency, Causes and Consequences. New York, Demos Publications, 1990, p 15.
3. Hauser WA, Kurland LT: The epidemiology of epilepsy in Rochester, Minnesota, 1935 through 1967. Epilepsia 16:1–66, 1975.
4. Mattson RH, Cramer JA, Collins JF, et al: Comparison of carbamazepine, phenobarbital, phenytoin, and primidone in partial and secondarily generalized tonic-clonic seizures. N Engl J Med 313:145–151, 1985.
5. Salazar AM, Jabbari B, Vance SC, et al: Epilepsy after penetrating head injury. I. Clinical correlates: A report of the Vietnam Head Injury Study. Neurology 35:1406–1414, 1985.
6. Sato S, White BG, Penry JK, et al: Valproic acid versus ethosuximide in the treatment of absence seizures. Neurology 32:157–163, 1982.
7. Simon D, Penry JK: Sodium di-*n*-propylacetate (DPA) in the treatment of epilepsy. A review. Epilepsia 19:379–384, 1989.
8. Spitz MC, Towbin JA, Shantz D: Risk factors for burns as a consequence of seizures in patients with epilepsy. Epilepsia (in press).
9. Temkin NR, Dikmen SS, Wilensky AJ, et al: A randomized, double-blind study of phenytoin for the prevention of post-traumatic seizures. N Engl J Med 323:497–502, 1990.
10. Treiman D: VA Cooperative Study (ongoing at the time of this writing).
11. Turnball DM, Rawlins MD, Weightman D, Chadwick DW: A comparison of phenytoin and valproate in previously untreated adult epileptic patients. J Neurol Neurosurg Psychiatry 45:55–59, 1982.
12. Wallace SJ, Aldridge-Smith J: Successful prophylaxis against febrile convulsions with valproic acid or phenobarbitone. BMJ 1:353–354, 1980.
13. Weiss GH, Salazar AM, Vance SC et al: Predicting posttraumatic epilepsy in penetrating head injury. Arch Neurol 43:771–773, 1986.
14. Young B, Rapp RP, Norton JLA, et al: Failure of prophylactically administered phenytoin to prevent late posttraumatic seizure. J Neurosurg 58:236–241, 1983.

XII. Common Disorders of the Chest

81. DYSPNEA

Jeffrey A. DesJardin, M.D.

1. How is dyspnea defined?
Dyspnea (breathlessness or shortness of breath) is defined as the sensation of labored breathing and a need to increase ventilation. This "awareness of breathing" is the major feature of dyspnea; because of its unpleasant and uncomfortable nature, the symptomatic individual often avoids situations that intensify it (e.g., exertion).

2. What basic principles are implicated in the pathophysiology of dyspnea?
The sensation of breathlessness arises through a complex series of steps; no single theory fully explains the pathophysiology of dyspnea. Chemoreceptors in the carotid body and brain; mechanoreceptors in airways, lung parenchyma, chest wall, and respiratory muscles; and input from the cerebral cortex transmit information to the brainstem, where dyspnea-producing stimuli are integrated. Dyspnea, a function of the effort expended in breathing or the "work of breathing," occurs in the following situations:

1. **Increased ventilatory requirements.** Work of breathing is related to the level of ventilation. Thus, even normal individuals experience dyspnea during extreme exercise. Other conditions that increase the level of ventilation and may be associated with dyspnea include hypoxemia, hypercapnea, anemia, acidemia, hyperthyroidism, pulmonary edema, and pulmonary vascular disease (pulmonary hypertension, pulmonary emboli).

2. **Increased effort necessary to overcome an imposed load.** Work of breathing consists of two components: work to produce airflow (i.e., to overcome airway resistance) and work to stretch the lung parenchyma and chest wall. Thus, dyspnea may develop in conditions associated with either increased airflow resistance (e.g., obstructive lung disease) or "stiff" lungs and chest wall (e.g., interstitial lung disease, pulmonary edema, pleural disease, or kyphoscoliosis).

3. **Increases in the proportion of respiratory muscle force required for breathing.** Neuromuscular weakness or impaired mechanical efficiency of the muscles of respiration increases respiratory effort and produces breathlessness.

4. **Psychological influences.** Dyspnea is a conscious perception and is strongly influenced by an individual's psychological state. Thus, psychological as well as neuroanatomic factors affect the level of dyspnea.

3. What conditions should be considered when a patient presents with sudden onset of dyspnea?
Exacerbations of asthma and chronic obstructive pulmonary disease (COPD), spontaneous pneumothorax, pulmonary edema, pulmonary embolism, and chest trauma (rib fractures, pulmonary contusions) should be considered in the acutely dyspneic patient. If objective findings do not correlate with subjective complaints, anxiety and hyperventilation should be suspected as other possible causes for sudden onset of dyspnea.

4. What is the differential diagnosis of the patient who presents with chronic or subacute dyspnea?

Respiratory disease
  Upper airway obstruction
  Asthma
  COPD
  Interstitial lung disease
  Pneumonia
  Malignancy
  Cystic fibrosis
  Pulmonary vascular disease
    Pulmonary hypertension
    Pulmonary embolus
    Vasculitis
    Arteriovenous malformations
    Venoocclusive disease
  Pleural disease
Cardiovascular disease
  Congestive heart failure
  Pericardial disease
  Right-to-left shunt

Neuromuscular disease
  Spinal cord transection (above C3–C5)
  Amyotrophic lateral sclerosis
  Poliomyelitis
  Guillain-Barré syndrome
  Myasthenia gravis
  Polymyositis
  Phrenic nerve dysfunction
Thoracic and abdominal wall abnormalities
  Kyphoscoliosis
  Obesity
  Ascites
  Pregnancy
Other
  Anemia
  Metabolic acidosis
  Hyperventilation syndrome
  Hyperthyroidism
  Deconditioning

From Mahler DA: Dyspnea: Diagnosis and management. Clin Chest Med 8:215–230, 1987.

5. What is the value of routine pulmonary function testing in evaluating the patient with chronic dyspnea?

If a careful history, physical examination, and chest radiograph point to lung disease as a cause of dyspnea, an abnormality in respiratory function should be demonstrable by pulmonary function testing. Testing is important not only to confirm the diagnosis, but also to determine the degree of impairment and response to therapy. Routine spirometry is often sufficient to diagnose obstructive airways disease (a ratio of $< 70\%$ between forced expiratory volume in one second [FEV_1] and forced vital capacity [FVC]). A decrease in both FEV_1 and FVC with an FEV_1/FVC ratio greater than 70% suggests restrictive lung disease. Furthermore, a reduction in single-breath diffusing capacity (DLCO) may be the first abnormality in lung function in patients with early interstitial lung disease and the only abnormality in patients with pulmonary vascular disease.

6. When should the patient with chronic dyspnea be referred for cardiopulmonary exercise testing?

1. When the exact cause of dyspnea remains unclear despite complete pulmonary function testing.

2. When the patient has both pulmonary and cardiac disease and the contribution of either needs to be determined.

3. When the patient's symptoms are out of proportion to the severity of physiologic impairment.

4. When obesity, deconditioning, or anxiety is suspected as a cause of chronic dyspnea.

7. What other medical illnesses should be considered in patients with COPD who present with worsening shortness of breath?

Bronchogenic carcinoma, pulmonary embolism, pneumonia, pneumothorax, congestive heart failure, and ischemic heart disease are common conditions that exacerbate dyspnea in patients with COPD. Respiratory muscle weakness from steroid myopathy, hypothyroidism, or polymyositis (e.g., paraneoplastic syndrome) also should be considered. Worsening dyspnea in patients with COPD also may occur because of increased ventilatory drive due to hyperthyroidism or anemia.

8. What is the hyperventilation syndrome?

Hyperventilation syndrome, or psychogenic hyperventilation, is primary hyperventilation that produces respiratory alkalosis. Symptoms associated with this condition are extremely varied but include dyspnea in 50–90% of patients. Dyspnea, however, is rarely related to exercise. Diagnosis of hyperventilation syndrome must exclude compensatory hyperventilation and hyperventilation caused by organic or physiologic factors.

9. Why is the hyperventilation syndrome of importance to the primary care provider?

Hyperventilation syndrome affects 6–11% of the general population. The majority of cases occur in the third or fourth decade of life; women are affected 2–4 times more often than men. Anxiety is the primary cause. Symptoms frequently produce further anxiety, thus creating a vicious cycle. Treatment involves psychotherapy, behavioral modification, tricyclic antidepressants, or beta-adrenergic blockers. Anxiolytic drugs should be used only as temporary treatment.

10. Are narcotics or anxiolytics useful in the treatment of profoundly dyspneic patients?

Treatment of the underlying disease is obviously the first choice in the therapy of dyspnea. Relief of breathlessness is often incomplete, however, leading to consideration of pharmacologic agents to improve symptoms of profound dyspnea. Narcotics and anxiolytics may alter the preception of breathlessness, although they do not treat the underlying cause. The concern about their use centers on their potential to depress respiratory function and to worsen gas exchange. Most of the knowledge about such agents results from treatment of patients with COPD (dyspnea refractory to standard medical therapy) or patients with terminal cancer and intractable dyspnea.

Narcotics. Opiates have been used with variable efficacy to relieve dyspnea. Their major mechanism of action is respiratory depression through direct effects on the respiratory center of the brainstem. They not only alter the perception of breathlessness but also may reduce ventilatory drive. Exercise tolerance may increase without increased sensation of breathlessness. However, because of their frequent side effects (e.g., nausea, vomiting, constipation, drowsiness) and potential for addiction, they should be used only for the most severe cases of dyspnea in preterminal patients.

Anxiolytics. Anxiety and panic are often confounding factors in severely dyspneic patients. Because benzodiazepines act as anxiolytics and reduce respiratory drive, they are potentially beneficial in the treatment of refractory dyspnea. Early reports showed a subjective improvement in both dyspnea and exercise tolerance. However, the majority of the literature has not demonstrated consistent benefit in improving symptoms of breathlessness, exercise tolerance, or arterial blood gas values. In general, benzodiazepines are not indicated in treatment of dyspnea and should be used with extreme caution in patients with profound breathlessness and anxiety.

11. When is oxygen therapy indicated in the treatment of dyspnea?

Oxygen therapy is indicated only in dyspneic individuals with documented hypoxia at rest or with exercise. If mild hypoxemia is present (55 torr < partial pressure of oxygen [pO_2] < 59 torr), oxygen therapy is appropriate only in the dyspneic patient with evidence of cor pulmonale or pulmonary hypertension. Patients with dyspnea and no evidence of hypoxia may experience subjective relief of symptoms, but the relief is postulated to be a placebo effect due to wearing a nasal cannula.

CONTROVERSIES

12. Is the disproportionate dyspnea seen in some patients with breathlessness psychological in origin?

In patients with COPD and comparable degrees of respiratory impairment, the severity of breathlessness may vary considerably. Such variations in the level of dyspnea probably occur because dyspnea is a subjective sensation dependent on numerous factors, including past behavioral influences, the situation in which breathlessness occurs, and the patient's ability to describe breathlessness. It has been suggested that depression, anxiety, and hysterical reactions may cause disproportionate symptoms.

For:

Comparisons between patients with and without disproportionate dyspnea found that significant numbers of patients with disproportionate breathlessness have depression (52%), anxiety (22%), and hysterical reactions (26%), whereas the other group suffers from no formal psychiatric disorder. Furthermore, successful treatment of the psychiatric disorder 2–3 years later revealed complete or partial resolution of dyspnea in patients with disproportionate symptoms. Finally, some data suggest that the threshold for detection of resistive ventilatory loads is greater in anxious individuals.

Against:

Differences among patients in perception of changes in respiratory effort, thoracic displacement, or respiratory muscle force offer a physiologic explanation for differences in the sensation of dyspnea. In addition, successful treatment of psychiatric symptoms with no improvement in disproportionate dyspnea has been reported. This suggests that the psychiatric disorders are a consequence and not a cause of dyspnea.

13. Is theophylline indicated in dyspneic patients with COPD?

For:

The bronchodilator effect of theophylline may relieve symptoms in patients with obstructive lung disease. It also may improve diaphragmatic contractility and decrease the likelihood of fatigue, resulting in less dyspnea. From a clinical standpoint, some studies have shown that theophylline improves subjective symptoms of dyspnea, pulmonary function, arterial blood gases, and exercise tolerance.

Against:

Not all studies have demonstrated significant improvement in arterial blood gases, lung function, or exercise tolerance. Furthermore, a higher dose of theophylline (serum levels near 15 μg/ml) is needed to show clinical benefit; because higher serum levels are associated with more side effects, the benefits do not clearly outweigh the risks.

BIBLIOGRAPHY

1. Brashiar RE: Hyperventilation syndrome. Lung 161:257–273, 1983.
2. Burns BH, Howell JBL: Disproportionately severe breathlessness in chronic bronchitis. Q J Med 38:277–294, 1969.
3. Cohen MH, Johnston-Anderson A, Krasnow SH, et al: Treatment of intractable dyspnea: Clinical and ethical issues. Cancer Invest 10:317–321, 1992.
4. Light RW, Muro JR, Sato RI, et al: Effects of oral morphine on breathlessness and exercise tolerance in patients with chronic obstructive pulmonary disease. Am Rev Respir Dis 139:126–133, 1989.
5. Liss HP, Grant BJB: The effect of nasal flow on breathlessness in patients with chronic obstructive pulmonary disease. Am Rev Respir Dis 137:1285–1288, 1988.
6. Mahler DA: Dyspnea: Diagnosis and management. Clin Chest Med 8:215–230, 1987.
7. Man GCW, Hsu K, Sproule BJ: Effect of alprazolam on exercise and dyspnea in patients with chronic obstructive pulmonary disease. Chest 90:832–836, 1986.
8. Murciano D, Auclair MH, Pariente R: A randomized, controlled trial of theophylline in patients with severe chronic obstructive pulmonary disease. N Engl J Med 320:1521–1525, 1989.
9. Roser R, Guz A: Psychological approaches to breathlessness and its treatment. J Psychosom Res 25:439–447, 1981.
10. Sweer L, Zwillich CW: Dyspnea in the patient with chronic obstructive pulmonary disease. Clin Chest Med 11:417–445, 1990.
11. Tobin MJ: Dyspnea: Pathophysiologic basis, clinical presentation, and management. Arch Intern Med 150:1604–1613, 1990.

82. HEMOPTYSIS

Jeffrey M. Sippel, M.D.

1. Define scant hemoptysis (blood streaking), frank hemoptysis, massive hemoptysis, and pseudohemoptysis.

Scant hemoptysis is sputum that contains trace amounts of blood but is composed primarily of mucus. Frank or gross hemoptysis is expectoration of blood that originates in the lower respiratory tract (lung parenchyma, bronchi, and trachea). Scant and frank hemoptysis are the most common types in the outpatient setting. Massive hemoptysis is expectoration of more than 600 cc of blood in 24 hours or any amount that causes respiratory distress, hemodynamic compromise, or anemia. Pseudohemoptysis is expectoration of blood that does not originate from the lower respiratory tract. Sources include hematemesis or blood aspirated from the gastrointestinal (GI) tract and blood that collects in the hypopharynx or trachea from the oral cavity, sinuses, or nasopharyngeal or tracheal source.

2. What is the differential diagnosis of hemoptysis based on the quantity of blood present?

Hemoptysis commonly arises from diseases affecting the lung parenchyma or tracheobronchial tree, which may be either focal, such as bronchogenic carcinoma, pneumonia, and tuberculosis, or diffuse, such as pulmonary vasculitis and collagen vascular diseases. Cardiovascular or hematologic disorders, such as mitral stenosis or thrombocytopenia, also may be implicated, although less commonly. Although the differential diagnosis may be rather large, certain patient populations are associated with a higher frequency of specific illnesses. For example, an elderly male cigarette smoker has a much higher prevalence of lung cancer than a young woman who is more likely to have pulmonary vasculitis or collagen vascular disease. In addition, the various causes of hemoptysis may produce different amounts of bleeding. The list below is not exhaustive but focuses on the more common etiologies of hemoptysis:

Scant hemoptysis (blood streaking)
- Bronchitis
- Bronchiectasis
- Lung cancer
- Tuberculosis

Frank and massive hemoptysis
- All of the above
- Arteriovenous malformations
- Bleeding diathesis or coagulopathy
- Cystic fibrosis
- Goodpasture's syndrome
- Mitral stenosis
- Necrotizing or cavitary pneumonia
- Pulmonary embolus or infarct
- Pulmonary vasculitis
- Systemic lupus erythematosus
- Wegener's granulomatosis
- Iatrogenic (pulmonary artery catheter, tracheoinnominate fistula)

Pseudohemoptysis
- Upper GI bleed with aspiration or expectoration of blood
- Sinus, oral, pharyngeal, or laryngeal bleeding site

3. What are the most common causes of hemoptysis in the outpatient setting?

The etiology of hemoptysis has changed over the last 50 years. Tuberculosis and bronchiectasis were the most common causes of hemoptysis before effective antimicrobial chemotherapy. According to recent studies, however, bronchitis (22–44%), bronchogenic carcinoma (6–29%), and idiopathic hemoptysis (22–33%), are now the three most common etiologies. Tuberculosis is seen in only 1.5–7% of patients and bronchiectasis in 1%. The populations in these epidemiologic studies were predominantly male, cigarette smokers, and over the age of 50 years; the etiologies may vary with the population studied.

4. What factors, in combination with hemoptysis, are risks for pulmonary malignancy?

Risk Factor	Prevalence with malignancy
Cigarette smoking	45–100% have more than 40 pack-year history
Age over 40 years	Nearly 100%
Abnormal chest roentgenogram	25–80%
Symptoms for over 1 week	50–80%
Male	58–99%

5. What should be included in the initial evaluation of hemoptysis in the outpatient setting?
A thorough history focuses on quantity and duration of hemoptysis, cigarette smoking, presence of cough and sputum production, fever or other constitutional symptoms, and cardiovascular symptoms. The physical examination focuses on the nares, sinuses, oropharynx, heart, lungs, and extremities. If available, mirror laryngoscopy should be performed; if laryngoscopy is negative, a chest roentgenogram is obtained. If history and physical examination suggest an etiology other than acute bronchitis or if symptoms are recurrent, appropriate tests include sputum cytology, arterial blood gases, blood and platelet counts, prothrombin time, partial thromboplastin time, tuberculin skin test, urinalysis, and creatinine level. Pending results of these studies, further evaluation may include fiberoptic bronchoscopy and other radiographic techniques.

6. What is the role of fiberoptic bronchoscopy in the evaluation of hemoptysis?
Bronchoscopy provides diagnostic information in 10–69% of cases, depending on the subset of patients. The diagnostic yield of bronchoscopy generally increases in patients who are smokers, male, or over the age of 40 years, or who have prolonged symptoms or an abnormal chest roentgenogram. Fiberoptic bronchoscopy is an integral part of the evaluation when malignancy is suspected because tissue biopsies can be performed. Bronchoscopy also permits collection of lavage or brush specimens for mycobacterial and fungal cultures and may be useful for localizing the anatomic site of bleeding if hemoptysis is ongoing.

7. What is the role of computed tomography (CT) in the evaluation of hemoptysis?
If the chest roentgenogram is normal or nonlocalizing, chest CT scans yield additional information that suggests an etiology in 39–68% of cases. Chest CT is a reasonable alternative if malignancy is suspected and bronchoscopy is not available. Chest CT findings are abnormal in nearly 100% of patients with bronchogenic carcinoma; however, chest CT scans do not obviate the need for tissue diagnosis if malignancy is suspected. Likewise, chest roentgenogram and fiberoptic bronchoscopy fail to suggest malignancy in only 3% or less of cases. CT scans are more sensitive than either roentgenogram or fiberoptic bronchoscopy for the diagnosis of bronchiectasis.

8. Do diffuse infiltrates on chest roentgenogram always imply a diffuse process as the cause of hemoptysis?
No. Although bilateral infiltrates suggest that the hemoptysis may be due to a more widespread process or systemic illness, a focal hemorrhage may cause the same radiographic appearance if the patient aspirates blood.

9. What is idiopathic hemoptysis? How should it be managed?
Idiopathic hemoptysis is a diagnosis of exclusion and should be made only after a thorough investigation has yielded no specific diagnosis. The incidence of idiopathic hemoptysis is estimated at 22–33%, and the disorder carries an overall favorable prognosis. Adelman et al.[1] followed 67 patients with hemoptysis, a normal or nonlocalizing chest roentgenogram, and

nondiagnostic fiberoptic bronchoscopy for 3 years. The hemoptysis resolved within 6 months in 90% of patients and recurred in only 5%. Bronchogenic carcinoma was diagnosed at 20-month follow-up in only 1 patient (1.5%). The average patient age was 54 years; 72% smoked or had smoked cigarettes; 39% had a diagnosis of COPD; and 46% were tuberculin skin test-positive. A study by Santiago et al.[10] confirmed the low rate of pulmonary malignancies: only 3 of 119 patients (2.5%) developed cancer within follow-up of 2–5 years.

10. What systemic illnesses may cause hemoptysis?

Amyloidosis	Mitral stenosis
Coagulation disorders	Pulmonary-renal syndromes
(iatrogenic and acquired)	Sarcoidosis
Congestive heart failure	Systemic lupus erythematosus
Metastatic cancer	Vasculitis

11. How do the initial evaluation and management differ in massive and frank hemoptysis?

Major complications of massive hemoptysis include hemodynamic instability and death from asphyxiation. Immediate management, therefore, must focus on hemodynamic stabilization and prevention of asphyxiation by aggressive airway control. The patient may require emergent endotracheal intubation. If hemorrhage is localized to one lung, either placement of a double-lumen endotracheal tube or bronchoscopic-directed selective mainstem intubation may help to isolate and preserve gas exchange in the nonhemorrhaging lung. The nonhemor-rhaging lung also may be protected by placing the patient in the decubitus position, bleeding side down; if the hemorrhage is of unknown or diffuse origin, the patient should be placed in the Trendelenburg position. Subsequent assessment should include a complete serologic evaluation, fiberoptic or rigid bronchoscopy, and surgical consultation.

CONTROVERSY

12. Should bronchoscopy be performed early (within 48 hours) in patients with hemoptysis?

For early bronchoscopy:
1. The procedure has minimal risk and is tolerated well by most patients.
2. The diagnostic yield for visualizing the site of bleeding is greater while the patient is actively hemorrhaging.
3. Therapeutic options after visualization include endobronchial tamponade, selective mainstem intubation, and surgical resection, all of which are facilitated by localizing the site of bleeding.

Against early bronchoscopy:
1. Early bronchoscopy induces coughing, which may worsen hemoptysis.
2. Although early bronchoscopy more frequently reveals a source of bleeding (40% early vs. 10% delayed), clinical management and outcome are not affected.

BIBLIOGRAPHY

1. Adelman M, et al: Cryptogenic hemoptysis: Clinical features, bronchoscopic findings, and natural history in 67 patients. Ann Intern Med 102:829–834, 1985.
2. Berger R, Rehm SR: Bronchoscopy for hemoptysis. Chest 99:1553, 1991.
3. Gong H, Salvatierra C: Clinical efficacy of early and delayed fiberoptic bronchoscopy in patients with hemoptysis. Am Rev Respir Dis 124:221–225, 1981.
4. Jackson CV, Savage PJ, Quinn DL: Role of fiberoptic bronchoscopy in patients with hemoptysis and a normal chest roentgenogram. Chest 87:142–144, 1985.
5. Johnston H, Reisz G: Changing spectrum of hemoptysis. Underlying causes in 148 patients undergoing diagnostic flexible fiberoptic bronchoscopy. Arch Intern Med 149:1666–1668, 1989.
6. Naidich DP, et al: Hemoptysis: CT-bronchoscopic correlations in 58 cases. Radiology 177:357–362, 1990.

7. O'Neil KM, Lazarus AA: Hemoptysis. Indications for bronchoscopy. Arch Intern Med 151:171–174, 1991.
8. Poe RH, et al: Utility of fiberoptic bronchoscopy in patients with hemoptysis and a nonlocalizing chest roentgenogram. Chest 92:70–75, 1988.
9. Santiago S, Lehrman S, Williams AJ: Bronchoscopy in patients with haemoptysis and normal chest roentgenograms. Br J Dis Chest 81:186–188, 1987.
10. Santiago S, Tobias J, Williams AJ: A reappraisal of the causes of hemoptysis. Arch Intern Med 151:2449–2451, 1991.
11. Weaver LJ, Solliday N, Cugell DW: Selection of patients with hemoptysis for fiberoptic bronchoscopy. Chest 76:7–10, 1979 [see also editorial 1–2].

83. COUGH AND SPUTUM PRODUCTION

Carlos E. Girod, M.D., and Michael E. Hanley, M.D.

1. What are the components of the cough reflex?

The cough reflex protects the lung from injury and infection by clearing large bronchial airways of foreign material or accumulated secretions. The cough reflex requires interaction of three components: sensory nerves, the cough center in the central nervous system, and motor nerves. The sensory component of the cough reflex includes cough receptors located not only in the respiratory system but also in extrapulmonary sites, including the pleura, ear canal, nose, paranasal sinuses, stomach, pericardium, and diaphragm.

2. What pathophysiologic stimuli contribute to cough?

Activation of the cough reflex occurs through inflammatory, mechanical, chemical, and thermal stimuli. Inflammation of the pharynx, upper airway, trachea, and bronchi activates the cough reflex by exposing superficial sensory nerves that are abundant throughout the epithelium of the respiratory system. Mechanical stimuli, such as foreign objects, impacted mucopurulent material, postnasal drip, and airway manipulation, activate the cough reflex through stimulation of myelinated or nonmyelinated sensory nerves in the larynx or the rapidly adapting stretch receptors in the lung. Examples of chemical stimuli that may activate the cough reflex include gastric acid from gastroesophageal reflux, chlorine gas, and other irritant reducing or oxidizing agents. Thermal stimuli (cold or hot air exposure) promote cough in patients with underlying reactive airway disease.

3. What are the four most common causes of chronic cough?

Cough is the fifth most common chief complaint encountered by office-based physicians. Chronic cough is defined as troublesome cough that lasts more than 3 weeks. More than 90% of patients with chronic cough have one or more of the following etiologies: postnasal drip, 41%; occult asthma, 24%; gastroesophageal reflux, 21%; and chronic bronchitis, 5%. A large percentage of patients have a nonpulmonary disorder as the main cause of cough. In most cases, therefore, the diagnosis of chronic cough can be made without referral to a pulmonologist.

4. What are the less common causes of chronic cough?

Less common causes of chronic cough include postviral cough, bronchiectasis, bronchogenic carcinoma, left ventricular failure, sarcoidosis, esophageal diverticuli, tuberculosis, and use of angiotensin-converting enzyme (ACE) inhibitors. Most of these conditions can be diagnosed by careful history, physical exam, and chest roentgenogram. Nevertheless, some authors report that even after extensive work-up for chronic cough 12% of patients remain undiagnosed.

Rare causes of chronic cough, such as vocal cord dysfunction, laryngeal polyps, foreign body aspiration, bronchostenosis, or broncholithiasis, may require invasive, specialized procedures for diagnosis (direct laryngoscopy or fiberoptic bronchoscopy). On the other hand, chronic cough may be due to a trivial diagnosis such as loose hair in the external ear canal that impinges on the tympanic membrane and stimulates cough receptors located in the auditory canal mucosa.

5. What drugs may be associated with chronic cough?

The awareness that certain drugs may promote cough has increased. Beta blockers were once the most common medications associated with chronic cough, especially in patients with underlying or previously asymptomatic bronchial hyperreactivity. The mechanism is broncho-constriction through direct blockade of beta-2 receptors in the airways.

More recently, a new class of widely used drugs with vasodilator and antihypertensive effects—the ACE inhibitors—have been associated with a high incidence (5–25%) of chronic cough. The pathophysiologic mechanism is believed to be the accumulation of prostaglandins, kinins, and/or substance P, which directly or indirectly excites cough receptors that initiate the cough reflex. The diagnosis can be eliminated or confirmed with a short 4-day trial of withdrawal of the medication and careful observation for resolution or improvement of cough. Therapy consists of removal of the offending medication. Attempts to treat ACE inhibitor cough with the addition of nonsteroidal inflammatory agents or change to another ACE inhibitor are not recommended.

6. What is psychogenic cough?

Psychogenic cough is a rare condition in which chronic cough is believed to be consciously or unconsciously mediated by the patient. It is usually seen in children or adolescents during periods of high emotional stress. Psychogenic cough is a diagnosis of exclusion. Clues to the diagnosis include complete absence of cough during sleep and ability to reproduce the cough pattern at the examiner's request. In most cases, psychogenic cough is self-limited and resolves in a few months. A unique therapeutic technique involves placement of a chest harness or folded bedsheet around the chest with a large knot over the sternum and negative reinforcement through sharp commands to stop coughing. This technique was successful in 31 of 33 pediatric patients.

7. How does a history of sputum production help in the evaluation of chronic cough?

Sputum production may promote cough through direct stimulation of cough receptors in the airways by accumulated secretions. A history of sputum production helps to narrow the differential diagnosis of chronic cough to primary pulmonary conditions, such as chronic bronchitis, emphysema, bronchiectasis, and cystic fibrosis. It is unlikely that cough accompanied by sputum production originates from an extrapulmonary source. Therefore, the cause of chronic cough accompanied by sputum production is easily diagnosed by obtaining a careful history, physical exam, chest roentgenogram, and, if needed, pulmonary function testing.

8. What are the roles of sinus radiographs, pulmonary function tests, and other laboratory evaluations in the diagnosis of chronic cough?

The most helpful parts of the evaluation of patients with chronic cough are the history and physical examination. In a recent study of 102 patients, Irwin et al.[6] delineated the clinical usefulness of the following tools in the diagnosis of chronic cough:

1. History	70%	5. Upper GI series	21%
2. Physical exam	49%	6. Esophageal pH monitoring	16%
3. Pulmonary function tests	26%	7. Sinus radiographs	15%
4. Methacholine inhalation challenge	23%	8. Chest radiograph	7%
		9. Bronchoscopy	4%

Sinus radiographs, pulmonary function tests, methacholine inhalational challenge, upper GI series, and ambulatory pH monitoring are helpful only if the initial history and physical examination suggest sinus disease, occult asthma, or gastroesophageal reflux, respectively. A useful diagnostic protocol for the evaluation of chronic cough is based on this strategy:

1. All patients must receive a careful history and physical examination focused on the anatomic location of cough receptors. Chest radiograph is recommended for all patients.

2. In smokers and patients with occupational or environmental exposures, initial steps include elimination of the irritant and observation, with no further diagnostic studies for at least 4 weeks.

3. Other imaging studies and pulmonary physiologic evaluation depend on the suspected cause after initial evaluation by history, physical examination, and chest radiograph. For example, if postnasal drip and chronic sinus disease are suspected, sinus roentgenogram and allergy evaluation should be ordered first. If occult asthma is suspected, pulmonary function tests and methacholine inhalation challenge are recommended. If no cause is suggested by the history and physical examination, the next appropriate step is pulmonary function testing before and after administration of a bronchodilator or methacholine.

4. If the above strategy suggests no cause, tests for the evaluation of gastroesophageal reflux are recommended, including esophagogram and, if available, ambulatory pH monitoring, even in the absence of symptoms. If these studies are negative, bronchoscopy and/or cardiac function imaging studies are recommended.

5. If one or more possibilities are discovered, specific therapy should be initiated to pinpoint the exact cause of the cough.

9. When does a cough that follows an upper respiratory tract illness warrant evaluation?
Viral infections of the upper respiratory tract may promote or activate the cough reflex by injuring the airway epithelium and exposing sensory nerves that represent the afferent loop of the cough reflex. Approximately 77% of patients affected by a viral upper or lower respiratory tract infection have a cough that lasts up to 3 weeks. In such patients, bronchial hyperactivity, as demonstrated with inhalational challenge, persists for up to 7 weeks after viral infection. In a significant number of patients, chronic cough may last longer than 8 weeks from the onset of viral infection. Therefore, full evaluation for chronic cough after viral upper and lower respiratory infection is not recommended unless the cough lasts longer than 8 weeks or is significantly troublesome to the patient.

10. When does a cough in a cigarette smoker require evaluation?
The evaluation of chronic cough in smokers may lead to multiple unnecessary and expensive diagnostic procedures. Useful guidelines for full evaluation of chronic cough in a smoker include (1) change in or development of sputum production, (2) increase in frequency of cough, (3) hemoptysis, or (4) constitutional symptoms, such as weight loss and fatigue. Evaluation should focus on exclusion of lung cancer, emphysema, and chronic bronchitis. The physician also must use this opportunity to reinforce the need for smoking cessation.

Evaluation should follow the diagnostic protocol described in question 7, focusing on history, physical exam, and chest radiograph. If the results are negative, no other diagnostic tests are recommended before complete cessation of smoking. If cough persists after 4 weeks of smoking cessation, fiberoptic bronchoscopy should be considered.

11. What complications are associated with cough?
1. Musculoskeletal: torn chest muscle, rib fractures
2. Pulmonary: pneumothorax, pneumomediastinum
3. Psychological: self-consciousness, fear of public appearances
4. Cardiovascular: syncope or near syncope
5. Neurologic: cough headache
6. Genitourinary: urinary incontinence

7. Constitutional: fatigue, poor appetite, weight loss
8. Miscellaneous: wound dehiscence, hoarseness

12. When and how should chronic cough be treated empirically?

The anatomic diagnostic protocol delineated by Irwin et al.[6] leads to a specific diagnosis and treatment for chronic cough in more than 90% of patients. Failure of specific therapy is likely due to incorrect diagnosis or undertreatment. Therefore, empirical therapy for chronic cough is seldom necessary.

When complications are serious or diagnostic tests are not available, chronic cough should be treated in the absence of a diagnosis. However, the cough reflex should not be suppressed if it benefits the patient by clearing the airway of purulent secretions. When empirical therapy is indicated, the most studied and efficacious nonspecific antitussives should be used: narcotics (codeine or codeine-derived cough suspensions), nonnarcotics (most commonly dextromethorphan), and inhaled ipratropium bromide.

Certain clinical scenarios of chronic cough also merit empirical therapy. In some patients diagnosis of gastroesophageal reflux may require 24-hour ambulatory pH monitoring, which is not readily available in most medical centers. Ing et al.[3] performed 24-hour ambulatory pH monitoring on 13 patients with chronic cough of unclear etiology. The majority had reflux episodes associated with onset of cough, and 11 of 13 patients responded to at least 2 weeks of therapy with histamine blockers. Therefore, in patients suspected of having gastroesophageal reflux, empirical therapy with histamine blockers and antireflux techniques should be instituted with careful observation of changes in the cough pattern.

Because of the high incidence of chronic cough due to occult asthma, many authors recommend a short course of oral corticosteroids for chronic cough with no obvious cause. Empirical steroids also may be helpful in treating postviral cough by relieving the associated airway inflammation and reactivity.

13. What is the role of mucolytic therapy in the management of chronic cough and sputum production?

Conditions associated with chronic cough and accompanied by sputum production include emphysema, chronic bronchitis, bronchiectasis, cystic fibrosis, and diseases of the large airways. Although its benefits have not been well documented, mucolytic therapy frequently is used in such clinical settings. Most common mucolytic agents work by thinning hyperviscous mucus. Examples include nebulized water and hypertonic electrolyte solutions, iodides and organic iodine compounds, guaifenesin, ipecacuanha, bromhexine, N-acetyl cysteine (Mucomyst), and proteolytic enzymes. Clinical studies have shown that many of these agents have no benefit in the treatment of chronic sputum-producing conditions, and most must be given at high, nauseating doses to achieve mucolytic action. Nevertheless, mucolytic agents may be helpful in short-course treatment of acute viral respiratory infections and in acute exacerbations of chronic sputum disorders.

14. Do patients with persistent cough after an upper respiratory illness require pulmonary function tests?

Persistent cough after an upper respiratory tract infection is common. Patients may develop obstruction of the small airways and increased bronchial reactivity, both of which can be documented by pulmonary function testing and methacholine challenge. In most patients the cough resolves without therapy in less than 3 weeks. If pulmonary function tests and methacholine inhalational challenge are performed too early ($<$ 7 weeks) after an upper respiratory tract infection, false-positive results may lead to the erroneous diagnosis of bronchial asthma. Therefore, persistent cough after upper respiratory viral illness is best treated by a short course of corticosteroid and/or inhaled ipratropium bromide. Pulmonary function testing is not recommended.

CONTROVERSY

15. Is fiberoptic bronchoscopy of value in the evaluation of chronic cough?
In the early 1970s, chronic, severe, unexplained cough was an indication for fiberoptic bronchoscopy. Most of the controversy surrounding bronchoscopy for chronic cough is due to this uncorroborated indication, which was based on anecdotal reports of high yields of endobronchial abnormalities or carcinoma. In the 1980s and 1990s, many careful studies of patients with chronic cough demonstrated that bronchoscopy in a patient with a normal chest radiograph results in a low yield (approximately 4%) of diagnoses. Irwin et al.[6] performed fiberoptic bronchoscopy in 51 of 109 patients with chronic cough and made a diagnosis of occult bronchogenic carcinoma in only one. Fiberoptic bronchoscopy is recommended if the chest roentgenogram is abnormal, but it should not be included routinely in the evaluation of chronic cough.

On the other hand, Sen and Walsh[12] performed bronchoscopy in 25 patients with undiagnosed chronic cough despite careful examination, chest radiograph, and trial of empirical therapy. Fifty percent of the patients were older (> 50 years) smokers with extensive prior work-up for cough. In approximately one-fourth, bronchoscopy yielded a diagnosis of broncholithiasis, tracheobronchopathia, tuberculous bronchostenosis, laryngeal dyskinesis, or laryngeal polyps. The authors recommend bronchoscopy in selected older patients with undiagnosed cough that lasts more than 2 months and is refractory to empirical therapy.

BIBLIOGRAPHY

1. Cohlan S, Stone SM: The cough and the bed sheet. Pediatrics 74:11–15, 1984.
2. Fuller RW, Jackson DM: Physiology and treatment of cough. Thorax 45:425–430, 1990.
3. Ing AJ, Mgu MC, Breslin ABX: Chronic persistent cough and clearance of esophageal acid. Chest 102:1668–1671, 1992.
4. Irwin RS, Curley FJ, Pratter MR: The effects of drugs on cough. Eur J Respir Dis 71(Suppl 153):173–181, 1987.
5. Irwin RS, Zawacki JK, Curley FJ, et al: Chronic cough as the sole presenting manifestation of gastroesophageal reflux. Am Rev Respir Dis 140:1294–1300, 1989.
6. Irwin RS, Curley FJ, French CL: Chronic cough: The spectrum and frequency of causes, key components of the diagnostic evaluation, and outcome of specific therapy. Am Rev Respir Dis 141:640–647, 1990.
7. Irwin RS, Curley FJ: The treatment of chronic cough: A comprehensive review. Chest 99:1477–1484, 1991.
8. Israili ZH, Hall WD: Cough and angioneurotic edema associated with angiotensin-converting enzyme inhibitor therapy: A review of the literature and pathophysiology. Ann Intern Med 178:234–242, 1992.
9. O'Connell EJ, Rojas AR, Sachs MI: Cough-type asthma: A review. Ann Allergy 66:278–282, 1991.
10. Poe RH, Israel RH, Utell MJ, Hall WJ: Chronic cough: Bronchoscopy or pulmonary function testing? Am Rev Respir Dis 126:160–162, 1982.
11. Poe RH, Harder RV, Israel RH, Kallay MC: Chronic persistent cough: Experience in diagnosis and outcome using an anatomic diagnostic protocol. Chest 95:728–732, 1989.
12. Sen RP, Walsh TE: Fiberoptic bronchoscopy for refractory cough. Chest 99:33–35, 1991.
13. Widdicombe JG: Mechanisms of cough and its regulation. Eur J Respir Dis 153(Suppl):173–181, 1987.
14. Zanjanian MH: Expectorants and antitussive agents: Are they helpful? Ann Allergy 44:290–295, 1980.

84. UPPER RESPIRATORY INFECTIONS AND SINUSITIS

Thomas R. Vendegna, M.D.

1. Define the spectrum of upper respiratory tract illness.
Upper respiratory illness (URI), which is responsible for a majority of the morbidity in the United States, consists primarily of the common cold, pharyngitis, otitis, and sinusitis.

2. Why has no cure been found for the common cold?
The common cold consists of five families of virus, each with different serotypes: parainfluenza, rhinovirus, respiratory syncytial virus, coxsackievirus, and coronavirus. It is extremely difficult to develop an agent or vaccine that is effective in preventing or treating all of the insulting agents.

3. When is an individual at most risk for a cold? How is the infection spread?
The peak incidence (6–8 colds/1000 population/day) coincides with the seasonal prevalence of the causative viruses, usually during the winter months. During an average year adults and children suffer 2–4 colds/year and 6–8 colds/year, respectively. Cigarette smokers experience the same incidence of common colds but have a more severe course.

The mode of transmission has been debated for many years. Airborne particles are suggested by transmission of clinical symptoms between infected and healthy individuals across a divided room, if airflow is maintained. Similarly, the rate of transmission between infected and healthy individuals playing cards was the same whether the healthy players were unable to touch their face if allowed to move their arms freely; thus direct contact may not be the most important mode of spread. Although research of this nature is difficult, primary transmission is probably through airborne particles, although other forms, such as direct contact, also may contribute.

4. What is the effect of vitamin C on the common cold?
Multiple studies have demonstrated no prophylactic effect of vitamin C against the common cold. However, vitamin C decreases duration of symptoms, mildly improves their objective severity, and greatly improves subjective measures of severity. Vitamin C appears to be quite safe even in high doses, but most individuals experience diarrhea at doses of 4–10 gm/day because of the excess that is not absorbed.

5. How does vitamin C work?
The beneficial effects of vitamin C may be due to its antioxidant properties. Most viruses that cause the common cold result in little epithelial damage; thus most of the symptoms are due to inflammatory response. Vitamin C may decrease the damage caused by oxygen free radicals that have escaped neutrophil phagosomes, where most of the virus is killed.

6. What is the treatment of the common cold?
Because so many medical therapies and home remedies have been tried, it is hard to gather information about effectiveness. An intense review of the literature, however, reveals that in adolescents and adults chlorpheniramine, pseudoephrine hydrochloride, oxymetazoline hydrochloride, phenylpropanolamine hydrochloride, ipratropium bromide, and atropine methonitrate improve nasal symptoms. Combination therapy using antihistamines and decongestants also relieves symptoms. Naproxen has no documented effect on shedding of rhinovirus but improves symptoms. Studies confirm that antihistamines, decongestants, and analgesics relieve symptoms but do not alter the course of viral infection.

7. What pathogens are involved in pharyngitis?
The infective agents in viral pharyngitis are similar to those that cause the common cold. Laryngitis with pharyngitis suggests a viral etiology. In addition, bacterial infection also is common (see chapter 27). Primary infection with the human immunodeficiency virus (HIV) may present as pharyngitis with adenopathy and should be considered in high-risk populations.

8. What conditions predispose to sinusitis?
Prolonged URI (> 7 days), smoking, allergies, mechanical difficulties (such as deviated septum or polyps), and certain diseases, such as HIV infection and cystic fibrosis.

9. When should fungal causes of sinusitis be considered?
Immunocompromised patients and patients with diabetes mellitus are at risk for fungal infections of the sinus, which may be rapidly invasive organisms.

10. When should the clinician treat for sinusitis?
The anatomic location determines the presenting complaints of sinusitis. However, maxillary sinusitis is the most common form after the common cold. Clinical symptoms include cough and purulent discharge; facial pain, fever, and headache are far less common. Confirmatory tests include opacification by transillumination. A single sinus radiograph (Waters' view) demonstrating opacification, air fluid levels, or thickening > 8 mm is the most sensitive, specific, and cost-effective diagnostic test.

11. How should sinusitis be treated?
A 10-day course of oral antibiotics, usually trimethoprin sulfamethoxazole, amoxicillin–clavu-lanate, or cefuroxime, is indicated for acute maxillary sinusitis. Symptoms should improve within days; persistent symptoms suggest mechanical obstruction or infection with resistant organisms. Although therapy for chronic maxillary sinusitis should be aimed at improving drainage, a trial of 4–6 weeks of antibiotics directed at anaerobic organisms is reasonable.

12. When should sinus radiographs be taken?
Radiographs are mandatory for the diagnosis of frontal, ethmoid, and sphenoid sinusitis. Computed tomography (CT) and consultation with an otolaryngologist are indicated for the evaluation of complications, often, serious. Infections in these sinuses should be suspected in the presence of the following symptoms or complications:

Sinus	Symptoms	Physical Examination	Complications
Frontal	Fever, purulent discharge	Tenderness over frontal sinus	Subperiosteal abscess (forehead edema)
Ethmoid	Fever, eye pain	Edema of eyelid Conjunctival injection	Orbital disease such as ophthalmoplegia, proptosis
Sphenoid	Fever, headache	Tenderness over vertex or mastoids	Cavernous sinus thrombosis, meningitis

13. When does a sinus radiograph return to normal?
After acute sinusitis, radiographs may remain abnormal for as long as 2 months. Thus, follow-up films are not routinely indicated; failure of therapy in the first few months is determined by clinical course.

14. Can a nasal swab be used to direct antibiotic therapy?
No. Organisms identified by nasal swab do not correlate with organisms identified by direct sinus puncture. Thus, when sinusitis is complicated, sinus puncture may be needed to determine the etiologic organism.

BIBLIOGRAPHY

1. Gwaltney JM, Scheld WM, Sande MA, Sydnor A: The microbial etiology and antimicrobial therapy of adults with acute community-acquired sinusitis: A fifteen-year experience at the University of Virginia and review of selected studies. J Allergy Clin Immunol 90:457–461, 1992.
2. Hemila H: Vitamin C and the common cold. Br J Nutr 67:3–16, 1992.
3. Herr RD: Acute sinusitis: Diagnosis and treatment update. Am Fam Physician 44:2055–2062, 1991.
4. Karma P, Palva T, Kouvalainen K, et al: Finnish approach to the treatment of acute otitis media. Report of the Finnish Consensus Conference. Ann Otol Rhinol Laryngol 129(Suppl):1–19, 1987.
5. Lloyd EL: Transmission of common cold. Lancet 1:597, 1988.
6. Mandell GL, Douglas RG, Bennett JE: Principles and Practices of Infectious Disease, 3rd ed. New York, Churchill Livingstone, 1990, pp 489–516.
7. Pichichero ME: Culture and antigen detection tests for streptococcal tonsillopharyngitis. Am Fam Physician 45:199–205, 1992.
8. Smith MBH, Feldman W: Over-the-counter cold medications: A critical review of clinical trials between 1950 and 1991. JAMA 269:2258–2263, 1993.
9. Sperber SJ, Hendley JO, Hayden FG, et al: Effects of naproxen on experimental rhinovirus colds. Ann Intern Med 117:37–41, 1992.
10. Woolbert LF: Do antihistamines and decongestants prevent otitis media? Pediatr Nurs 16:265–267, 1990.

85. ASTHMA AND CHRONIC OBSTRUCTIVE PULMONARY DISEASE

John E. Fitzgerald, M.D., and Michael E. Hanley, M.D.

1. What are the important historical considerations in asthma?

Asthma is usually easy to diagnose by its periodicity and characteristic symptoms. Chest tightness, breathlessness, and wheezing are reported most commonly. In some patients, especially children and adolescents, cough may be the only symptom. Once the diagnosis is made, emphasis should turn to identification of triggers that may be avoidable or treatable. Patients with extrinsic asthma usually have a personal or family history of atopy, high serum IgE levels, and symptoms triggered by inhalation of readily identifiable allergens. Exercise, cold air, and inhaled irritants or fumes are other common triggers. Esophageal reflux and chronic sinusitis may worsen asthma; a history of such disorders should be pursued aggressively. Some patients may have poor control because of concomitant use of beta blockers or nonsteroidal drugs. Others may experience symptoms after exposure to metabisulfite in wines and salad bars. If the patient works in a high-risk occupation[3] or reports improvement in symptoms during holidays and weekends, occupational asthma should be suspected.

2. Is there a difference in the pathophysiology of intrinsic and extrinsic asthma?

No. Asthma is an inflammatory disease of the airways characterized by reversible airflow limitation. The pattern of inflammation is similar in allergic (extrinsic) and nonallergic (intrinsic) asthma. The airways are infiltrated with eosinophils and lymphocytes. Release of inflammatory mediators results in airway edema, smooth muscle hypertrophy, and mucus secretion. Mast cell activation and histamine release are probably important in the early bronchoconstrictor response to allergens and other stimuli but not critical in the more chronic late-phase inflammatory reaction, which causes bronchial hyperresponsiveness.

3. Why may bronchoprovocation testing be useful in the diagnosis of asthma?

Spirometry that reveals obstruction with substantial improvement after inhalation of a bronchodilator is highly suggestive of the diagnosis of asthma. However, asthma is an episodic condition in most patients, and many have normal spirometry between exacerbations. In this setting, bronchoprovocation testing should be performed; a patient with unexplained cough or dyspnea also may be diagnosed by bronchoprovocation. Testing involves measuring spirometry after inhalation of escalating doses of methacholine, histamine, or specific substances such as metabisulfites (if the history suggests possible sensitivity). It also may involve exercise testing or inhalation of cold, dry air. The sensitivity of bronchial challenge testing is quite high, but the specificity is low. Other possible diagnoses include chronic obstructive pulmonary disease (COPD), viral respiratory tract infections, smoke inhalation or exposure to chemical irritants, cystic fibrosis, hay fever, and sarcoidosis. Patients who survive the adult respiratory distress syndrome (ARDS) also may demonstrate the same phenomenon.

4. Should patients with asthma undergo inhalation challenge to identify offending allergens?
The majority of patients with asthma demonstrate immediate skin-test reactions to common airborne allergens. Inhalation of allergens is an important mechanism by which asthmatic symptoms are maintained. Perennial symptoms are most often related to house dust mites. Pet dander and cockroaches produce other common aeroallergens, and seasonal asthma is usually related to pollens or molds. Identification of offending allergens by inhalation challenge generally should not be performed because of the potential to induce life-threatening, refractory bronchospasm.

5. When may patients benefit from immunotherapy for asthma?
Immunotherapy may have a role in treating extrinsic asthma when the patient's history correlates well with skin-test results, when avoidance of the allergen is not possible, or when symptoms are difficult to control with inhaled corticosteroids and bronchodilators. If desensitization therapy is selected, higher doses of antigen and longer duration of treatment probably produce the best results. However, evidence that some asthmatics improve with desensitization therapy is limited.

6. When should occupational asthma be considered?
Occupational asthma is a condition characterized by reversible airflow limitation that results from exposure to certain chemicals and antigens in the workplace. Over 200 substances are known to produce the syndrome.[3] Symptoms usually develop within a few years of steady exposure. The typical patient experiences relief outside the workplace (e.g., over the weekend or during vacations) but relapses on return to work. Frequent peak-flow monitoring throughout the workday and on weekends for 3–4 weeks may be necessary to make the diagnosis, because patients with predominantly late-phase asthmatic reactions do not become symptomatic until hours after exposure, typically when they are at home. Patients with preexisting asthma who experience exacerbations due to nonspecific irritants in the workplace do not qualify for the diagnosis of occupational asthma. Treatment hinges on avoidance of the antigen; continued exposure may translate into progressive disease. If changing jobs is not an option, the use of a respirator and standard asthma therapy must be strongly considered.

7. What are the goals of therapy in asthma?
Treatment of asthma varies depending on its severity. Patients with mild asthma have infrequent exacerbations and may be managed adequately with bronchodilators as needed. Moderate and severe asthma are characterized by more frequent or severe exacerbations. The principal goals in such patients are to prevent the majority of attacks by limiting airway hyperresponsiveness and to maintain near-normal lung function while avoiding the unwanted effects of polypharmacy. Patients with moderate asthma should be treated with prophylactic anti-inflammatory pharmacotherapy with inhaled steroids (200–1600 μg/day) or cromolyn (2 puffs 4 times/day). Aerosolized corticosteroid therapy should begin after an exacerbation when prednisone is tapered to 10 mg/day. Dosing 4 times/day is generally preferred when asthma is clinically active. If symptoms (or peak flows) suggest inadequate control or if the patient requires more frequent use of beta agonists, the dose of inhaled steroid should be increased up

to 1600 μg/day. Patients must be educated about the disease and allowed to participate actively in tailoring treatment. For chronic severe asthma characterized by daily symptoms and severe limitation of physical activity, regularly scheduled beta agonists (e.g., albuterol, 1–2 puffs every 4–6 hr) and oral steroids may be required. Before beginning sustained treatment with oral glucocorticoids, inhaled steroid and beta-agonist therapy should be maximized, metered dose inhaler (MDI) technique should be checked, and a careful search for reversible triggers (e.g., avoidable allergens, chronic sinusitis) should be made. Theophylline also may be considered at this stage, but it always should be initiated at a low dose (200–400 mg/day) with gradual titration upward until a good response is achieved. The dose required to achieve the usual therapeutic target of 12–20 μg/ml varies greatly from patient to patient. Toxicity increases markedly when serum levels exceed 20 μg/ml.

8. How should patients with asthma be educated?
Education involves helping patients to understand the disease and to practice the skills necessary to manage it. Information should include the pathophysiology of asthma, especially signs and symptoms, and the need to identify and avoid triggers. In addition, the importance of close monitoring of airway function with peak-flow meters and early intervention when attacks begin must be stressed. Finally, patients must be educated about therapeutic approaches, including the mechanism of action of medications, potential side effects with acute and chronic use (including misconceptions), proper use of inhalers, indications for emergency care, and written plans for managing acute exacerbations.

9. Is peak-flow monitoring useful in asthma?
Studies have suggested a reduction in the severity of asthma and reduced airflow variability when peak flows are monitored for several months and therapy is adjusted accordingly. Peak-flow meters simply measure the maximal rate of expiratory airflow after inspiration to total lung capacity. Because peak flows are highly dependent on personal effort, patients must be well motivated. If effort is good, serial peak flows provide an objective measurement of airway function and are useful in monitoring respiratory trends in moderate and severe asthma. Such monitoring is important because some patients can subjectively detect changes in airflow, whereas others cannot. Optimal benefit from peak-flow monitoring therefore requires keeping a diary that records simultaneous symptoms. The patient should record peak flows each morning and evening (before and after use of a bronchodilator), and whenever chest symptoms occur. Normally, some diurnal variation is seen, with morning values less than evening values. The degree of hyperresponsiveness in asthmatics has been shown to correlate with early morning peak flows, the gap between morning and evening values (normally < 15%), and the amount of improvement in flow rates after bronchodilator use. If a trend toward increased hyperresponsiveness is seen, the dose of inhaled steroid may be augmented. The converse also may be true.

10. How does magnesium work in acute asthma?
Intravenous magnesium, 1–2 gm administered over 20 minutes, is helpful in treating patients with moderate-to-severe attacks who do not respond to beta agonists. Magnesium is believed to interfere with calcium-dependent contraction of smooth muscles and release of histamine from mast cells; it also may potentiate the effects of beta-adrenergic agents on the airways. In addition, magnesium decreases release of bronchoconstricting acetylcholine from nerve terminals.

11. Does heparin have a therapeutic role?
Recent evidence suggests that inhaled heparin may prevent exercise-induced bronchospasm (EIB). By interfering with inosine triphosphate-mediated release of calcium, heparin may reduce mast-cell degranulation and the release of bronchoconstricting substances. Inhaled heparin may prove to be even more effective than cromolyn or preexertion bronchodilators in blocking EIB.

12. When should a patient with asthma be hospitalized?

The decision to hospitalize an asthmatic patient depends on several factors, including the nature and persistence of the inciting stimulus and the severity of prior attacks (history of hospitalizations, intubation, steroid dependence). Indicators of severe obstruction include tachycardia ($>$ 110 bpm), extensive use of accessory muscles of respiration, pulsus paradoxus $\geq$ 15, and inability to complete a sentence. The initial forced expiratory volume in 1 second (FEV_1) is generally $<$ 40% of the predicted value. Impending arrest is suggested by cyanosis, altered mental status, normal-to-high $PaCO_2$, low pH, exhaustion, bradycardia, or a silent chest. If signs and symptoms do not improve within 20–30 minutes of aggressive beta-adrenergic therapy, the patient should be admitted. If discharge from the emergency department (ED) is considered, improvement in symptoms and spirometry must be significant and sustained with a rise in FEV_1 to at least 40% of the predicted value after 60–90 minutes. With a history of brittle asthma, relapsing course over the previous weeks or months, or prior ED visits during the current exacerbation, the patient should be considered for admission, regardless of the acute response to bronchodilators and steroids.

13. What is the proper way to use an MDI?

After shaking the inhaler, the patient should exhale normally to functional residual capacity (FRC), place the device about 4 cm in front of the mouth, simultaneously depress the canister, and begin a slow inhalation. Inspiration continues to total lung capacity (TLC), at which point the breath is held for at least a few seconds. Inspiration faster than 4–5 seconds causes excessive deposition of particles in the oropharynx and large airways. Breath-holding is also crucial to allow aerosolized particles to settle on the mucosal surface of the targeted small airways. When used properly, MDIs are at least as effective as nebulizers. Spacers decrease the amount of medication lost to the air or deposited in the oropharynx and should be used routinely during severe exacerbations when slow inspiration and prolonged breath-holding are difficult to perform. They also are useful if proper MDI technique cannot be mastered.

14. What is chronic obstructive pulmonary disease (COPD)?

COPD has no precise definition. To some physicians, it simply refers to any condition associated with chronic airflow limitation. The long list of such disorders includes refractory asthma, cystic fibrosis, and various granulomatous lung diseases. By most physicians, however, COPD is used as a synonym for chronic bronchitis and emphysema. Chronic bronchitis is a clinical diagnosis defined as the presence of a productive cough for three or more months in at least 2 consecutive years without a known underlying cause. Histologically, inflammation of the airway mucosa and hypertrophy of submucosal glands occurs as a result of chronic exposure to inhaled irritants. Emphysema is a pathologic diagnosis defined as the irreversible enlargement of airspaces distal to terminal bronchioles with destruction of gas-exchanging surfaces. As alveolar septae are destroyed, radial traction on small airways is lost. This loss of elastic recoil results in hyperinflation, excessive collapse of airways during expiration, and chronic airflow limitation. Cigarette smoking is by far the most important risk factor in the development of COPD, but only 10–15% of smokers develop clinically significant disease.

15. Is it important to differentiate clinically or physiologically between the blue bloaters and pink puffers?

Patients with chronic bronchitis, often referred to as "blue bloaters," present with cough and copious sputum production. They are typically overweight and tend to have more upper respiratory infections as well as worse matching of ventilation and perfusion than patients with emphysema. Hypoxemia and hypercapnia are worse, and complications such as cor pulmonale and polycythemia are more prevalent. Because patients with predominant bronchitis are not markedly hyperinflated and have a tendency toward superimposed hypoventilation, dyspnea (which is related to work of breathing) may not be a major complaint.

Patients with predominant emphysema, often referred to as "pink puffers," are typically thin. Lung volumes are considerably elevated due to air trapping, and dyspnea is a major complaint. Pursed lip breathing and use of accessory muscles of respiration are common, and breath sounds are markedly diminished. In contrast to patients with chronic bronchitis, diffusing capacity may be severely reduced, indicating a major disturbance at the alveolar-capillary interface. Ventilation and perfusion deficits are relatively balanced, however, resulting in only mild or moderate hypoxemia. Hypercapnia usually occurs only during acute exacerbations or in endstage disease. Consequently, the emphysematous patient experiences fewer complications of chronic hypoxia and hypercapnia and generally lives longer but has more disability related to breathlessness.

Although pure examples exist, chronic bronchitis and emphysema typically coexist in varying proportions within the same patient. In the endstage patient, it is particularly difficult to distinguish between the two.

16. What concerns arise in administering oxygen therapy in patients with COPD?

A common worry associated with administering oxygen in patients with COPD is that it will suppress the patient's hypoxic ventilatory drive and result in dangerous hypoventilation. In reality, several studies have shown that, even while breathing 100% oxygen, the reduction in overall ventilation is generally minimal. When oxygen is administered, hypoxic bronchocon-striction is reduced throughout the lung, including areas which are poorly perfused due to destruction of septal capillaries. The result is increased dead-space ventilation, usually accompanied by a modest rise in carbon dioxide tension. Some patients show an *increase* in minute ventilation as a result of the rising $PaCO_2$. When oxygen therapy is instituted, the flow rate should be titrated gradually upward to maintain a PaO_2 of 60 and an oxygen saturation of 90% without overcorrection. Any adjustment should be accompanied by measurement of arterial blood gases. Oxygen must not be withheld from a hypoxic patient because of fear of a rising $PaCO_2$.

17. Are bronchodilators indicated in patients with COPD if spirometry does not improve acutely after their administration?

Unfortunately, many patients with COPD are labelled as nonresponders in the pulmonary testing laboratory when, on one occasion, they fail to show improvement after beta-adrenergic treatment. Although patients with COPD rarely respond to bronchodilators as dramatically as patients with asthma, most have a component of airway hyperreactivity that improves with treatment. Benefit may be indicated over a few weeks of treatment by improvement in FEV_1, decreased hyperinflation (with or without improved flow rates), reduction in dyspnea, or improved exercise tolerance. Additionally, in patients with stable COPD, anticholinergic agents such as ipratropium bromide produce more bronchodilation than conventional doses of beta agonists and do not lose efficacy over time. Anticholinergics are especially useful in patients with chronic bronchitis, because they reduce the volume of sputum without changing its viscosity. However, because maximal benefit is not achieved for 30 minutes or more after use, these agents are less convenient for testing and often are not used in the pulmonary function laboratory.

18. Are corticosteroids effective in patients with COPD?

Although corticosteriod therapy in some form is essential in managing all patients with moderate or severe asthma, it is often ineffective in patients with COPD. However, 10–20% of stable outpatients with COPD benefit from steroids. Although such patients also tend to have the greatest responses to bronchodilators, it is difficult to predict exactly who will respond to steroids. A clinical trial is therefore warranted in patients with moderate-to-severe disease after cessation of smoking and institution of maximal bronchodilator therapy. Pulmonary function testing should be performed before and after the trial to assess objectively the effect on airflow limitation. Prednisone, 40 mg/day (or the equivalent) for 4 weeks, is a reasonable trial. If the patient shows significant objective improvement, the dose should be tapered to the lowest effective maintenance level. No solid evidence indicates that patients with COPD can be helped with inhaled corticosteroids.

19. What can be done to improve quality of life in patients with severe COPD?

Despite cessation of smoking and optimal medical therapy (including oxygen), patients with severe COPD often continue to complain of breathlessness. Patients begin to avoid physical activity because of anticipated dyspnea and their level of conditioning worsens. Some patients reap great benefits from a program of education and rehabilitation that addresses these issues. After screening for heart disease and exercise-induced hypoxia, daily exercise training may be initiated (e.g., stationary bicycle, walking) to build endurance and to increase the patient's ability to perform activities of daily living. Instruction in diaphragmatic and pursed-lip breathing may be of further assistance. Occupational therapists often suggest energy-saving devices and help to plan daily schedules that include rest periods. Furthermore, mental health professionals may play a key role in managing the reactive depression that is common in patients with severe COPD.

CONTROVERSIES

20. Should anticholinergic agents be used with beta agonists in patients with asthma?

For:

1. By inhibiting cholinergic tone and dilating the large airways, anticholinergic agents theoretically may improve penetration of beta agonists into the lungs.

2. Occasionally patients who respond poorly to beta agonists respond well to ipratropium or combination therapy (especially older patients).

3. Anticholinergics are preferred in the treatment of psychogenic asthma, because they block the parasympathetically mediated bronchospasm triggered by emotional factors.

Against:

1. No synergistic effect has been proved.

2. Combination therapy results in substantially greater cost and inconvenience to the patient.

3. In most patients, anticholinergic agents are clearly less effective than beta agonists in producing bronchodilation.

21. Are inhaled steroids completely safe?

For:

1. Because systemic absorption is slight, hypercortisolism does not occur.

2. Suppression of the pituitary-adrenal axis has not been reported in adults, even with high doses.

3. Worsening of diabetes mellitus has not been reported.

4. Oral candidiasis is a local complication that can be prevented with use of spacers and rinsing/gargling after use.

Against:

1. Some studies in children have documented measurable suppression of the pituitary-adrenal axis, possibly related to the higher dose/kg of body weight.

2. Increased bone turnover (as measured by bone metabolites) occurs with doses that do not suppress cortisol production. It is not known whether this effect will translate into significant osteoporosis after sustained use.

3. It is not known whether long-term use of inhaled steroids may increase the risk of developing cataracts.

4. Use may be associated with the development of thrush and dysphonia.

22. Is theophylline beneficial in the management of patients with asthma and COPD?

For:

1. Patients with prominent nocturnal symptoms may be greatly helped by 24-hour theophylline preparations given once daily in the early evening.

2. Theophylline may be used as a steroid-sparing measure in patients with chronic severe asthma.

3. Theoretical benefits include reduced diaphragmatic fatigability, positive inotropy, and improved mucociliary clearance.

4. Theophylline is a central respiratory stimulant and may benefit a subset of patients with COPD who hypoventilate even though their resistive loads are not extreme (i.e., blue bloaters).

5. Some studies suggest improved performance and quality of life not necessarily related to improved spirometry.

Against:

1. During acute exacerbations, no improvement in spirometry or symptoms results when theophylline is added to maximal beta-agonist therapy, but side effects usually increase.

2. Theophylline has a narrow therapeutic window and levels may be affected by many commonly prescribed drugs as well as by smoking.

3. The theoretical benefits are modest at best and of uncertain clinical importance.

23. Are oral beta agonists indicated in patients with asthma?

For:

1. Long-acting preparations are particularly useful for relief of nocturnal asthma.

2. Many small children and some adults cannot be trained to use MDIs effectively.

Against:

1. Oral beta agonists are less effective than the inhaled drug for both treating and preventing bronchospasm.

2. Oral agents have more systemic side effects.

3. For patients who cannot use MDIs properly, spacer devices, nebulizers, and rotacaps are available.

4. New ultra-long-acting inhaled beta agonists, such as salmeterol, soon will be available for the treatment of nocturnal symptoms.

BIBLIOGRAPHY

1. Ahmed T: Preventing bronchoconstriction in exercise-induced asthma with inhaled heparin. N Engl J Med 329:90, 1993.
2. Braman SS, Corrao WM: Bronchoprovocation testing. Clin Chest Med 10:165, 1989.
3. Chan-Yeung M, Lam S: State of the art: Occupational asthma. Am Rev Respir Dis 133:686, 1985.
4. Chapman KR: Therapeutic algorithm for COPD. Am J Med 91:4A–17S, 1991.
5. Clark NM, Evans D, Mellins RB: Patient use of peak flow monitoring. Am Rev Respir Dis 145:722, 1992.
6. Ferguson GT, Cherniack RM: Management of COPD. N Engl J Med 328:1017, 1993.
7. Gross NJ: COPD: Current concepts and therapeutic approaches. Chest 97:19S, 1990.
8. Groth ML, Hurewitz AN: Diagnosing and managing bronchial asthma. Emerg Med Sept 19, 1992.
9. Idris AH, et al: Emergency department treatment of severe asthma. Chest 103:665, 1993.
10. Li JT, Reed CE: Proper use of aerosol corticosteroids to control asthma. Mayo Clin Proc 64:205, 1989.
11. Listello D, Glauser F: COPD: Primary care management with drug and oxygen therapies. Geriatrics 47:28, 1992.
12. Make B: COPD: Management and rehabilitation. Am Fam Physician 43:1315, 1991.
13. Middleton E, Reed CE, et al: Allergy: Principles and Practice. St. Louis, Mosby, 1993.
14. Murray JF, Nadel JA: Textbook of Respiratory Medicine. Philadelphia, W.B. Saunders, 1992.
15. National Asthma Education Program: Guidelines for the Diagnosis and Management of Asthma. Bethesda, MD, National Heart, Lung, and Blood Institute, 1991.
16. Weiss EB, Stein M: Bronchial Asthma, 3rd ed. Boston, Little, Brown, 1993.

86. PULMONARY FUNCTION TESTS

Michael E. Hanley, M.D.

1. When are pulmonary function tests (PFTs) indicated?

The primary purposes of PFTs are diagnostic (to uncover clinically undetected disease and to determine the nature of physiologic dysfunction), quantitative (to determine severity of dysfunction), and monitory (to follow response to therapy or progression of disease). Common indications for pulmonary function testing in the primary care setting include evaluation of patients with unexplained dyspnea, cough, hypoxemia, right-sided congestive heart failure, or abnormal chest roentgenogram suggestive of diffuse lung disease. Pulmonary function tests are particularly useful for chronic monitoring of patients with conditions characterized by infiltrative processes or airflow limitation.

2. Describe the myriad of PFTs.

Simple spirometry, lung volumes, diffusion capacity of the lungs for carbon monoxide (DLCO), flow-volume loops, and arterial blood gases are available in most laboratories. More extensive tests, including pressure-volume curves, airway resistance and conductance, inhalational challenge, exercise testing, ventilatory drive studies, maximum inspiratory and expiratory pressures (PI_{max} and PE_{max}), and polysomnography, are available in specialty laboratories.

3. What constitutes simple spirometry?

Simple spirometry consists primarily of forced vital capacity (FVC), forced expiratory volume in one second (FEV_1), FEV_1/FVC ratio, forced expiratory flow between 25 and 75% of vital capacity ($FEF_{25-75\%}$), and peak expiratory flow rate (PEFR). Simple spirometry also includes measurement of these parameters after bronchodilator treatment. Additional flow rates, such as forced expiratory flow at 25%, 50%, and 75% of vital capacity ($FEF_{25\%}$, $FEF_{50\%}$, and $FEF_{75\%}$) are occasionally reported but do not add significantly to the sensitivity of the other tests.

4. How is simple spirometry interpreted?

The patient's ability to perform the tests must be evaluated first. Abnormal results are occasionally obtained because patients are either unable (because of poor comprehension of instructions, altered mental status, or abnormal oral anatomy that precludes a good spirometer interface) or unwilling to cooperate with testing. Clues to poor patient cooperation include inability to reproduce results (spirometry is generally measured at least 3–5 times during a test session) and written comments of the technician performing the tests. Although all parameters measured in simple spirometry depend on patient effort, the FEV_1 and FVC are the most reproducible and therefore offer the most reliable information.

If patient cooperation is good, the next step is to determine if the results are normal. Absolute PFT values obtained in normal subjects are influenced by several factors, including age, height, and sex. Regression equations are used to calculate published predicted normal values for a given patient on the basis of these factors. Other factors, in particular race, also influence predicted normal values but are not routinely considered in published standards. In general, predicted values for patients of African or Asian heritage tend to be 8–13% lower than those for Caucasians, but the optimal correction factors are controversial and not well defined.

Finally, if the results of FEV_1 or FVC are not within the normal range, the pattern of dysfunction should be determined by consideration of the FEV_1/FVC ratio and other flow rates (see questions 5 and 6).

5. Define "obstructive" lung diseases. How are they diagnosed?

Obstructive lung diseases are characterized anatomically and physiologically by obstruction of airflow (airflow limitation). Airflow depends on the lung volume at which it is measured (lower rates occur at smaller lung volumes), resistance of the airways, and pressure that generates flow (driving force determined by elastic recoil of the lung-thoracic cage unit). Common obstructive lung diseases caused primarily by increased airway resistance include asthma, chronic bronchitis, and chronic bronchiectasis; airflow limitation in emphysema is largely secondary to decreased elastic recoil. Because the FEV_1 depends on the rate of airflow more than the FVC, the FEV_1 is generally decreased out of proportion to the FVC in obstructive lung processes. Thus, the FEV_1/FVC ratio is decreased, usually below 0.7.

6. What are restrictive lung diseases?

Restrictive lung diseases are characterized by a reduced total lung capacity (TLC). The differential diagnosis is complex but can be simplified by organizing restrictive disorders into four categories: (1) parenchymal infiltrative disease (interstitial and/or alveolar); (2) chest wall abnormalities; (3) pleural disease; and (4) neuromuscular weakness involving ventilatory muscles.

Restrictive diseases are characterized by decreased lung volumes and, with the exception of neuromuscular weakness, increased elastic recoil of the lung-thoracic cage unit. Thus, although absolute measures of airflow are decreased (because of lower lung volumes), airflow corrected for lung volume is normal or increased. The FEV_1/FVC ratio is therefore normal or increased in patients with restrictive lung disease.

7. Define lung volumes.

Lung volumes measure the absolute volumes of the lungs at various points in the respiratory cycle. Commonly reported volumes include total lung capacity (TLC; volume of gas in the lungs after total inspiration), residual volume (RV; volume of gas in the lungs after total expiration), and function residual capacity (FRC; volume of gas remaining in the lungs at end expiration during tidal volume breathing). When FRC is measured by body plethysmography (body box), it is referred to as thoracic gas volume (TGV).

As with simple spirometry, normal values are influenced by age, height, sex, and race. Thus, results are reported as both absolute values and as a percentage of the predicted normal value.

8. What approach is used in interpreting lung volumes?

Measurement of lung volumes is especially sensitive to patient effort. Of the three commonly measured volumes, FRC (or TGV) is the least effort-dependent and the most reliable; thus it should be considered first. In obstructive lung diseases, all three volumes are usually increased, whereas in restrictive diseases, they are usually decreased. Demonstration of a decreased TLC and an increased RV (regardless of FRC) suggests poor patient effort (inability or unwillingness to perform maneuver).

9. When are lung volumes indicated?

Simple spirometry differentiates obstruction from restriction in most patients. Similarly, spirometry alone is adequate to monitor most patients' clinical condition and response to therapy over time. Therefore, lung volumes, which add significant expense to PFTs, are seldom required. Lung volumes are indicated (1) to evaluate patients with pulmonary symptoms and normal spirometry; (2) to quantitate more accurately the severity of restriction or obstruction; (3) to evaluate patients with both obstruction and restriction; and (4) to evaluate patients with severe obstruction and a markedly reduced FVC. In patients in the fourth category, lung volumes can clarify whether the decrement in FVC is due to obstruction alone or a coexistent restrictive process.

10. What does DLCO measure?

DLCO measures the diffusion of carbon monoxide (CO) across the alveolar-capillary membrane and is thought to reflect the efficiency of gas exchange. Although the permeability (and therefore thickness) of the membrane affects the value of DLCO, other factors are also important, including the surface area of the membrane (and therefore the lung volume at which it is measured), the hemoglobin (Hb) concentration in blood (Hb binds CO), and matching of ventilation and perfusion. Absolute values for DLCO are usually corrected for some of these factors. Specifically, DLCO-Hb corrects DLCO for hemoglobin concentration, and DLCO-volume alveolar (VA) corrects for the lung volume at which it is measured.

11. What diseases are associated with an abnormal DLCO?
DLCO is decreased in lung diseases characterized by thickening of the alveolar-capillary membrane (pulmonary infiltrative disorders), destruction of the membrane (emphysema or pulmonary vasculopathies), and mismatching of ventilation and perfusion. Thus, an abnormal DLCO is nonspecific.

Conditions characterized by increased DLCO include congestive heart failure (prolonged capillary blood transit time increases the time for absorption of CO) and significant alveolar or airway hemorrhage.

12. Should PFTs be obtained in the acutely ill patient?
The timing of PFTs depends on the clinical scenario. Physiologic evaluation during an acute exacerbation of a chronic illness may be valuable to diagnose the cause of previously unexplained dyspnea, hypoxemia, or cough or to monitor response to therapy in exacerbations of chronic obstructive disease. However, if the diagnosis is already known or readily apparent from other clinical data, PFTs in the acutely ill patient add little useful information but considerable unnecessary expense. For comparative purposes it is generally more valuable to determine severity of illness when patients are at baseline function. Return to baseline may require up to 6 weeks of convalescence after an acute exacerbation of obstructive disease. In addition, response to therapy in acutely ill patients is more efficiently and economically accomplished by monitoring PEFR alone.

13. Is the diagnosis of asthma confirmed by demonstration of improved airflow after administration of bronchodilators?
One of the clinical hallmarks of asthma is reversibility of airflow obstruction. Reversibility is indicated by significant improvement in FEV_1 and/or FVC after administration of an inhaled bronchodilator, usually a beta-2 agonist. Significant is defined as an increase > 15–20% in either parameter. However, other obstructive lung diseases, such as chronic bronchitis and emphysema, occasionally demonstrate similar improvement. Furthermore, PFTs in patients with severe asthma may not demonstrate acute reversibility until parenteral corticosteroids have been administered for several months. Thus, the diagnosis of asthma requires thorough consideration of all available clinical, physiologic, radiographic, and pathologic data and not solely the response to bronchodilator therapy.

BIBLIOGRAPHY

1. Bates DV: Respiratory Function in Disease, 3rd ed. Philadelphia, W.B. Saunders, 1989.
2. Clausen JL: Pulmonary Function Testing Guidelines and Controversies. Equipment, Methods, and Normal Values. New York, Academic Press, 1983.
3. Crapo RO, Gardner RM: Single breath carbon monoxide diffusion capacity (transfer factor): Recommendations for a standard technique. Am Rev Respir Dis 136:1299–1307, 1987.
4. Crystal RG, Fulmer JD, Roberts WC, et al: Idiopathic pulmonary fibrosis: Clinical, histologic, radiographic, physiologic, scintigraphic, cytologic, and biochemical aspects. Ann Intern Med 85:769–788, 1976.
5. Englert M, Yernault JC, de Coster A, Clumeck N: Diffusing properties and elastic properties in interstitial disease of the lung. Prog Respir Res 8:177–185, 1975.
6. Gardner RM, Hankinson JL, Clausen JL, et al: Standardization of spirometry—1987 update. Am Rev Respir Dis 136:1285–1298, 1987.
7. Goldman HI, Becklake MR: Respiratory function tests: Normal values at median altitudes and the prediction of normal results. Am Rev Tuberc 79:457–467, 1959.

8. Jelek V, Ficik J, Michaljanic A, Jezkova L: The prognostic significance of functional tests in kryptogenic fibrosing alveolitis. Bull Physiopathol Resp 16:711–720, 1980.
9. Knudson RJ, Burrows B, Lebowitz MD: The maximal expiratory flow-volume curve: Its use in the detection of ventilatory abnormalities in a population study. Am Rev Respir Dis 114:871–879, 1976.
10. Knudson RJ, Lebowitz MD, Holberg CJ, Burrows B: Changes in the normal maximal expiratory flow-volume curve with growth and aging. Am Rev Respir Dis 127:725–734, 1983.
11. Rodenstein DO, Stanescu DC: Reassessment of lung volume measurement by helium dilution and by body plethysmography in chronic air-flow obstruction. Am Rev Respir Dis 126:1040–1044, 1982.
12. Rossiter CE, Weill H: Ethnic differences in lung function: Evidence for proportional differences. Int J Epidemiol 3:55–61, 1974.
13. Tisi GM: Pulmonary Physiology in Clinical Medicine, 2nd ed. Baltimore, Williams & Wilkins, 1985.

87. HYPOXEMIA AND OXYGEN THERAPY

Eugene J. Sullivan, M.D., and Michael E. Hanley, M.D.

1. List the pathophysiologic causes of hypoxemia.

There are six major causes of hypoxemia: reduction in inspired partial pressure of oxygen (PO_2), hypoventilation, diffusion impairment, ventilation-perfusion (V-Q) mismatch, shunting, and reduced mixed venous oxygen tension.

2. When does decreased inspired PO_2 contribute to hypoxemia?

1. In patients receiving an inadequate concentration of oxygen in inspired gas (FiO_2) on mechanical ventilation

2. In persons who travel to or live at an altitude at which inspired PO_2 is decreased because of lower barometric pressure

3. How does hypoventilation cause hypoxemia?

Arterial PO_2 is determined in part by the partial pressure of oxygen in the alveolus (P_{AO_2}). P_{AO_2}, in turn, is determined by the total pressure in the alveolus (essentially barometric pressure) and the proportion of oxygen in alveolar gas. Hypoventilation results in increased alveolar carbon dioxide (CO_2). As alveolar CO_2 increases, the proportion of oxygen in alveolar gas falls. Therefore, P_{AO_2} is lower, and hypoxemia develops.

4. Define diffusion impairment. Why is isolated diffusion impairment unlikely to cause hypoxemia?

In disease such as pulmonary fibrosis, an abnormally thickened alveolar-capillary membrane may impair oxygen diffusion. However, blood in the pulmonary capillaries of normal persons is in contact with the alveolus approximately three times longer than is necessary to reach oxygen equilibrium. Thus, abnormalities in the alveolar-capillary membrane must be quite severe before hypoxemia results from diffusion impairment alone.

5. What is the most common cause of hypoxemia?

V-Q mismatch is the most common cause of clinically noted hypoxemia. Optimal gas exchange requires balanced ventilation and perfusion throughout the lung. Blood passing through poorly ventilated areas of the lung is inadequately oxygenated and contributes to hypoxemia. Because of the characteristics of the oxygen dissociation curve, hyperventilation of normal areas of the lung cannot correct the hypoxemia.

6. When does shunt occur?

Shunt occurs when blood crosses from the venous to the arterial circulation without receiving ventilation. Anatomic defects such as atrial or ventricular septal defects, patent ductus arteriosus, or arteriovenous malformations result in shunting. More common causes of shunting include atelectasis and airspace-filling disorders, such as pneumonia or pulmonary edema.

7. When should acute hypoxemia be suspected?
Clinically, acute hypoxemia is manifest by abnormal function in some organs and compensatory changes in others. Disturbance of the central nervous system (CNS) is usually the first clinical sign of hypoxemia. Initially, malaise and impairments of short-term memory and judgment are detectable. As hypoxemia worsens, cognitive and motor function become more compromised until eventually the patient loses consciousness. Cardiovascular compensation for mild-to-moderate hypoxemia includes tachycardia and increased stroke volume, but as hypoxemia worsens, rhythm disturbances develop. Hypoxic stimulation of the carotid body results in increased minute ventilation. Severe hypoxemia results in declining renal function and urine output and development of metabolic acidosis due to anaerobic metabolism. Many patients who are hypoxemic appear cyanotic. Cyanosis, a bluish discoloration of the skin and mucous membranes, is present when the concentration of reduced hemoglobin in capillary blood reaches 5 g/100 ml.

8. What are pitfalls in the observation of cyanosis?
Because the detection of cyanosis is determined by the amount of reduced hemoglobin in capillaries, a severely anemic patient may not appear cyanotic despite significant hypoxemia, because of insufficient hemoglobin. Conversely, a patient with polycythemia may have hemoglobin in excess of oxygen-carrying needs and appear cyanotic despite a normal blood oxygen content. Furthermore, cyanosis may be caused by disorders other than systemic hypoxemia, such as peripheral vasoconstriction (e.g., Raynaud's disease) and methemoglobinemia.

9. What physical signs and laboratory results suggest chronic hypoxemia?
Hypoxemia results in pulmonary vasoconstriction, which, when chronic, causes pulmonary hypertension. Pulmonary hypertension increases right ventricular workload and eventually leads to right heart failure. In addition, chronic hypoxemic states result in elaboration of erythropoietin, which causes polycythemia. A patient with chronic hypoxemia may manifest signs of pulmonary hypertension and right heart failure, depending on the extent and duration of hypoxemia. Such signs include a right ventricular heave, loud pulmonic component to the second heart sound, right ventricular S3, murmur of tricuspid regurgitation, jugular venous distension, hepatojugular reflux, and lower extremity edema. Laboratory tests reveal polycythemia. The electrocardiogram shows signs of right ventricular hypertrophy.

10. What is critical hypoxemia? How is it managed?
When a patient is found to be hypoxemic, the first issue to be addressed is whether the hypoxemia is an acute or subacute event or a chronic process. In acute events (e.g., pneumonia, pulmonary embolus, congestive heart failure), hospitalization often is indicated to diagnose and treat the underlying problem. A $PaO_2 < 50$ (because of precarious hemoglobin saturation due to the physicochemical characteristics of the O_2 saturation curve) places the patient at risk for arrhythmias and further decompensation. Hospitalization also should be considered for patients with clinical signs of organ dysfunction, such as tachypnea, tachycardia, or CNS disturbance. Chronic hypoxemia, if severe enough, has long-term detrimental effects but usually does not require urgent intervention.

11. What factors may lead to false readings of arterial blood gas (ABG) analysis?
Air bubbles in the syringe, if greater than 5% of the sample size, may artifactually lower PO_2 and PCO_2 readings toward ambient air values. In addition, if ABGs are not processed promptly, gas may diffuse through plastic syringe walls, altering readings. Lastly, extreme

leukocytosis may result in pseudohypoxemia because of oxygen consumption by the white blood cells in the syringe.

12. How is the alveoloarterial oxygen (A-a O_2) gradient calculated? When is it useful?

The A-a O_2 gradient is the difference between the alveolar PO_2 (P_{AO_2}) and the arterial PO_2 (PaO_2). The arterial PO_2 is measured on routine blood gas analysis, but the alveolar PO_2 must be calculated. P_{AO_2} is calculated with the following equation:

$$P_{AO_2} = FiO_2(P_B - P_{H_2O}) - \frac{Pa_{CO_2}}{0.8}$$

where FiO_2 is the proportion of oxygen in inspired air, P_B is barometric pressure, P_{H_2O} is water vapor pressure (47 mmHg), and Pa_{CO_2} is the CO_2 tension in arterial blood. The A-a O_2 gradient in normal room air is 5–15, depending on the patient's age. The gradient helps to distinguish hypoxemia due to cardiopulmonary disorders from other causes and to identify patients with significant lung pathology but a "normal" arterial oxygen tension because of hyperventilation.

13. How does the A-a gradient differentiate the various pathophysiologic causes of hypoxemia?

An elevated A-a O_2 gradient reflects an abnormality in gas transfer between alveoli and pulmonary capillaries. The A-a O_2 gradient is normal if hypoventilation or decreased FiO_2 is the cause of hypoxemia but elevated if diffusion abnormalities, V-Q mismatching, or shunt is present. Hypoventilation is distinguished from decreased inspired O_2 by the presence of elevated PCO_2. Most patients with V-Q mismatch, diffusion impairment, or shunt are able to increase minute ventilation sufficiently to normalize PCO_2 in acute or subacute settings. Therefore, as long as the increased minute ventilation is maintained, blood gases reveal hypoxemia with normal or low PCO_2. V-Q mismatch and shunt can be distinguished by assessing the effect of supplemental O_2 on hypoxemia. Increasing the FiO_2 improves hypoxemia if V-Q mismatch is the cause but does not significantly change hypoxemia caused by shunting.

14. What are the limitations of pulse oximetry?

Pulse oximetry uses optical differences between saturated and nonsaturated hemoglobin to assess the percentage of oxygen saturation. Because it is rapid, noninvasive, and simple to perform, it has become commonly used in emergency departments, intensive care units, and office practices as a method of assessing patients for hypoxemia. It is accurate within 3–5% in patients with saturations above 70%. The biggest limitation of pulse oximetry is that it provides no measure of the patient's PCO_2, a value that is critical both diagnostically and therapeutically. For example, an oxygen saturation of 96% is considered normal unless it is associated with a reduced PCO_2, indicating that the patient must hyperventilate to maintain normal saturation. In addition, carboxyhemoglobin, methemoglobin, abnormal acid-base status, poor perfusion, and bright external light may complicate the interpretation of pulse oximeter readings.

15. When is oxygen therapy indicated?

Supplemental oxygen is used for treatment of tissue hypoxia. Clinical scenarios characterized by presumed tissue hypoxia include acute myocardial infarction, acute anemia, carboxyhemo-globinemia, methemoglobinemia, conditions in which oxygen transport is compromised, and hypoxemia with a $PaO_2 < 60$ mmHg or arterial O_2 saturation $< 90\%$.

In chronic settings, long-term oxygen therapy should be initiated if a clinically stable patient on an optimal medical regimen demonstrates a $PaO_2 \leq 55$ mmHg or a $PaO_2 \leq 59$ mmHg in the presence of cor pulmonale or polycythemia.

16. Should all patients with chronic obstructive pulmonary disease (COPD) who are newly diagnosed with hypoxemia be placed on chronic supplemental oxygen?

As many as 50% of patients with COPD who are hypoxic but not on medical therapy no longer will be hypoxic once proper therapy is established. Therefore, only patients who are clinically stable and receiving appropriate medical therapy should be considered for supplemental oxygen. Such patients should be placed on long-term supplemental oxygen if the criteria listed in question 15 are met. Studies have shown a clear survival advantage with the use of chronic supplemental oxygen. Improvements in hemodynamics and neuropsychological function also have been demonstrated. In patients with continuous hypoxemia, maximal benefit is achieved with continuous oxygen delivery (i.e., 19–24 hr/day). Although the exact mechanism of benefit from long-term oxygen therapy is not known, it is the only therapy that has been shown to improve survival in patients with COPD.

17. How severe must COPD be before hypoxemia results?
In general there is a poor correlation between the severity of COPD as determined by spirometry and alterations in blood oxygen tension. Patients with severely reduced FEV_1 may maintain normal oxygen tension, whereas others with less severe airflow limitations may be hypoxic. This poor correlation is due to two factors:

1. Although the primary mechanism of hypoxemia in patients with COPD is V-Q mismatch, alterations in airflow as measured by spirometry do not necessarily parallel alterations in V-Q balance. Emphysema and chronic bronchitis, which contribute to airflow limitation to varying degrees, do not result in equivalent degrees of V-Q mismatching. Thus a patient whose obstruction is primarily emphysematous may not have as severe a V-Q disturbance as a patient with equal obstruction due primarily to chronic bronchitis.

2. Individual patients have varying abilities to compensate for hypoxemia related to pulmonary parenchymal abnormalities by recruiting minute ventilation or cardiac output.

18. What is transtracheal oxygen therapy? List its benefits and risks.
Transtracheal oxygen therapy is a relatively new system of oxygen delivery in which a catheter is placed transcutaneously, usually under local anesthesia, into the trachea at the level of the second or third tracheal ring. The transtracheal delivery system has been shown to have several benefits: improved cosmesis and comfort, decreased oxygen flow rate requirement, improved exercise tolerance, improved patient compliance, and fewer hospitalizations. The most common complications include accidental catheter displacement, obstruction of the end of the catheter with a mucus plug, and mild local cellulitis.

19. What issues are involved with air travel in patients with pulmonary disorders?
Although commercial aircraft cruise between 22,000 and 44,000 feet, passenger cabins are maintained at pressures equivalent to altitudes of 5,000–8,000 feet. It is difficult to estimate the PaO_2 of a particular patient at these altitudes because of varying abilities to compensate (i.e., increased minute ventilation and cardiac output). However, in a stable normocapneic patient with COPD, a sea level $PaO_2 > 72$ mmHg usually results in a $PaO_2 > 50$ at 8,000 feet. The patient's expected PaO_2 at a particular altitude can be determined more exactly with the Hypoxia Altitude Simulation Test (HAST), which uses normobaric hypoxic breathing to simulate altitude and may be performed in PFT laboratories.

20. How does altitude affect blood oxygen level? What advice should be given to a pulmonary patient who wishes to travel to the mountains?
Atmospheric oxygen is fairly constant at 21% of total barometric pressure at any altitude. However, barometric pressure decreases as altitude increases, resulting in a lower partial pressure of inspired oxygen (PO_2). The inspired PO_2 is 149 at sea level but decreases by approximately 4 mmHg/1,000 feet of elevation. Normal persons respond to the acute hypoxia of altitude by increasing minute ventilation (by increasing tidal volume) to maximize alveolar PO_2. A healthy person can maintain a PaO_2 of 50–60 mmHg at 8,000–10,000 feet. In addition, mild tachycardia develops, thus increasing cardiac output and maintaining oxygen delivery to tissues. Blood flow to the brain is maintained as hypoxic vasodilatation overcomes the vasoconstrictor effect due to respiratory alkalosis. Such issues should be kept in mind when counseling a pulmonary patient about travel to high altitudes. Patients with borderline

oxygenation at sea level may become hypoxic, depending on the altitude to which they travel. Such patients may require supplemental oxygen, especially if they have a history of co-morbid conditions such as angina pectoris, congestive heart failure, or cerebrovascular disease. In addition, patients already receiving supplemental oxygen may require an increase in the oxygen flow rate.

21. Is chronic supplemental oxygen therapy indicated for patients who desaturate only with exercise?

Many patients with COPD have normal or near-normal oxygen tension at rest but desaturate with exercise. No clinical trials have evaluated the benefits of oxygen therapy in such patients. Therefore the role of supplemental oxygen in this setting is not well defined. Because patients with COPD generally spend only a small percentage of their day participating in exercise, it may be unlikely that exercise desaturation contributes significantly to morbidity or mortality. However, some patients report an increase in exercise tolerance with supplemental oxygen. To the extent that supplemental oxygen improves quality of life, it may be reasonable to prescribe supplemental oxygen for such patients. However, before doing so, a blinded trial should be performed to document an improvement in exercise tolerance.

BIBLIOGRAPHY

1. Anthonisen NR: Home oxygen therapy in chronic obstructive pulmonary disease. Clin Chest Med 7:673–678, 1986.
2. Dantzker DR: Pulmonary gas exchange. In Bone RC, et al (eds): Pulmonary and Critical Care Medicine. Boston, Mosby, 1993.
3. Fulmer J, Snider GL: ACCP-NHLBI National Conference on Oxygen Therapy. Chest 86:234–247, 1984.
4. Gong H: Air travel and oxygen therapy in cardiopulmonary patients. Chest 101:1104–1113, 1992.
5. Hoffman LA, et al: Nasal cannula and transtracheal oxygen delivery: A comparison of patient response after 6 months of each technique. Am Rev Respir Dis 145:827–831, 1992.
6. Nocturnal Oxygen Therapy Trial Group: Continuous or nocturnal oxygen therapy in hypoxemic chronic obstructive lung disease. Ann Intern Med 93:391–398, 1980.
7. Wagner PD: Effects of COPD on gas exchange. In Cherniak NS (ed): Chronic Obstructive Pulmonary Disease. Philadelphia, W.B. Saunders, 1991.

88. SOLITARY PULMONARY NODULE

Michael E. Hanley, M.D.

1. Why is it important to distinguish between a pulmonary nodule and a pulmonary mass?

A solitary pulmonary nodule (SPN) is a well-circumscribed, approximately round lesion on chest roentgenogram that is less than 4–6 cm in diameter. By definition it is completely surrounded by aerated lung, thus excluding pleural- or mediastinal-based lesions. It is distinguished from a pulmonary mass by size (mass > 4–6 cm in diameter). Although this distinction is arbitrary, it has clinical significance in that the probability of malignancy increases with the size of the lesion.

2. Does a coin lesion differ from an SPN?

No. SPN and "coin lesion" are synonymous terms. Coin lesion, however, is a misnomer, because it implies a two-dimensional lesion, whereas SPNs are three-dimensional.

3. What is the differential diagnosis of an SPN?

The differential diagnosis of SPNs is quite extensive. The major diagnostic consideration is to distinguish benign from malignant processes.

Neoplastic lesions

Malignant
1. Primary lung
   - Bronchogenic carcinoma
   - Alveolar cell carcinoma
   - Adenoma
   - Sarcoma
   - Lymphoma
   - Hodgkin's disease
2. Solitary metastases

Benign
1. Hamartoma
2. Teratoma

Nonneoplastic lesions

Infection
1. Tuberculosis
2. Coccidioidomycosis
3. Histoplasmosis
4. Blastomycosis
5. Nocardiosis
6. Actinomycosis

Inflammatory process
1. Wegener's granulomatosis
2. Organizing pneumonia
3. Rheumatoid necrobiotic nodule
4. Pulmonary infarct

Vascular lesions
1. Arteriovenous malformations
2. Pulmonary vein varix

Miscellaneous
1. Bronchial cyst
2. Bronchopulmonary sequestration
3. Pulmonary hematoma
4. Lipoid pneumonia
5. Other

4. Which three constellations of factors favor a benign nodule?

Calcification of the lesion, absence of a history of tobacco use, and age less than 35 years are important factors that strongly correlate with benign nodules. Noncalcified lesions may be benign or malignant. Absence of smoking history does not entirely exclude a malignant process because of potential exposure to other carcinogens (e.g., radon gas, asbestos, chromium) and second-hand smoke (passive smoking). Indeed, 15% of primary lung cancers occur in non-smokers. Patients under age 35 years are more likely to have a benign lesion; however, this association is not absolute. A diagnostic work-up may be necessary in the presence of other malignant risk factors, such as enlarging lesions or heavy tobacco use beginning at an early age.

5. Why is regular follow-up of a calcified pulmonary nodule important?

Six common patterns of calcification of SPNs are recognized: diffuse, central, popcorn, laminar, stippled, and eccentric. The first four are almost always benign, whereas the latter two may be either benign or malignant. However, even benign calcification does not exclude the presence of coincidental malignancy in adjacent tissue or the subsequent degeneration of a previously benign process into a malignant lesion ("scar" carcinoma). For this reason, close observation with serial chest roentgenograms every 6 months for at least 2 years is prudent for nodules with benign patterns of calcification.

A. Diffuse   B. Central   C. Popcorn   D. Laminar,   E. Stippled   F. Eccentric
                                                    Concentric

Six common patterns of calcification occur in SPNs. Patterns A–D are associated with benign conditions; patterns E and F occur in both benign and malignant conditions. (Adapted from Webb WR: Radiologic evaluation of the solitary pulmonary nodule. AJR 154:701–708, 1990, with permission.)

6. What other radiographic clues help to differentiate between benign and malignant lesions?
Cavitating lesions, lesions with multilobulated or spiculated contours, and lesions with shaggy or extremely irregular borders tend to be malignant. However, none of these associations is strong enough to determine accurately the nature of a lesion.

7. What is the most valuable test in evaluating an SPN?
The most valuable diagnostic test is comparison with an old chest roentgenogram. Benign nodules tend to grow at either very slow or very rapid rates. In contrast, malignant processes grow at steady, predictable, exponential rates. The growth rate of a nodule is conventionally defined as the doubling time (i.e., the time required for its *volume* to double) and corresponds to an increase in diameter by a factor of 1.26. In general, doubling times > 16 months or < 1 month (20–25 days) are associated with benign processes. Intermediate doubling times require additional evaluation to determine the nature of the lesion. If a nodule has not increased in size over a 2-year period, the probability that it is benign is greater than 99%.

8. Does sputum cytology aid in the diagnosis of an SPN?
Sputum cytology has a low yield (5–20%) and is of limited value.

9. What are the pros and cons of the invasive tests available for diagnosing an SPN?
Absolute determination of the true nature of an SPN necessitates obtaining tissue for histologic evaluation. Three options are available:

   1. Resection of the nodule by either **open thoracotomy or video-assisted thoracoscopy** (VAT) unequivocally determines the nature of the lesion but is associated with significant perioperative morbidity and occasional mortality.

   2. **Fiberoptic bronchoscopy with transbronchial biopsy** is relatively safe (incidence of pneumothorax and significant hemorrhage < 3%), but its sensitivity in diagnosing malignancy depends on the size of the lesion. Overall, the yield is approximately 10–40% for lesions 1–2 cm in diameter, 60% for lesions 2–3 cm, and 80% for lesions > 3 cm. These figures, however, depend heavily on the operator's skill. Addition of transbronchial brushing, washing, and needle aspiration improves the yield.

   3. **Percutaneous transthoracic needle aspiration** has a higher sensitivity in diagnosing malignancy than transbronchial biopsy but is associated with more morbidity. The diagnostic yield exceeds 90% for malignancy. However, subsequent pneumothorax occurs in 25% of patients, one-half of whom require tube thoracostomy. In addition, the sensitivity for diagnosing benign lesions is even lower than that for transbronchial biopsy. Because the specific yield of both transbronchial biopsy and transthoracic needle aspiration for benign lesions is low, nonmalignant but nonspecific results do not exclude malignancy with certainty.

10. When should a patient with an SPN be referred for invasive tests?
Initial evaluation of an SPN by the primary care provider consists of a thorough history and physical examination, laboratory tests to screen for potential metastases, and comparison with previous chest roentgenograms. If the presence or pattern of calcification is not readily apparent on a plain chest roentgenogram, computed tomography (CT) of the chest should be obtained. Patients with a high probability of malignancy should be referred for invasive tests. Patients with a low probability of malignancy (based on characteristics of the nodule and risk factors) should have a repeat chest radiograph in 1 month. If no change is seen, the patient should be followed closely with serial chest roentgenograms (every 6 months) until radiographic stability of the nodule has been demonstrated for at least 2 years.

CONTROVERSIES

11. Do all patients undergoing thoracotomy for an SPN require CT of the chest before surgery?
For:
Potential benefits of CT scans include identification of a benign pattern of calcification not

evident on the plain chest roentgenogram, identification of additional nodules, and identification of mediastinal pathology (lymphadenopathy or direct metastases).

Against:

Demonstration of additional peripheral nodules or mediastinal lymphadenopathy by CT does not confirm that such lesions are malignant (especially when mediastinal lymph nodes are less than 1 cm in diameter). Furthermore, the probability that chest CT will reveal previously unrecognized mediastinal pathology is low if the mediastinum appears normal on the plain chest roentgenogram.

12. Should patients who have an SPN with a high risk of cancer and who also are good surgical candidates be managed by immediate resection of the nodule by either open thoracotomy or VAT rather than subjected to invasive, exclusively diagnostic procedures?

For:

Diagnosis of malignancy by transbronchial biopsy results in subsequent referral for therapeutic thoracotomy, whereas nonmalignant results are usually nonspecific, do not exclude malignancy, and result in referral for a diagnostic thoracotomy.

Against:

Prethoracotomy fiberoptic bronchoscopy allows staging of the major airways by screening for metachronous endobronchial malignancies that may preclude or alter the extent of subsequent surgery. In addition, 5% of malignant SPNs are small-cell carcinomas that are not treated with surgery. Finally, morbidity and mortality are much lower for transbronchial biopsy and percutaneous transthoracic needle aspiration than for thoracotomy; although the yield for benign lesions is low, the higher risk of thoracotomy justifies an attempt at diagnosis by less invasive approaches, especially for patients who are psychologically reluctant to undergo surgery or at high risk from thoracotomy or VAT.

BIBLIOGRAPHY

1. Cummings SR, Lillington GA, Richard RJ: Estimating the probability of malignancy in solitary pulmonary nodules. A Bayesian approach. Am Rev Respir Dis 134:449–452, 1986.
2. Cummings SR, Lillington GA, Richard RJ: Managing solitary pulmonary nodules. The choice of strategy is a "close call." Am Rev Respir Dis 134:453–460, 1986.
3. Garland LH, Coulson W, Wollin E: The rate of growth and apparent duration of untreated primary bronchial carcinoma. Cancer 16:694–707, 1963.
4. Khouri NF, Meziane MA, Zerhouni EA, et al: The solitary pulmonary nodule: Assessment, diagnosis, and management. Chest 91:128–133, 1987.
5. Levine MS, Weiss JM, Harrell JH, et al: Transthoracic needle aspiration biopsy following negative fiberoptic bronchoscopy in solitary pulmonary nodules. Chest 93:1152–1155, 1988.
6. Nathan H: Management of solitary pulmonary nodules. An organized approach based on growth rates and statistics. JAMA 227:1141–1174, 1974.
7. O'Keefe ME, Good CA, McDonald JR: Calcification in solitary nodules of the lung. AJR 77:1023–1033, 1957.
8. Siegelman SS, Khouri NF, Leo FP, et al: Solitary pulmonary nodule: CT assessment. Radiology 160:307–312, 1986.
9. Steele JD: The solitary pulmonary nodule: Report of a cooperative study of resected asymptomatic solitary pulmonary nodules in males. J Thorac Cardiovasc Surg 46:21–39, 1963.
10. Webb WR: Radiologic evaluation of the solitary pulmonary nodule. AJR 154:701–708, 1990.

XIII. Common Disorders of the Skin

89. ECZEMATOUS DERMATITIS

Mark Fogarty, M.D., and Loren E. Golitz, M.D.

1. Define eczema.

Eczema is the final common manifestation of dermatitis of several etiologies, including atopic dermatitis, allergic and irritant contact dermatitis, and various other clinical forms of dermatitis. Papules, macules, and vesicles often coalesce with weeping and crusting. Eventually, thickening and scaling, called lichenification, result.

2. What rules should be considered in using topical steroid therapy?

1. Topical steroid preparations of low, mid, and high potency must be carefully distinguished. Examples: desonide 0.05% (low), triamcinolone acetonide 0.1% (mid), fluocinonide 0.05% (high).

2. Ointments may be more effective in dry, thickened skin than creams.

3. Potent topical steroids (especially fluorinated) should not be applied to intertriginous areas or to the face and neck.

4. Potent topical steroids should be avoided in young children because of the possibility of systemic absorption.

5. Potential side effects from prolonged use of potent topical steroids include cutaneous atrophy, development of striae, and suppression of the hypothalamus-pituitary-adrenal (HPA) axis. The risk of systemic absorption and suppression of the HPA axis is increased by high-potency preparations, prolonged use, application to large areas, and occlusive dressings.

3. When are systemic corticosteroids indicated?

In general, systemic steroids are indicated in self-limited, steroid-responsive disorders that present acutely with severe symptoms in an otherwise healthy patient. For example, prednisone may be started at a dose of 40 mg/day and tapered over 3 weeks in acute, severe cases of contact dermatitis. Systemic steroids should be avoided, if possible, in chronic illnesses such as psoriasis and atopic dermatitis.

4. What is the most common dermatologic disease seen in the primary care clinic?

Acute allergic contact dermatitis is the most common dermatologic disease in the primary care clinic. Poison ivy is a good example, but many other materials in the environment may stimulate an allergic cutaneous reaction. Swelling and itching of the eyelids and genitalia should suggest a diagnosis of allergic contact dermatitis.

5. What substances are the most common causes of allergic contact dermatitis?

Poison ivy, poison sumac, and poison oak are the three most common plants that cause contact dermatitis in the United States. Topical medications, including neomycin, ethylenediamine, topical anesthetics, and thimerosal, are commonly implicated. Nickel is a common culprit because of its ubiquitous use in jewelry. Chromium may be implicated in patients with industrial exposures to substances such as cement. Rubber, epoxy glues, cosmetics, perfumes, and formaldehyde also may cause allergic contact dermatitis. Paraphenylenediamine in permanent black hair dyes may cause severe scalp dermatitis.

6. How is contact dermatitis diagnosed?
The clinical history, including exposures at work and at home, is the most important element in making the diagnosis. The acute episode often follows contact with the allergen by approximately 48 hours. Hobbies are an important source of contact allergens. Any chemical that gets on the hands is readily transferred to the eyelids and genitalia.

7. Describe the classic presentation of poison ivy.
Poison ivy presents with a mixture of vesicles, bullae, and crusting. The blisters often appear in a linear arrangement at points where the broken stem or leaf of the plant has touched the skin. The rash is associated with intense pruritus.

8. Which parts of the hands and feet are commonly affected by contact dermatitis?
Contact dermatitis of the hands and feet usually involves the dorsal aspects, because the palms and soles are relatively protected by the thick layer of keratin.

9. What treatments are effective for contact dermatitis?
Treatment of allergic contact dermatitis includes cool compresses with a Burow's solution (a 1:20 solution is made by diluting 1 package of powder in 1 pint of cool water). The area should be soaked for 10–15 minutes and then patted dry with a towel. A topical steroid in the form of a cream, lotion, or spray may be applied to the skin 2–4 times/day. The topical application of phenolated Calamine lotion may provide some drying and relief from pruritus. Once a patient is allergic to a specific chemical, the allergy is maintained throughout life; thus avoidance of contact with the agent is important.

10. In what instances are patch tests useful?
Patch testing may establish the specific cause of an allergic contact dermatitis. Screening trays allow testing of multiple potential allergens. Tests normally are read 48 or 72 hours after application. Patch tests may be used to support the diagnosis of contact dermatitis, to identify the specific allergen, or to exclude the diagnosis. Difficulties include false-positive and false-negative results as well as positive results with unclear clinical significance. Test results must be correlated with the patient's exposures. A common cause of false-negative testing is a delayed reaction after the usual 48-hour reading. A second reading 4–7 days after the application is recommended. Patch tests should not be used during an episode of severe extensive dermatitis.

11. Does atopic dermatitis affect adults?
Usually atopic dermatitis is a disease of infancy and childhood, beginning before age 6 months and diminishing in adulthood. However, up to 60% of patients with childhood atopic dermatitis have some form, albeit more limited, in adulthood. Pruritus, the major symptom, is accompanied by dry, lichenified patches on the flexor surfaces of elbows, knees, wrists, ankles, and the periorbital region. The condition is usually idiopathic; exacerbating factors include extreme temperature, soaps, and irritating clothing.

12. What is the relationship of atopic dermatitis to other atopic states?
Up to 70% of patients have a personal or family history of asthma, hay fever, or dermatitis. Severe atopic dermatitis is seen in the hyperimmunoglobulin E (IgE) syndrome. Thus, diagnosis is usually made by the clinical and family history, examination of the lesions, and, in severe cases, assessment of the IgE level.

13. What is the mainstay of treatment of atopic dermatitis?

The mainstays of treatment are skin hydration and topical steroids. Patients should apply emollients to damp skin after bathing and repeatedly during the day. Topical steroids should be applied 2–4 times each day; ointments of mid-to-high potency, such as triamcinolone acetonide 0.1%, may be required. Occlusive dressings may be used to treat stubborn lesions.

14. What possibilities should be considered when atopic dermatitis fails to respond to therapy?

1. The patient is not meticulous about the frequency of therapy.

2. The patient is allergic (sensitized) to the topical agent. This possibility is especially likely when the treated area coincides with worsening disease.

3. Superinfection with *Staphylococcus aureus* is present. True infection is difficult to determine in the absence of cellulitis. However, vesicles, pustules, and large exudative lesions may warrant therapy with systemic antistaphylococcal agents.

4. The diagnosis is allergic contact dermatitis rather than atopic dermatitis, and the patient continues to be exposed to the allergen. Patch testing may be diagnostic.

15. What causes a pruritic, dry, and scaly dermatitis in elderly patients?

Pruritic, dry, and scaly dermatitis in elderly patients, usually called asteatotic eczema or "winter itch," is related to decreased skin lipids. Drying climate, frequent bathing, and diuresis exacerbate the areas of dryness. Skin fissuring and erythema, most commonly on the anterior legs, dorsum of the hands, and interscapular region, are accompanied by pruritus. Emollients to hydrate the skin, low-potency topical steroids, and decreased bathing usually provide relief.

16. Who is at risk for irritant hand dermatitis?

Irritant hand dermatitis, as opposed to allergic contact dermatitis, appears on the palmar aspect of the hand. Persons at risk include (1) patients with a history of atopic dermatitis or other skin disease and (2) housekeepers, health care professionals, and others who chronically expose hands to water and detergents.

17. Describe the therapy for irritant hand dermatitis.

Hand dermatitis may prove particularly difficult to clear, but the following steps usually are helpful:

1. Use of mild soap and vinyl gloves with avoidance of water
2. Use of cool compresses and mid-potency steroids
3. Aggressive treatment of secondary bacterial infection

In addition, dermatophophyte infection should be ruled out with a potassium hydroxide (KOH) preparation and culture.

BIBLIOGRAPHY

1. Fitzpatrick TB, et al (eds): Dermatology in General Medicine, 4th ed. New York, McGraw-Hill, 1993.
2. Moschella SL, Hurley HJ (eds): Dermatology, 3rd ed. Philadelphia, W.B. Saunders, 1992.
3. Phillips TJ, Dover JS: Recent advances in dermatology. N Engl J Med 326:167–178, 1992.
4. Sulzberger MB: The patch test: Who should and should not use it and why. Contact Dermatitis 1:117, 1975.

90. MACULOPAPULAR ERUPTIONS

Mark Fogarty, M.D., and Loren E. Golitz, M.D.

1. What is meant by the terms morbilliform and scarlatiniform?

Erythematous macules and papules are referred to as morbilliform, whereas diffuse erythematous macular lesions are scarlatiniform. A morbilliform rash is due to either a viral exanthem or a drug eruption. A scarlatiniform rash, classically seen in scarlet fever, is also seen in patients with toxic shock syndrome and Kawasaki's disease.

2. Describe the typical appearance of a drug eruption.

The most common drug eruption is a morbilliform rash on the trunk, extremities, palms, and soles. The rash may become confluent and is usually quite pruritic. Mild fever may accompany the eruption. The reaction usually begins within a week of starting the drug and may last up to 2 weeks. Drug eruptions also may manifest as urticarial or photosensitive eruptions. Most drugs are suspect, but common etiologic agents include penicillin, barbiturates, allopurinol, and trimethoprim-sulfamethoxazole (a common cause of drug rashes in patients infected with the human immunodeficiency virus [HIV]).

3. How are drug rashes treated?

Treatment involves discontinuation of the drug and avoidance of further exposure. Desensitization is effective in some cases and may be considered when alternative regimens are ineffective. Pruritus is treated with antihistamines such as hydroxyzine hydrochloride, 25 mg 4 times/day. Severe, generalized drug eruptions may be treated with a short course of oral prednisone.

4. Which three classic childhood exanthems result in a predominant morbilliform rash?

1. **Measles.** A rash beginning on the forehead and hairline follows a prodrome of coryza, cough, and development of small white lesions with blue centers on the oral mucous membranes (Koplik's spots).

2. **Rubella.** Pale maculopapular lesions start on the face and spread downward; lymphadenopathy (occipital and postauricular) is a consistent finding.

3. **Fifth disease** (erythema infectiosum). This parvovirus infection presents with a slapped-cheek appearance and often is accompanied by a mild fever, followed by a diffuse, reticular rash that spreads to the extremities.

5. What diagnosis is suggested when a morbilliform rash develops in a patient treated with ampicillin for pharyngitis?

The probable diagnosis is infectious mononucleosis, which is caused by Epstein-Barr virus. In this instance, a drug-virus interaction results in the eruption. This interaction occurs with much greater frequency (up to 95% of patients treated) than a reaction to ampicillin alone.

6. What diagnosis should be considered when a maculopapular eruption of palms, soles, ankles, and wrists follows a febrile syndrome?

The initial eruption of **Rocky Mountain spotted fever** follows this distribution. Although lesions eventually become classically purpuric, early recognition of this tick-borne infection is important to appropriate management. **Atypical measles** also may present in this manner, especially in immunized adults.

7. What other viral entities cause a morbilliform exanthem?

Epstein-Barr virus, coxsackievirus, echovirus, and adenovirus.

8. Why is it important to think of Kawasaki's disease in a child with a morbilliform or scarlatiniform rash?

Kawasaki's disease is a multisystem disorder of young children that results in coronary artery aneurysms in as many as 25% of patients. Early recognition of the disease may permit appropriate therapy (high-dose intravenous gamma globulin and aspirin) to reduce the incidence of coronary arteritis. Hallmarks of the disease include rash (often leading to desquamation), conjunctival injection, nonsuppurative cervical lymphadenopathy, oral erythema with strawberry tongue, and fever.

9. When should the provider consider scabies as a diagnosis?

Scabies is caused by a mite and characteristically presents with linear burrows 1–2 mm wide and < 1 cm long. Papules are typically located in skinfolds, between the fingers, on the male genitalia, and on the buttocks. Burrows are often replaced by excoriations. Family members and close contacts are often affected. Severe pruritus is usually the presenting feature and often worsens at night.

10. What is appropriate therapy for scabies?

Treatment must include all household and sexual contacts in addition to the patient. Gamma benzene hexachloride (lindane: Kwell) is applied to the dry skin of the entire body below the neck for a period of 4 hours and then washed off. This application may be repeated once in 5 days to eliminate hatching ova. All family members should be treated simultaneously. Patients should be instructed that the pruritus may persist for 3–4 weeks after treatment is completed. Pruritus can be managed with medium-potency topical steroids (triamcinolone cream, 0.025%) and oral hydroxyzine hydrochloride, 25 mg 4 times/day. Gamma benzene hexachloride should not be used in children younger than 1 year. Alternatives include permethrin (Elimite) or sulfur ointment, 5%.

BIBLIOGRAPHY

1. Fitzpatrick TB, et al (eds): Dermatology in General Medicine, 4th ed. New York, McGraw-Hill, 1993.
2. Moschella SL, Hurley HJ (eds): Dermatology, 3rd ed. Philadelphia, W.B. Saunders, 1992.
3. Phillips TJ, Dover JS: Recent advances in dermatology. N Engl J Med 326:167–178, 1992.

91. PAPULOSQUAMOUS SKIN LESIONS

Mark Fogarty, M.D., and Loren E. Golitz, M.D.

1. What characterizes papulosquamous skin lesions?

This major category of skin disorders is characterized by raised (papular) lesions with scales. They may or may not be pruritic.

2. Name the three most common diseases seen in primary care practice that present with a generalized papulosquamous rash.

Psoriasis, pityriasis rosea, and lichen planus.

3. Describe the presentation of psoriasis.

Psoriasis is usually a slowly progressive inflammatory disease that manifests as demarcated erythematous plaques covered with silvery scales and symmetrically distributed over extensor surfaces of elbows and knees, the gluteal cleft, and scalp.

4. When is the Koebner phenomenon seen?
The Koebner phenomenon, which refers to the development of plaques in areas of previous trauma, is commonly seen in patients with psoriasis and lichen planus.

5. What other findings are associated with psoriasis?
Nail-pitting is found in over 50% of patients, along with onycholysis and thickened nails. Joint manifestations are typically rheumatoid factor negative, asymmetric, and often limited to distal interphalangeal joints.

6. What should be the initial therapy for psoriasis?
Skin hydration and mid-potency steroids are standard therapy for limited skin plaques. A kerolytic agent (salicylic acid) or a tar gel may enhance steroid effectiveness. When the disease becomes less responsive or widespread (especially if erythroderma is present), more aggressive treatment with ultraviolet light or systemic methotrexate may be required. Such patients should be seen by a dermatologist to consider the most appropriate mode of therapy.

7. What is a herald patch?
A herald patch is an annular lesion 2–6 cm in size that "heralds" the onset of pityriasis rosea by a few days.

8. What causes pityriasis rosea?
The cause of this self-limited, seasonal disease (seen in spring and fall) is unknown. A truncal papulosquamous eruption of oval brown lesions parallel to skinfolds follows the herald patch. Treatment for pruritus is symptomatic; topical steroids may be used, if needed. Resolution is expected by 6–8 weeks.

9. What disease may pityriasis rosea mimic?
The lesions of pityriasis are similar to those of secondary syphilis. However, pityriasis rosea does not involve the palms and soles, both of which are commonly involved in secondary syphilis.

10. Where do lesions of lichen planus occur?
The pruritic, violaceous, papulosquamous lesions of lichen planus favor the wrists, shins, lower back, and genital area. Such lesions also commonly involve the oral mucosa, presenting as a white reticulated patch in the buccal area. Scalp involvement may lead to hair loss.

11. What causes lichen planus?
The cause of lichen planus is unknown. Similar lichenoid eruptions may result from a reaction to several drugs, including diuretics, antimalarials, and phenothiazines. Most cases, however, are idiopathic and spontaneously remit within 2 years. Topical steroids are usually helpful.

12. What disease is characterized by severe dandruff and greasy, scaly, erythematous plaques over the central area of the face?
Seborrheic dermatitis, which also affects the eyelids, eyebrows, external ear, and glabella and occasionally is even more widespread.

13. What types of individuals are particularly susceptible to seborrheic dermatitis?
1. Infants—"cradle cap"
2. Patients with Parkinson's disease
3. Patients who previously suffered a cerebrovascular accident
4. Patients infected with the human immunodeficiency virus (HIV)

14. How should seborrheic dermatitis be treated?
1. Nonfluorinated topical steroid solutions of low-to-mid potency (fluocinolone acetonide solution, 0.01%)
2. Shampoos with salicylic acid or coal tar

15. Why should a chronic scaly patch or plaque in the swimming-trunk distribution be considered for biopsy?

Such nonspecific lesions, which often appear psoriatic, may be a prodromal or heralding lesion of mycosis fungoides (a T-cell lymphoma). Although the trunk distribution is common, lesions also may appear on extremities. Biopsy initially may be nonspecific, but eventually a mononuclear cell infiltrate with Pautrier's abscesses may be found.

BIBLIOGRAPHY

1. Fitzpatrick TB, et al (eds): Dermatology in General Medicine, 4th ed. New York, McGraw-Hill, 1993.
2. Moschella SL, Hurley HJ (eds): Dermatology, 3rd ed. Philadelphia, W.B. Saunders, 1992.
3. Phillips TJ, Dover JS: Recent advances in dermatology. N Engl J Med 326:167–178, 1992.

92. VESICULAR AND BULLOUS SKIN ERUPTIONS

Mark Fogarty, M.D., and Loren E. Golitz, M.D.

1. What is the difference between a vesicle and a bulla?

Both are blisters of the skin filled with serous fluid, but vesicles are < 0.5 cm and bullae > 0.5 cm in diameter. Some diseases are predominantly vesicular or bullous, whereas others involve a spectrum of lesions.

2. What is the differential diagnosis of a disseminated vesicular rash in children?

A vesicular rash is varicella (chickenpox) until proved otherwise. The diagnosis is suggested by history of exposure (90% attack rate in seronegative individuals) and crops of maculopapular lesions that progress to vesicles within hours, beginning on the trunk and face, and are accompanied by pruritus. Patients are contagious 48 hours before eruption and until all vesicles are crusted.

Other less likely possibilities, often distinguished by the appropriate history and setting, include (1) infections with coxsackie- or echovirus, (2) rickettsialpox (which may be distinguished by a herald spot at the site of the mite bite), and (3) disseminated herpes simplex infection (which may be seen in patients with atopic dermatitis).

3. What advice should the provider give to patients with chickenpox infections?

1. Lukewarm soaks and compresses relieve pruritus and prevent secondary infection.
2. Close clipping of fingernails prevents excoriations.
3. Aspirin should be avoided because of the risk of Reye's syndrome.
4. Oral acyclovir should be given to adolescents and adults with chickenpox of < 24 hours' duration.
5. New-onset respiratory symptoms require medical assessment.

4. What is shingles?

Shingles or herpes zoster disease results from varicella virus that has been latent in the dorsal root or cranial nerve ganglia. It presents as isolated pain followed by a unilateral vesicular eruption in a dermatomal distribution. Shingles occurs sporadically in the elderly population but rarely recurs. Cranial nerves may be involved, leading to mucosal, ear, and eye lesions.

5. What can be done to decrease the incidence of postherpetic neuralgia?
Up to 50% of older patients have dermatomal pain months after resolution of the vesicular lesions of zoster infection. This pain may be prevented by treatment with 7–10 days of acyclovir; the efficacy of steroids is less clearly established. Symptomatic relief with analgesics and amitriptyline may be attempted.

6. Which patients are at high risk of dissemination from varicella infections?
Immunocompromised patients, including those with Hodgkin's and non-Hodgkin's lymphoma; patients who receive bone marrow transplant; and newborns are at risk of dissemination from varicella virus. Immune prophylaxis should be given to exposed patients; intravenous acyclovir is indicated for evidence of disease.

7. What four classic diseases should be considered in the differential diagnosis of a bullous eruption?
The four classic bullous diseases are pemphigus vulgaris, bullous pemphigoid, erythema multiforme, and dermatitis herpetiformis, which often can be diagnosed by clinical appearance. Diagnosis is confirmed by routine biopsy or by immunofluorescence microscopy of frozen tissue. Because treatment is somewhat different in each, correct diagnosis is crucial.

8. What is the typical appearance of erythema multiforme?
Erythema multiforme, the most common of the four classic bullous diseases, affects predominantly children and young adults. Cutaneous lesions vary from erythematous papules and plaques to annular and bullous lesions. The classic lesion is the target (also termed an iris lesion), which most often occurs on the distal extremities and is characterized by a dusky gray center and an erythematous rim. Involvement of mucous membranes, especially the oral mucosa, is common. Less often the ocular and genital mucosa are affected.

9. What are the most common causes of erythema multiforme?
The most common cause of erythema multiforme minor is recurrent herpes simplex infection (about 90% of patients). The rash of erythema multiforme occurs 7–10 days after a lesion of herpes simplex. Because herpes simplex is frequently recurrent, erythema multiforme also may recur. The second most common cause of erythema multiforme minor is drugs, especially sulfa drugs, barbiturates, and antibiotics such as tetracycline.

10. What is Stevens-Johnson syndrome?
Erythema multiforme major, a more severe form of erythema multiforme, also is known as Stevens-Johnson syndrome. The majority of cases are caused by drugs, particularly sulfa drugs. Patients with Stevens-Johnson syndrome are often very ill and may require hospitalization. Mucous membranes often show severe involvement. If the ocular mucous membranes are involved, an ophthalmologist should be consulted to prevent permanent eye damage.

11. How are erythema multiforme and Stevens-Johnson syndrome treated?
The treatment of erythema multiforme minor is generally symptomatic, because the condition is self-limited. Triamcinolone creams (0.025%, applied 2–4 times/day) and hydroxyzine hydrochloride (for pruritus) are usually effective in relieving the symptoms. In patients with frequent recurrences of herpes simplex and erythema multiforme, long-term suppressive therapy with oral acyclovir may be indicated. If the etiologic agent is a drug, it should be discontinued. The management of Stevens-Johnson syndrome often includes hospitalization.

12. What diagnosis does a recurrent, severely pruritic vesicular eruption suggest?
Dermatitis herpetiformis is characterized by extremely pruritic vesicles grouped on the elbows, interscapular areas, lower back, and knees. Excoriations are often evident. Approximately 80%

of patients have a gluten-sensitive enteropathy, but most are asymptomatic. A routine biopsy of a fresh blister confirms the diagnosis. Mucous membranes are not involved.

13. Describe the treatment of dermatitis herpetiformis.

Therapy with dapsone, 50–100 mg/day, produces a dramatic improvement in the pruritus. The vesicles rapidly heal, and patients usually become asymptomatic. If the patient can maintain a gluten-free diet, the dose of dapsone often may be reduced or eliminated. However, because patients usually do not have bowel symptoms, it is difficult to keep them on a gluten-free diet. Dapsone often needs to be maintained for a long duration at the lowest possible dose. Before initiating dapsone therapy, patients should be evaluated for deficiency of glucose-6-phosphate-dehydrogenase because of the risk of methemoglobinemia. Dapsone causes a mild hemolysis of red blood cells in most patients. Rarely, bone marrow suppression or hepatitis may result. Therefore, patients on dapsone should be monitored with appropriate laboratory tests.

14. How is pemphigus vulgaris treated?

Before the development of systemic corticosteroids, pemphigus vulgaris was considered to be a uniformly fatal disease. Therefore, treatment needs to be relatively aggressive to control the disease as quickly as possible. Once the correct diagnosis is established, patients should be treated with prednisone, 60–80 mg in a single daily dose. Antacids and H_2 blockers should be used in patients with a history of peptic ulcer disease. In most cases, a steroid-sparing drug, such as azathioprine, should be started at the initiation of prednisone therapy. The full steroid-sparing effect of azathioprine requires approximately 6 weeks. Once the cutaneous lesions of pemphigus vulgaris show complete healing, the dosage of prednisone is slowly reduced. The goal should be to keep the patient on the lowest dose of alternate-day prednisone that controls the disease. It may require several months before the prednisone and azathioprine can be completely discontinued.

15. Describe the presentation and treatment of bullous pemphigoid.

Bullous pemphigoid is typically a disease of middle-aged and elderly patients. At one time, it was referred to as bullous disease of the aged. It is characterized by large tense blisters with a predilection for the intertriginous areas such as the inner thighs and axillae. The blisters show much less tendency to rupture than those of pemphigus vulgaris. Blisters may occur in the mouth but, unlike pemphigus vulgaris, mucosal lesions usually follow the onset of skin disease. Often the tense blisters of bullous pemphigoid are situated on red urticarial plaques. Bullous pemphigoid is less likely to be a life-threatening disease than pemphigus vulgaris. Therefore, the dose of oral prednisone and steroid-sparing agents, such as azathioprine, may be more conservative. An initial prednisone dose of 40–60 mg/day is usually adequate. The disease responds to treatment more quickly than pemphigus vulgaris.

BIBLIOGRAPHY

1. Fitzpatrick TB, et al (eds): Dermatology in General Medicine, 4th ed. New York, McGraw-Hill, 1993.
2. Moschella SL, Hurley HJ (eds): Dermatology, 3rd ed. Philadelphia, W.B. Saunders, 1992.
3. Phillips TJ, Dover JS: Recent advances in dermatology. N Engl J Med 326:167–178, 1992.

93. URTICARIA

Mark Fogarty, M.D., and Loren E. Golitz, M.D.

1. What is acute urticaria?

Acute urticaria is a localized, transient, white or erythematous swelling of the skin of less than 6 weeks' duration. Individual lesions, also called hives or wheals, are frequently annular or poly-cyclic. The swelling is due to a localized increase in capillary and venule permeability mediated by histamines and other cytokines. Individual wheals usually resolve within 24 hours but may be present in multiple stages of evolution. Lesions are commonly associated with pruritus or a stinging sensation. Papular urticaria, which is caused by hypersensitivity to arthropod bites, begins as umbilicated red papules and may progress to annular lesions or plaques.

2. What is the difference between angioedema and urticaria?

Urticaria involves the superficial aspect of the skin, whereas angioedema involves the deeper layers, including the subcutaneous tissue. Both may occur separately or together. Demarcation of lesions is less evident in angioedema, which also may involve the upper respiratory tract, presenting as bronchospasm, and the gastrointestinal tract, manifesting as gastrointestinal colic. Thus the caregiver should ask about such symptoms in patients with the complaint of urticaria.

3. When should the provider suspect acute urticaria as a manifestation of anaphylaxis?

Anaphylaxis is a life-threatening response of the sensitized individual to a specific antigen. Respiratory distress followed by vascular collapse may be heralded by or accompanied by pruritus and urticaria, with or without angioedema. The most important aspect in ascertaining the diagnosis of anaphylaxis is an acute history documenting the onset of signs and symptoms within minutes of exposure to an antigen. Early recognition is paramount, because death from anaphylaxis may occur within minutes to hours.

4. Name the most common causes of acute urticaria.

Urticaria with or without angioedema may be immunoglobulin E (IgE)-dependent, complement-mediated, or due to direct release of histamine from mast cells. The most common identifiable causes are medications, arthropod bites, and infections. However, in the majority of patients, a definite cause is not identified.

5. What is the mainstay of treatment for acute urticaria?

Treatment involves elimination of the cause, if known. The mainstays of medical therapy are histamine-1 (H_1) receptor blockers, including classic H_1 antihistamines (e.g., diphenhydramine and hydroxyzine) and nonsedating H_1 antihistamines (terfenadine, astemizole, and loratadine). Such agents should be initiated at standard doses and titrated as tolerated. Doxepin hydro-chloride, a tricyclic antidepressant with powerful H_1 antagonist activity, also may be useful. H_2 antihistamines administered in combination with H_1 blockers may be more effective than H_1 antihistamines alone in some patients. Disodium cromoglycate, terbutaline, and calcium channel blockers also may have a role in the treatment of some patients. In rare patients, a 1- to 2-week course of systemic corticosteroids may be needed.

6. Is epinephrine ever indicated in the treatment of acute urticaria?

Yes. In severe cases of urticaria or when anaphylaxis is suspected, subcutaneous epinephrine (0.3 cc of a 1:1000 solution) should be administered and may be repeated at 30-minute intervals for severe reactions. Intravenous or intramuscular administration of epinephrine is required in patients with airway involvement, anaphylaxis, or cardiovascular collapse.

7. What should be done for patients who manifest urticaria to bee stings?

It is important to determine the patient's potential risk of anaphylaxis. If no history is easily obtainable to assess risk, a skin test should be considered. Potential for anaphylaxis correlates with a positive skin test. After assessing the risk for anaphylaxis, the following steps should be provided:

1. **Instruction in prevention.** Lifestyle should be modified to avoid exposure to bees (wearing of shoes, avoidance of eating or wearing perfume in high-risk areas, limitation of unnecessary yard work, especially hauling trash).

2. **Instruction in emergency measures.** Unexpired epinephrine kits should be readily available at home and in the car, and informational bracelets and tags should be used.

3. **Desensitization.** In patients with a history or serious risk of anaphylaxis, venom immunotherapy may be undertaken until the skin test is negative. Desensitization is not required for children who experience a systemic reaction limited to the skin, because progression to anaphylaxis is unlikely.

8. Define chronic urticaria.

Chronic urticaria is defined as urticaria lasting longer than 6 weeks. It may be continuous or episodic.

9. Which conditions may be mistaken for chronic urticaria?

Systemic or subacute lupus erythematosus
Erythema multiforme
Erythema annulare centrifugum
Bullous pemphigoid
Drug eruptions
Urticarial vasculitis, a form of leukocytoclastic vasculitis
    associated with hypocomplementemia

10. What are the most common causes of chronic urticaria?

Causes of chronic urticaria include chronic infections (e.g., sinusitis, vaginitis, otitis, hepatitis), drugs, neoplasia, mastocytosis, collagen-vascular diseases, hyperthyroidism, contact urticaria, pressure urticaria, and psychogenic urticaria. Urticaria may be prominent in skin disorders such as bullous pemphigoid. In most cases of chronic urticaria, the specific cause cannot be determined.

11. Describe the initial evaluation of patients with chronic urticaria.

A thorough history and physical examination are the most important parts of the work-up. Key historical features include the pattern of occurrence and relationship to medications, diet, and activity. Medication usage, including nonprescription drugs and home remedies, should be reviewed. Physical examination should rule out signs of systemic disease and physical urticaria. Screening laboratory tests should include complete blood count, liver and renal function tests, erythrocyte sedimentation rate, and urinalysis. Further testing is usually not necessary, unless suggested by positive findings from the history or physical examination (e.g., antinuclear antibodies, stool for ova and parasites, hepatitis-B serology, thyroid function studies, thyroid antibodies).

12. When is a skin biopsy indicated?

If individual lesions of urticaria are purpuric or persist for days, a skin biopsy should be considered to rule out urticarial vasculitis.

13. What common disease is associated with urticaria?

Urticaria may be associated with sinusitis. If symptoms of sinusitis are present with urticaria, sinus radiographs are a cost-effective diagnostic procedure. Chronic sinusitis may require an extended course of antibiotics (see chapter 84).

14. How is dermatographism diagnosed and treated?

Dermatographism is the most common cause of physical urticaria. Linear wheals develop rapidly after blunt, firm stroking of the skin and resolve within 1 hour. About 5% of the population has asymptomatic simple dermatographism; symptomatic dermatographism is much less common. Patients with atopic dermatitis have an increased incidence of dermatographism. For symptomatic patients, the pruritic wheals may last for several hours. Treatment consists of oral antihistamines and avoidance of trauma to the skin. Delayed dermatographism presents with linear, red nodules that develop 3–6 hours after stimulation and persist for 24–48 hours.

BIBLIOGRAPHY

1. Bush RK (ed): Clinical allergy. Med Clin North Am 76:805–840, 1992.
2. Cooper KD: Acute and chronic urticaria and angioedema. J Am Acad Dermatol 25:146–154, 1991.
3. Fitzpatrick TB, et al (eds): Dermatology in General Medicine, 4th ed. New York, McGraw-Hill, 1993.
4. Kennard CD, Ellis CN: Pharmacologic therapy for urticaria. J Am Acad Dermatol 25:177–189, 1991.
5. Moschella SL, Hurley HJ (eds): Dermatology, 3rd ed. Philadelphia, W.B. Saunders, 1992.
6. Phillips TJ, Dover JS: Recent advances in dermatology. N Engl J Med 326:167–178, 1992.
7. Yecies LD, Kaplan AD: Urticaria. In Parker CW (ed): Clinical Immunology. Philadelphia, W.B. Saunders, 1980, pp 1283–1315.

94. SKIN INFECTIONS

Mark Fogarty, M.D., and Loren E. Golitz, M.D.

1. Describe the presentation and treatment of impetigo contagiosa.

Impetigo contagiosa is an infectious disorder of the skin that begins as small vesicles and progresses rapidly to erosions covered by a thick, honey-colored crust. Exposed parts of the body, such as the face and arms, are commonly involved. Most patients are children. Over the past decade *Staphylococcus aureus* has replaced beta-hemolytic streptococci as the most common organism and accounts for approximately 85% of positive cultures. Treatment includes regular cleansing with antibacterial soap and treatment with oral erythromycin, cephalosporin, or dicloxacillin. Topical antibiotics such as mupirocin may be used instead of systemic antibiotics if skin involvement is not extensive.

2. What is ecthyma?

Ecthyma is similar to impetigo but is deeper and produces a shallow ulcer covered by crust. The causative organisms are the same as for impetigo contagiosa. The lower legs are most commonly affected and the condition is more prevalent in warm, humid climates. Low-grade fever and lymphadenopathy commonly occur. Treatment includes warm compresses to remove the crust and oral erythromycin, cephalosporin, or dicloxacillin. With appropriate therapy the lesions of impetigo and icthyma usually heal within 1 week.

3. What is secondary pyoderma?

Secondary pyoderma is a bacterial infection of skin associated with preceding dermatologic disorders such as atopic dermatitis, neurodermatitis, scabies, or traumatic lesions. *Staphylococcus aureus* is the causative organism in approximately 80–85% of cases; in the bulk of the remaining cases, the infectious agents are streptococci. Gram-negative organisms, including *Proteus* sp., *Pseudomonas* sp., and *Escherichia coli*, may colonize the skin in patients with other debilitating conditions, such as diabetes mellitus.

4. How is secondary pyoderma treated?

Treatment includes systemic antibiotics based on culture results and removal of crust and purulent drainage. Abscesses may need to be surgically drained. Antipruritic agents, such as hydroxyzine hydrochloride (25 mg 4 times/day), are useful in the presence of extensive excoriations. Once the infection is under control, the underlying dermatosis should be treated with topical corticosteroids, such as triamcinolone acetonide cream.

5. Describe the typical appearance and treatment of dermatophyte infection of the scalp.

Tinea capitis is a fungal infection of the scalp most commonly seen in children between the ages of 4 and 14 years. *Trichophyton tonsurans* is the most common causative organism in the United States. Infection begins as a small erythematous papule around a hair shaft and then spreads to involve surrounding hairs. Involved hairs often break off at the scalp surface, producing the appearance of black dots. Kerion, an inflammatory plaque associated with hair loss and purulent drainage, also may be caused by *T. tonsurans.*

6. Which simple clinical tests help to make the diagnosis of tinea capitis?

Wood's lamp examination of lesions caused by *Microsporum* sp. shows bright green fluorescence of hair shafts just above the skin surface of the scalp. Hair shafts and scale should be obtained for microscopic examination and culture on Sabouraud's agar. Infected areas may be scraped with a scalpel, or hairs in the infected areas may be plucked. The specimen should be examined microscopically after the addition of 20–25% potassium hydroxide (KOH) solution. Hyphae and spores are seen on or within the hair shaft. The differential diagnosis includes seborrheic dermatitis, atopic dermatitis, psoriasis, alopecia areata, trichotillomania, and secondary syphilis.

7. How should tinea capitis be treated?

Systemic antifungal agents are required for the treatment of tinea capitis. Adults should receive 1 gm/day of microsize griseofulvin in divided doses with meals; 6 weeks to 3 months of therapy is usually required to produce clinical resolution and negative cultures. In children, the dose of microsize griseofulvin is 10–20 mg/kg/day. Adjunctive therapy with selenium sulfide shampoo may reduce the transmission of tinea capitis to others. Inflammatory tinea capitis (kerion) should be treated with the same dose of griseofulvin plus systemic corticosteroids to reduce the inflammation that often results in areas of permanent hair loss and scarring. Although kerion resembles a purulent bacterial infection, systemic antibiotics are not effective.

8. How do dermatophyte infections of the hands and feet present?

Tinea pedis and tinea manuum are fungal infections of the feet and hands, respectively. Tinea pedis occurs most commonly in the summer months. Infections are transmitted from one person to another by the use of communal pools and baths. The most common etiologic fungi include *Trichophyton rubrum* (which causes a dry, moccasin-type eruption), *Trichophyton mentagrophytes* (which may cause vesicles), and *Epidermophyton floccosum* (which is rare and usually limited to the toe webs). Cases of tinea pedis with prominent interdigital maceration and hyperkeratosis may have a secondary bacterial infection. Occasionally, a dermatophyte may involve both feet and one hand (the two-feet, one-hand syndrome). Diagnosis is based on the clinical appearance, positive culture, and a KOH preparation showing branching, septate hyphae.

9. How are tinea pedis and tinea manuum treated?

Treatment includes reduction of excessive moisture with talcum or antifungal powders. Eradication can be achieved with a systemic antifungal agent, such as griseofulvin (1 gm/day) in divided doses with meals), but recurrence is common. Topical agents for tinea pedis or tinea manuum include tolnaftate, clotrimazole, miconazole, ketoconazole, and terbinafine. An economic topical treatment for chronic tinea pedis of the dry, moccasin type is 10% salicylic acid ointment, applied twice daily.

10. Describe the appearance of tinea corporis.

Tinea corporis includes fungal infections of glabrous skin, except the hands, feet, and groin. The most common etiologic organisms are *T. rubrum, Microsporum canis,* and *T. mentagrophytes.* Infection may be acquired from contact with infected humans or animals. Tinea corporis most commonly presents as annular lesions with an erythematous scaly border and central clearing. Animal ringworm (i.e., *M. canis*) is often inflammatory or pustular. The differential diagnosis includes other ringlike eruptions, such as erythema annulare centrifugum, nummular eczema, and granuloma annulare.

11. Can dermatophyte infections involve the face?

Yes. Dermatophyte infection of the face, called tinea faciei, may mimic lupus erythematosus, seborrheic dermatitis, and contact dermatitis. Microscopic examination of a KOH preparation of scrapings obtained from the border of the lesions shows branching, septate hyphae. A positive KOH examination may be difficult to demonstrate in the inflammatory variants of tinea. Combining fungal culture and KOH examination increases the likelihood of making the definitive diagnosis.

12. How are tinea corporis and tinea faciei treated?

Localized cases are treated with topical antifungal agents (see question 9), whereas inflammatory and widespread lesions often require treatment with griseofulvin. Because treatment of tinea corporis with griseofulvin usually requires a course of at least 6–8 weeks, the drug should be prescribed only for patients with a positive KOH examination or culture.

13. What is tinea cruris?

Tinea cruris, commonly referred to as "jock itch," begins in the groin fold and progresses with a raised, scaly border. In contrast to inguinal candidiasis, the scrotum and labia are rarely involved, the color is rarely beefy red, and satellite vesicopustules are usually absent. Scrapings of scales are usually positive for hyphae with the KOH examination. Reduction of moisture with talcum powders and application of topical antifungal agents (see question 9) are generally effective. Extensive cases may require 6–8 weeks of therapy with oral griseofulvin.

14. Describe the differentiation of cutaneous candidiasis and tinea cruris.

Infections caused by *Candida albicans* most commonly involve skinfolds, including the axilla, genitocrural, gluteal, submammary, and perianal areas. Candidiasis of the skinfold has a beefy red color and often shows satellite pustules. Obesity, diabetes mellitus, and chronic occupational exposure to excessive moisture are the most common accompanying factors. Presentation may be atypical in immunocompromised patients and may not be limited to intertriginous areas. Other manifestations of candidal infection include thrush, vulvovaginitis, and balanitis. The diagnosis is based on a KOH preparation, which shows round- or oval-budding yeast and pseudohyphae. The organism is easily cultured on Sabouraud's medium.

15. How is cutaneous candidiasis treated?

Treatment of cutaneous candidiasis includes correction of predisposing conditions such as heat and moisture and use of topical antifungal creams or ointments. Powder or cream containing nystatin may be helpful in the treatment of moist intertriginous areas. Occasionally, treatment of the gastrointestinal tract with oral nystatin, in combination with topical agents, is helpful for treating candidiasis of the anogenital area. Oral nystatin is not absorbed and is not useful alone in treating cutaneous candidiasis.

BIBLIOGRAPHY

1. Fitzpatrick TB, et al (eds): Dermatology in General Medicine, 4th ed. New York, McGraw-Hill, 1993.
2. Moschella SL, Hurley HJ (eds): Dermatology, 3rd ed. Philadelphia, W.B. Saunders, 1992.
3. Phillips TJ, Dover JS: Recent advances in dermatology. N Engl J Med 326:167–178, 1992.

95. ISOLATED SKIN LESIONS

Mark Fogarty, M.D., and Loren E. Golitz, M.D.

1. How do common warts present?
Common warts (verrucae vulgaris) appear as sharply marginated keratotic papules with a rough surface. They may appear anywhere on the skin but are most common on the dorsal surfaces of the hand and fingers. Common warts are a neoplasm caused by the human papillomavirus.

2. Describe the two common treatments for warts.
1. Twice daily application of 17% salicylic acid solution (Compound W, Wart-Off) results in sloughing of keratin. Prolonged therapy is usually required.

2. Cryotherapy with liquid nitrogen may be applied with a probe, pressurized spray, or cotton swab. The wart and a narrow rim of normal skin should be frozen for 20–30 seconds, allowed to thaw, and frozen a second time. The treatment is associated with mild burning pain. The double freeze-thaw method should be repeated at 7–10-day intervals until the warts are eliminated. Patients should be told that formation of a blister is an expected effect. The fluid should be drained and the area kept clean.

3. What topical agents are useful in the treatment of genital warts?
For most genital warts (condylomata acuminatum), 25% podophyllin in tincture of benzoin may be applied in the office. Petroleum jelly then should be applied to the normal skin to protect it from irritation. The podophyllin must be washed off in 4 hours. The treatment is repeated weekly until the condylomata are gone. Podophyllin should not be given to patients for home treatment because of the potential for severe reactions. Podofilox may be used topically on genital condylomata and has the advantage that the patient may apply it at home. Less commonly used therapies include 5-fluorouracil and intralesional interferon or bleomycin.

4. How does basal cell carcinoma present?
Basal cell carcinoma, the most common cutaneous malignancy, is found predominantly in patients with a history of chronic sun exposure; 80–90% of lesions are found on the head and neck. Lesions typically are nonkeratinized papules with a smooth translucent surface and telangiectatic vessels. Large lesions commonly have central ulceration and crusting. Basal cell carcinomas may be heavily pigmented and difficult to differentiate from malignant melanoma.

5. Describe the appearance of actinic keratosis.
Actinic keratosis is an isolated macule or papule in a sun-exposed area that is red-brown in color and often has a dry, rough adherent scale.

6. Why should actinic keratosis be distinguished from seborrheic keratosis?
Actinic keratosis is a premalignant lesion that leads to squamous cell carcinoma of the skin and thus should be removed. Seborrheic keratosis, which appears both on the face and trunk, is a brownish papule with a "stuck-on" appearance and has no particular implication (other than cosmetic).

7. Describe the typical appearance of squamous cell carcinoma.
Squamous cell carcinomas also arise in sun-damaged skin such as the head, neck, or arms. Lesions appear as firm skin-colored or slightly erythematous nodules with a distinct margin. The surface is rough or verrucous, and ulceration is common. Squamous cell carcinomas of the skin often develop from preexisting actinic keratoses.

8. How does the clinical course of squamous cell carcinoma of the lip differ from that of typical squamous cell carcinoma?

Squamous cell carcinomas that develop on the lower lip, in burn scars, or in areas of prior radiation therapy tend to behave in a more aggressive manner and may metastasize.

9. How are basal and squamous cell carcinomas diagnosed and treated?

The definitive diagnosis is based on histologic examination of a biopsy specimen. Metastases are rare in basal cell carcinomas and squamous cell carcinomas in chronically sun-damaged skin. However, both tumors may be locally aggressive. Treatments include surgical excision, curettage and electrosurgery, micrographic surgery, and radiotherapy. Referral to a dermatologist is appropriate.

10. Who is at risk for the development of melanoma?

- Individuals who are fair-skinned, blue-eyed, red-haired, and freckled
- Individuals with dysplastic nevi (atypical moles)
- Patients with a family history of melanoma
- Individuals with a congenital melanocyte nevus
- Immunocompromised individuals

11. What features of a pigmented skin lesion suggest the diagnosis of malignant melanoma?

The ABCD rule can be used to evaluate a pigmented lesion for the possibility of melanoma or melanoma precursor (dysplastic nevus):

Asymmetry	Color variegation or dark color
Border irregularity	**D**iameter > 0.6 cm

The ABCD features are more common in melanomas than in benign pigmented lesions. Ulceration, pruritus, pain, new lesions, or changes in existing pigmented lesions also should arouse suspicion.

12. How can a hemangioma be distinguished from a nodular melanoma?

Both lesions may appear as a reddish, bluish dome-shaped nodule. However, compression of a hemangioma (with a glass microscopic slide) results in blanching.

13. How is the prognosis of melanoma established?

Definitive diagnosis of a suspicious lesion is made by excisional biopsy. Prognosis of localized melanoma (localized to the skin) is based largely on tumor thickness, which is measured histopathologically. Lesions less than 0.76 mm in thickness are associated with a favorable 5 year survival rate.

14. What treatment and follow-up are indicated?

Stage I melanoma is treated with surgical excision. Recent studies have shown that wide surgical margins usually are not necessary. Lesions up to 1 mm thick can be treated with 1-cm margins, whereas 2-cm margins may be indicated for thicker lesions. Prospective, randomized studies of prophylactic regional lymph node dissection have shown no survival benefit. Patients should have regular follow-up for local recurrence, metastases, and second primary melanomas. Patients with melanoma are best followed by oncologists, dermatologists, or other specially trained physicians.

BIBLIOGRAPHY

1. Fitzpatrick TB, et al (eds): Dermatology in General Medicine, 4th ed. New York, McGraw-Hill, 1993.
2. Koh HK: Cutaneous melanoma. N Engl J Med 325:171–182, 1991.
3. Moschella SL, Hurley HJ (eds): Dermatology, 3rd ed. Philadelphia, W.B. Saunders, 1992.
4. Preston DS, Stern RS: Nonmelanoma cancers of the skin. N Engl J Med 327:1649–1662, 1992.

96. ACNE

Mark Fogarty, M.D., and Loren E. Golitz, M.D.

1. Describe the pathogenesis of acne vulgaris.
Follicular orifices become filled with debris and may or may not become inflamed, pustular, or even cystic. Inflammation is due to colonization with lipophilic bacteria.

2. Do adults experience acne?
Yes. Although acne vulgaris is usually a disease of young adults, up to 20% of adults may experience some form of acne. In addition, acne rosacea, characterized by central facial erythema and pustules (without comedones), is an adult-onset disease more common in women. Acne rosacea may lead to connective tissue overgrowth (rhinophyma) and inflammatory lesions of the eye.

3. What external factors aggravate acne?
  1. Trauma from overvigorous skin scrubbing or irritant contact (scarf, strap)
  2. Topical agents (cosmetics and industrial compounds that are comedone-forming, such as petrolatum, lanolin, parfarin oil, and oleic acid)

4. What drugs may cause an acneiform eruption or exacerbate underlying acne?
Glucocorticoids (topical or systemic), phenytoin, phenobarbital, and isoniazid.

5. What topical agents are effective therapies for acne vulgaris?
The treatment of acne vulgaris includes various topical agents, which may be more effective when used in combination. Benzoyl peroxide formulations function as topical antibacterial agents. Classic topical antibiotic agents include clindamycin and erythromycin. Topical vitamin A (tretinoin) interferes with the hyperkeratinization that plugs pilosebaceous units to produce comedones. The combination of 5% benzoyl peroxide in the morning and tretinoin (0.05% cream) at bedtime seems to work better than a single topical agent in many patients.

6. What are the indications for oral antibiotics?
Oral antibiotics are indicated in patients with moderate-to-severe acne or mild-to-moderate acne that does not respond to topical therapy. Oral antibiotics decrease the number of *Propionibacterium acnes* in the pilosebaceous units. The organisms break down triglycerides to free fatty acids, thus increasing inflammation. The oral antibiotics most commonly used are tetracycline and erythromycin at doses of 500–1000 mg/day in divided doses. The dose may be decreased to 250 mg/day after 1–2 months.

7. Are there contraindications to the use of tetracycline?
Yes. Tetracycline is contraindicated in pregnant women and in children under 10 years of age because of its effects on developing teeth and bones. Tetracycline may interfere with the effectiveness of oral contraceptive agents. Dairy products reduce the absorption of tetracylcine, which is best taken on an empty stomach.

8. What are the indications for second-line antibiotics in the treatment of acne?
In patients who fail to improve after 2–3 months of oral tetracycline or erythromycin, other antibiotics, such as minocycline, should be considered.

9. When should isotretinoin (Accutane) be used?
Isotretinoin is indicated for severe nodulocystic acne refractory to standard therapy. Because of potential severe side effects, patient reliability is important. Doses usually range

from 0.5–1.0 mg/kg/day with doses up to 2.0 mg/kg/day for severe truncal involvement. Therapy should be continued for 15–20 weeks and discontinued after 70–80% improvement is achieved.

10. What are the most common side effects of isotretinoin therapy?
Cheilitis occurs in almost every case. Other side effects include dry mouth, xerosis, conjunctivitis, vertebral hyperostoses, elevated serum lipids, mental depression, and hepatic toxicity. The most important side effect is severe fetal malformation.

11. What precautions should be taken before prescribing isotretinoin to women of childbearing age?
Women of childbearing age should receive isotretinoin only after reading the educational material provided by the manufacturer and giving informed consent, because it has been associated with a 25-fold increase in the risk of severe fetal abnormalities. Women of childbearing age should practice a reliable method of birth control continuously, starting at least 1 month before initiation of therapy. A negative serum pregnancy test should be obtained before initiating therapy, and patients should receive counseling on contraception. Pregnancy should be avoided for approximately 1 year after completing therapy with isotretinoin.

BIBLIOGRAPHY

1. Fitzpatrick TB, et al (eds): Dermatology in General Medicine, 4th ed. New York, McGraw-Hill, 1993.
2. Moschella SL, Hurley HJ (eds): Dermatology, 3rd ed. Philadelphia, W.B. Saunders, 1992.
3. Phillips TJ, Dover JS: Recent advances in dermatology. N Engl J Med 326:167–178, 1992.

97. DISORDERS OF THE NAILS AND HAIR

Mark Fogarty, M.D., and Loren E. Golitz, M.D.

1. How does fungal infection of the nail present?
Onychomycosis, which is most commonly caused by *Trichophyton rubrum* and *Trichophyton mentagrophytes,* usually begins at the distal edge of the nail and causes hyperkeratosis beneath the nailplate and distal separation of nailplate from the nailbed. The fungus grows proximally, leading to thickening and crumbling of the nailplate. Usually some nails are spared. Concomitant tinea pedis or tinea manuum is common. As a general rule, the feet should be examined when a patient presents with a rash of the hands or fingernails.

2. When is treatment of onychomycosis indicated?
Onychomycosis usually has only cosmetic sequelae, making treatment of toenail infection unnecessary in most patients. The appearance of infected fingernails may be more bothersome and may warrant therapy. Treatment must be continued until the entire nail grows out, which may require 1 year or more. Griseofulvin is the most commonly used agent. The usual adult dose is 1000 mg/day in the microsize form. Ketoconazole is also effective but more costly; furthermore, prolonged use may be associated with gynecomastia and/or hepatotoxicity. A positive fungal culture of nails is necessary before initiation of prolonged therapy, because other disorders such as psoriasis may mimic onychomycosis. Topical therapy is usually ineffective for fungal infections of nails or hair.

3. What diseases are associated with pitting of the nailbeds?

Psoriasis causes pitting of the surface of the nailplate due to involvement of the nail matrix. Discoloration, thickening, and distal onycholysis also may be seen. Dermatitis of the posterior nailfold skin may cause pitting or irregularity of the nailplate. Alopecia areata, a form of patchy nonscarring hair loss, also may be associated with nail pitting.

4. What do Beau's lines signify?

Acute illness, such as systemic infection or thyrotoxicosis, may cause temporary malfunction of the nail matrix, leading to development of transverse grooves called Beau's lines. The distance of Beau's lines may date the patient's illness; nails grow at the rate of approximately 1 mm/month.

5. How specific are splinter hemorrhages for subacute bacterial endocarditis (SBE)?

Splinter hemorrhages are seen in patients with SBE but also may be caused by local trauma in otherwise normal individuals. Splinter hemorrhages also have been reported with mitral stenosis, glomerulonephritis, vasculitis, cirrhosis, and various other diseases. Rheumatoid arthritis may cause excessive ridging and beading of the nails; systemic sclerosis (scleroderma) causes abnormalities in the capillary arcade of the nailbed, resulting in telangiectatic dilatations that can be seen with a hand-held magnifying glass.

6. What are the common causes of scarring and nonscarring alopecia?

The first distinction to make in a patient with alopecia is whether the hair loss is scarring or nonscarring. In nonscarring alopecia, the skin appears and feels normal. Examination of the skin in patients with scarring alopecia reveals atrophy, lack of visible follicular openings, and often erythema and hyperpigmentation or hypopigmentation. Causes of nonscarring alopecia include alopecia areata, androgenic alopecia (common baldness), and telogen effluvium (hair loss often seen in women 2–3 months after childbirth). Examples of scarring alopecia include discoid lupus erythematosus, lichen planopilaris (a form of lichen planus), and folliculitis decalvans.

7. Name three common causes of patchy alopecia.

The second major question to be answered in the clinic is whether the alopecia is patchy or diffuse. Three examples of patchy alopecia are alopecia areata, trichotillomania, and discoid lupus erythematosus. Alopecia areata shows round areas of hair loss without scarring. At the periphery of the patches, one may identify small hair shafts (approximately 3–4 mm long) that taper toward the skin surface (exclamation point hairs). Trichotillomania, which may be difficult to distinguish from alopecia areata, often occurs in children and adolescents. Hair loss is patchy, usually without scarring. However, careful examination of the patch of hair loss reveals broken hairs of variable length and often superficial excoriations and areas of scale. In addition to the scalp, eyebrows and eyelashes also are commonly involved. Invariably the patient denies pulling out the hair. Discoid lupus erythematosus is a form of patchy alopecia with scarring. A round or disklike area typically shows central hypopigmentation and atrophy with a hyperpigmented active margin. The surface is scaly, and often hair follicles are plugged with keratin, resembling the open comedones seen in acne. Other forms of patchy alopecia include trauma, radiation therapy, and metastatic carcinoma, particularly breast cancer in women.

8. What causes alopecia at the periphery of the scalp, usually in women?

Occasionally alopecia involves primarily the periphery of the scalp in the areas of the temples and above the ears. This form of alopecia is almost always secondary to traction, such as ponytails, corn-rowing, or tight hair curlers.

9. Which systemic illnesses may result in diffuse alopecia?

Telogen effluvium is the term given to the diffuse alopecia that results when many scalp follicles suddenly enter a resting phase, leading to fall-out of hair shafts. Typically this change occurs 2–3 months after an acute illness, major surgery, childbirth, or severe emotional breakdown. Systemic diseases such as hyper- and hypothyroidism and systemic lupus erythematosus also may cause telogen effluvium. The skin appears normal. Patients can be assured that the hair will grow back, although regrowth may take several months.

10. What nutritional deficiencies may result in hair loss?
Biotin, iron, protein, and zinc.

11. Characterize androgenic alopecia.
Androgenic alopecia (male- and female-pattern baldness) is usually classified as diffuse alopecia, although hair loss is accentuated in the areas of the temples and crown. The thickness of hair behind the ears usually appears normal. Most patients have a family history of first-degree relatives with significant androgenic alopecia. Androgen-producing tumors are a relatively rare cause of androgenic alopecia. On rare occasion, alopecia areata may present as diffuse alopecia.

BIBLIOGRAPHY

1. Fitzpatrick TB, et al (eds): Dermatology in General Medicine, 4th ed. New York, McGraw-Hill, 1993.
2. Moschella SL, Hurley HJ (eds): Dermatology, 3rd ed. Philadelphia, W.B. Saunders, 1992.

98. DERMATOLOGIC MANIFESTATIONS OF SYSTEMIC DISEASES

Loren E. Golitz, M.D., and Jeanette Mladenovic, M.D.

1. What conditions should be considered when a patient complains of pruritus but no rash is present?
Chronic renal disease. Up to 80% of patients undergoing hemodialysis have pruritus. The cause is unclear, and pruritus has no clear relationship to renal function tests. Patients undergoing dialysis have an increased number of intradermal mast cells and increased pruritus in response to histamine injection. Treatment with antihistamines is usually ineffective. A recent study demonstrated a marked improvement of pruritus in patients treated with erythropoietin. In some patients with secondary hyperparathyroidism, the pruritus may resolve after parathyroidectomy. Therapy with oral psoralen and long-wave ultraviolet light (PUVA) has been effective in some cases of pruritus related to renal failure, possibly through an effect on cutaneous mast cells.

Cholestatic liver disease. Although itching is correlated with increased levels of unconjugated bilirubin, the amount of pruritus is not. Biliary drainage or treatment wtih bile salt binders (colestipol or cholestyramine) often improves the pruritus.

Endocrine diseases. Thyrotoxicosis may present with generalized itching. Pruritus in hypothyroidism is probably related to dryness of the skin. Diabetes mellitus is usually not a cause of itching, although it may be associated with candidiasis or folliculitis.

Malignancy. With the exceptions of Hodgkin's lymphoma and polycythemia vera (P. vera), malignancies rarely cause significant pruritus. One study of 360 patients with Hodgkin's lymphoma found that 5.8% presented with generalized pruritus. "Bath itch" is a diffuse prickling sensation that occurs in 50% of patients with P. vera 30–60 minutes after a bath or shower. The occurrence of pruritus may precede the development of P. vera by several years.

Senescence. Itching occurs in many older patients. Most cases are not associated with systemic disease and are believed to be related to dry skin. The mainstay of treatment is hydration of the skin with water and moisturizing creams and avoidance of drying soaps.

Psychogenic disorders. Generalized or localized pruritus (commonly anogenital) may be a manifestation of anxiety. The diagnosis is made after primary skin diseases and systemic disorders are excluded. Extensive excoriation may produce areas of neurodermatitis. Patients with severe psychiatric illnesses may present with parasitophobia manifested by the sensation of worms crawling on or under the skin.

2. Describe the evaluation of patients who have pruritus without rash.

The history should focus on medications, underlying diseases, and dry skin. The physical examination should evaluate for adenopathy and organomegaly. Screening laboratory tests may include complete blood count, chest radiograph, and liver, renal, and thyroid function tests. Patients who have pruritus without a rash should be followed for evaluation of symptoms. Therapy is based on treatment of the underlying disorder. In idiopathic cases, a trial of emollients and oral antihistamines, such as hydroxyzine hydrochloride, is indicated.

3. Why is it important to distinguish palpable purpura from purpura?

Palpable purpura is always a manifestation of systemic disease, whereas purpuric lesions may result from abnormalities in the clotting system or, less commonly, may be isolated cutaneous lesions, with the exception of fat or cholesterol emboli.

4. What types of diseases should be considered in patients with palpable purpura?

Palpable purpura results from vasculitis or embolic disease. Lesions due to vasculitis are seen in patients with polyarteritis nodosa and leukocytoclastic vasculitis. Embolic diseases include meningococcemia, disseminated gonococcemia, ecthyma gangrenosum (due to *Pseudomonas* sp. or other gram-negative organisms), and Rocky Mountain spotted fever.

5. Describe erythema nodosum.

Erythema nodosum presents as red subcutaneous nodules, most commonly on the shins. The nodules become bluish in color as they resolve. Erythma nodosum is often idiopathic; however, the most common systemic associations are streptococcal infection, sarcoidosis, inflammatory bowel disease, and, less commonly, fungal infections (e.g., coccidioidomycosis, tuberculosis, histoplasmosis) and drug toxicity.

6. What is the significance of acanthosis nigricans?

Acanthosis nigricans is an acquired velvety hyperpigmentation in the axilla and groin. It is most often associated with obesity, although it may be associated with other endocrinopathies as well as malignancy, usually of the gastrointestinal tract. Thus, in patients with idiopathic onset and no clearly ascribable cause, a search for malignancy (with attention to appropriate screening for age) should be considered.

7. What does vitiligo imply?

Patients with vitiligo have an increased incidence of autoimmune disorders, especially hypothyroidism, Graves' disease, and pernicious anemia. Less frequently, a variant of melanoma may present with truncal vitiligo.

8. What systemic diseases should be considered in patients with nonhealing ulcers?

In addition to evident vascular diseases (arterial insufficiency of any etiology, microvascular disease of diabetes, venous insufficiency), nonhealing ulcers may be associated with (1) local malignancy, (2) hemoglobinopathies and blood dyscrasias (spherocytosis, cryoglobulin), (3) pyoderma gangrenosum (although the appearance of this entity is characteristic), and (4) vasculitis (rheumatoid vasculitis, Raynaud's phenomenon, Behçet's disease).

9. What diseases are characterized by photosensitivity reactions?

A number of skin diseases, lupus erythematosus, and dermatomyositis are aggravated by the sun. However, true acquired photosensitivity reactions evidenced by erythema, fragility, telangiectasias, recurrent blistering, bullae, and desquamation in sun-exposed areas is limited to a short differential diagnosis: drug sensitization (both topical and systemically administered), acquired porphyria cutanea tarda, and, on rare occasions, acquired metabolic defects. Photoallergy differs in that an eczematous picture develops, again most commonly in response to drug sensitization.

10. What disorder is associated with yellow plaques surrounded by erythematous halos on extensor surfaces of the extremities?

Such lesions, called xanthomas, are associated with hypertriglyceridemia. They erupt with elevated triglycerides and involute as levels fall.

BIBLIOGRAPHY

1. Fitzpatrick TB, et al (eds): Dermatology in General Medicine, 4th ed. New York, McGraw-Hill, 1993.
2. Isselbacher KJ, Brownwald E, Martin JB, et al (eds): Harrison's Principles of Internal Medicine, 13th ed. New York, McGraw-Hill, 1994.
3. Moschella SL, Hurley HJ (eds): Dermatology, 3rd ed. Philadelphia, W.B. Saunders, 1992.

XIV. Care of Special Patients

99. THE ADOLESCENT PATIENT

Roberta K. Beach, M.D., M.P.H.

1. What is special about adolescence?

Adolescence is a time of dramatic physical and developmental changes that challenge the coping skills of adolescents, families, health professionals, and communities to a greater degree than any other age. For convenience, the age range of 13–19 years is often specified as adolescence, but this transition phase between childhood and adulthood lasts for over a decade, beginning around age 10 years and extending through age 21 years or later. Dynamic changes in three areas are of special interest:

    1. **Physical changes:** The growth spurt, development of adult body physique, hormonal changes, sexual development, and ability to reproduce come with puberty, although there is marked variation in timing and progression of physical growth.

    2. **Psychosocial (developmental) changes:** Essential tasks of adolescence include emancipation from family, development of peer relationships and sexual intimacy, determination of educational and vocational goals, and establishment of identity and self-responsibility. Major social milestones are achieved. The legal rights to drive, vote, drink, and the cultural rites of passage such as leaving school, leaving home, first sexual relationship, and first job have immense social significance to the adolescent.

    3. **Cognitive changes:** The adolescent progresses from concrete operational thinking ("here and now") to abstract operational thinking, with a maturing ability to engage in deductive reasoning, to understand risk and benefit, and to appreciate future consequences of current choices.

2. Characterize the adolescent personality.

Although adolescents are frequently portrayed as hostile, rebellious, and alienated, in fact they have many positive attributes. Adolescents are intensely idealistic and often have a passion for fairness and social justice. They are energetic and enjoy peak physical health. They tend to be optimistic about the future and excited about dreams, plans, and goals. They have a tremendous resilience and capacity for growth, and even serious problems can be converted into learning experiences and opportunities for change. The majority (about 80%) of adolescents progress through this stage of life with only modest difficulty and without serious social problems.

3. How do I get an adolescent patient to talk to me?

Although caregivers often consider them difficult to interview, adolescents are actually eager to find someone "safe" to talk to about their concerns. Because they often believe that "no one understands me," they are highly sensitive to disapproval or negative judgment. Several techniques help to establish a sense of trust that promotes the therapeutic alliance:

- Privacy: Interview the adolescent alone and with full attention in a setting free of interruptions.
- Confidentiality: Clarify the policy on confidentiality, and assure the patient that nothing will be shared without permission, unless it is of a life-threatening nature (such as a suicide attempt) or legally required (such as child abuse).

- Listening skills: Listen much more than you talk, interrupt rarely, do not lecture, and pay attention to body language, both yours and the patient's.
- Nonjudgmental approach: Avoid assumptions, respect differences, and show genuine interest.
- Use open-ended, nonthreatening questions early in the interview ("Tell me what a typical day in your life is like.").
- Lead into sensitive questions by using third person examples ("Have any of your friends experimented with drugs?").
- Once rapport is established, ask direct questions for specific information ("Have you had sex in the last 3 months? Do you think you could be pregnant?").
- Look for the hidden agenda: Although the chief complaint is the "entrée to care," frequently an underlying concern motivates the visit. ("Hidden agendas" often relate to sexual concerns.)
- If the adolescent is unwilling to talk, reflective listening techniques are the most helpful approach ("You seem very unhappy," "You said you hate being here . . . hate?"). Wait patiently for answers.
- Use positive reinforcement whenever possible; adolescents are hungry for honest praise and support. ("It took a lot of courage for you to talk about this. Thank you.")

4. What are the three developmental stages of adolescence?

Psychosocial development is a dynamic process that continues throughout the lifespan. Adolescence is commonly divided into three developmental stages: **early** (11–14 years), **middle** (15–17 years), and **late** (18–21 years). Age ranges are approximate, and girls tend to progress through the stages earlier than boys. At each stage, characteristic changes take place in cognitive thinking, behaviors, typical health concerns, and most effective caregiver approach to the patient. Behavioral issues are usually subdivided into the four task areas: family, peers, school/vocation, and self-perception/identity. The following table briefly summarizes the characteristics for each stage.

Adolescent Developmental Stages

	EARLY ADOLESCENCE (11–14 YRS)	MIDDLE ADOLESCENCE (15–17 YRS)	LATE ADOLESCENCE (18–24 YRS)
Cognitive thinking	Concrete thinking: here and now; appreciate immediate reactions to behavior but no sense of later consequences.	Early abstract thinking: inductive/deductive reasoning; ability to connect separate events, understand later consequences.	Abstract thinking: adult ability to think abstractly; philosophical; intense idealism about love, religion, social problems.
Psychosocial task areas			
1. Family— independence	Transition from obedient to rebellious; Ambivalence about wishes (dependence/ independence); Hero worship of other adults	Insistence on independence, privacy; May have overt rebellion or sulky withdrawal; Much testing of limits	Emancipation (leave home); Reestablishment of family ties; Become legally responsible for care
2. Peers— social/sexual	Same-sex "best friend"; "Am I normal?" concerns; Sexual intercourse not normal at this age; indicates family dysfunction	Dating; Sexual experimentation; Risk-taking actions; Need to please significant peers (of either sex)	Partner selection ("serial monogamy"); Mature friendships; True intimacy possible only after own identity is established

Table continued on following page

Adolescent Developmental Stages (Continued)

	EARLY ADOLESCENCE (11–14 YRS)	MIDDLE ADOLESCENCE (15–17 YRS)	LATE ADOLESCENCE (18–24 YRS)
Psychosocial task areas *(Cont.)*			
3. School— vocation	Middle school Need structured setting Goals unrealistic, changing Want to copy favorite role models	High school Need choices, electives, more flexibility Beginning to identify skills, interests Start part-time jobs	Full-time work or college Identify realistic career goals Watch for apathy (no future plans) or aliena-tion: correlated with unplanned pregnancy, juvenile crime, etc.
4. Self-perception— identity	Poor self-image Losing child's role but do not have adult role; hence low self-esteem Tend to use denial (it can't happen to me)	Confusion about self-image Seek group identity Very narcissistic Impulsive, impatient	Realistic, positive self-image Able to consider others' needs, less narcissistic Able to reject group pressure if not in self-interest
5. Values	Stage II values (backscratching): good behavior in exchange for rewards	Stage III values (conformity): behavior that peer group values	Stage IV values (social responsibility): behavior consistent with laws and duty
Chief health issues (other than acute illness)	Psychosomatic symptoms Fatigue and growing pains Concerns about normalcy Screening for growth and development problems	Outcomes of sexual experimentation (prevention of preg-nancy, STDs, AIDS) Health-risk behaviors (smoking, drugs, alcohol, driving) Crisis counseling (run-aways, acting-out, family problems)	Health promotion/ healthy lifestyles Contraception and STD–AIDS prevention Self-responsibility for health and health care Transition to adult care settings
Professional approach	Firm, direct support Convey limits—simple, concrete choices Do not align with parents, but do be an objective, caring adult Encourage parental presence in clinic, but interview teen alone	Be an objective sounding board (but let them solve own problems) Negotiate choices Ensure confidentiality Adapt system to walk-ins, impulsiveness, testing of limits	Allow mature partici-pation in decisions Act as a resource Idealistic stage, so convey "professional" image Can expect patient to examine underlying wishes, motives regarding behavior

5. What are the physical stages of adolescent growth?

Compared with the complexities of psychosocial development, physical development during adolescence tends to be orderly and straightforward. Growth is divided into five stages from prepubertal to adult. Called Tanner stages, after John Tanner's classic descriptions, they are now referred to as sexual maturity ratings (SMR) 1–5. The onset of puberty is highly variable, but in girls normally begins between 8 and 14 years of age and in boys between 9 and 16 years of age. Physical growth continues for 5–6 years, until adult stature is achieved. In girls, the progression usually begins with breast budding at **thelarche** (SMR 2), followed by pubic hair at **pubarche** (SMR 3), first menses at **menarche** (SMR 4), and completion of pubic hair and breast growth (SMR 5). The average age of menarche in American girls is 12.3 years. The peak female growth spurt occurs immediately before menarche (SMR 2–3). Bone epiphyses close approximately 2 years after menarche, and growth is completed. In boys, the progression begins with early enlargement of the testes (SMR 2), followed by growth of pubic hair (SMR 3), penile growth (SMR 3–4), peak growth spurt (SMR 3–4), and facial hair and completion of genital and pubic hair growth (SMR 5). The average age of first nocturnal emission (wet dream) in boys is 13–14 years. In both boys and girls, pubic hair extends onto the thighs during SMR 5 and heralds the completion of physical growth.

6. When is puberty considered precocious?
Pubertal development that is out of phase with peers is a cause of great concern to early adolescents. Early pubertal development (too soon) is usually a concern of girls. Delayed pubertal development (too late) is typically a concern of boys.

Breast budding in girls is normal from age 8 years. It may be unilateral, causing concern about a "breast tumor" when noted in an 8- or 9-year-old girl. However, a breast bud should **not** be biopsied (removal destroys future breast growth). Menarche may occur as early as 9 or 10 years, especially in overnourished girls. Complete puberty in girls before the age of 8 years is termed "precocious puberty" and is caused by the presence of gonadotropins and sex hormones (estrogens and androgens). The differential diagnosis includes hormone-secreting tumors (brain, liver, adrenal glands, ovaries); exogenous administration of estrogen, anabolic steroids, or androgens; and hypothyroidism, neurofibromatosis, congenital adrenal hyperplasia, and other rare disorders. Virilization of a young girl indicates an endocrine disorder.

7. When should delayed puberty be evaluated?
If there are no signs of puberty by age 16 years, delayed puberty should be evaluated. The most common causes of delayed puberty include familial short stature, constitutional growth delay, and chronic illness. Boys with genetic short stature tend to grow at a rate below but parallel to the third percentile throughout childhood and adolescence. They often begin puberty at the same time as their peers. They will always be short. In constitutional growth delay, the onset of puberty is delayed, but the patient eventually catches up in growth.

8. Which chronic illnesses are responsible for delayed puberty?
In delayed puberty, the most important aspects of evaluation are the family history, past growth pattern, SMR stage, medical history, and bone-age radiographs. Chronic illnesses that may delay puberty include severe asthma, other pulmonary disorders, renal disease, cardiac disorders, and inflammatory bowel disease. Growth hormone deficiency should be considered if height is 3–4 standard deviations below the mean.

9. What are the primary health issues of adolescents?
Major morbidity and mortality during adolescence relate to risk-taking behaviors and experimentation. Health concerns resulting from complex behavioral decisions include adolescent pregnancy, substance abuse, sexually transmitted diseases, infection with human immunodeficiency virus (HIV), depression, suicide, violence, and motor vehicle injuries.

10. How do health supervision visits for adolescents differ from traditional health maintenance visits for adults?
Primary care providers must respond to the health consequences of risk-taking behavior by making preventive services a major component of the clinical approach to adolescents. The American Medical Association, in cooperation with the Centers for Disease Control and Prevention, has published *Guidelines for Adolescent Preventive Services* (GAPS), a comprehensive set of recommendations that provide a framework for the organization and content of preventive health services. Health supervision visits for adolescents differ from traditional health maintenance visits in six ways:

1. The provider actively complements the health guidance that adolescents receive from school, family, and community.

2. Preventive interventions target "new morbidities," such as alcohol, drugs, and sexual risk-taking, rather than emphasize biomedical problems.

3. The provider screens for co-morbidities, which are clusters of risk-taking behaviors, rather than treats categorical health conditions.

4. Annual health supervision visits are recommended to provide anticipatory guidance and early intervention rather than episodic visits, such as those for immunizations or sports exams.

5. Comprehensive physical examinations are recommended at each of the three stages of development: early, middle, and late adolescence. Sexually active adolescents need annual screening for sexually transmitted diseases, including an annual Papanicolaou test in sexually active young women.

6. Parents of adolescents should receive specific counseling on parental concerns and adolescent needs at least twice during their child's adolescence.

11. What are the most important positive health behaviors to stress?
Primary care givers have a critical role in ensuring that all adolescents are competent and motivated to make wise choices as they form life-long health habits. The Centers for Disease Control/Division of Adolescent and School Health selected six priority health behaviors for youth based on risk factors that are a major source of morbidity and mortality, highly prevalent, modifiable, and measurable (see table below). Other areas of great concern for mortality, such as suicide and homicide, are difficult to reduce to a single, achievable behavioral goal and therefore are not addressed in the six priority behaviors.

Priority Health Behaviors for Adolescents

1. Use seat belts
2. Do not drink (or use drugs) and drive
3. If you have sex, use condoms
4. Do not smoke
5. Eat a low-fat diet
6. Get regular aerobic exercise

These six "golden rules" are the most effective and achievable lifetime behaviors that will reduce years of potential life lost to the major killers: motor vehicle accidents, AIDS, cardiovascular disease, and cancer.

12. How can anticipatory guidance (office counseling) be given without lecturing?
Office counseling is most effective if it actively engages the adolescent in problem-solving. Four steps are involved:

1. **Define the problem.** Ask the adolescent to describe the situation and his or her feelings and fears about it. ("What if your pregnancy test were positive today?")

2. **Explore the options.** Ask the adolescent to describe the ways in which he or she has considered solving the problem. The provider simply listens. ("Tell me at least three choices you would have if you were pregnant.") Suggest other options if appropriate.

3. **Analyze the consequences.** Ask the adolescent to review the most likely positive and negative consequences of the best solutions that he or she has considered. ("What will be the best thing and the worst thing for you if you placed your baby for adoption?") Then mention any major consequences or responsibilities that the adolescent overlooked.

4. **Develop an action plan.** Ask the adolescent to identify the specific steps to take after leaving your office. Include a plan for follow-up.

13. List the most common causes of adolescent medical visits.
Common causes of adolescent medical visits include acne, asthma, headache, abdominal pain, fatigue, and musculoskeletal pain.

14. List four common principles applicable to the care of adolescents with symptomatic complaints.
1. Adolescents may have excessive concerns related to the question, "Am I normal?"; therefore they need large amounts of reassurance.

2. Adolescents often have underlying anxiety that they are to blame for the condition because of some behavior about which they feel guilty, such as experimenting with sex or drugs.

3. Adolescents may be very concerned about confidentiality and often want to obtain care independently, without parental involvement.

4. Adolescents may need extra support to achieve compliance with treatment plans. They frequently test limits, act impulsively, and discontinue treatment in an effort to "be like everyone else." In general, adolescents require extra time, more education, and closer follow-up than other age groups.

15. Why is there so much concern about adolescent sexuality?

The medical consequences of adolescent sexual activity, particularly unintended pregnancy, sexually transmitted disease, and HIV infection are a national health concern. One million American adolescents become pregnant each year, although only 400,000 are age 17 years and under. Over 3,000,000 cases of sexually transmitted diseases occur in adolescents annually. It is estimated that the number of adolescents with HIV infection doubles every 14 months, and acquired immunodeficiency syndrome (AIDS) is now the 7th leading cause of death in the 15–24-year-old age group.

16. When do adolescents become sexually active?

Middle to late adolescence has always been the average age for initiation of sexual intercourse. Since the late 1960s ("the sexual revolution"), greater numbers of younger adolescents have become sexually active. The 1992 National Youth Risk Behavior Survey of 11,631 students in grades 6–12 reported that 54% of all high school students had begun sexual intercourse, with 39% having sex in the 3 months prior to the survey. Rates increase rapidly during high school, with 25% of 8th graders, 40% of 9th graders, and 72% of 12th graders reporting sexual intercourse. The median age of first intercourse reported by students is 16.1 years for boys and 16.9 years for girls.

17. Should the primary care provider support contraceptive use?

Yes. Health promotion goals for adolescents include postponement of sexual activity until psychosocial maturity is achieved, with consistent use of condoms and contraceptives by those who do engage in sexual intercourse. Abstinence is highly effective in preventing pregnancies and STDs if used consistently and correctly; in actual use, however, abstinence has a failure rate of 24% in adolescent couples who attempt to use it for 1 year. The level of condom use by adolescents has doubled between 1979 and 1988; nearly half report use of condoms with their first coitus. The actual pregnancy rate in sexually active adolescents has decreased by 12% since 1976, reflecting an increased use of contraception. If the social environment is supportive, adolescents can be effective contraceptive users, as demonstrated in other Western countries. Caregivers must ensure that all adolescents receive anticipatory guidance on safer sex practices and have access to condoms and contraceptives when needed. Despite the perception of crisis, responsible sexual behavior by adolescents has increased.

18. Where do adolescents go for health care?

Of adolescents who have seen a physician in the last 2 years, approximately one-third see pediatricians, one-third see family practice or internal medicine providers, and one-third use local emergency rooms.

Adolescents have long been recognized as an underserved population who are particularly difficult to reach with health services. Issues of emancipation, independence, and desire for confidential care create significant barriers for adolescents in the traditional health care system. Adolescents in general have less than 1 visit every 2 years to a health care provider, and such visits tend to be primarily for episodic illness or emergency care. With five million uninsured adolescents in America, many have no regular source of health care. Even insured adolescents underutilize care. In one large study in New York state, upper-middle-class adolescents who could identify a private physician stated that they would be unwilling to consult the physician for many sensitive concerns, such as sexual or drug-related problems, for fear that their parents would find out.

CONTROVERSY

19. Consent and confidentiality: Should adolescents receive health care without parental involvement?

The ability to provide confidential care to adolescents, with the minor's own consent, has been an essential concept of adolescent medicine for a quarter of a century. Although parental involvement is generally beneficial and should be strongly encouraged, the adolescent's preferences about the degree of involvement are respected to the greatest possible extent.

Consent and confidentiality are separate legal issues. Consent is a basic legal requirement for the provision of health care to patients of all ages. In general, minors under the age of 18 years require parental consent for medical treatment. However, because of the compelling interest of the state in encouraging adolescents to seek early health care for pregnancy, sexually transmitted diseases, and substance abuse, courts and legislatures have created numerous exceptions to parental consent that enable adolescents to obtain care independently for specific types of health concerns.

Confidentiality refers to maintaining privacy of medical information. Numerous studies have documented that many adolescents are reluctant or completely unwilling to seek care without the assurance of confidentiality. Many require privacy as part of the normal process of developing autonomy; others may face hostile or abusive reactions from alienated or dysfunctional families if sensitive information is disclosed. Even when general parental consent for treatment has been obtained, medical record information is usually not released without the patient's permission in accordance with the adolescent's constitutional right to privacy. Every state has specific statutes related to a minor's access to health care.

Recently legislative initiatives to require parental consent or notification for issues related to sexuality, particularly birth control and abortion, have been increasing. Proponents argue that parents have a legal right and obligation to be involved in their child's health care, that adolescents are too immature to make decisions on their own, and that parental involvement enhances family communication and support for troubled adolescents. Although parental notification legislation typically is initiated by conservative religious groups, it is often supported by a much wider spectrum of parents who believe that knowledge of their adolescent's activities will allow them to play a protective or beneficial role.

Careful analyses of the impact of such legislation in states where it has been passed show no beneficial effect on family communication. Adolescents who are unwilling to share private information with parents do not change their attitude simply because of a law. Instead, they tend to delay or avoid care, to seek clandestine care, or to use judicial bypass mechanisms to access medical care under their own consent. The major documented effects of such legislation are delay in timely diagnosis and treatment and increased medical risk. Numerous studies have shown that adolescents 14 years and older are as competent as adults to make informed choices about reproductive health care. Other studies demonstrate that adolescents willingly involve their families (even without the legal requirement to do so) if they believe that their families will be supportive and nonjudgmental. The most effective means for parents to ensure involvement in their adolescent's health care decisions is by establishing open, trusting communication from early childhood forward.

BIBLIOGRAPHY

1. American Medical Association, Department of Adolescent Health: Guidelines for Adolescent Preventive Services. Chicago, IL, American Medical Association, 1992.
2. Centers for Disease Control: Sexual behavior among high school students. MMWR 40:885–888, 1992.

3. Coupey SM, Klerman LV (eds): Adolescent sexuality: Preventing unhealthy consequences. Adolescent Medicine: State of the Art Reviews. Philadelphia, Hanley & Belfus, June 1992.
4. Elster AB: Confronting the crisis in adolescent health: Visions for change. J Adolesc Health 14:505–508, 1993.
5. Friedman HL: Promoting the health of adolescents in the United States of America: A global perspective. J Adolesc Health 14:509–519, 1993.
6. Friedman SB, Fisher M, Schonberg SK (eds): Comprehensive Adolescent Health Care. St. Louis, Quality Medical Publishing, 1992.
7. Greydanus DE: Contraception in adolescence: An overview for the pediatrician. Pediatr Ann 19:223–240, 1992.
8. Hofmann AD, Greydanus DE: Adolescent Medicine, 2nd ed. Norwalk, CT, Appleton & Lange, 1989.
9. McAnarney ER, Kreipe RE, Orr DP, Comerci GD (eds): Textbook of Adolescent Medicine. Philadelphia, W.B. Saunders, 1992.
10. Neinstein LS: Adolescent Health Care: A Practical Guide, 2nd ed. Baltimore, Urban & Schwarzenberg, 1991.
11. Slawkowski DJ: Adolescent medicine and law. Adolescent Medicine: State of the Art Reviews. Philadelphia, Hanley & Belfus, 1993, pp 204–218.
12. Stout JW, Kirby D: The effects of sexuality education on adolescent sexual activity. Pediatr Ann 22:120–126, 1993.

100. THE ELDERLY PATIENT

Evelyn Hutt, M.D.

1. What is functional assessment? Why is it important?

Functional assessment is a formalized way of paying attention to how a patient manages the details of daily life. We assume that most young patients are cognitively intact, can get around in their homes, get into and out of the bathroom and bath tub safely, and do their own cooking, shopping, and eating. However, because the prevalence of disabilities in performing activities of daily living (ADL) is so high among elders (10% of community-dwelling elders have at least one deficit in ADL performance) and because neither patients nor careproviders are accustomed to thinking of such matters as part of medical care, we need a more formal way of including such information in our review of systems. Several brief questionnaires are available for use in clinical practice. Consistent use of any one will provide insight into how the patient functions in daily life.

As the physician manages more incurable or chronic disease, it becomes increasingly important to improve the quality and independence of a patient's life. If we have not asked how well a patient is managing (by performing a functional assessment) when he or she presents, we (1) miss significant treatable problems and (2) do not know whether we have affected the patient's day-to-day function positively or negatively.

2. Which special aspects of the physical exam need evaluation during the assessment of an elder?

Perceptual function
Cognitive and emotional function
Gait

3. When a patient presents to the clinic with a new change in mental status, how do you know whether the patient is delirious, depressed, or demented?

The difference between delirium and dementia can be recognized clinically. Delirious patients have an altered level of consciousness (either depressed or agitated), whereas simply demented patients are awake, alert, and calm. Ascertaining the patient's baseline status from a reliable source is crucial.

A patient who presents with abnormal mental status should be presumed to be delirious rather than demented. Delirium is a serious but often treatable manifestation of disease. Patients known to be demented by reliable history or chart documentation often present with acute worsening of mental status as the only sign of infection, myocardial infarction, or central lesion from a fall.

Distinguishing between depression and dementia can be difficult. Paradoxically, patients who present with complaints of memory problems are more likely to be depressed than demented. Other clues to depression include difficulty with concentration out of proportion to other deficits in the mental status exam; recent major losses (family members, friends, health, independence); sleep disturbance; and weight loss. Even after brief formal screening for both depression and cognitive deficits (for example, with the Geriatric Depression Scale and Mini-mental Status Exam), the diagnosis may not be clear. Referral for neuropsychiatric testing or a trial of antidepressants may be helpful.

4. What major derangements should be considered in the etiology of delirium?
The mnemonic **DELIRIUM** is a helpful reminder of the many treatable causes of delirium.

D = Drugs. Unfortunately the list of potential offenders is extensive. Most important are anticholinergics, which are very common in over-the-counter medications and often impair cognitive function. Other side effects particularly bothersome to older people include dry mouth, constipation, and urinary retention. All psychoactive medications may induce delirium. A thorough drug history is therefore the first step in sorting out the cause of delirium. Elimination of as many agents as possible and reduction of the remainder to the lowest possible dose are helpful.

E = Electrolytes. Electrolyte imbalance and other metabolic disturbances may impair cognitive function. Examples include hypo- and hypernatremia, hypo- and hyperkalemia, hypo- and hypercalcemia, hypo- and hypermagnesemia, hypo- and hyperglycemia, hypoxia, and hypercarbia.

L = Low temperature (hypothermia) and Lunacy. High temperature, of course, may also induce delirium. Acute psychosis is uncommon in elders without a prior history.

I = Intoxication and Intracranial processes. Alcoholism is no less prevalent among elders than among younger populations. The diagnosis of alcoholism is particularly easy to overlook in elderly women. Intracranial processes include subdural hematomas, neoplasms, and infection. If no other cause for delirium is apparent, the elder presenting with an acute or subacute change in cognitive function should have a brain imaging study.

R = Retention, either urinary or fecal. Prevalence of retention as a true cause of delirium is difficult to ascertain, but the problem is easy to relieve. It should be considered causal only if the patient improves and other, more serious, causes have been considered.

I = Infection. Infection is the most important treatable cause of delirium. The *only* presenting sign of infection in an older person may be a change in mental status. Because immune function declines with age, elders may have pneumonia, urosepsis, or an abdominal catastrophe without pain, fever, or an elevated white blood cell count.

U = Unfamiliar surroundings with decreased sensory input. In this disorder, often described as the sundowning phenomenon, patients with subclinical dementia function well until a strange environment combines with impaired vision and hearing to induce confusion. Simple expedients may ameliorate the problem: well-lit room, undisturbed sleep, clock, calendar, familiar pictures and visitors, and easy access to food, water, and toilet.

M = Myocardial infarction and other causes of decreased central perfusion. Like infection, acute cardiovascular events may present without localizing signs.

5. Which tests should be used to evaluate a patient with dementia? Why?
About 10% of dementia cases are at least partially reversible, including those caused by hypothyroidism, B12 deficiency, syphilis, and depression. Thus, evaluation should be directed at reversible etiologies. Although normal pressure hydrocephalus can be treated, the associated

dementia generally does not reverse. Subdural hematomas may cause a subtle and subclinical decline in mental status without localizing neurologic findings and should be investigated in anyone with a history of both associated symptoms and a recent fall.

A reasonable laboratory work-up for dementia, once delirium has been excluded, includes levels of thyroid-stimulating hormone and B12, venereal disease research laboratory test, liver function tests, and a complete blood count. Whether a computed tomographic (CT) or magnetic resonance imaging (MRI) scan of the head is necessary remains controversial and depends on the unique presentation of the patient (e.g., possibility of subdural hematoma).

6. Discuss the major options for the treatment of depression in an older patient.
Three major modalities are available for the treatment of depression: psychotherapy, medication, and electroconvulsion.

Psychotherapy has the clear advantage of fewer side effects, but it may be difficult to persuade an older person to begin such treatment because of their cultural bias against expression of affect and "complaining." The cognitive behavioral model offers a more acceptable and less embarrassing style of therapy. The primary care provider should be aware of who in the psychotherapeutic community offers this approach and is comfortable treating older patients.

Medications are readily available for treatment and may be divided into roughly four groups: tricyclics, serotonergics, psychostimulants, and others (see table). Use of tricyclics entails the risks of anticholinergic side effects, which may be decreased by choosing the metabolite compounds, nortriptyline or desipramine. Nortriptyline is somewhat more sedating than desipramine. If respiratory depression is a concern, protriptyline can be used. An electrocardiogram should be obtained to look for underlying conduction delay, and dosing should begin at 25 mg. It is useful to measure drug levels at this dose, particularly in the presence of renal insufficiency. A 4–6 week trial at adequate levels is needed to produce benefit.

There are no controlled studies of the use of the newer serotonergic agents (fluoxetine, sertraline, and paroxetine) in an older population. Fluoxetine commonly causes gastrointestinal distress and anorexia. It has a long half-life and should be used cautiously if a major symptom of the depression has been weight loss. Psychostimulants, chiefly methylphenidate, have been shown to be useful when a more rapid response is needed to gauge whether the patient is likely to respond to medication. The beginning dose is 5 mg 2 or 3 times/day. Other agents include trazodone and bupropion. Trazodone may be particularly useful in patients with underlying lung disease. Bupropion is newer, more expensive, and not well studied in older populations.

Antidepressants in the Elderly

	ADVANTAGES	DISADVANTAGES
Tricyclics	Short-acting Inexpensive	Anticholinergic side effects Overdose Cardiac conduction delays Monitoring
Serotonergics	Fewer side effects of drowsi- ness, dry mouth, constipation	Long half-life (days) Expensive
Psychostimulants	Rapid response	Tremor Sleeplessness
Other Trazadone	Little respiratory depression Few cardiac effects	Orthostatic hypotension Sedating

Electroconvulsive therapy (ECT) is a highly effective treatment for older depressed patients. It probably is safer and has fewer side effects than tricyclic antidepressants. Because of the fear and horror that it engenders in many people, it is an underused modality. Primary care providers should know which psychiatrists in their area are comfortable using ECT in older patients.

7. Why do elderly patients fall?

A combination of extrinsic (environmental) and intrinsic (to the patient) factors increase the risk of falling. Extrinsic factors such as clutter in the home, poor lighting, throw rugs, and slippery bathtubs are probably the most easily correctable. Intrinsic precipitants include (in decreasing order of importance) drugs, cognitive impairment, disability of the lower extremities, abnormal balance and gait, and foot problems. The risk of falling increases linearly with the number of risk factors.

8. Which particular type of drug is associated with morbidity from falls?

All classes of sedatives (anxiolytics, antidepressants, and neuroleptics) are associated with falls and with hip fractures. Both dosage and half-life of the medication are related to incidence of falls.

9. What are the consequences of falls for the elderly?

Only 5% of falls result in a fracture. Serious soft-tissue injury occurs in another 10%. Such injuries account for 9,500 deaths/year. Falls that do not result in injury may have the serious consequence of fear, leading to reduced activity. Of patients who decide to enter nursing homes, 40% say that falls and instability contributed to that decision.

10. What are the most important causes of visual impairment in the elderly?

The majority of visual impairment in older patients is due to three conditions:

Cataracts affect 13% of people 65–74 years of age and over 40% of those over 75. Early in the course, decline in distant visual acuity and difficulty in tolerating glare may be the presenting complaints. In most patients cataract removal and lens implantation can be done on an outpatient basis. A common late complication is delayed opacification of the posterior capsule, which occurs in up to 50% of patients. It can be managed in 90% of patients with yttrium aluminum garnet (YAG) laser treatment.

Macular degeneration affects 6.4% of people 65–74 years of age and about 20% of those over 70. Two types are identified clinically: nonexudative, which is managed expectantly, and exudative, which is managed with argon laser photocoagulation. Ninety percent of patients have the nonexudative type.

Glaucoma affects 3% of people over 65 years of age. Prevalence rates are higher among African-Americans.

11. How common is hearing impairment among the elderly?

About one-third of people over the age of 65 years are hearing-impaired. Close to one-half of those over age 80 are affected. Men are more commonly affected than women. Given this prevalence, when you interview an older patient, be sure that he or she can see your face. Speak clearly, reduce background noise, use gestures, and check often for comprehension. Inexpensive amplifiers ($40) are available for office use. Drugs that are ototoxic should be used sparingly: aminoglycosides, erythromycin, vancomycin, loop diuretics, and nonsteroidal anti-inflammatories.

12. How are pharmacokinetics altered by the usual aging process?

As people age, the proportion of body water to fat shifts toward fat. This shift changes the volume of distribution as well as the half-life for all drugs. Lipophilic agents, which affect the central nervous system, tend to have much longer half-lives in older people. In general, drug absorption is not affected by age, nor is liver metabolism if the liver is healthy. Whether renal function necessarily declines with age is controversial, but practically speaking, it usually does. A simple formula for calculating creatinine clearance—(140 – age) (× 0.85 for women) divided by the serum creatinine—can be used to adjust dosing intervals in renally excreted drugs.

13. What is an advance care directive?

An advance care directive is a written and witnessed document specifying treatment preferences in the event that a patient becomes incompetent. Two forms exist: living wills generally become effective when the patient is both terminally ill and incompetent; durable powers of attorney for health care appoint a surrogate decision maker and express treatment preferences, whether or not a terminal condition exists. Laws on the formulation and enactment of both directives vary from state to state, but all older patients, as well as patients with serious chronic illness, should be provided the opportunity to discuss end-of-life options.

14. When should elder abuse be suspected?

Although hard data are lacking, abuse is thought to affect at least 3% of the elderly population (1–2 million elders/year). As with the problem of child abuse, neglect is probably much more common. In general, the physician should screen for abuse when the patient fits the "typical victim" profile, when the caregiver fits an "abuser profile," and when certain symptom complexes are found.

The **typical victim profile** includes patients with multiple frailties and behavioral problems, such as dementia, incontinence, nocturnal shouting, wandering, and paranoia.

The **abuser profile** includes over-burdened caregivers who live with the elder, are sleep-deprived, and/or have marital and work-related stresses of their own. Abusers also may be socially isolated and have a history of substance abuse, psychopathology, or other domestic violence.

Symptom complexes that should arouse suspicion include unexplained weight loss, signs of trauma (multiple fractures, falls, dislocations, bruises of varying ages, burns in unusual places, genital pain, or bleeding), and decubitus ulcers. Psychosocial manifestations include excessive fear, depression, infantile behavior, confusion over or ignorance of the patient's own financial situation, and the caregiver's refusal to let the patient see the doctor alone. The physician should persist in repeated screening, even in the face of denial. Fear may keep the victim from reporting abuse.

15. Which vaccines should be routine?

All people over 65 years of age should have yearly influenza vaccine, pneumococcal vaccine polyvalent (Pneumovax) at least once, and tetanus booster every 10 years. Whether Pneumovax should be repeated every 10 years is controversial; there is no clear evidence in either direction. Because vaccination rates are so low, from a public health point of view efforts should focus on one Pneumovax per elder.

Changes in Preventive Care for the Elderly

Vaccines	Yearly influenza
	1 Pneumovax
	Tetanus booster every 10 years
Lipid profiles	In the absence of cardiovascular disease, discontinue at age 70–75 years
Papanicoloau smears	If routinely negative, discontinue at age 70 years

16. When can you stop checking cholesterol?

The answer depends on whether there is known cardiovascular disease. For patients with known disease, no upper age limit applies, and treatment guidelines are no different for elders than for middle-aged patients. In the absence of cardiovascular disease, screening probably may end at age 70 or 75 years. This guideline takes into account the 10 years needed to show an effect of cholesterol reduction on the incidence of myocardial infarction and life expectancy. Virtually no data are available about the utility of lowering cholesterol in women. Consideration should be given to treating people with LDL levels greater than 100 plus age; the approach needs to be individualized.

17. Should elders continue to be screened for breast, cervical, and colon cancer?
The incidence of breast and colon cancer rises continously with age, whereas the incidence of cervical cancer reaches a plateau. Therefore, it makes sense to set no upper limit on screening for breast and colon cancer, but Papanicoloau smears may be stopped in the early 70s if the patient has had several negative exams.

18. How and why should you skin-test for tuberculosis in the elderly?
Tuberculosis (TB) screening should be performed. TB is more common among the elderly, who are at greater risk of reactivation as they age and become less immunocompetent. Skin testing is an important part of baseline data so that TB may be appropriately considered when the patient becomes ill. A control skin test should be placed simultaneously to distinguish anergy from a negative response. The purified protein derivative (PPD) test should be repeated in 2–4 weeks if it is negative to allow for anamnestic response. This practice prevents the false diagnosis of recent conversion, if the patient undergoes TB testing in the future.

BIBLIOGRAPHY

1. American Geriatric Society: Hearing and visual impairment. In Geriatric Review Syllabus. New York, American Geriatric Society, 1989.
2. Anetzberger GJ, Lachs MS, O'Brien JG, et al: Elder mistreatment: A call for help. Patient Care 1993, June 15, pp 93–130.
3. Council on Scientific Affairs: Elder abuse and neglect. JAMA 257:966–971, 1987.
4. Francis J, Kapoor WN: Delirium in the hospitalized elderly. J Gen Intern Med 5:65–79, 1990.
5. Kane RL, Ouslander JG, Abrass IB: Essentials of Clinical Geriatrics, 2nd ed. New York, McGraw-Hill, 1989.
6. Lachs MS, Feinstein AR, Cooney LM, et al: A simple procedure for general screening for functional disability in elderly patients. Ann Intern Med 112:699–706, 1990.
7. Lipowski ZJ: Delirium in the elderly patient. N Engl J Med 320:578–582, 1989.
8. McGreevey JF, Franco K: Depression in the elderly. J Gen Intern Med 3:498–507, 1988.
9. Ray WA, Griffin MR, Schaffner W, et al: Psychotropic drug use and the risk of hip fracture. N Engl J Med 363–369, 1987.
10. Roose SP, Glassman AH: Cardiovascular effects of tricyclic anti-depressants in depressed patients with and without heart disease. J Clin Psychiatry 7:1–18, 1989.
11. Satel SL, Nelson JC: Stimulants in the treatment of depression: A critical overview. J Clin Psychiatry 50:241–249, 1989.
12. Thompson LW, Gallagher D, Breckenridge JS: Comparative effectiveness of psychotherapies for depressed elders. J Consult Clin Psychol 55:385–390, 1987.
13. Tinetti ME, Speechley M: Prevention of falls among the elderly. N Engl J Med 320:1055–1060, 1989.
14. Tinetti ME, Speechley M, Ginter SF: Risk factors for falls among elderly persons living in the community. N Engl J Med 319:1701–1708, 1988.
15. United States Public Health Service: Prevention and control of tuberculosis in facilities providing long-term care to the elderly. MMWR 39:7–20, 1990.
16. Woolf SH, Kamerow DB, Lawrence RS, et al: The periodic health examination of older adults: The recommendations of the U.S. Preventive Services Task Force. J Am Geriatr Soc 38:933–942, 1990.

101. THE OBESE PATIENT

Jeanette Mladenovic, M.D., and Daniel H. Bessesen, M.D.

1. What is medically significant obesity?
A recent Health Technology Assessment Conference at the National Institutes of Health identified a paradox related to body weight. On the one hand, many people who do not need

to lose weight are trying to do so, whereas most Americans who need to lose weight are not succeeding. In 1990, 45% of Americans (37% of men and 52% of women) considered themselves to be overweight. In a recent survey a surprising 44% of female and 15% of male high school students reported trying to lose weight. At a time when they should be growing, 14% of female and 4% of male high school students reported using self-induced vomiting as a weight-loss strategy. At the same time, the prevalence of obesity among adults continues to increase and now averages 30%, despite an expenditure of almost 30 billion dollars on weight loss products. Most Americans are concerned about body weight for cosmetic rather than health reasons. Medically significant obesity is a degree of obesity associated with excessive morbidity or mortality. Although visual inspection and total body weight may give an estimate of the degree of obesity, a simple but more sophisticated measurement of fatness is the body mass index (BMI), which is calculated as follows: BMI = weight (kg)/height^2 (meters). The table below uses the height (inches) and weight (lbs) of the patient to estimate BMI. An ideal BMI is less than 25. BMIs above this level appear to correlate with increases in morbidity and mortality.

*Body Weights in Pounds According to Height and Body Mass Index**

HEIGHT	BODY MASS INDEX, kg/m^2													
	19	20	21	22	23	24	25	26	27	28	29	30	35	40
IN	←						BODY WEIGHT, *lb*							→
58	91	96	100	105	110	115	119	124	129	134	138	143	167	191
59	94	99	104	109	114	119	124	128	133	138	143	148	173	198
60	97	102	107	112	118	123	128	133	138	143	148	153	179	204
61	100	106	111	116	122	127	132	137	143	148	153	158	185	211
62	104	109	115	120	126	131	136	142	147	153	158	164	191	218
63	107	113	118	124	130	135	141	146	152	158	163	169	197	225
64	110	116	122	128	134	140	145	151	157	163	169	174	204	232
65	114	120	126	132	138	144	150	156	162	168	174	180	210	240
66	118	124	130	136	142	148	155	161	167	173	179	186	216	247
67	121	127	134	140	146	153	159	166	172	178	185	191	223	255
68	125	131	138	144	151	158	164	171	177	184	190	197	230	262
69	128	135	142	149	155	162	169	176	182	189	196	203	236	270
70	132	139	146	153	160	167	174	181	188	195	202	207	243	278
71	136	143	150	157	165	172	179	186	193	200	208	215	250	286
72	140	147	154	162	169	177	184	191	199	206	213	221	258	294
73	144	151	159	166	174	182	189	197	204	212	219	227	265	302
74	148	155	163	171	179	186	194	202	210	218	225	233	272	311
75	152	160	168	176	184	192	200	208	216	224	232	240	279	319
76	156	164	172	180	189	197	205	213	221	230	238	246	287	328

* Each entry gives the body weight in pounds (lb) for a person of a given height and body mass index. Pounds have been rounded off. To use the table, find the appropriate height in the left-hand column. Move across the row to a given weight. The number at the top of the column is the body mass index for the height and weight. (From NIH Technology Assessment Conference Panel: Methods for voluntary weight loss and control. Ann Intern Med 116:942–949, 1992.)

2. What is meant by the term "regional adiposity"? What is its significance?

The health consequences of obesity are a function not only of body weight but also of the distribution of adipose tissue. Adipose tissue located around the hips and thighs, as is common in women (gynoid pattern), carries fewer health risks than adipose tissue located in the abdominal region, as is common in men (android pattern). Women who carry excessive adipose tissue in the abdominal region have substantially increased risk for diabetes mellitus, hypertension, and hyperlipidemia. Because they are more likely to distribute adipose tissue in an android pattern, obese men are at increased risk for the same diseases. Adipose tissue located within the abdominal cavity (intra-abdominal fat) may be correlated most strongly with adverse health consequences. The distribution of adipose tissue can be estimated by the waist/ hip ratio, which is calculated by measuring the minimal waist circumference and the maximal hip circumference with a tape measure. Central obesity is defined as a waist-to-hip ratio of more than 1.0 for men and 0.8 for women. Thus, the BMI and the waist-to-hip ratio are the two most important indices of medically significant obesity.

3. What causes obesity?

Obesity results when caloric intake exceeds energy expenditure. In addition to a positive caloric balance, obesity develops in the presence of a positive "fat balance"; that is, the individual consumes more fat calories than he or she burns. Several processes play important roles in the development of obesity:

Genetics. Twin and adoption studies have indicated that an individual's genotype is important in determining the rate of energy expenditure and fat distribution. The specific genes that cause obesity have not been identified, but this is an area of active investigation. Genetic factors, however, explain only 25–30% of weight variation within a population.

Dietary influences. Perhaps the most important factor in the increasing incidence of obesity is the consumption of a high fat diet. The prevalence of obesity in the United States has risen simultaneously with the average fat content of the diet. In a number of cultures, such as the Pima Indians of Arizona and the Nahru people of Polynesia, obesity was unknown when the people ate a native diet. With the introduction and subsequent easy access to high fat foods, the prevalence of obesity among adults in these groups is now 70–80%. This "Western" or "modern" diet promotes a positive fat balance, in part because the body does not adjust with sufficient accuracy the oxidation of fat to its increased consumption.

Decreases in energy expenditure. Because weight gain occurs when caloric intake exceeds caloric expenditure, another important factor in the development of obesity is decreased energy expenditure. Energy expenditure has three components: (1) basal metabolic rate (BMR), or amount of energy required to keep the body warm, to keep sodium (Na^+) out of cells and potassium (K^+) in cells, to breathe, and to keep the heart beating; (2) the thermic effect of food (TEF), or amount of energy expended during digestion; and (3) the energy of activity, or amount of energy expended during physical activity or exercise. BMR is strongly related to lean body mass, almost no evidence suggests that obesity is caused by decreases in BMR. Whether TEF decreases in obese individuals is controversial. Increasing evidence, however, suggests that decreased physical activity may play an important role in the development and maintenance of obesity. When immigrants came to the United States, many went from working in labor-intensive agricultural jobs to more sedentary office jobs. Obesity soon followed.

Appetite. The understanding of the neurobiology of appetite is rapidly expanding. Various neurotransmitters, such as norepinephrine, serotonin, and the peptides neuropeptide Y and cholecytokinin, play important roles in regulating not only total food intake but also preference for fat, carbohydrate, and protein. Recent data suggest that obese individuals may have increased preference for high fat food and that with weight loss they may acquire a preference for foods with high caloric density.

Metabolism. A growing body of scientific evidence suggests that obesity is determined by the number and size of fat cells. Once the number of fat cells increase, they may not decrease. As a result, only their size decreases during weight loss. Factors that determine the number of fat cells are not clear. In addition, some evidence suggests that obesity is regulated by homeostatic mechanisms surrounding a set weight; the set point can be only marginally modified by external factors such as diet and exercise. Moreover, some individuals may preferentially oxidize carbohydrate and store fat. In the setting of increased fat intake and decreased activity levels, such individuals are predisposed to obesity.

4. What are the economic and health consequences of obesity?

Economic impact. In 1980, 34 million Americans were obese. The overall costs in 1986 dollars was estimated to be $39.3 billion or 5.5% of annual health costs in the United States, including $22.2 billion for cardiovascular disease, $11.3 billion for diabetes, $1.5 billion for hypertension, and $1.9 billion for breast and colon cancer. This estimate does not include costs of musculoskeletal disorders, which could almost double the total figure. In addition, the loss in wages and productivity attributed to obesity approaches $20 billion/year.

Psychosocial manifestations. Situational depression and anxiety related to obesity are frequent. The obese person may suffer from discrimination, which contributes further to difficulties with poor self-image and social relationships. In a recent study, obese adolescents were compared with adolescents with other chronic health problems. Both groups were followed for 7 years. At the end of this period, obese women were 20% less likely to be married, made $6,700/yr less, and had 10% more poverty than lean controls. This effect was independent of baseline aptitude test scores and socioeconomic status.

Greater prevalence and incidence of medical diseases:

Coronary artery disease (CAD)	Sleep apnea	Left ventricular hypertrophy
Type II diabetes mellitus	Pulmonary emboli	with congestive heart failure
Hypertension	Cholesterol stones	Osteoarthritis

In the Nurses' Health Study, which examined 115,886 women, those with a BMI of 25–29 were 1.8 times more likely to have coronary heart disease than those with a BMI < 21 (the lowest risk group). Women with a BMI > 29 were 3.3 times more likely to have CAD. Although a relative risk of 1.8 may not seem large, millions of women have a moderate level of obesity. The actual number of cases of CAD attributable to moderate obesity (attributable risk = relative risk × population at risk) is therefore substantial. For this reason, the largest public health impact of obesity lies not with the morbidly obese, but with the millions of moderately obese individuals seen by primary providers for other medical problems.

Death. Increased mortality is correlated with the severity of obesity, as defined by the body mass index (BMI). The exact nature of this relationship, however, is complex. Early studies by life insurance companies established a relationship between weight and mortality and formed the basis of the widely used "ideal body weight tables." These studies suggest that an underweight individual also has increased mortality. When the studies were reanalyzed, however, the excessive mortality in the lightest individuals was found to be due to cancer or complications of smoking (the average weight of smokers is significantly lower than that of nonsmokers). This finding suggests that the excessive mortality in the lightest individuals was not due to reduced weight. Instead, both reduced weight and excessive mortality were due to a third factor, either preexisting cancer or cigarette smoking. In a recent study of Seventh Day Adventists, overall mortality decreased with body weight so that the lowest overall mortality occurred in persons with a BMI < 21.

To establish firmly the role of obesity in overall mortality, a study needs to examine individuals over a long period of time and to control for confounding variables. Two such studies are the Framingham Study and the Harvard Growth Study. In the Framingham Study the relative risk of nonsmoking men who were 10–20% above ideal body weight was twice as high as the risk of men of ideal body weight. In the Harvard Growth Study, 500 lean or obese (BMI > 25) adolescents were followed for 55 years. Mortality among obese men was 1.8 times higher than among lean controls. Obesity in adolescence predicted a broad range of adverse health effects. Again, the relative risk of moderate obesity may not be large, but given the millions of Americans who are moderately obese, the mortality attributable to moderate obesity is likely to be substantial.

5. Which malignancies have shown an increased incidence in obese patients?

Obese women have an increased incidence of endometrial cancer, postmenopausal breast cancer, and gallbladder and biliary cancers. Obese men have a higher mortality from cancers of the prostate, rectum, and colon.

6. What common metabolic abnormalities are found in obese patients?

Insulin resistance. Obesity is associated with a decrease in the ability of insulin to stimulate peripheral glucose disposal and to suppress hepatic glucose output. The body then increases insulin secretion to compensate. Insulin resistance and hyperinsulinemia may be caused by increased delivery of free fatty acids to the liver from the adipose tissue located within the abdomen. This theory explains why abdominal obesity is associated with more metabolic complications.

Lipid abnormalities. Plasma triglycerides are frequently elevated in obese individuals. This elevation leads to decreases in HDL cholesterol levels because of increases in HDL clearance. An increase in LDL cholesterol concentration also may be present.

Hyperuricemia. Hyperuricemia is due to both decreased clearance and increased production of uric acid.

Sex hormone abnormalities. Obese men show evidence of decreased levels of testosterone and follicle-stimulating hormone (FSH). Obese women may have high estrogen levels after menopause that predispose to endometrial cancer. An increased level of androgens is seen in women with upper body obesity and may lead to hirsutism, anovulatory menstrual cycles, and dysfunctional uterine bleeding. Increased androgen levels appear to be causally related to the hyperinsulinemia seen in obese women.

7. What disease is only seen in obese patients?

The pickwickian syndrome, named for the fat boy Joe in Dickens' *Pickwick Papers,* is characterized by obesity, hypoventilation, somnolence, secondary polycythemia, right ventricular failure, and in some instances, sleep apnea. All symptoms showed marked improvement with weight loss. Surprisingly the pulmonary problems may improve markedly with only a 20–30-lb weight loss.

8. When do organic causes of obesity need to be considered?

Rarely. Less than 1% of obese patients have underlying medical disorders as the primary cause of obesity. Cushing's syndrome, with excessive cortisol production, results in central obesity and the associated risks of hypertension and diabetes. Hypothyroidism also may cause an individual to gain 10–15 lbs, and patients with recent weight gain should be screened. Hypothyroidism and hypercortisolism, however, virtually never cause massive obesity independently.

Although typically we think of weight loss as a sign of major depression, some individuals manifest depression as weight gain. Signs of depression should be carefully sought, because depression may result from and contribute to the weight-control difficulties of the obese patient.

9. How does one take a nutritional history from an obese patient?

As with any medical condition, the evaluation should begin with a complete history. To make a dietary intervention, one must first know what the patient is currently eating. Many physicians are not comfortable taking a nutritional history and defer this task to the dietitian. In fact, taking a nutritional history is no more difficult than taking any other kind of history, and discussion by the primary care provider of the details of the patient's diet reinforces the importance of diet in overall health.

Dietitians often use two tools in taking a nutritional history: the diet recall and food frequency. The nutritionist asks the patient to record all foods eaten for 2–5 days. Although this approach is far more accurate than a 1–2-day oral recall history, it is also more time-consuming. For a primary caregiver, it is easier to ask patients what they ate the day before and the day of the clinic visit. Although this information is limited, the caregiver learns a great deal about how the patient eats. Many obese individuals do not eat breakfast, occasionally eat lunch, then snack on high-fat foods through much of the late afternoon and early evening. They may eat while doing other things. This makes it difficult for them to assess what they actually eat. Such information allows the caregiver to make simple nutritional suggestions. To take a food frequency history the nutritionist may use a questionnaire to ascertain how often certain foods are eaten. A simpler approach for the primary caregiver is to ask about the frequently eaten meals. Many people have a limited repertoire of meals that are eaten repetitively. They eat the same breakfast and lunch 3–5 times per week. If you can help patients to modify frequently consumed meals, you have substantially modified their diet.

History-taking tools are then combined with dietary advice. Such steps do not replace good nutritional counseling, but they are a powerful adjunct to the work done by a registered dietitian. They demonstrate that the primary care provider is committed to dietary therapy and interested in working with the patient in this important area.

10. What are the major components of a weight-loss program?
Numerous issues are important.

1. **What is the goal?** The patient may want to lose 40 lbs in 40 days. This approach is guaranteed to fail in the long run. A better goal is mild, sustained weight loss. A more realistic goal may be prevention of further weight gain. Perhaps the best goal is to improve eating and activity habits. These are the only factors that most individuals can influence in the long run. A shift in focus from weight to personal habits allows patients to succeed today if they change their habits and to fail next month if habits revert, even if the weight target has been achieved.

2. **Habits change slowly and gradually.** It is not realistic to expect anyone to go from a 50% fat diet to a vegetarian diet overnight. It is neither reasonable nor appropriate to have an obese patient become an aerobic athlete in 2 weeks. Patience on the part of both the primary care provider and the patient is a cornerstone of success.

3. **Any meaningful change in behavior must be lifelong.** Because there is a biological basis for obesity, as soon as the individual stops the weight-loss strategy, weight tends to return to its previous level. Therefore the changes must be simple and fit into the patient's lifestyle. More extensive, radical, and labor-intensive techniques probably will not be sustained, and the weight lost will return. The four Es should be remembered in counseling obese patients:

- **Eating.** The usual problem with the eating habits of obese individuals is not that they do not know what to eat, but that they do not pay attention to what they eat. A major goal of diet therapy for novice dieters is to get them to pay more attention to what they eat. The primary care provider should encourage the individual to eat 3 meals per day; to eat only at mealtimes; and to eat only one serving at each meal. Patients who follow these three recommendations have to make active decisions about the food that they eat. The primary caregiver can work with the dietitian to prescribe a flexible and balanced intake restricted to approximately 1200 calories, which will result in consistent and appropriate weight loss. The diet should try to minimize fat intake. Habits change slowly and need to be changed for the long term. Anyone who has switched from whole milk to 1–2% milk has experienced personally how a gradual, incremental change is far more tolerable than a radical one. Patients who eat at fast-food restaurants 5 times a week perhaps can initially change to 4 times per week; once a week, they eat something lower in fat that they find palatable. Over time they can replace more and more of the "usual meals" with new meals. Another approach is not to eliminate foods but simply to reduce portion size or frequency of consumption.

- **Exercise.** Exercise plays an important role in a successful weight-loss program. Studies that look at the effect of exercise in addition to diet show that exercise does not produce a great deal of added weight loss, but individuals who succeed in long-term weight reduction usually exercise regularly. Studies that examine body composition show that diet alone reduces total body weight, fat mass, and lean body mass. On the other hand, diet plus exercise may produce a similar decrease in total weight but a much greater decrease in fat mass, because lean body mass actually increases. This increase in lean body mass may allow the individual to liberalize an otherwise unacceptably restricted diet. Many patients who are too focused on total weight loss and engage in a vigorous exercise program are frustrated that they do not lose enough weight. It may help to measure body composition by underwater weighing to demonstrate that they have lost substantial fat mass and gained lean body mass. Although most experts have advocated aerobic training, recent evidence suggests that a balanced program of strength training along with aerobic exercise may be better than either alone.

- **Education.** The patient should be encouraged to become educated about nutrient content of foods, individual caloric intake, and trigger patterns that lead to increased eating. Often the failure of a dietary program occurs during periods of high stress. Eating is a pleasurable experience for most people, and when life is difficult, it may be an activity that they use for comfort.
- **Emotional support.** One of the most important components of a weight-loss program is follow-up by a physician, health care team, and/or weight-loss group. Education and emotional support form the bases of the highly significant impact of behavior modification on weight-loss efforts. Groups like Weight Watchers and TOPS have worked well for many individuals. A recent article in *Consumer Reports,* listed in the bibliography, is well written for laypersons and reviews the efficacy, cost, advantages, and disadvantages of several proprietary and nonproprietary weight-loss programs.

11. What medicines should be prescribed to aid in weight loss?
Various medications have been used to induce weight loss. Amphetamines, thyroid hormone, and diuretics, which were used in the past, should not be used for weight loss. They have far too many side effects to be acceptable. Phenylpropanolamine (PPA) (Dexatrim, Acutrim) is an over-the-counter weight-loss aid. Controlled data suggest that PPA has a statistically significant but quantitatively small effect on body weight. In a recent survey by *Consumer Reports,* less than 5% of those who used PPA were satisfied with the effects. One-half were dissatisfied, and many experienced troubling side effects. Numerous drugs that affect serotonin metabolism have been used in clinical trials. Fenfluramine is perhaps the best studied, and it has been shown to afford a greater degree of weight loss than diet alone. Weight loss is maintained as long as the drug is continued, but weight returns when the drug is discontinued.

A number of new medications—including pancreatic lipase inhibitors, which inhibit the absorption of dietary fat; atypical beta agonists, which increase thermogenesis, and neurotransmitter reuptake blockers, which reduce appetite—are in clinical trials. Each shows some promise, although none is without side effects. The central problem with drug therapy for obesity is that therapy must be lifelong; to date, the long-term risk-benefit ratio of such compounds has not been established. At this time, therefore, drug therapy for obesity cannot be advocated.

12. Should liposuction be advocated for obese patients?
In the only controlled trial, weight lost by liposuction was regained. Sometimes the adipose tissue reaccumulated in the same site; at other times it reaccumulated elsewhere. Liposuction cannot be advocated as a weight-loss strategy for patients with medically significant obesity.

13. What is morbid obesity?
Morbid obesity has been variably defined as weight that is 100% or 100 lbs above ideal. Another definition is obesity that results in substantial compromise of health. Most morbidly obese people have sleep apnea and hypoventilation, with or without right-heart failure. The relative risk of sudden death is 15–30 times higher than in lean controls. Morbidly obese individuals have a significant medical problem with a high risk of dying in the short term. Although it is controversial, many experts advocate aggressive weight-loss therapy in morbidly obese individuals, including very low calorie diets (VLCDs) and surgical treatments.

14. Define VLCD. When should it be considered?
A very low caloric diet (VLCD) is a diet of 800 kcal/day, which produces rapid weight loss. Most patients lose 1.5–2.5 kg/wk on a VLCD. Such diets should be administered by an experienced team in a supervised manner. When given in this manner, serious complications are unusual; the most common is cholelithiasis. General physicians probably should not be involved in the administration of VLCDs unless they are prepared to work with someone with more experience or to engage in such therapy regularly. The long-term results with VLCDs are

no better than with other diet programs. For this reason VLCDs have limited usefulness and should be used only in patients with a BMI > 30.

15. What mechanical methods are available for treatment of morbidly obese individuals?
For morbidly obese patients who suffer severe medical complications from obesity, various methods may be available. Gastric operations, resulting in small gastric pouch (gastroplasty) or gastric bypass (to bypass absorption of food) may be undertaken. For patients with a BMI > 40, surgical therapy may offer the best long-term chance for a reduced body weight. However, surgery should be considered only after more traditional approaches have failed and after the patient has been evaluated by an experienced multidisciplinary team. The surgeon must have extensive and ongoing experience for the patient to have the optimal chance for a good outcome. Placing the patient on a VLCD preoperatively may allow improved surgical outcome by reducing hepatic volume and thereby improving visualization of the stomach and also by reducing perioperative pulmonry complications.

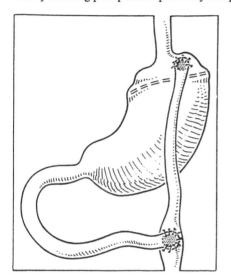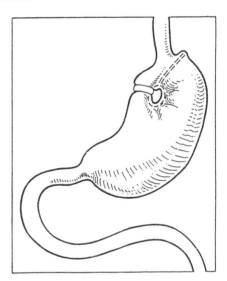

Gastroplasty (*left*) and gastric bypass (*right*).

CONTROVERSY

16. Does weight loss reduce the morbidity and mortality associated with obesity?
Although increased body weight is associated with adverse health consequences, it is not clear that weight loss is accompanied by a concurrent decrease in the same adverse health consequences. Clearly successful weight loss lowers blood pressure, improves insulin action and blood glucose control, puts less stress on joints, and improves the lipid profile. However, the effects on overall mortality and morbidity are less clear. Large population-based studies, including NHANES, MRFIT, and the Framingham Study, surprisingly show that weight loss is associated with a higher mortality rate than weight stability. The explanation may be that weight loss is usually associated with weight regain; thus the real culprit may be weight cycling (yo-yo dieting). Unfortunately, despite the billions of dollars spent on weight-loss products, we still do not have a single trial designed to evaluate the long-term health effects of weight loss in a prospective and randomized manner. Until such a trial is done, a reasonable approach is to encourage patients to develop good eating habits and engage in regular exercise, to discourage inappropriate weight-loss strategies, and to focus less on the cosmetics of obesity and more on a healthy lifestyle.

BIBLIOGRAPHY

1. Bray GA: Drug treatment of obesity. Am J Clin Nutr 55:538S–544S, 1992.
2. Gortmaker SL, Must A, Perrin JM, et al: Social and economic consequences of overweight in adolescence and young adulthood. N Engl J Med 329:1008–1012, 1993.
3. Grundy SM: Gastrointestinal surgery for severe obesity. Ann Intern Med 115:956–961, 1991.
4. Kuczmarski RJ: Prevalence of overweight and weight gain in the United States. Am J Clin Nutr 55:495S–502S, 1992.
5. Losing weight: What works, what doesn't. Consumer Reports June 347–357, 1993.
6. Manson JE, Colditz GA, Stampfer MJ, et al: A prospective study of obesity and risk of coronary heart disease in women. N Engl J Med 322:882–889, 1990.
7. Must A, Jacques PF, Dallai GE, et al: Long-term morbidity and mortality of overweight adolescents. N Engl J Med 327:1350–1355, 1992.
8. National Institutes of Health Consensus Development Panel on the Health Implications of Obesity: Health implications of obesity. Ann Intern Med 103:147, 1985.
9. National Task Force on the Prevention and Treatment of Obesity: Very low-calorie diets. JAMA 270:967–974, 1993.
10. Technology Assessment Conference Panel: Methods for voluntary weight loss and control: Technology Assessment Conference statement. Ann Intern Med 116:942–949, 1992, and 119(7 pt 2):641–764, 1993.
11. Wadden TA, Van Itallie TB, Blackburn GL: Responsible and irresponsible use of very-low-calorie diets in the treatment of obesity. JAMA 263:83, 1990.
12. Wing RR: Behavioral treatment of severe obesity. Am J Clin Nutr 55:545S–551S, 1992.

102. THE PATIENT WITH ACQUIRED IMMUNODEFICIENCY SYNDROME

David Lehman, M.D., Ph.D.

1. When does a patient have acquired immunodeficiency syndrome (AIDS)?

AIDS is the clinical syndrome of acquired immunodeficiency resulting from infection with the human immunodeficiency virus (HIV). When a patient who is HIV-positive develops an opportunistic infection, a specific neoplasm, or other specified conditions, the patient has AIDS. The most common opportunistic infections are *Pneumocystis carinii* pneumonia (PCP), *Mycobacterium avium* complex (MAC), cytomegalovirus (CMV), *Mycobacterium tuberculosis* infection, *Candida* esophagitis, coccidioidomycosis, and other fungal infections. The most common neoplasms are Kaposi's sarcoma and non-Hodgkin's lymphomas, but invasive cervical carcinoma is also AIDS-defining. Other specific AIDS-defining conditions include a CD4 count < 200, pulmonary tuberculosis, recurrent pneumonia, HIV encephalopathy, and wasting syndrome.

Relative Risk of AIDS-defining Conditions as a Function of CD4 Count

Higher CD4 Counts (increased risk with lower counts)	**Rare, unless CD4 < 200**
Tuberculosis	*Pneumocystis carinii* pneumonia
Herpes	**Rare, unless CD4 < 50**
Kaposi's sarcoma	*Mycobacterium avium* complex
HIV encephalopathy	Cytomegalovirus disease
Systemic fungal infection	
Lymphoma	

2. What risk factors for HIV disease should be assessed in primary care practice?
A complete history includes an assessment of HIV risk: male homosexual practices, intravenous (IV) drug use (specifically needle sharing), sex with IV drug users, prostitution, sex with prostitutes, history of blood transfusion between 1978 and 1985, history of sexually transmitted diseases, and history of multiple sexual partners. Potential may be clarified by determining the frequency of safe/unsafe sexual practices. The risk assessment process also may be used to educate patients about risk reduction, including safer sex and safer drug use.

3. When should the physician encourage the patient to be tested for HIV?
HIV testing should be recommended if a history of more than minimal risk is obtained. Patients should be counseled about confidentiality issues and consent to testing. Some patients choose to be tested anonymously at an alternate test site.

4. How can the physician judge the patient's risk of transmission?
Parenteral transfusion of blood products and receptive rectal intercourse have the highest rate of transmission, although the rate has not been quantified. Men are also at risk, albeit somewhat lower, via insertive rectal sex. The risk of heterosexual (male-to-female) transmission has been studied by evaluating the proportion of infected women among the steady partners of infected men. The rate varies from 7–10% for the partners of hemophiliac men to 18% for the partners of transfusion recipients and 22–33% for the partners of bisexual men. Female-to-male transmission is probably lower, although the low prevalence in women has limited the collection of suitable data.

5. How accurate is HIV testing?
The joint false-positive rate of sequential ELISA and Western blot testing is about 0.1%, depending on the experience of the laboratory. In a population with a low prevalence of HIV infection, this may correspond to positive predictive values of < 50%. False-negative tests in low prevalence populations are rare and result mainly from the window between infection and development of antibodies (usually < 3 mos, but rarely up to 6 mos).

6. What are the natural history and prognosis of HIV infection?
On average, about 50% of HIV-infected patients progress to AIDS in 10 years. Patients often gain a more positive outlook by learning that this also means that one-half of patients will *not* progress to AIDS after 10 years. The natural history of progression to AIDS has been studied in several populations:
- San Francisco City Clinic Cohort, with 54% progression after 11 years;
- Transfusion recipients, with 49% progression after 7 years; and
- Hemophiliacs, with 25% progression after 9 years.

Mathematical models predict that > 95% of HIV patients will eventually progress to AIDS, but the data do not allow us to conclude that every HIV-positive individual will inevitably develop AIDS. The median survival after development of an AIDS-defining condition has increased to about 24–30 months with current therapy.

7. How should the newly diagnosed HIV-positive patient be evaluated?
The complete history and physical examination for HIV-positive patients includes special emphasis on risk factors (timing seroconversion, if possible), psychosocial issues, systemic issues (fever and weight loss), and targeted organs: skin, oropharynx, lungs, gastrointestinal (GI) tract, and lymph nodes. Routine laboratory evaluation includes chest radiograph; complete blood count with differential and platelet count; levels of serum glutamate oxaloacetate transaminase (SGOT), lactate dehydrogenase (LDH), bilirubin, alkaline phosphatase (AP), albumin, total protein, and creatinine; serologic test for syphilis and hepatitis B surface antigen (HBsAg); and assessment of T cells with subsets. For patients who have lived in coastal areas, a toxoplasmosis titer is included. Vaccinations (including diphtheria-tetanus,

Pneumovax, and influenza) are updated, and purified protein-derivative (PPD)-skin testing is done immediately for patients with > 500 CD4 cells. Hepatitis B vaccine is recommended for HBsAg-negative patients with ongoing risk behavior. Patients with < 500 CD4 cells who choose to take zidovudine (AZT; see question 9) receive vaccinations and skin testing after 4 weeks of AZT therapy because of data suggesting an improved response. Risk-reduction behavior (tobacco cessation, alcohol moderation, IV drug cessation) should be encouraged. A nutritional evaluation helps patients to maintain a healthy weight.

8. What treatment is available for HIV-positive patients?
Current treatment falls into two areas: **antiretroviral therapy** and **prophylaxis against opportunistic infections.** The timing and choice of antiretroviral agents are areas with rapidly evolving data about which physicians disagree. Well-informed patients often state their own preferences, which should be a major factor in therapeutic decision making. Prophylaxis against PCP has been shown to prolong life for HIV-positive patients. Several agents are available: trimethoprim/sulfamethoxazole (first-line), dapsone, and aerosolized pentamidine. Patients should be monitored for side effects, which may require a change to a different agent. Ongoing trials are attempting to determine the relative benefit of prophylaxis against MAC with rifabutin, clarithromycin, or combination chemotherapy.

9. What facts may the physician share with the patient in evaluating the risks and benefits of therapy with AZT?
The physician may share the following facts with patients to help in the decision process:
   1. AZT prolongs life for patients who have already progressed to AIDS.
   2. AZT cuts in half the rate of progression to AIDS in the first year for patients with CD4 counts < 500.
   3. At 3 years the Concorde study showed no difference in progression between patients who took AZT early and those who took it later.
   4. Patients who switched to ddI after a short course of AZT therapy did better than patients who stayed on AZT, although the survival rate was the same.
   5. All drugs have side effects, some of which are dangerous and some of which are annoying symptomatically.
   6. AZT causes irreversible bone marrow suppression in about 1/10,000 patients, and reversible anemia in 3–5% of patients. Symptomatic side effects include GI distress and headaches.
   7. Side effects of ddI include pancreatitis, which on occasion is fatal, and peripheral neuropathy, which may be irreversible. The most common side effect is diarrhea.
   8. Because HIV develops resistance to drugs over time, the best long-term course is not known.
   9. Research is ongoing; a better drug may be available in the next 1–5 years.

10. Describe the common skin problems in HIV infection.
Up to 90% of HIV-positive patients have a skin disease. Kaposi's sarcoma is discussed below with other malignancies. The prevalence of skin infections is high. Among bacterial etiologies, *Staphylococcus aureus* is the most common, usually presenting as a folliculitis or less frequently as bullous impetigo, ecthyma, abscesses, or cellulitis. Among viral etiologies, herpes viruses (zoster and simplex) are the most common. The suggestion to assess HIV risk factors in all adults aged 18–50 years is especially applicable if the patient (even up to 65 yrs) presents with zoster. *Molluscum contagiosum* is common and especially difficult to eradicate in HIV-positive patients.

By virtue of taking more drugs, HIV-positive patients and patients with AIDS are at increased risk of drug reactions. The most common reaction is due to trimethoprim-sulfamethoxazole (TMP-SMX) and presents as a diffuse maculopapular eruption. Other antibiotics, notably penicillins, are also common offenders. Zidovudine and acyclovir are implicated only rarely.

11. What mouth problems are common in HIV infection?
Common oral lesions in HIV-positive patients have fungal, bacterial, viral, or neoplastic etiologies. The two most common types are hairy leukoplakia (white thickening of mucosal surfaces, often with vertical corrugations) and thrush (pseudomembranous candidiasis). Both conditions have been shown to predict progression to AIDS independently of CD4 counts. Candidal infection also may present as angular cheilitis, candidal leukoplakia, or the erythematous form. Gingivitis and periodontitis are common bacterial complications of HIV disease. Kaposi's sarcoma may produce oral lesions.

12. What entities should be considered when an HIV-positive patient complains of dysphagia?
Candidal esophagitis is the most common cause of dysphagia; odynophagia and retrosternal chest pain are other frequent symptoms. Less common etiologies are CMV, herpes virus, and Kaposi's sarcoma. Response to empiric treatment for candidal infection with ketoconazole sometimes provides a presumptive diagnosis. Endoscopy with biopsies is needed for a definitive diagnosis.

13. Describe the neuropsychiatric complications of HIV infection.
The common neurologic manifestations may be due directly to HIV (e.g., AIDS dementia complex and peripheral neuropathy) or secondary to opportunistic disease, including fungal (*Cryptococcus* sp.), protozoan (toxoplasmosis), mycobacterial, and viral infections. Peripheral neuropathy presents as a painful sensation with limited sensory or motor deficits. *Cryptococcus neoformans* meningitis is the most common fungal infection of the central nervous system in HIV-positive patients. Other fungal pathogens are histoplasmosis and coccidioidomycosis. *Toxoplasmosa gondii* causes encephalitis and focal intracerebral lesions, which are ring-enhancing on computed tomographic (CT) scan. Progressive multifocal leukoencephalopathy (PML), caused by the human polyomavirus JC, commonly presents insidiously over weeks with focal neurologic deficits. AIDS dementia complex is an organic mental disorder with cognitive deficits (confusion, memory loss, impaired concentration, or mental slowing), behavioral manifestations (depressed affect or agitation), and motor symptoms (weakness, unsteady gait, or decreased coordination). Other common psychiatric manifestations include adjustment, affective, and anxiety disorders. An increased prevalence of substance abuse is self-evident among intravenous drug users, but also has been described empirically in the male homosexual population.

14. When should the primary care physician seek hematologic consultations for HIV disease?
Anemia, leukopenia, and thrombocytopenia may occur singly or in combination, either as a direct manifestation of HIV disease or as a result of opportunistic infections or neoplasms, drug effects, or nutritional deficiencies. In many instances, the primary care physician may diagnose and manage the penias of HIV infection.

Anemia is the most common abnormality, occurring in up to 85% of patients with AIDS. Isolated anemia is associated with *Mycobacterium avium* or parvovirus infection. Hemolytic anemia may occur in patients who are deficient in glucose 6-phosphate-dehydrogenase and treated with dapsone. Zidovudine may cause anemia that requires transfusions as well as neutropenia and thrombocytopenia. Ganciclovir, pentamidine, trimethoprim, and cancer chemotherapeutic agents commonly cause neutropenia.

Isolated immune thrombocytopenia may occur as a manifestation of HIV infection or AIDS. Diagnosis and treatment of immune thrombocytopenia may require bone marrow biopsy and hematologic consultation. In some instances, treatment of appropriate patients (CD4 counts < 500) with AZT may lead to marked improvement of the thrombocytopenia. In addition, the administration of growth factors (erythropoietin and granulocyte colony-stimulating factor [G-CSF]) may be helpful in some instances.

15. Contrast the clinical presentations and management of the various forms of pneumonia in HIV-positive patients.
PCP is the most common AIDS-defining condition and usually occurs only in severely immunocompromised patients (CD4 < 200). Clinical presentation includes fever, nonproductive

cough, and progressive shortness of breath; pleuritic chest pain is uncommon. Supportive evidence includes an elevated LDH, hypoxia, or at least an increased alveoloarterial oxygen gradient and a diffuse interstitial infiltrate on chest radiograph. Diagnosis is made by fluorescent antibody stain of induced sputum (64% sensitive) or, if necessary, of bronchoalveolar lavage specimens (97% sensitive). Treatment options include TMP/SMX, pentamidine, TMP/dapsone, clindamycin/primaquine and atovaquone, and the addition of steroids for acute disease.

Bacterial pneumonia, which is AIDS-defining if recurrent, occurs with increased frequency in all HIV-positive patients. The most common pathogens include *Pneumococcus pneumoniae, Haemophilus influenzae,* and *Moraxella catarrhalis.* The presenting symptoms, fever, productive cough, and dyspnea, are often acute and of short duration. The chest radiograph more often shows lobar or segmental infiltrates. Blood cultures are positive in 40–80% of cases. The sputum Gram stain sometimes gives an immediate diagnosis. Empirical treatment with TMP/SMX provides excellent coverage of the common bacterial agents as well as PCP, pending definitive diagnosis.

Mycobacterial infection, which occurs with pulmonary as well as systemic manifestations, is discussed in question 17. The herpes family also causes pneumonia as well as infects other organs or presents as systemic disease (see question 18). Fungal agents include cryptococci, *Histoplasma,* and coccidioidomycosis.

16. Should HIV-positive patients be screened regularly for tuberculosis?

Yes. *Mycobacterium tuberculosis* has been found in 3.8% of patients with AIDS, with a disproportionate increase in extrapulmonary sites. Intravenous drug users and ethnic minorities are at especially increased risk. The 1993 revised case definition added pulmonary tuberculosis as an AIDS-defining condition. Annual screening with PPD (a > 5 mm reaction is positive) is recommended for all HIV-positive patients who are not already known to be anergic. Because of frequent anergy, some physicians also recommend a screening chest radiograph, depending on local prevalence of tuberculosis. PPD-positive patients, of whatever age, should take prophylactic isoniazid. Initial empiric treatment for active tuberculosis includes isoniazid, rifampin, and pyrazinamide, with further adjustment depending on the presence of extrapulmonary tuberculosis and the local prevalence of multidrug-resistant strains.

17. Which patients are susceptible to MAC?

Disseminated MAC is a frequent late complication of HIV infection (up to 53% in one autopsy series). It usually occurs in patients with < 100 CD4 cells (usually < 50). Its common clinical manifestations are fever, malaise, weight loss, anemia, neutropenia, chronic diarrhea, abdominal pain, and malabsorption. Diagnosis is made by special blood culture techniques. Because of their low sensitivity and low positive predictive value, stool cultures are not recommended. Various multidrug regimens have been tried with only limited success.

18. List the three most common viral infections in HIV-positive patients.

Herpes simplex infection has a high prevalence (95% seropositivity in homosexual men with AIDS), and sometimes has severe manifestations in HIV-positive patients, including esophagitis, pneumonia, and encephalitis. Some patients require chronic acyclovir suppression. *Herpes zoster* (recurrent varicella zoster infection) occurs frequently in HIV-positive patients, and the new diagnosis of zoster in any patients younger than 65 years should prompt a risk assessment and consideration of testing for HIV. Patients may experience multiple recurrences and systemic dissemination. **Active CMV** is a frequent late complication of AIDS (CD4 < 50). Clinical manifestations include retinitis, pneumonia, encephalitis, and severe diarrhea.

19. How should an HIV-positive patient with diarrhea be evaluated and treated?

First, a diagnosis should be sought to identify treatable etiologies of diarrhea. Stool should be cultured for bacteria and examined microscopically for parasites. *Mycobacterium avium intracellulare* (MAI) is best identified by blood cultures (see question 17). Common bacterial etiologies include *Salmonella, Shigella,* and *Campylobacter* spp., *Giardia lamblia, Entamoeba histolytica,* and, less commonly, *Cryptosporidium* and *Isospora belli* are common parasitic agents. A toxin for *C. difficile* should be considered when the patient has been on antibiotics. In one series, CMV colitis was the most common cause of diarrhea; diagnosis requires identification of CMV and biopsy of mucosal ulcers. If no specific cause is identified, symptomatic treatment with nonspecific antidiarrheal drugs may provide significant benefit to patients.

20. Which malignancies are associated with HIV infection?
The AIDS-defining opportunistic malignancies are Kaposi's sarcoma (most common), non-Hodgkin's lymphoma, and invasive cervical carcinoma. Kaposi's sarcoma usually presents as violaceous, palpable nodules of the skin or oral mucosa; it also may involve the GI tract, lungs, and lymph nodes. About 70% of non-Hodgkin's lymphoma is B-cell lymphoma and usually presents as advanced extranodal disease. Two-thirds of patients with non-Hodgkin's lymphoma have CD4 counts below 200; the disease may present as primary lymphoma of the central nervous system, but usually not until patients are severely immunocompromised (CD4 < 50). Invasive cervical carcinoma was added as an AIDS-defining condition in the revised case definition of 1993.

21. Describe the special issues associated with HIV in women.
The rising frequency, epidemiology, and severity of HIV infection in women present special issues. The fastest growing AIDS group is women. Intravenous drug use (IDU) is responsible for 68% of AIDS cases in women, either directly (50%) or indirectly (18%) through sex with an intravenous drug user. Minorities are disproportionately represented; 74% of women with AIDS are black or Hispanic. AIDS is now the most common cause of death in women aged 25–44 years in seven American cities on the East Coast. Women tend to present in more advanced stages of disease, in part because up to 50% with heterosexual sex as a risk factor were unaware of the risk. As in men, PCP is the most frequent AIDS-defining diagnosis. Candida vaginitis is the most frequent symptom of early immunodeficiency and may occur in patients with CD4 counts > 500. HIV-infected women also appear to have vaginal warts and cervical dysplasia (associated with human papilloma virus) more frequently and more severely.

22. When and how should advance care directives be discussed with HIV-positive patients?
The 100% mortality rate associated with an AIDS diagnosis compels a discussion of advance care directives so that the extent and type of endstage care complies with the patient's wishes. This is best done by a caring provider within a long-term provider/patient relationship. Postponing the discussion until emergent hospital admission is a disservice to the patient; the admitting physician (unfamiliar with the patient and subject to frequent distractions) is less qualified to help the patient understand the issues needed to make an appropriate decision. Physicians must accept the responsibility to anticipate situations in which a clear advance directive will improve patient care and to initiate discussion of this issue in a timely manner.

BIBLIOGRAPHY

1. Cockerell CJ: Human immunodeficiency virus infection and the skin. Arch Intern Med 151:1295–1303, 1991.
2. Cohn DL: Bacterial pneumonia in the HIV-infected patient. Infect Dis Clin North Am 5:485–507, 1991.
3. Haas JS, et al: Discussion of preferences for life-sustaining care by persons with AIDS. Arch Intern Med 153:1241–1248, 1993.
4. Horsburgh CR: *Mycobacterium avium* complex infection in the acquired immunodeficiency syndrome. N Engl J Med 324:1332–1338, 1991.
5. Kahn JO, et al: A controlled trial comparing continued zidovudine with didanosine in human immunodeficiency virus infection. N Engl J Med 327:581–587, 1992.
6. Lagakos S, et al: Effects of zidovudine therapy in minority and other subpopulations with early HIV infection. JAMA 266:2709–2712, 1991.

7. Minkoff HL, DeHovitz JA: Care of women infected with the human immunodeficiency virus. JAMA 266:2253–2258, 1991.
8. Nightingale SD, et al: Logarithmic relationship of the CD4 count to survival in patients with human immunodeficiency virus infection. Arch Intern Med 153:1313–1318, 1993.
9. Pantaleo G, Graziosi C, Fauci AS: The immunopathogenesis of human immunodeficiency virus infection. N Engl J Med 328:327–335, 1993.
10. Peterman TA, et al: Risk of human immunodeficiency virus transmission from heterosexual adults with transfusion-associated infections. JAMA 259:55–58, 1988.
11. Rabkin CS, et al: Incidence of lymphomas and other cancers in HIV-infected and HIV-uninfected patients with hemophilia. JAMA 267:1090–1094, 1992.
12. Sande MA, Volberding PA (eds): The Medical Management of AIDS, 3rd ed. Philadelphia, W.B. Saunders, 1992.
13. Selik RM, Chu SY, Buehler JW: HIV infection as leading cause of death among young adults in US cities and states. JAMA 269:2991–2994, 1993.

103. THE PATIENT WITH ANOREXIA AND/OR WEIGHT LOSS

Lawrence Smith, M.D.

1. What is medically important weight loss?

Any degree of weight loss can be significant, but most experts define loss of 5% of body weight over 6 months as medically important, if the patient was not on a reduced calorie diet or undergoing diuretic therapy. Greater amounts of weight loss are more often associated with serious disease.

2. When does anorexia need to be evaluated?

Anorexia without weight loss is rarely the consequence of serious disease. Side effects of medication, changes in taste, gastrointestinal (GI) and liver disease, or psychiatric conditions need to be considered. However, the basic evaluation of serious anorexia parallels that of unintentional weight loss.

3. Is it important to verify weight loss?

Weight loss is a common complaint to primary care physicians. Over one-half of such patients have been found not to have sustained significant weight loss and need no evaluation. Verifying weight loss is essential; methods include comparison with earlier weights, demonstration of a change in clothing size, clear confirmation from friends or relatives, or visible signs of cachexia.

4. What are the major causes of weight loss?

The data in the table below combine several studies in the literature. Of note is that studies of inpatients showed a higher percentage of serious organic disease, whereas studies of outpatients show a higher percentage of psychiatric disease.

Causes of Weight Loss*

CAUSE	RELATIVE FREQUENCY	CAUSE	RELATIVE FREQUENCY
Psychiatric disease	24%	Hyperthyroid disease	2%
Malignancy	22%	Other severe physical disease	10%
Gastrointestinal disease	11%	Medication effects	3%
Food intake disorders	4%	No cause found	24%

* Estimates compiled from four studies with a total of 407 patients.

5. Do serious illnesses often present only as weight loss?

Although most serious illnesses, such as cancer, endstage heart disease, chronic obstructive pulmonary disease, arthritis, or renal failure, are associated with significant involuntary weight loss, this usually occurs long after the disease is diagnosed. It is rare for someone to have weight loss from a serious organic illness that is not obvious at the time of evaluation.

6. Does occult malignancy present as weight loss?

Most studies have shown that malignancy is an uncommon cause of weight loss, and occult malignancy is very rare. In all series, most malignancies were obvious at initial visits, and all were diagnosed by 6 months after the first evaluation. Extensive evaluations searching for occult malignancy are not appropriate in patients with weight loss.

7. What causes weight loss and increased appetite?

Few conditions truly produce the combination of weight loss and increased appetite. Possibilities include hyperthyroidism, diabetes mellitus, and perhaps malabsorption syndromes. Psychiatric disorders, such as schizophrenia or a primary eating disorder, also need to be considered.

8. Why do patients not maintain adequate food intake?

Anorexia is not the only reason for inadequate food intake. Pain associated with eating, as in esophageal and gastric disease, may lead to aversion of food. Dental problems, taste disorders, neurologic difficulties, social conditions, financial problems, and many other factors may contribute to poor nutrition. In evaluating poor food intake, an open-minded approach is important.

9. How extensive should the initial evaluation be?

Serious organic disease is usually obvious at the time of presentation. All studies emphasize the high sensitivity of a good history and physical examination. The table below shows a typical initial screening panel of laboratory studies.

Initial Screen for Weight Loss

Complete history
Complete physical examination, including mental status and functional assessment
Complete blood count
Sequential multiple analysis—12 tests
Urinalysis
Chest radiograph
Stool—occult blood
Upper GI series if abdominal symptoms are present
Thyroid tests if symptoms are suggestive or patient is elderly

10. When should the physician look extensively for occult disease?

The answer is probably never. Occult serious disease is rare and usually becomes evident quickly on follow-up. Specifically, CT scans to discover unsuspected problems have not proved useful in the setting of weight loss. The exception may be the patient with a high level of alkaline phosphatase and low level of serum albumin; in one study, the incidence of positive findings was high in such patients.

11. Approximately 25% of patients with weight loss have no specific diagnosis. How long does follow-up need to be continued?

If no illness is obvious at 6 months, it is highly unlikely that the weight loss is due to undiagnosed organic disease. Serious social or psychiatric problems, however, may have been missed.

12. What psychiatric disorders are associated with weight loss?
Most studies show depression as the most common psychiatric disorder in all patients with weight loss and the most common diagnosis overall in outpatients with weight loss. In addition, schizophrenia, conversion disorder, and the primary eating disorders of anorexia nervosa and bulimia are seen occasionally. Addiction to drugs and alcohol also may present with profound weight loss.

13. How are primary eating disrders recognized?
Patients with eating disorders are typically young adult white women of middle-to-upper socioeconomic class. Bulimic patients present at an older age than patients with anorexia nervosa. Symptoms are vague and usually result from weight loss (e.g., amenorrhoea, fatigue, weakness) or from vomiting (e.g., electrolyte abnormalities). Patients rarely seek help on their own and, despite being thin, perceive themselves as overweight. They are at risk for life-threatening problems from weight loss and vomiting. Bulimics frequently also abuse laxatives and diuretics. A team approach with psychiatric evaluation and nutritional support is essential.

14. What social conditions may present as weight loss?
Poverty, isolation, lack of transportation, and inability to cook or shop for food are only some of the social problems associated with significant weight loss. If suspicion is high, a social service referral and a home visit may be valuable.

15. Are elderly patients of special concern?
Decreasing functional states, dementia, stroke, and decreasing taste for and interest in food are some of the geriatric problems accounting for weight loss. A careful neurologic exam, minimental status evaluation, functional assessment, and screening for depression are particularly useful in the elderly. Because hypothyroidism may present in its apathetic form in elderly patients, routine thyroid function studies are probably in order. The elderly are also particularly susceptible to the anorectic side effects of medication.

CONTROVERSY

16. Does forced feeding benefit the patient when weight loss is due to serious organic illness?
Despite many clinical trials, especially among patients with terminal cancer, attempting to reverse cachexia with forced feeding, including total parenteral nutrition, has shown little evidence of overall benefit. Transient weight gain has been reported but without consistent benefit to functional status or survival.

BIBLIOGRAPHY

1. Garfinkel P, Garner D, Kaplan A, et al: Differential diagnosis of emotional disorders that cause weight loss. Can Med Assoc J 129:939–945, 1983.
2. Marton K, Sox H, Krupp J: Involuntary weight loss: Diagnostic and prognostic significance. Ann Intern Med 95:568–574, 1981.
3. Rabinovitz M, Pitlik S, Leifer M, et al: Unintentional weight loss. Arch Intern Med 146:186–187, 1986.
4. Thompson M, Morris L: Unexplained weight loss in the ambulatory elderly. J Am Geriatr Soc 39:498–500, 1991.

104. THE PATIENT WITH CANCER

Kathleen Ogle, M.D.

1. What pitfalls should be avoided when telling a patient that he or she has cancer?

The clinician who makes a diagnosis of cancer bears the brunt of the patient's initial emotional reaction. Thus, in most instances a certain diagnosis must be made before informing the patient or consulting the oncologist. A presumed surprise or error in diagnosis only adds additional suffering to the patient and disrupts the trust of the physician/patient relationship. Compassionate communication of the diagnosis and reassurance that all appropriate measures will be taken are important. It is crucial to avoid the pitfall of attempting to estimate the duration of remaining life: such estimates are frequently proved wrong or, worse yet, become self-fulfilling prophecy.

The patient's cultural background, socioeconomic status, education level, and personal experience influence psychological response to a diagnosis of cancer. A large difference between the provider's cultural beliefs and those of the patient and family may lead to difficulties. An example is the taboo, common in some Asian cultures, that forbids telling the patient of the diagnosis. A compromise between biases of the provider and the patient must be sought.

Patients with testicular cancer or Hodgkin's disease frequently recall with bitter resentment having been told soon after diagnosis that they are "lucky" to have such a curable neoplasm. In fact, considering the strenuous treatment that they face, such a comment, however well-meaning, is quite cruel and obviously should be avoided.

2. Should an attempt at antineoplastic treatment be made at the time of diagnosis of all cancers?

No. Some cancers are so indolent that in essence they "coexist" with the patient and may never require treatment. In other circumstances, the general health of the patient precludes attempts at treatment of the malignancy. Numerous randomized trials of anticancer treatment demonstrate that patients confined to bed for $\geq 50\%$ of an average day (i.e., poor performance status) are unlikely to benefit from treatment. This seems to be true whether or not the poor performance status is due to malignancy.

3. Which cancers can be cured with current therapy?

Around 50% of new cancer diagnoses can be successfully treated, and early diagnosis improves the chance of cure by surgery or local irradiation. Advanced cancers frequently curable with chemotherapy include some leukemias, Hodgkin's disease, some lymphomas, testicular and germ-cell cancer in adults, and many childhood malignancies. Chemotherapy or hormone therapy adds years of life often without signs of active malignancy in patients with certain other cancers, such as small-cell lung cancer, breast cancer, prostate cancer, colorectal cancer, and ovarian cancer. When other malignancies spread beyond the local site, treatment is palliative.

4. When a patient presents with a metastatic cancer of unknown primary site, what are the appropriate diagnostic tests to consider?

For the majority of patients who present with widespread carcinoma for which no obvious primary site is apparent, a complete history and physical examination (including pelvic and rectal exams) should be followed by a chest radiograph, a mammogram in women, and laboratory tests and radiographs designed to investigate symptoms or abnormal signs. Meticulous screening for intra-abdominal cancers or occult bronchogenic tumors does not affect outcome and is unnecessary in most cases. Following this evaluation, the patient should be referred to an oncologist for further therapy.

5. What are the most common symptoms of advanced cancer?

Pain is a major symptom in cancer; up to 70% of patients with advanced cancer experience significant pain. Most studies indicate that undertreatment of cancer-related pain is a pervasive problem in the United States. Other common symptoms of advanced malignancy are fatigue, loss of appetite, weight loss, dyspnea, and excessive somnolence.

6. What are the greatest fears expressed by patients with cancer?

When questioned about beliefs and fears surrounding dying and death, persons of all ages identify several areas of concern. Loss of autonomy and dignity, disfigurement, and loss of body control and mental awareness are cited frequently. Fear of abandonment by family and friends as well as by health care providers is often high on the list. However, fear of a painful death is paramount; cancer and pain are inextricably linked in the minds of patients.

Acknowledgment of common fears and concerns by the physician accomplishes a great deal in alleviating them. Patients are rarely confident or self-aware enough to verbalize their anxieties about death, and the health care professional should raise the topic. In particular, reassurance that the patient will not be abandoned in the dying process is crucial and should take place early in the discussion of terminal illness.

7. What is the best approach to the management of pain in a patient with cancer?

Pain in the terminally ill should be managed as if it were a separate problem from the underlying disease. Physical pain in a patient with cancer may be related to the malignancy, to debility resulting from cancer, or to treatment; it also may be unrelated to cancer. An effort should be made to diagnose and treat more readily reversible causes of pain (such as constipation, stomatitis, headache from brain edema, infection in locally advanced tumors). If a focal site of cancer metastasis is found to cause pain, local radiation is useful to alleviate the symptom. When it is determined that the cause of the pain is not reversible or is unknown, analgesic therapy should be appropriate to the level of pain, as perceived by the patient.

8. What pain syndromes occur in patients with cancer? How do they affect therapy?

Three types of pain can be recognized as separate syndromes requiring somewhat different management strategies.

Somatic or musculoskeletal pain results from pressure on peripheral nerves by masses and organ infiltration. This type of pain is generally more localized and intense; it may be intermittent and tends to be the most responsive to narcotic analgesics. When somatic pain originates from bone metastases, the frequently associated inflammation may respond well to anti-inflammatory drugs.

Visceral pain may result from compression of autonomic nervous pathways, as in deep-seated tumors of the abdomen, or from obstruction of bowel or other visceral organs. This pain is less localized by the patient and often associated with other unpleasant sensations, such as nausea; in addition, it often has a component that is constant and a component that is intermittent but much more severe. Visceral pain may be associated with hyperesthetic areas on overlying skin. It usually responds to narcotic analgesics, but higher doses may be required.

Neuropathic pain results from destruction of nerves and causes associated burning and hyperesthesia in the affected region. Episodes of associated lancinating pains may be excruciating but very brief. Neuropathic pain is the least responsive to opioids. Adjunctive medications such as tricyclic antidepressants or anticonvulsants are often needed. Corticosteroids as an adjunct to analgesics may be useful in both somatic and neuropathic pain syndromes.

9. How should analgesics by used in the terminally ill patient?

The most important tenets of pain control in the terminally ill patient are the following five rules:

1. **Use scheduled doses** of analgesics, in addition to "as needed."
2. **Adjust the dose frequently.** The goal is to control the pain to a tolerable level within a few hours, if possible.

3. **Allow the patient to control dosing** and dose adjustment as much as possible.

4. **The oral route** for analgesics is preferred.

5. **Use a sufficient dose** to control the pain. It is better to "overshoot" and titrate downward.

An occasional patient with pain due to cancer may require only acetaminophen, aspirin, or some other nonsteroidal anti-inflammatory agent. However, the majority of patients with cancer who experience pain require more potent analgesics at some point.

10. When does the physician switch to a narcotic for pain control? How are narcotics safely used?

For moderate pain or pain that is not controlled with nonnarcotic analgesics, it is appropriate to use mild opioids such as codeine or oxycodone. As soon as the mild opioids fail to control pain, or if a patient presents with severe pain, it is appropriate to begin a potent opioid such as morphine sulfate. The tables below present the oral and parenteral dose-equivalencies to morphine sulfate of common narcotic analgesics and compare three common potent opioids.

Narcotic Dose Equivalents for Chronic Pain Control

ORAL DOSE (mg)	ANALGESIC	PARENTERAL DOSE (mg)
15	Morphine	5
150	Meperidine	50
100	Codeine	60
10	Oxycodone*	10
10	Methadone	5
4	Hydromorphone	2
2	Levorphanol	1
NA	Fentanyl patch	25 μg/hr[†]

* Oxycodone is available primarily in combination with acetaminophen or aspirin; a recently reformulated product is available as oxycodone alone.

[†] Fentanyl patch dose equivalent to 10–20 mg/day of morphine given parenterally or 30–60 mg/day of oral morphine.

NA = not applicable.

Potent Narcotic Analgesics

Morphine sulfate (MS)
  Available routes of administration
  Oral, buccal, sublingual
  Slow-release oral pill
  Rectal
  IV, IM, subcutaneous
  Intrathecal
  Intraventricular
  Slow release pills (MS-Contin, Oramorph-SR)
  8–12-hour duration of analgesia
  Ease of administration, dosing
  Can be given rectally
  Expensive

Methadone
  Available only orally
  Variable duration of analgesia
  Duration of analgesia not equivalent to duration of sedating effects because of accumulation of metabolites
  Cheap
  Not cross-reactive in morphine-allergic patients

Fentanyl
  Routes: topical (dermal absorption) or IV
  New product (Duragesic–fentanyl): transdermal patch
  Excellent alternative to MS infusion in patient unable to swallow
  Very expensive (but not as much as IV morphine)
  Slow onset of action, depot effect in subcutaneous tissue, and variable rate of absorption

IV = intravenous; IM = intramuscular

Morphine sulfate has several advantages over other potent opioids: (1) it is available by any route of administration; (2) it is well absorbed orally; (3) the potency ratio of oral to parenteral dosage is predictable; and (4) it is relatively less expensive than many potent opioids. It is also available in two slow-release formulations that allow dosing every 8–12 hours. Rapid-onset morphine for oral dosing is available in low- or high-concentration liquids as well as in far less expensive pills. Rapid-onset morphine can be used for breakthrough pain in a patient on slow-release tablets or as a means to achieve rapid pain control in a patient with severe pain.

Anticipatory management of the side effects of opiates is required for effective pain control. All patients on narcotic analgesics have some decrease in gut motility, which results in constipation in the majority and nausea in a significant proportion. Stool softeners and a mild antiemetic should be prescribed along with the first prescription for a narcotic, even codeine. A bowel program to prevent constipation should be taught to patients and caregivers.

Other less frequent but sometimes distressing narcotic side effects include urinary retention, pruritus, excessive sweating, and myoclonic jerking. Reassurance may be all that is necessary for the last three; urinary retention occasionally requires use of an indwelling catheter.

11. What is the maximal dose of narcotics?

The dose required to achieve analgesia in an individual patient is *whatever dose is necessary. No evidence suggests that a maximal dose of narcotic analgesic exists.* Physiologic tolerance is an expected outcome of chronic opiate use and should be anticipated. Patients may require hundreds, even thousands, of milligrams of morphine per day, yet remain awake, even ambulatory. Respiratory depression and somnolence are rarely significant problems because of the rapid development of tolerance in the vast majority of patients. However, even if respiratory depression does occur, it may be viewed as a secondary effect and should not lead to hesitation on the part of the provider to use whatever dose is needed to control terminal pain or discomfort. Naloxone should be avoided in patients on chronic narcotics, because it precipitates immediate narcotic withdrawal symptoms and causes extreme pain and suffering.

12. What special problems relate to treatment of cancer pain in infants and children?

One needs a high index of suspicion for pain when dealing with children, along with observational techniques and parental reporting for infants and facial scales or other visual aids in young children. Children express chronic pain through rapid (within days) behavioral changes, such as apathy, depression, and withdrawal, rather than by overt crying. Initial doses of opioids need to be adjusted downward for infants under 6 months of age but are otherwise used in doses proportional to weight. Infants and children develop narcotic tolerance the same as adults and may require high doses for pain control.

13. How are pharmacologic adjuncts to analgesics used to improve pain control in patients with malignancy?

1. Nonsteroidal anti-inflammatory agents may be used at standard doses as part of the treatment of bone pain due to malignancy.

2. Nortriptyline, desipramine, amitriptyline, imipramine, and doxepin at one-tenth to one-half the doses used for antidepressant effects may be prescribed for neuropathic pain, sleep, and depression associated with a diagnosis of cancer.

3. Lancinating pains and neuropathic pain may be treated with carbamazepine at 100–200 mg orally 2 or 3 times daily. Other anticonvulsants also have been used successfully.

4. Corticosteroids have been used at high doses (e.g., dexamethasone, 8–40 mg/day) for control of brain edema and resultant headaches, or for nerve root or spinal cord compression symptoms. At low doses (e.g., dexamethasone, 0.75 mg/day, or prednisone, 10–20 mg/day) corticosteroids are sometimes helpful in treating pain from diffuse bone metastases or visceral pain from deep-seated intraabdominal tumors.

5. Antihistamines, cannabinoids, and amphetamines have been reported anecdotally to help alleviate pain.

6. Topical drugs, such as local anesthetics applied to ulcers or capsaiacin cream to painful or dysesthetic intact skin, may be helpful.

14. Should any drugs be avoided in the management of cancer pain?

Mixed narcotic agonist/antagonist drugs, such as pentazocine (Talwin), should be avoided. Meperidine given orally has poor bioavailability. Parenteral meperidine is somewhat useful for acute pain, but the duration of action is too short for chronic pain; long-acting metabolites may cause confusion and, on rare occasions, precipitate seizures. Methadone, although much cheaper than morphine, has long-acting metabolites that accumulate and cause sedation, even after the analgesic effect has worn off; thus it is much less useful for chronic pain management. Benzodiazepines as an adjunct to cancer pain may paradoxically sedate the patient enough to prevent the expression of pain but do little to abate the sensations. Heroin has no role in the management of cancer pain. Heroin is hydrolized to morphine in the body, and its analgesic effects are identical; however, the metabolites of heroin have neurostimulatory effects that may lead to its extreme abuse.

15. What nonpharmacologic adjuncts are useful in the management of cancer pain?

Unquestionably, the emotional state of a patient with cancer vastly affects perception of pain. Anxiety about approaching death, uncertainty, anger, loss of control, and fear of abandonment exacerbate perception of pain. Recognition of fears and sometimes simply naming them may dissipate anxiety. Treatment of overt depression by pharmacologic means should be considered.

Relaxation and self-hypnosis techniques can be taught to patients. Distraction plays an important role in lessening perception of pain. Humor, music, pets, travel, fulfilling long-desired wishes—even a return to work or a long-neglected hobby—may help individual patients to be less aware of pain. Sometimes merely suggesting such an alternative allows patients to find their own options. Spiritual support provides others with a powerful alleviating factor.

Acupuncture, chiropractic treatments, and therapeutic massage may be beneficial to individual patients. The practitioner of such treatments must be given sufficient information about the patient's malignancy so that injury is avoided.

16. How should the cancer patient with back pain be assessed?

Rapidly. A frequent complication of cancer is spinal cord or cauda equina compression from metastases. Such compression is a medical emergency, because any delay in diagnosis and therapy may result in permanent loss of neurologic function. The patient's neurologic function at the time of discovery of spinal cord compression is the most important factor in predicting outcome. Patients who develop neurologic compromise without appropriate evaluation after initial reports of back pain or, worse yet, progress neurologically under direct observation of health care workers are grossly mismanaged. It is extremely important to make every effort to diagnose and treat spinal cord compression before abnormal neurologic findings appear.

In 90% of patients with spinal cord or cauda equina compression, pain in the back is the primary symptom. The pain may be exacerbated by movement, coughing, straining, or lying down. The pain also may have a radicular component, sometimes only with the exacerbating maneuver. Radicular pain allows fairly precise localization of the lesion. Pain usually proceeds neurologic symptoms by weeks to months. Weakness and sensory loss are next, followed rapidly first by urinary retention and constipation, then by paraplegia and loss of bowel and bladder continence. Once neurologic symptoms begin, progression to complete and permanent paraplegia may take only a few hours.

17. Which malignancies most commonly metastasize to the spine?

The malignancies that most commonly metastasize to the spine are cancers of the lung, breast, and prostate, myeloma, lymphoma, and renal-cell carcinoma. Most often, spinal cord compression occurs in a patient with a known cancer; but it is not uncommonly the presenting symptom of malignancy. The location of cord compression is most often the thoracic spine (70%), followed by the lumbar (20%), and cervical (10%) spines. More than one area of spine may be involved, and several locations may threaten the cord. Compression most often results from a mass that begins in the vertebral body or neural arch and extends into the spinal canal, compressing the epidural space. More rarely a tumor may form in the epidural or intradural spaces without bone involvement.

18. What should you do if a patient with cancer develops signs of cord compression?

Any patient with cancer and signs of cord compression requires immediate treatment, followed by imaging of the suspected area of involved spine and spinal cord. Intravenous dexamethasone should be given (10–20 mg) with a 4-mg dose repeated every 4–6 hours while immediate neurologic, neurosurgical, and oncologic consultations are arranged and before imaging studies are done.

19. What should be considered in a patient with cancer and change in mental status?

The patient with cancer who presents with a mental status change, either directly or by corroborative history from the caregiver, should undergo a careful neurologic examination. In the presence of focal abnormalities or complaints of headache, a structural cause should be assumed; however, many patients with stuctural central nervous system lesions have no focal findings on exam. Evaluation consists of metabolic screening laboratory tests, review of drug therapy, and an imaging study of central nervous system (lumbar puncture, if indicated).

Causes of Changes of Mental Status in Patients with Cancer

Structural	Metastasis, carcinomatosis hemorrhage, or stroke
Infectious	Meningitis
Metabolic	Hypercalcemia, hyponatremia, hyperglycemia, or hypoglycemia
Drugs	Sedatives, antiemetics, anxiolytics, antineoplastics: ifosfamide, high-dose cytosine arabinoside, 5 fluorouracil (rare), interferons, and interleukin-2
Miscellaneous	Pain, constipation, depression, psychosis

20. What is the most common metabolic paraneoplastic syndrome? How is it treated?

Hypercalcemia is the most frequent metabolic abnormality due to paraneoplastic syndrome. It is commonly associated with lung tumors, breast cancer, multiple myeloma, and renal-cell cancer. It may be due to production by the tumor of a parathyroid hormone-like molecule, to direct lysis of bone by metastases, or to both. Symptoms of a high level of serum calcium include confusion, nausea, constipation, polydipsia, and polyuria.

Urgent treatment is required for calcium > 12 mg/dl or if the patient is symptomatic. Normal saline and diuresis should be used when calcium is extremely high (e.g., > 14 mg/dl), followed by the institution of the appropriate drug treatment. Pamidronate is the treatment of choice for most patients and may be safely given on an outpatient basis over 3–5 hours at a dose of 60–90 mg by vein. Its effects begin within 24–48 hours and last 3–6 weeks. Other less successful or more toxic options include gallium nitrate, plicamycin, calcitonin, or oral diphosphonates. Corticosteroids work only in hypercalcemia due to hematologic malignancy—and then often only transiently. Nonsteroidal anti-inflammatory agents are ineffective except in a few very mild cases.

21. What are the common causes of dyspnea in a patient with cancer?

Patients with cancer are at risk for **pulmonary embolus**. A hypercoagulable state accompanies adenocarcinomas, particularly carcinoma of the prostate, pancreas, and breast. Patients with breast cancer who undergo chemotherapy are at especially high risk for thromboembolic events. Other patients at extremely high risk are adults with primary brain tumors, probably because of an association with hemiparesis, but even in the absence of paralysis, pulmonary emboli are seen with high frequency in patients with glioma.

The **superior vena cava (SVC) syndrome** usually presents with dyspnea as well as facial and arm swelling, conjunctival edema, venous engorgement on the chest wall or in the neck, and, on rare occasions, somnolence. The SVC may be blocked by extrinsic pressure, intravascular invasion, or thrombosis from an indwelling catheter, usually in association with lung carcinoma, mediastinal lymphomas, germ-cell cancer, and occasionally breast cancer. SVC syndrome is a diagnosis easily made by physical examination and chest radiograph; invasive studies are rarely necessary, and it is rarely a true emergency. Maintaining the patient in an upright posture is the most important initial step in management; some patients temporarily feel better with corticosteroids or mild diuresis. Depending on the underlying tumor type, treatment may be radiation or chemotherapy; anticoagulation is recommended only in catheter-induced thrombosis.

Pleural and pericardial effusions caused by malignant studding of the serosal surface or by mediastinal lymphatic obstruction are also common causes of dyspnea. Lung, breast, and ovarian cancers are common causes of effusions, but lymphomas, leukemias, and many other tumors may involve the pleura or pericardium. A pleural effusion large enough to cause dyspnea is usually quite apparent on exam and chest radiograph. A pericardial effusion requires a higher index of suspicion. Patients with dyspnea and tachycardia with no other explanation should be carefully evaluated for both pericardial effusion and the equally insidious pulmonary embolus.

22. How may the patient with cancer be potentially immunocompromised?

1. Altered cellular immunity may develop, as in patients receiving corticosteroids and patients with lymphoid malignancies.

2. Cancer patients may be anatomically or functionally asplenic and thus at risk of early death from bacterial infections.

3. Many hematologic cancers cause decreased or absent production of normal immunoglobulins.

4. Insufficient numbers of granulocytes may result from treatment or from the disease process.

5. Macroscopic host defenses may be impaired as a result of breaks in the skin or mucous membranes, visceral or bronchial obstruction, or indwelling catheters.

23. What information is necessary to evaluate the urgency of fever in the patient with cancer?

Several important questions should be asked about every febrile cancer patient:

1. What is the patient's leukocyte and granulocyte count?

2. What is the relationship of the fever to the patient's last session of chemotherapy and most recent blood product transfusion?

3. Is the patient receiving antibiotics? What type? For how long?

4. What is the fever pattern? Is this the first fever, or has the patient been febrile for some time?

The patient who is granulocytopenic may not have sufficient white blood cells to produce pus and therefore may have no localizing findings at all. Similarly, patients receiving corticosteroids may not show fever or other symptoms, even in the presence of active infection.

24. When are empirical antibiotics used in patients with cancer? What is the rationale for their use?

The febrile granulocytopenic patient, who is both at greatest risk for and least likely to present with obvious evidence of serious infections, requires immediate empirical coverage. Granulocytopenia is defined as less than 500 granulocytes per cubic microliter of blood. The absolute granulocyte count (AGC) is calculated by multiplying the total leukocyte count by the added percentage of neutrophils plus bands; it is also often referred to as the absolute neutrophil count (ANC). Granulocytopenic patients are at particular risk for spontaneous bacteremia, especially from gram-negative organisms. Because of observations in patients and animal studies of granulocytopenia and infection, empirical antibiotics are now considered standard treatment for the febrile granulocytopenic patient.

25. Which empirical antibiotics are appropriate?

Antibiotic combinations designed to provide the broadest spectrum of bacterial coverage for staphylococci and gram-negative organisms (including *Pseudomonas* sp.) are appropriate if the patient has no localizing symptoms or signs. Additional coverage should be considered in unique clinical situations. Acceptable combinations include:

1. Aminoglycoside plus antipseudomonal penicillin (APsP) or APsP plus clavulanic acid or

2. Antipseudomonal cephalosporin with or without aminoglycoside.

Other broad-spectrum antibiotics that may prove useful include the quinolones, the new erythromycin derivatives, and the carbopenems and monobactams. The first two are good choices in persons with both penicillin and cephalosporin allergies.

26. What is the practical approach to the outpatient who is undergoing treatment for cancer and whose white blood cell counts are dropping?

The vast majority of cancer therapy is safely given in an outpatient setting. One result is that many patients experience iatrogenic myelosuppression at home. Most chemotherapy regimens have a predictable peak time of cell death, which usually starts 7–10 days after drug administration and lasts for a few days. If a patient develops absolute granulocytopenia (< 500) but feels well and remains afebrile, no intervention is needed. Patients should be instructed to check their temperature twice a day and to report fevers or symptoms of infection. The counts should be repeated daily or every other day until the AGC rises above 1000. Patients with moderate fever and moderately low granulocyte counts (i.e., 500–1000) or patients who are "on the rise" probably can be safely placed on a broad-spectrum oral antibiotic but should be checked frequently.

27. When should patients with cancer be transfused?

Anemia caused by chemotherapy is likely to be slow in onset and slow to reverse. Packed red blood cell transfusions should be cautiously considered. There is no absolute hemoglobin level at which all patients require blood transfusions. A young person may tolerate a hemoglobin of 7 gm/dl or lower with only mild fatigue, whereas a patient with angina or congestive heart failure may require a hemoglobin of 9 or 10 gm/dl to avoid severe symptoms. Erythropoietin injections, now approved for cancer-related anemia, improve the hematocrit, but their expense and slow onset of action must be balanced against the benefits of decreasing transfusions.

Thrombocytopenia caused by chemotherapy in an outpatient is rarely severe enough to require transfusions. For several decades the standard cut-off that indicated a need for prophylactic platelet transfusions to prevent spontaneous bleeding has been 20,000 platelets/μ^3. Recently this time-honored criterion has been seriously questioned. It may be safe and reasonable to wait until the level is 10,000 or less. This controversy awaits further study.

28. What is the role of nutritional support in the management of patients with cancer?

For the most part studies of nutritional support in patients with cancer do not show any benefit. Both total parenteral nutrition (TPN) and oral or enteral concentrated feedings fail to achieve increases in lean body mass. Indeed, in two randomized trials of TPN vs. supportive care, patients with metastatic cancer who were treated with nutritional supplementation actually had a shortened survival. When a specific mechanical problem prevents normal eating or when severe treatment-associated mucositis prevents eating because of pain, TPN may be of value for a limited time. Under such circumstances the goal is specific: temporary support until relief of mechanical obstruction by surgery or healing of mucosa and return to a normal diet.

Food and water have great symbolic significance to patients and especially to family members, representing a life-prolonging basic function. It is a source of tremendous emotional distress for family members to be asked to sit by and watch their loved one apparently starve. In a survey of hospice workers, however, death associated with malnutrition and dehydration was observed to be peaceful and not accompanied by pain. Denial on the part of family members also may influence their inability to accept the patient's lack of nutritional support. A commonly expressed concern is that "if only he could gain some weight, he'd be strong enough to fight the cancer." Yet for the patient with profound anorexia due to advanced cancer, being forced to eat is often burdensome and intrusive. This common end-of-life symptom may be an adaptive mechanism. Education of patients and family members as well as health care workers is crucial. Families must be helped to understand the lack of benefit and the potential harm of forced nutrition in a terminally ill patient. No effective appetite stimulant has yet been identified for cancer-associated anorexia.

29. What is hospice care?
Hospice care is intended simply to control symptoms of terminal conditions, to alleviate pain, and to allow a peaceful death. The first hospice was opened in 1967 by Dr. Cicely Saunders in London. A hospice may be in the home or in a specially designed facility. After death, bereavement counseling is an important part of a hospice program.

30. How should the primary care physician follow a patient with cancer after treatment is successfully completed?
The intention of follow-up after antineoplastic treatment is to detect problems that can be treated successfully, whether complications or recurrences of cancer. Only a handful of cancers can be cured or adequately treated after a relapse: testicular cancer, Hodgkin's disease, certain lymphomas, some leukemias, and occasionally breast cancer recurrence. Such patients should be aggressively followed, according to instructions from the treating oncologist. No other cancers in adults can be successfully eradicated a second time, except in rare circumstances. Thus there is no real justification for routine radiographic and laboratory screening in posttreatment phase; yet this is precisely what many patients have undergone and have been "taught" to expect. Certainly screening with costly imaging studies such as computerized scans or nuclear medicine scans has been shown to have virtually no impact on patient survival or even on palliation; indeed, the anxiety surrounding the testing may be antipalliative. Great controversy exists over the value of routine serum tumor markers (except in testicular cancer) during follow-up.

31. What are the major types of problems to expect in long-term survivors of successful cancer treatment?
1. **Social adjustments** are frequent in survivors of cancer. Many report problems with obtaining employment and with eligibility for health or life insurance. Many patients experience long-term anxiety about the possibility of relapse, especially at the time of visits to the doctor.

2. **Persistent physical problems** include sexual dysfunction manifesting as ejaculatory disturbances in men and vaginal dryness that leads to dyspareunia in women; infertility in both men and women; sensory peripheral neuropathies; xerostomia; skin dryness or thinning in irradiated areas; fibrosis or inflammation in irradiated areas or surgical scars; growth retardation and learning problems in children; cataracts in recipients of head or whole-body radiation; cardiomyopathy in persons treated with cardiotoxic drugs or chest radiation; accelerated atherosclerosis in radiation fields; and hypertension, Raynaud's phenomenon, and hypercholesterolemia in survivors of testicular cancer.

3. **Higher risk for the development of another cancer** or for second malignancies that are treatment-induced. Early after chemotherapy (< 5 years) for various cancers (best described after Hodgkin's disease), about 5% of patients develop chemotherapy-induced acute myelogenous leukemia or a myelodysplastic disorder.

BIBLIOGRAPHY

1. Bilezikian JP: Management of acute hypercalcemia. N Engl J Med 326:1196–1203, 1992.
2. Blatt J, Olshan A, Gula MJ, et al: Second malignancies in very-long-term survivors of childhood cancer. Am J Med 93:57–60, 1992.
3. Boring CC, Squires TS, Tong T: Cancer statistics, 1993. Cancer 43:7–26, 1993.
4. Byrne TN: Spinal cord compression from epidural metastases. N Engl J Med 327:614–619, 1992.

5. Foley KM: The treatment of pain in cancer. N Engl J Med 313:84–95, 1985.
6. Hainsworth JD, Greco FA: The treatment of patients with cancer of an unknown primary site. N Engl J Med 329:257–263, 1993.
7. Kanner R: Recent advances in cancer pain management. Cancer Invest 11:80–87, 1993.
8. Loescher JL, Welch-McCaffrey D, Leigh SA, et al: Surviving adult cancers. I. Physiologic effects. Ann Intern Med 111:411–432, 1989.
9. Miller RJ, Albright PG: What is the role of nutritional support and hydration in terminal cancer patients? Am J Hospice Care Nov/Dec:33–38, 1989.
10. Pizzo PA: Management of fever in patients with cancer and treatment-induced neutropenia. N Engl J Med 328:1323–1332, 1993.
11. Raghavan D, Cox K, Childs A, et al: Hypercholesterolemia after chemotherapy for testis cancer. J Clin Oncol 10:1386–1389, 1992.
12. Rhymes JA: Clinical management of the terminally ill. Geriatrics 46(2):57–67, 1991.
13. Welch-McCaffrey D, Hoffman B, Leigh SA, et al: Surviving adult cancers: Psychological and social effects. Ann Intern Med 111:517–524, 1989.
14. Yellen SB, Cella DF, Bonomi A: Quality of life in people with Hodgkin's disease. Oncology 7(8):41–45, 1993.

105. THE PREOPERATIVE PATIENT

Jeffrey Pickard, M.D.

1. What test(s) must be done before surgery?

The simple answer is that no test is considered essential for preoperative evaluation. In general, tests should be based on the type of surgery (e.g., urinalysis before urologic surgery) and the patient's current and past medical history (e.g., chest radiograph for patients with chronic obstructive pulmonary disease [COPD]). Practically speaking, however, certain tests are ordered almost routinely, because they can be obtained relatively easily and cheaply (e.g., complete blood count, urinalysis, electrocardiogram [EKG], and chest radiograph in the elderly).

2. How does age affect the outcome of surgery?

The answer is somewhat controversial. Some studies consider age over 70 years to be an independent risk factor. Recent studies, however, have challenged this notion, suggesting that the patient's underlying physiology is much more important than age alone. Age may be a risk factor only in that the elderly are more likely to have underlying disease.

3. What type of anesthesia is the safest?

There is a fairly common misconception that spinal anesthesia is safer and better tolerated than general anesthesia. However, both confer equal risks of postoperative fatal and nonfatal myocardial infarctions. Regional or local anesthesia may be less risky than general or spinal anesthesia. The type of anesthesia should be determined by the anesthesiologist.

4. Which types of surgery are inherently riskier than others?

As indicated above, vascular surgery appears to carry the greatest risk, both because the procedures are physiologically stressful and because patients who require such procedures have a high incidence of coronary artery disease. Intrathoracic, intraperitoneal, and emergency procedures are also high risk.

5. What is meant by a patient's preoperative cardiac risk index?

The preoperative cardiac risk index refers to a quantitative assessment of a patient's risk of adverse cardiac outcome intra- or postoperatively; it is based on various preoperative clinical, historical, and laboratory variables. The first, and probably most widely used, of these indices was published by Goldman et al. in 1977.

Computation of the Cardiac Risk Index

CRITERIA*	MULTIVARIATE DISCRIMINANT-FUNCTION COEFFICIENT	"POINTS"
1. History		
Age > 70 yr	0.191	5
MI in previous 6 mo	0.384	10
2. Physical examination		
S_3 gallop or JVD	0.451	11
Important VAS	0.119	3
3. Electrocardiogram		
Rhythm other than sinus or PACs on last preoperative EKG	0.283	7
> 5 PVCs/min documented at any time before operation	0.278	7
4. General status		
Po_2 < 60 or Pco_2 > 50 mmHg K < 3.0 or HCO_3 < mEq/liter BUN > 50 or Cr > 3.0 mg/dl, abnormal SGOT, signs of chronic liver disease or patient bedridden from noncardiac causes	0.132	3
5. Operation		
Intraperitoneal, intrathoracic or aortic operation	0.123	3
Emergency operation	0.167	4
Total possible		53 points

* MI denotes myocardial infarction, JVD = jugular-vein distention, VAS = valvular aortic stenosis, PACs = premature atrial contractions, EKG = electrocardiogram, PVC's = premature ventricular contractions, Po_2 = partial pressure of oxygen, Pco_2 = partial pressure of carbon dioxide, K = potassium, HCO_3 = bicarbonate, BUN = blood urea nitrogen, Cr = creatinine, and SGOT = serum glutamic oxaloacetic transaminase.

Cardiac Risk Index

CLASS	POINT TOTAL	NO OR ONLY MINOR COM-PLICATION (N = 943)	LIFE-THREATENING COMPLICATION* (N = 39)	CARDIAC DEATHS (N = 19)
I (N = 537)	0–5	532 (99)[†]	4 (0.7)	1 (0.2)
II (N = 316)	6–12	295 (93)	16 (5)	5 (2)
III (N = 130)	13–25	112 (86)	15 (11)	3 (2)
IV (N = 18)	> 26	4 (22)	4 (22)	10 (56)

* Documented intraoperative or postoperative myocardial infarction, pulmonary edema, or ventricular tachycardia without progression to cardiac death.
[†] Figures in parentheses denote percent.
From Goldman L, Caldera DL, Nussbaum SR, et al: Multifactorial index of cardiac risk in noncardiac surgical procedures. N Engl J Med 297:845–850, 1977, with permission.

6. How accurate are indices in assessing preoperative cardiac risk?

In general, preoperative cardiac risk indices appear to have a fairly high positive predictive value, but their negative predictive value may be less helpful, especially in patients who are undergoing vascular surgery. Patients who appear to be at high risk for perioperative complications on the basis of risk scores have a higher percentage of adverse outcomes than patients with low risk scores. However, patients with low scores may still be at substantial risk and may benefit from further study.

7. How does a history of a myocardial infarction affect a patient's perioperative risk?

Most investigators and clinicians believe that within the first 3–6 months after myocardial infarction, perioperative cardiac morbidity and mortality is significantly increased. Therefore, nonemergent surgery should be delayed, if possible, until after this time period. After 6 months, perioperative risk remains relatively stable, assuming the absence of sequelae (e.g., congestive heart failure, rhythm disturbances). Some authors believe that the level of risk returns to preinfarct levels ($< 1\%$ in the general population), whereas others believe that the risk remains somewhat elevated (2–8%).

8. Which patients should be evaluated for coronary artery disease (CAD) before surgery?

Patients who undergo high-risk procedures such as those listed above (especially vascular procedures that require cross-clamping of the aorta) may require additional evaluation for CAD, such as an exercise treadmill test (ETT). Patients with unstable angina, new EKG changes (especially ischemic), or high cardiac risk indices also should be considered for further cardiac evaluation. Patients who are unable to exercise (e.g., patients with peripheral vascular disease) or who have baseline EKG abnormalities may require a dipyridamole-thallium scan to detect ischemia.

Patients with evidence of ischemic disease on noninvasive testing may require coronary angiography with an eye toward coronary artery bypass grafting (CABG) before high-risk surgery. CABG, of course, carries its own operative risks, but patients who have had successful CABG reduce their perioperative cardiac risk to approximately that of the normal population.

9. How does the presence of hypertension affect perioperative risk?

Hypertension as an independent risk factor is notably absent from both Goldman's and Detsky's scoring systems. Mild-to-moderate hypertension appears to be generally well-tolerated during and after surgery. However, patients with diastolic blood pressure > 110 mmHg or systolic blood pressure > 170 mmHg are at increased risk of perioperative morbidity and should have their blood pressure controlled before going to surgery, if possible.

10. How should antihypertension medications be adjusted in patients who are undergoing elective surgery?

Assuming adequate control of blood pressure, most antihypertensive medications should be continued until surgery and restarted postoperatively when the patient resumes oral intake. Guanethidine and monoamine oxidase (MAO) inhibitors are rarely used and probably should be avoided perioperatively. Earlier case reports suggested that abrupt withdrawal of both clonidine and beta blockers was associated with rebound hypertension and ischemia and recommended that both agents should be tapered before surgery. According to current recommendations, however, these medications are continued during the perioperative period. If necessary, transdermal clonidine and intravenous beta blockers may be used while oral intake is prohibited.

11. Describe the perioperative management of patients on medication for diabetes.

Ideally, patients should be euglycemic perioperatively, but this goal is often not practical, because the risks of hypoglycemia may be substantial. Therefore, patients generally are allowed to be somewhat hyperglycemic. Patients on insulin should be given approximately one-half of the usual morning dose of neutral protamine Hagedorn (NPH), or Lente, insulin on the morning of surgery and should be maintained on a continuous infusion of dextrose until oral intake is resumed. Fingerstick glucoses should be obtained at regular intervals during prolonged procedures. Levels of blood sugar should be checked, either by fingerstick or phlebotomy, every 4–6 hours postoperatively until the patient is able to resume normal oral intake. Small doses of subcutaneous regular insulin may be used to maintain blood glucoses ≤ 250 mg/dl, if possible. Patients with type I diabetes or patients who are difficult to control may require insulin drips. Patients on oral hypoglycemic agents usually do not require significant adjustment of medications. Some authors recommend discontinuing chlorpropamide

2–3 days before surgery because of its prolonged half-life and risk of hypoglycemia. However, this is an issue only in the rare patient with type II diabetes who is euglycemic on oral medications.

12. What is the value of preoperative pulmonary function tests (PFTs)?
In patients with no history of pulmonary problems, PFTs are of little or no value and should not be routinely ordered. Although some authors believe that severely obese patients are at risk for postoperative pulmonary complications, few data support the use of PFTs as part of the preoperative evaluation. Patients with a history of lung disease (COPD, asthma, smokers with productive cough) or signs and symptoms of pulmonary dysfunction (wheezing, dyspnea) may be at risk for postoperative pulmonary complications. In such patients, PFTs may be helpful in identifying patients with severe disease (FEV ≤ 0.5L; hypercapnia) but otherwise are of little help in quantifying the risk of postoperative pulmonary complications.

13. How should patients with potential pulmonary problems be evaluated before surgery?
As stated above, patients with pulmonary disease are at increased risk for postoperative pulmonary complications, and their respiratory status should be optimized before surgery. Chest radiographs are usually obtained for baseline values but rarely change management. Other risk factors may include length of surgery (> 3.5 hours), surgical factors (intrathoracic surgery and intraabdominal procedures, especially those close to the diaphragm), and smoking (> 20 years or > 1 pack/day actively). There is no difference in risk between general and spinal anesthesia, although procedures done under regional or local anesthesia may have lower risk.

14. How should cigarette smokers be counseled before surgery?
Although only a small percentage of smokers will quit when advised to do so by their physicians, all smokers should be advised to quit before elective surgery. Abstinence for at least 2 months is necessary to decrease postoperative pulmonary complications significantly.

15. What patients should be placed on prophylactic antibiotics perioperatively?
The goal of prophylactic antibiotics is to decrease the potential morbidity of postoperative infections when the procedure is likely to contaminate normally sterile areas or when the potential for infection of a prosthetic device exists (e.g., heart valve, artificial joint, vascular graft).

Most surgical procedures (75%) are **clean** and normally require no antibiotic prophylaxis. Approximately 15% are **clean-contaminated** procedures, in which gastrointestinal, genitourinary, or respiratory mucosa are invaded. Likelihood of infection in such cases is about 10%. The remaining procedures are either **contaminated** (e.g., fresh trauma) or **dirty** (e.g., trauma more than 4 hours old); rates of infection in these cases are 20% and $\geq 40\%$, respectively.

16. What regimens are recommended for perioperative antibiotic prophylaxis?
Although there are about as many antibiotic regimens as there are surgical procedures, general recommendations are provided in the table below.

Recommended Regimens for Perioperative Antibiotic Prophylaxis

PROCEDURE	POSSIBLE INDICATIONS	ANTIBIOTIC REGIMEN
Cardiovascular (e.g., CABG, valve replacement, pacemaker)	Transthoracic wires	Cefazolin, 1 gm IV preoperatively; alternative vancomycin
Upper GI tract	Age, local infection	Cefazolin, 1 gm IV preoperatively; alternative clindamycin, metronidazole
GU tract (e.g., TURP)		Cefazolin, 1 gm, IV preoperatively; alternative clindamycin, ciprofloxacin
GU (e.g., hysterectomy)	Prolonged procedure	Cefazolin, 1 gm, IV preoperatively

Table continued on following page.

Recommended Regimens for Perioperative Antibiotic Prophylaxis (Continued)

PROCEDURE	POSSIBLE INDICATIONS	ANTIBIOTIC REGIMEN
Orthopedics (e.g., joint arthroplasty)		Cefazolin, 1 gm, IV preoperatively with q6h × 24 hours; alternative vancomycin
Peripheral vascular (e.g., AAA repair)		Cefazolin, 1 gm, IV preoperatively and q6h × 24 hours
Thoracic surgery		Same as above

CABG = coronary artery bypass graft, IV = intravenously, GI = gastrointestinal, GU = genitourinary, TURP = transurethral prostatectomy, AAA = abdominal aortic aneurysm.

CONTROVERSY

17. How should patients on chronic anticoagulation be managed perioperatively?
There is no standard regimen to prepare patients on chronic warfarin therapy for surgery. Patients with prothrombin time (PT) < 20 and international normalized ratio (INR) < 2.9 rarely have significant postoperative bleeding problems. However, most patients on warfarin therapy can safely be taken off their medications 3–4 days before surgery and restarted postoperatively when oral intake is resumed. Patients at high risk for thromboembolic disease (e.g., patients with mechanical valves or mitral stenosis or patients who have had recurrent thromboembolisms in the past) may be switched to full-dose heparin (preferably by continuous intravenous infusion) 3–4 days before surgery. The heparin may be stopped approximately 6 hours before the procedure and restarted as soon as adequate postoperative hemostasis has been attained (usually the evening after surgery or 12 hours after the procedure). Patients requiring dental surgery rarely bleed while on warfarin; thus discontinuance is usually unnecessary. Likewise, routine cataract surgery is avascular and does not necessitate reversal of anticoagulation.

BIBLIOGRAPHY

1. Cygan R, Waitzin H: Stopping and restarting medications in the perioperative period. J Gen Intern Med 2:270–283, 1987.
2. Freeman WK, Gibbons RJ, Shub C: Preoperative assessment of cardiac patients undergoing noncardiac surgical procedures. Mayo Clin Proc 64:1105–1117, 1989.
3. Jackson CV: Preoperative pulmonary evaluation. Arch Intern Med 148:2120–2172, 1988.
4. Kroenke K: Preoperative evaluation: The assessment and management of surgical risk. J Gen Intern Med 2:257–269, 1987.
5. Lawrence VA, Page CP, Harris GD: Preoperative spirometry before abdominal operations: A critical appraisal of its predictive value. Arch Intern Med 149:280–285, 1989.
6. Mohr DH, Jett JR: Preoperative evaluation of pulmonary risk factors. J Gen Intern Med 3:277–287, 1988.
7. Nicholas GC: Evaluation of surgical patients with peripheral vascular disease. Surg Clin North Am 63:993–1002, 1983.
8. Schade DS: Surgery and diabetes. Med Clin North Am 72:1531–1543, 1988.
9. Walts LF, Miller J, Davidson MB, Brown J: Perioperatve management of diabetes mellitus. Anesthesiology 55:104–109, 1981.

106. THE PREGNANT PATIENT

Jeffrey Pickard, M.D.

1. At 37 weeks' gestation, a 20-year-old primigravida who has received optimal prenatal care is noted to have proteinuria, edema of both upper and lower extremities, and a 5-pound weight gain over the preceding week. Her blood pressure, which has been normal for pregnancy, now measures 136/92. What is the diagnosis?

The triad of hypertension, edema, and proteinuria occurring late in pregnancy is a classic presentation of preeclampsia. Preeclampsia occurs 6–8 times more commonly in primigravidas than in multigravidas. It is almost never seen before 20 weeks' gestation (except with trophoblastic diseases) and usually occurs near term.

2. How is preeclampsia managed?

The only definitive treatment of preeclampsia is delivery. Hypertension is only a sign of preeclampsia, and treatment of the blood pressure does little to alter the course of the disease. Diuresis for edema likewise does not alter the underlying pathophysiology and in fact may be counterproductive and adversely affect fetal outcome, because intravascular volume is already depleted in women with preeclampsia.

The triad of proteinuria, edema, and hypertension is not specific for preeclampsia. Edema may be seen during normal pregnancy, as may low levels of proteinuria. Hypertension late in pregnancy may be previously unrecognized chronic hypertension, or it may be transient hypertension of pregnancy. If the fetus is not yet mature, it may be appropriate to monitor the pregnancy closely in hope of delaying delivery.

3. What laboratory evaluations should be done in a woman who presents with hypertension during the second half of pregnancy?

A complete blood count should be obtained. Hemoglobin and hematocrit may be elevated, because hemoconcentration may occur in preeclampsia. Thrombocytopenia and evidence of hemolysis on the smear may suggest severe preeclampsia. Liver function tests (transaminase, lactate dehydrogenase, uric acid, and creatinine also may be elevated in cases of severe preeclampsia.

4. Describe the evaluation of a woman who presents with hypertension before week 20 of gestation.

In addition to obtaining the laboratory data mentioned above, a careful history should be obtained with emphasis on duration of elevated blood pressure, blood pressure in previous pregnancies, previous diagnostic evaluation, and symptoms associated with secondary causes of hypertension. Pregnant women, especially young pregnant women, with chronic hypertension or hypertension during the first half of pregnancy are more likely than other patients to have secondary causes of hypertension. Pheochromocytoma, although rare, is associated with high maternal mortality, and appropriate screening should be done with even minimal suspicion.

5. What is HELLP?

H = Hemolysis
E = Elevated
L = Liver enzymes, and
L = Low
P = Platelets

This syndrome, associated with severe preeclampsia, is rapidly progressive and life-threatening to both mother and baby. Regardless of the stage in pregnancy at which it occurs, the HELLP syndrome is an emergency and requires immediate termination of pregnancy.

6. How does the nonpharmacologic management of hypertension differ in pregnant and nonpregnant patients?

As in nonpregnant patients, mild-to-moderate hypertension should be treated with nonpharmacologic modalities first, especially when the diastolic blood pressure is between 90 and 99 mmHg. However, nonpharmacologic strategies for blood pressure control during pregnancy differ from those used in nonpregnancy.

Weight reduction is frequently recommended for blood pressure control in nonpregnant patients but should not be recommended during pregnancy. Salt (sodium) restriction should not be recommended during pregnancy unless the patient has been on a sodium-restricted diet before becoming pregnant. Volume status may be important for maintaining uteroplacental perfusion in the pregnant hypertensive patient, whose intravascular volume is usually lower than that in normotensive patients.

Because of its unknown effect on uteroplacental blood flow, exercise should be discouraged in pregnant women with hypertension. Whereas its effectiveness has not been well-studied in chronic hypertension, bed rest during pregnancy enhances uteroplacental blood flow, reduces premature labor, lowers blood pressure, and promotes diuresis in women with hypertension.

7. How should drugs be used to treat hypertension during pregnancy?

The goal of treating hypertension during pregnancy is to minimize short-term risks of elevated blood pressure to the mother without compromising fetal well-being. Pharmacologic therapy may be necessary if nonpharmacologic maneuvers are unsuccessful in lowering blood pressure or if diastolic blood pressure exceeds 99 mmHg.

First-line therapy for hypertensive pregnant women not already on medication is methyldopa, the only drug that is both efficacious for lowering maternal blood pressure and unquestionably safe for the fetus. Second-line therapy is usually hydralazine, because, other than methyldopa, it is the drug with most frequent use during pregnancy and generally is considered safe for the fetus. However, it is not highly effective as a single agent because of the reflex tachycardia and increased cardiac output that it causes. Other agents used to treat hypertension during pregnancy are beta blockers, labetolol, and nifedipine. Because of their theoretical effect on uteroplacental perfusion, thiazides are usually not begun during pregnancy but may be continued when already in use by a hypertensive woman who becomes pregnant. Angiotensin-converting enzyme inhibitors are relatively contraindicated during pregnancy because of their association with high rates of fetal loss in animals and because of several case reports of anoxic renal failure, sometimes fatal, in neonates exposed in utero.

Antihypertensive Medications in Pregnancy

MEDICATION	DAILY DOSE	COMMENTS
Methyldopa	500 mg–2 gm	Drug of choice during pregnancy
Hydralazine	40–200 mg	Second-line therapy; associated with reflex tachycardia
Hydrochlorothiazide	25–50 mg	Potentially decreases uteroplacental perfusion, may be continued during pregnancy if patient already taking it
Beta blockers (e.g., propranolol)	40–240 mg	Case reports of neonatal hypoglycemia, bradycardia, ? mild intrauterine growth retardation
Calcium channel blockers (e.g., nifedipine)	30–120 mg	Limited data in humans
Labetalol	200–1000 mg	Probably safe; limited data in humans
Angiotensin-converting enzyme inhibitors	—	Contraindicated; teratogenic in animals; anoxic renal failure in human neonates

8. What is the long-term prognosis of women who have hypertension during pregnancy?

Women with transient hypertension during one pregnancy have recurrent hypertension in up to 90% of subsequent pregnancies as well as a high likelihood of developing chronic hypertension in the future. In contrast, women who do not have hypertension during pregnancy, especially after age 25 years, have a low likelihood of developing chronic hypertension.

Women who develop preeclampsia–eclampsia during their first pregnancy have about a 10% chance of having preeclampsia in subsequent pregnancies. Their risk of developing chronic hypertension is no different from that of the general population. Women with chronic hypertension have an increased risk of developing preeclampsia when they become pregnant.

9. Describe normal maternal carbohydrate metabolism during pregnancy.

Early in pregnancy, usually at about 10 weeks' gestation, fasting glucose levels fall to as low as 60 mg/dl and either remain at this level or continue to decrease slightly throughout gestation. This early drop in maternal glucose levels occurs before the conceptus is large enough to have an effect and probably is due to an enhancement (increased sensitivity) of insulin-mediated glucose assimilation related primarily to the large rise in placental hormones (especially estrogen).

Basal insulin levels, normal during the first half of pregnancy, rise sharply (50–100%) during the second half of pregnancy. Throughout most of pregnancy, the stimulation of insulin in response to glucose load increases. Overall, insulin sensitivity in pregnancy is about 20% of that in the nonpregnant state. The mechanism for the decreased tissue responsiveness to insulin is not completely understood but probably relates to hormonal changes of pregnancy, such as elevated levels of prolactin, cortisol, and other counterregulatory hormones. The human placenta produces placental lactogen, an insulin antagonist, in increasingly larger amounts after 20 weeks. In addition to a decrease in insulin-receptor binding, postreceptor response to insulin at the tissue level also may be diminished.

10. How do the metabolic changes in a diabetic pregnancy affect the fetus?

Glucose crosses the placenta by facilitated diffusion so that fetal glucose levels are only slightly lower than the mother's. Maternal insulin does not cross the placenta. Maternal hyperglycemia, therefore, leads to fetal hyperglycemia. The fetal pancreas, which starts producing insulin between weeks 9 and 11, secretes large amounts of insulin to control glucose levels. Studies of fetal and infant pancreases exposed to diabetes in utero have documented beta-cell hypertrophy and hyperplasia. Amino acids are actively transported across the placenta and also stimulate fetal secretion of insulin. These and other substrates are stored in adipose and other insulin-responsive tissues and lead to macrosomia as well as organomegaly of heart, lung, spleen, liver, and adrenal glands. Hyperinsulinemia at birth leads to neonatal hypoglycemia in as many as 75% of infants of diabetic mothers. Other consequences of poor metabolic control include neonatal hypercalcemia, polycythemia, hyperbilirubinemia, and respiratory distress syndrome (RDS).

11. What is the White classification?

This classification schema was devised by Priscilla White to categorize women with pregestational diabetes on the basis of duration of disease, age at onset, mode of therapy, and presence of vascular complications. Current modifications now include gestational diabetes, either as a separate category or as defined by treatment (diet vs. insulin). Classes A–D correlate with slight increases in fetal mortality, whereas classes F and higher are also associated with increased maternal risk.

White Classification

CLASS	AGE AT ONSET*	DURATION*	INSULIN
A₁	Any	Any	–
A₂	Any	Gestational	+
B	≥ 20 years	< 10 years	+
C	10–19 years	10–19 years	+

Table continued on following page.

White Classification (Continued)

CLASS	AGE AT ONSET*	DURATION*	INSULIN
D	< 10 years	≥ 20 years	+
R	Proliferative retinopathy or vitreous hemorrhage		+
F	Nephropathy		+
RF	Retinopathy and nephropathy		+
H	Heart disease, usually coronary artery disease		+
T	Renal transplant recipient		+

* Either age at onset or duration determine class.
[†] Gestational diabetes mellitus (GDM) is often classified separately. In the original White classification, class A was diabetes of any age or duration that did not require insulin.

12. Discuss the other possible adverse outcomes of pregnancy in a woman with diabetes.

The incidence of major congenital anomalies associated with type I diabetes is as high as 10% in some studies, an overall risk of 2–4 times that of control populations. Patients in poor metabolic control and patients with vascular disease are at higher risk. Most likely, metabolic disturbances (hyperglycemia, hypoglycemia) during the period of organogenesis (weeks 3–8) are responsible for the malformations (mostly sacral agenesis and complex cardiac defects). Women who are in good metabolic control at the time of conception and through the first trimester appear to be at much lower risk of having either infants with congenital anomalies or first-trimester spontaneous abortions. Women in class F, R, or RF of the White classification are more likely to have infants with intrauterine growth retardation as well as premature infants.

Maternal morbidity is increased in diabetic pregnant women with retinopathy or nephropathy. Nephropathy (defined by proteinuria) may worsen during pregnancy, but the worsening is rarely permanent. Retinopathy (especially proliferative changes) worsens in a substantial number of women during pregnancy and may not completely regress after delivery.

13. What is gestational diabetes mellitus (GDM)? How is it diagnosed?

GDM is diabetes that is first diagnosed during pregnancy (although it may have existed before pregnancy). Every woman should be screened for GDM, usually between 24 and 28 weeks of gestation, with a randomly administered 50-gram glucose load. Plasma glucose ≥ 140 mg/dl 1 hour after ingestion indicates the need for further diagnostic testing, which consists of administering a 100-gram glucose load to a fasting woman and then measuring hourly glucose levels for 3 hours (see criteria below). If any two values are abnormal or if the fasting glucose is elevated, the patient has GDM and is followed accordingly.

Three-hour Glucose Tolerance Test

TIME	PLASMA GLUCOSE LEVEL (mg/dl)
Fasting	≥ 105
1 hour	≥ 190
2 hours	≥ 165
3 hours	≥ 145

14. What are the criteria for beginning insulin therapy in women with GDM?

Some authors advise starting prophylactic insulin in all women diagnosed with GDM. Most clinicians, however, assess control of diabetes by regularly checking fasting and 2-hour postprandial levels of serum glucose. Adequate control is indicated by a fasting level < 105 and a 2-hour postprandial level < 120. If either value is exceeded twice within 1 week, insulin is usually begun.

15. Describe the changes in respiratory physiology during pregnancy.

Normal pregnancy is a state of mild, compensated respiratory alkalosis. During the first trimester, the pregnant woman hyperventilates by increasing tidal volume by up to 50%. Respiratory rate stays fairly constant. Arterial pH is normal (7.40–7.45) because of renal compensation so that levels of serum bicarbonate fall. Such changes probably occur because of progesterone effects and remain constant throughout pregnancy. Both expiratory reserve volume (ERV) and residual volume (RV), which together make up the functional residual capacity (FRC), fall by a total of 20%, mostly during the third trimester. Vital capacity (VC) is essentially unchanged.

16. How should asthma be managed during pregnancy?

Pregnancy changes the management of asthma very little. Medications used to treat asthma in the nonpregnant patient also may be used during pregnancy. The one possible exception is saturated solution of potassium iodide (SSKI), which occasionally has been used as a mucolytic. The iodine crosses the placenta easily and theoretically may cause fetal thyroid abnormalities.

17. Describe the hemodynamic changes of pregnancy.

By early in the third trimester, cardiac output is increased by up to 50% over prepregnancy levels because of a marked increase in plasma volume (40–50%) and a lesser increase (20–30%) in red cell mass. This increased output causes a physiologic anemia of pregnancy. Despite the marked increase in cardiac output, however, blood pressure falls during pregnancy because of arteriolar vasodilation and a marked decrease in systemic vascular resistance. Pulmonary pressures are largely unchanged. Organs with the largest increase in perfusion are the kidneys, breasts, skin, and uterus.

18. How does pregnancy affect thyroid function?

Despite earlier reports to the contrary, the size of the normal thyroid gland usually does not change significantly during pregnancy when iodine intake is adequate. Because of the effects of estrogen, thyroid-binding globulin level rises 2–3 times above normal, and levels of total thyroxine (T4) and total triiodothyronine (T3) rise concomitantly. Levels of free T4 and free T3 stay within the normal to low-normal range. Levels of thyroid-stimulating hormone (TSH) may fall slightly during early pregnancy because of the weak thyroid-stimulating activity of beta human chorionic gonadotropin (hCG) but return to normal during the second and third trimesters.

19. How should a woman with seizures be treated during pregnancy?

A patient whose seizures are controlled by medication generally should continue medication during pregnancy. Although no antiepileptic agent is safe during pregnancy, uncontrolled seizures are harmful to both the mother and the fetus. If a woman has been seizure-free for 2 years, she may attempt to discontinue medication before becoming pregnant. If withdrawal is successful, she may be followed expectantly during gestation.

If possible, women taking valproic acid should change to another medication before becoming pregnant. Although published data in humans are not completely clear, valproic acid has been implicated in a number of congenital anomalies, but the major concern is neural tube defects. Trimethadione is clearly associated with a constellation of congenital anomalies and should be avoided during pregnancy.

20. How does infection with the human immunodeficiency virus (HIV) affect pregnancy?

Because HIV-infected women are part of a high-risk population (many are poor, urban, intravenous drug abusers), it is hard to ascertain what risks are specifically due to HIV. Although low birth weight, preterm birth, premature rupture of membranes, and intrauterine growth retardation are seen with higher frequency in HIV-infected women than in the normal population, the frequencies are no higher than in a high-risk seronegative control group.

The incidence of perinatal transmission is also unclear. It is probably less than 50% and may be less than 30%. Transmission may occur in one of three ways:

1. In utero transmission has been documented by isolating the virus from electively aborted second-trimester fetuses.

2. Transmission may occur at the time of birth by exposure to maternal blood and body fluids.

3. HIV has been found in breast milk. According to case reports, breastfeeding infants have contracted the disease from mothers who were infected by postpartum blood transfusions.

It is not clear why vertical transmission occurs in some cases but not in others.

Although the risks of zidovudine (AZT) to the fetus are not known, limited studies have shown that it is well-tolerated by pregnant women and has not been associated with congenital malformations or other adverse fetal outcomes. At the present time, AZT is recommended for HIV-infected women whose CD4 counts are < 200. An ongoing multicenter prospective trial sponsored by the AIDS Clinical Trials Group is evaluating the use of AZT during pregnancy. Interim analysis of the data has concluded that AZT also should be offered to all HIV-infected pregnant women with CD4 counts > 200.

21. What is the significance of asymptomatic bacteriuria during pregnancy?

Asymptomatic bacteriuria may occur in up to 5–10% of pregnant women. Unlike their nonpregnant counterparts, up to 40% of these women may develop infections. These infections may have a deleterious effect on pregnancy, especially if pyelonephritis ensues. Therefore, all pregnant women with asymptomatic bacteriuria should be treated with antibiotics. In women with recurrences, daily suppressive doses of antibiotics may be indicated until after delivery.

22. How should a pregnant woman with deep venous thrombosis be treated?

In general, warfarin should be avoided during pregnancy, because it crosses the placenta and has been associated with fetal malformations as well as neurologic dysfunction. In a pregnant woman with a documented blood clot, acute therapy should be given with intravenous heparin followed by intermittent (2 or 3 times/day) subcutaneous heparin for several weeks in doses adequate to keep the midinterval partial thromboplastin time at 1.5–2 times control. Thereafter, she should be maintained on low-dose subcutaneous heparin (5,000–10,000 U twice daily) until delivery. Warfarin is then generally substituted until 4–6 weeks after delivery. A woman taking warfarin may breastfeed her baby.

Women who have had thrombosis in a prior pregnancy are generally considered to be at risk if they again become pregnant. They are treated with low-dose subcutaneous heparin throughout gestation. Although opinions differ as to the proper dose, heparin levels apparently fall as pregnancy proceeds, if the amount is not increased accordingly. We therefore recommend 5,000 U subcutaneously twice daily in the first trimester; 7,500 U twice daily in the second trimester; and 10,000 U twice daily in the third trimester. Because the risk of thromboembolic events may persist in the early postpartum period, warfarin is used as above.

Low-molecular-weight heparin may have some advantages during pregnancy because of its longer half-life, which may allow once daily dosing with fewer bleeding complications. Low-molecular-weight heparin does not cross the placenta and has been used safely during a few pregnancies, although data are limited.

BIBLIOGRAPHY

1. Bares VA: Diabetes and pregnancy. Med Clin North Am 73:685–700, 1989.
2. Gianopoulos JG: Cardiac disease in pregnancy. Med Clin North Am 73:639–651, 1989.
3. Glinoer D, de Nayer P, Bourdoux P, et al: Regulation of maternal thyroid during pregnancy. J Clin Endocrinol Metab 71:276–287, 1990.
4. Greenberger PA, Patterson R: Management of asthma during pregnancy. N Engl J Med 312:897–902, 1985.

5. Jovanonic-Peterson C, Petersen CM: Pregnancy in the diabetic woman: Guidelines for a successful outcome. Endocrinol Metab Clin North Am 21:433–455, 1992.
6. Moreno JD, Minkoff H: Human immunodeficiency virus infection during pregnancy. Clin Obstet Gynecol 35:813–820, 1992.
7. National High Blood Pressure Education Program Working Group: Report on High Blood Pressure During Pregnancy. Am J Obstet Gynecol 163:1684–1712, 1990.
8. Patterson RM: Seizure disorders in pregnancy. Med Clin North Am 73:661–665, 1989.

XV. Abnormalities of Routine Screening Tests*

107. ASYMPTOMATIC FINDINGS ON THE HEMOGRAM

Jeanette Mladenovic, M.D.

1. What value on the complete blood count (CBC) is helpful when the mean corpuscular volume (MCV) is disproportionately low in comparison with the mildly low hemoglobin (Hb)? The major consideration is whether the low MCV results from disordered iron metabolism or globin-chain abnormality. Clues may be provided by the red cell distribution width (RDW). In iron deficiency the RDW is usually high (16.3 ± 1.8%), whereas in thalassemia minor it is normal (13.6 ± 1.6%). Thus a value < 14% suggests thalassemia, whereas a value > 15.3% suggests iron deficiency:

	Hb (g/dl)	MCW	RDW
Iron deficiency	8	74	> 15.3%
Chronic disease	10	86	Variable
Thalassemia syndromes	12	68	< 14%

2. What causes an elevated platelet count?
Thrombocytosis may result from primary or secondary causes. In primary thrombocytosis, an intrinsic defect in the stem cell leads to abnormally increased platelets, often irregular in size with variable granularity. Diseases such as polycythemia vera, chronic myelogenous leukemia, and essential thrombocythemia fall into this category. Secondary thrombocytosis is seen in patients with chronic inflammatory states, hemolysis, iron deficiency, gastrointestinal bleeding, and postsplenectomy syndrome. Chronic inflammatory states include malignancies in addition to conditions that result in a cellular immune response, such as chronic infections and autoimmune disease. Patients with primary thrombocytosis may be at risk from bleeding or clotting with platelet counts higher than 1 million, whereas patients with secondary thrombocytosis rarely develop such high counts.

3. Besides infection, what causes leukocytosis?
Leukocytosis may be secondary or due to primary bone marrow abnormalities. Secondary leukocytosis may be due to demargination, accelerated release of cells from the marrow, increased production of white cells, or even decreased removal. Demargination may be seen with sepsis or any stress-mediated response, such as hypotension or hypoxia. Increased release and production, indicative of infection, also may be seen with inflammation (such as blood in a closed space) or even with tumors that produce stimulatory factors (lung carcinoma).

---

*These chapters are meant to address the question of the "starred" abnormal laboratory values that return unexpectedly from the lab for otherwise healthy patients, or, in the case of commonly ordered serologic tests, the first level of interpretation to be considered within the clinical context. The answers are brief and superficial. The majority should be committed to the practitioner's intrinsic (not reference) knowledge base.

Primary leukocytosis occurs with leukemia. If the differential white blood cell count shows young white blood cells in circulation (blasts or cells of earlier differentiation than metamyelocytes), a primary marrow disorder (leukemia) is more likely.

4. Define lymphocytosis. With what disorders is it associated?

Lymphocytosis is defined as an absolute lymphocyte count $> 3.5 \times 10^9/L$. Lymphocytosis or a lymphoid leukemoid reaction may be seen in viral infections, such as infectious mononucleosis, cytomegalovirus (CMV), measles, and pertussis (in children). Lymphocytes may be atypical in appearance, variable in size, and reactive. In an adult without evidence of infection, a persistent lymphocytosis $> 5 \times 10^9/L$ suggests the diagnosis of chronic lymphocytic leukemia. Typing to determine that all lymphocytes are B-lymphocytes confirms the diagnosis.

5. What is significant leukopenia?

Leukopenia is defined as white blood cell count $< 4 \times 10^9/L$. Usually, as the count falls, cells of the neutrophil series are most affected. The percentage of the white blood cell count of granulocytic lineage (bands and mature cells) determines the absolute neutrophil count and the risk of life-threatening infection. Patients with granulocyte counts $< 1 \times 10^9/L$ are at risk of sepsis. Fever $> 38.3°$ C should be evaluated aggressively to determine the cause and treated with broad-spectrum antibiotics that cover gram-negative (including *Pseudomonas* sp.) and gram-positive (including staphylococci) organisms. As the absolute count falls, the association of fever with bacteremia increases.

6. What test should be ordered first to determine the cause of a prolonged prothrombin time (PT) and/or partial thromboplastin time (PTT)?

The first test that should be requested is a 1:1 mix, in which normal plasma is mixed with the patient's plasma and both PT and PTT are repeated. Complete correction suggests that prolongation is due to factor deficiency. Failure to correct suggests the presence of inhibitors in the patient's plasma. Patients with liver disease often have two defects; thus correction is incomplete. Alternatively, a prolonged PTT with evidence of inhibition is consistent with a lupus inhibitor.

7. What is the appropriate response when the hematocrit is elevated above normal?

An increased hematocrit may be due to decreased plasma volume (relative erythrocytosis) or a true increase in the red cell mass (primary polycythemia vera or secondary erythrocytosis). At a hematocrit of 55%, the odds of a true increase are only 50/50, whereas at a hematocrit of 60%, the red cell mass almost certainly is increased. Thus, at levels between 52–60%, the red cell mass should be determined to evaluate a persistently elevated hematocrit. Patients with elevated hematocrits should not undergo surgery or dye loads without evaluation because of the risk of thrombosis.

8. With new automated counters, which abnormalities may cause a false change in CBC values?

Erythrocytosis: lipids	Pseudothrombocytopenia: clumped platelets
Pseudoanemia: cold agglutinins	Pseudoleukocytosis: giant platelets
Pseudothrombocytosis: red cell fragments or microcytic red cells	Pseudoleukopenia: leukoagglutination

Thus, unexpected values should be evaluated visually and usually are flagged for further laboratory analysis.

9. What is the significance of polychromatophilia and nucleated red blood cells on the peripheral blood smear?

Such findings suggest early release of cells from the marrow in response to erythropoietin or secondary to displacement of the marrow with other elements (myelophthisis). A reticulocyte count is required to determine which process caused the increase in early circulating red cells.

10. Define significant eosinophilia and significant basophilia.

Mild eosinophilia (0.2–1.5×10^9 cells/L) may be seen with mild skin disease, atopy, and allergic reactions. Marked eosinophilia occasionally is seen in patients with asthma (especially in the presence of *Aspergillus* sp.) or angioneurotic edema. Extremely high or progressively increasing numbers of eosinophils also may suggest tissue helminthic infection or eosinophilic syndromes related to any organ of the body or secondary to malignancies. Prolonged, marked elevation of eosinophils may lead to tissue damage due to the eosinophils themselves. Eosinophilic leukemia is exceedingly rare.

Basophilia ($> 0.1 \times 10^9$) is seen in myeloproliferative diseases of all types. In the presence of leukocytosis or thrombocytosis, basophilia of any degree supports a diagnosis of primary myeloproliferative disease. Mild transient basophilia also is seen with ulcerative colitis and allergic systemic or skin diseases.

BIBLIOGRAPHY

1. Diagnostic hematology. Hematol Oncol Clin North Am 8:1–34, 1994.
2. Lee GR, Bithell TC, Foerster J, et al (eds): Wintrobe's Clinical Hematology, 9th ed. Philadelphia, Lea & Febiger, 1993.

108. ASYMPTOMATIC FINDINGS ON THE CHEMISTRY PROFILE

Jeanette Mladenovic, M.D.

1. May hyponatremia be an artifactual finding?

In the past, artifactual, asymptomatic hyponatremia was reported in patients with hyperlipidemia and extremely elevated protein levels. Now most laboratories have adopted methods that measure sodium selectively; thus the sodium measurement is true. Asymptomatic mild hyponatremia in patients whose volume should be normal (i.e., patients who are healthy and not on diuretics) suggests an early stage of the syndrome of inappropriate secretion of antidiuretic hormone (SIADH), endocrine deficiencies, or essential hyponatremia due to chronic disease.

2. What causes an elevation of uric acid?

Increased uric acid is due to undersecretion or overproduction. Occasionally the cause is identifiable (e.g., increased cell turnover in patients with hematopoietic disease or renal failure). However, most cases of hyperuricemia are idiopathic or due to drugs. The most common drugs that raise the level of uric acid are diuretics and alcohol. Although elevated levels of uric acid predispose the patient to gouty attacks, they should not be treated unless the patient has recurrent gout, tophi, or nephrolithiasis. Before treatment, a 24-hour urine collection should be ordered in patients with normal renal function to determine overproduction (> 800 mg/dl) or undersecretion so that the appropriate intervention can be determined.

3. What leads to hyperkalemia?

Mild laboratory hyperkalemia (pseudohyperkalemia) may result from hemolysis due to a difficult blood draw or to thrombocytosis or leukocytosis. However, values in excess of laboratory norms require repeat testing if hemolysis is suspected. If the value is < 6 mmol/L and the electrocardiogram (EKG) is normal or limited to questionable peaked T waves, elimination of potential causes is usually adequate. Moderate hyperkalemia (> 6 mmol/L) requires aggressive evaluation, and therapy is probably needed.

4. What is the most likely cause of hypercalcemia?

Isolated mild hypercalcemia found in asymptomatic patients during routine laboratory testing has led to increased frequency of the early diagnosis of hyperparathyroidism, which accounts for up to 60% of hypercalcemia in ambulatory patients. To determine that a mild increase in calcium is not due to protein binding, an ionized calcium test should be ordered at least once. Further work-up follows confirmation of an elevated value with repeated testing. In patients with no clearcut evidence of malignancy or renal failure, a parathormone level is useful.

5. What may cause an elevation in the total protein level?

The increased component of the total protein is likely to be the gamma globulin fraction. Total increase in the gamma globulins may occur in inflammatory states, in which case the increase is polyclonal, or secondary to clonal production of an immunoglobulin (monoclonal protein). A serum protein electrophoresis determines whether the increase is likely to be polyclonal (and even suggests a specific cause, such as liver disease) or monoclonal. A monoclonal protein requires further identification by type, both heavy and light chain. A monoclonal protein is seen not only in multiple myeloma but also in lymphoid malignancy and amyloidosis; alternatively, it may be a monoclonal gammopathy of uncertain significance (MGUS) ($<$ 2 gm/dl), which occurs with increasing age (up to 10% of individuals over age 75 years).

6. What may cause an asymptomatic mild elevation in bilirubin?

In a healthy individual without evidence of other liver test abnormalities, an elevated level of bilirubin may be due to pigment overload, as in mild circulating or intramedullary hemolysis, or to defects in conjugation, as in Gilbert's syndrome. Usually the hyperbilirubinemia is mild (1.2–3 mg/dl) and does not exceed 4 mg/dl, even in the presence of severe hemolysis, if liver function is normal. Mild unconjugated hyperbilirubinemia in an otherwise recuperating postoperative patient with normal liver function tests may be due to transfusions, hemolysis, or hematoma resorption. In pregnancy, the bilirubin normally should not exceed 2 mg/dl. Higher levels may be due to cholestasis, usually accompanied by changes in the alkaline phosphatase, as in drug-induced cholestasis.

7. What is the significance of an exceedingly low cholesterol level?

Low cholesterol may be consistent with poor dietary intake or malabsorption. Other tests, such as low levels of serum albumin, calcium, magnesium, and even iron, or a prolonged prothrombin time (PT) may support further evaluation for malabsorption.

8. What causes elevation of the serum amylase?

Besides pancreatitis or pancreatic disease, an elevation in serum amylase may be due to macroamylasemia, an inconsequential finding that results in no disease. The diagnosis is made by the finding of high serum amylase in the absence of urinary amylase or elevated serum lipase. In addition, increases may be due to entrance of amylase into the circulation from salivary (rare and usually clinically evident) or other gastrointestinal disorders, such as intestinal obstruction, infarction, or ectopic pregnancy. Asymptomatic hyperamylasemia also may be due to tumors, such as carcinoma of the lung, esophagus, breast, or ovary.

9. What conditions may lead to an unsuspected elevation in the creatinine phosphokinase (CPK)?

CPK is released not only from cardiac muscle but also from brain and skeletal muscle and thus may be elevated in any type of muscle injury, either traumatic or inflammatory. Even prolonged immobilization and myopathies may lead to a rise in CPK. In addition, an elevated level of CPK may be a clue to hypothyroidism.

10. Is asymptomatic elevation of lactic dehydrogenase a helpful finding?

Elevation of serum lactic dehydrogenase is often nonspecific because of the broad tissue distribution of the enzyme. Elevation may be due to hemolysis or tumors, especially lymphomas or pulmonary diseases.

11. What may cause a mild, isolated elevation of alkaline phosphatase (AP)?
AP arises from liver (hepatocytes and biliary epithelium), intestine, placenta (pregnancy), and bone and occasionally is made as a separate isoenzyme by some tumors. In asymptomatic patients, the source may be determined by evaluating either isoenzymes or associated enzymes (gamma-glutaryl transpeptidase or 5' nucleotidase), elevations of which correlate with a biliary source of AP. Levels that are 1–2 times greater than normal and arise from the liver may be seen in patients with parenchymal and infiltrative disease. However, elevation of AP also may be the first manifestation of Paget's disease. Occasionally, no cause for a minimal elevation of AP is found.

BIBLIOGRAPHY

Isselbacher KJ, Braunwald E, Wilson JD, et al (eds): Harrison's Principles of Internal Medicine, 13th ed. New York, McGraw-Hill, 1994.

109. SEROLOGY INTERPRETATION

Jeanette Mladenovic, M.D.

1. When is elevation of the erythrocyte sedimentation rate (ESR) a helpful finding?
Increases in the ESR are due to increases in inflammatory proteins or paraproteins (as in multiple myeloma) that hasten the rapidity of red cell sedimentation. Values over 100 mm/hr suggest the likely diagnoses of vasculitis (polymyalgia rheumatica or giant cell arteritis) or malignancy. Acute disease or physiologic states with a large cellular response and an increase in acute-phase globulins may cause a mild-to-moderate elevation in the ESR months after injury. Chronic disease with inflammation is also likely to be accompanied by moderate elevations in the ESR.

2. Does anemia affect the ESR?
Yes, but not significantly or predictably. Therefore, anemia is probably not a serious factor in clinical interpretation of the ESR, especially when newer methods are used.

3. What is the rheumatoid factor?
Rheumatoid factors are autoantibodies reactive with the Fc portion of immunoglobulin G (IgG). Most laboratory tests detect IgM antibodies.

4. When may rheumatoid factors be detected?
The test for rheumatoid factor is positive in up to 80% of patients with rheumatoid arthritis; it is routinely positive in patients with rheumatoid nodules. However, these autoantibodies are found in 5% of normal individuals, and the incidence increases with age (10–20% of individuals older than 65 years). Rheumatoid factor is also seen in other inflammatory or autoimmune diseases:

Chronic inflammation	Autoimmune diseases
Subacute bacterial endocarditis	Sjögren's syndrome (> 70%)
Osteomyelitis	Mixed connective tissue disease (> 35%)
Granulomatous infections or diseases	Systemic lupus erythematosus (> 20%)

5. How does the test for antinuclear antibody (ANA) help in the diagnosis of systemic lupus erythematosus (SLE)?
A positive ANA test is seen in the majority of patients with SLE, mixed connective tissue disease (MCTD), and drug-induced SLE (sensitivity = > 95%). Its specificity, however, is low. A negative test helps to exclude the above entities.

6. **List specific ANAs that are helpful in diagnosing specific diseases.**

Antidouble-stranded DNA   SLE
    Present in > 50% of patients with active disease (high specificity)
Anti-SM (Smith)   SLE
    Present in > 30% of patients with active disease (high specificity)
Antiribonuclear protein (RNP)   MCTD
    High sensitivity, but low specificity; a negative test excludes MCTD.
Anti-Ro (SSA)   Aggressive Sjögren's syndrome
                                             Neonatal SLE
    Present in > 60% of patients with Sjögren's syndrome (low specificity)

7. **What pattern of the fluorescent ANA is specific?**

A speckled pattern, which is the most common and nonspecific, is present even in individuals without rheumatic diseases. A homogeneous pattern is also common, often low-titer, and nonspecific but more characteristic of patients with drug-induced SLE. A rim pattern is rare and specific for SLE.

8. **What is an ANCA?**

ANCA refers to an antineutrophil cytoplasmic antibody, which is seen in Wegener's granulomatosis (> 85%), both generalized and limited. Its high specificity (95%) makes a positive test helpful in the diagnosis of this disease.

9. **What may cause a false-positive result on the Venereal Disease Research Laboratory (VDRL) test for syphilis?**

The VDRL measures a nonspecific reaginic antibody seen in response to any stage of syphilis (100% positive in secondary syphilis). False-positive tests may occur transiently after viral or mycoplasma infections. Chronically positive tests (> 6 months) may occur in intravenous drug abusers (< 15%) and patients with SLE (up to 20%), in whom it may be associated with other autoantibodies, such as a lupus inhibitor. Biologically false-positive tests also increase with age. A truly negative result excludes syphilis.

10. **Does a positive Lyme titer mean Lyme disease?**

In endemic areas, the titer is high in patients with subacute and chronic Lyme disease. However, the test has low specificity and thus is not useful in screening. It is helpful only when a high titer accompanies clinical manifestations of the disease.

BIBLIOGRAPHY

1. Isselbacher JK, Braunwald E, Wilson JD, et al (eds): Harrison's Principles of Internal Medicine, 13th ed. New York, McGraw-Hill, 1994.
2. Lee GR, Bithell TC, Foerster J, et al (eds): Wintrobe's Clinical Hematology, 9th ed. Philadelphia, Lea & Febiger, 1993.
3. Shmerling RH, Delbanco TL: The rheumatoid factor: An analysis of clinical utility. Am J Med 91:528, 1991.
4. Sox HC, Liang MH: The erythrocyte sedimentation rate: Guidelines for rational use. Ann Intern Med 104:515, 1986.

XVI. Drug Interactions

110. COMMON DRUG INTERACTIONS AND TOXICITY

Donald B. Hansen, B.S. Pharm, Pharm D., and Julie Rifkin, M.D.

1. List five levels at which drug interactions may occur.
1. Gastrointestinal absorption interactions
2. Plasma protein-binding interactions
3. Metabolic enzyme interactions
4. Renal excretion interactions
5. Pharmacodynamic interactions

2. If a pair of drugs is stated to interact, must one be stopped?
Not necessarily. Interactions range from effects that are detectable only with laboratory testing to effects that are clinically significant—and predictably so. If an interaction is known to produce clinically significant effects, it can be tracked as it occurs, and dosages can be adjusted to compensate. If other agents are available and the potential for adverse outcome is great, alternative therapy should be offered.

3. Does all drug interaction result in an adverse drug reaction (ADR)?
A drug interaction does not necessarily result in an ADR, even with documentable changes in drug level or physiologic parameters. The specific definition of an ADR varies but usually addresses the following issues: severity of outcome; whether the drug met therapeutic indications; and whether the adverse reaction occurred after an overdose, on withdrawal, or as a failure of the expected pharmacologic action.

4. What is a reportable ADR?
A reportable ADR is defined as a reaction that is (1) suspected to be secondary to drug therapy, (2) uncommon or not described in the package insert, or (3) severe in nature, requiring treatment or prolonging hospitalization. All ADRs should be recorded in the progress notes of the patient's medical record, along with outcome and treatment. ADRs that fit the above criteria should be reported to the institution through the mechanism approved by the local Pharmacy and Therapeutics Committee. If the institution does not have a mechanism for forwarding the information to the Food and Drug Administration (FDA), the individual may call the FDA directly at 1-800-FDA-1088. Such reports contribute to postmarketing surveillance of the drug.

5. Do drug interactions occur with alcohol and caffeine?
Yes. Alcohol abuse in patients taking warfarin prolongs the prothrombin time and predisposes to gastric microbleeding. Alcohol also disturbs glycemic control, adding to the hypoglycemia produced by drugs such as sulfonylureas. Metronidazole inhibits the metabolic oxidation of alcohol and may produce the disulfiram reaction of nausea, vomiting, and malaise in the presence of alcohol. The effect varies highly among the population.

Caffeine blocks the antiarrhythmic effects of adenosine IV; like theophylline, it is a competitive agonist for the adenosine receptor. Because the antagonism is competitive, the effect varies and may be clinically important only in the heavy coffee drinker. Ciprofloxacin and enoxacin (but probably not ofloxacin) inhibit the metabolism of caffeine and theophylline, resulting in higher levels than anticipated and requiring dosage adjustment.

6. Define steady-state concentration.

Steady state is achieved when the dosage intake per unit of time equals the elimination rate and fluctuations between peak and trough plasma levels remain fairly constant. Most drugs are eliminated by first-order kinetics. The time required to achieve steady state for first-order kinetic medications can be determined by the half-life of the drug. Steady-state levels generally are achieved at the end of 3–4 half-lives.

7. When is a loading dose used?

A loading dose is used when it is necessary to provide a rapid therapeutic concentration of a drug, often in the presence of a long half-life. Classes of drugs for which loading doses are used include aminoglycosides, antiarrhythmics, and anticonvulsants.

8. What are the pitfalls in the interpretation of plasma drug concentration?

Drug levels must be interpreted in light of the patient's clinical status. The major pitfall in interpreting drug assays probably relates to timing of the blood level. A rule of thumb is that 5.5 drug half-lives are needed before steady-state concentrations are achieved. Accurate peak and trough levels cannot be measured except at steady-state concentrations. Sample timing is critically important. Thus, the best time to draw drug levels is immediately before the next dose, during a steady-state infusion, or at least 8 hours after a dose when the drug is taken twice daily. Renal and hepatic alterations of half-life must be considered. The patient's age, height, and sex as well as possible alterations in drug absorption, binding, and active metabolites may have unpredictable effects on plasma drug levels.

9. Which drugs commonly require monitoring by serum levels? Why?

1. **Aminoglycosides** may cause nephrotoxicity and/or ototoxicity at high levels and are significantly affected by changes in creatinine clearance. Serum peak and trough levels are therefore useful for monitoring. Optimum sampling strategies for single daily dose aminoglycosides have yet to be determined.

2. **Tricyclic antidepressants** display great variations in blood level, depending on dosage. Afro-Americans usually have 50% greater blood levels than Caucasians for the same dose schedule. In geriatric patients conventional doses may lead to toxic levels. Furthermore, symptoms of overdose may mimic the symptoms for which the drug was prescribed. Steady-state plasma levels are achieved after about 2 weeks on a given dosage.

3. Serum levels of **anticonvulsant medications** are helpful in assessing compliance and during use of more than one anticonvulsant. Plasma concentrations of a given drug may increase or decrease when a second agent is added.

4. Serum levels of **digoxin** are useful to confirm or prevent toxicity. Advanced patient age, renal insufficiency, and/or concomitant use of quinidine elevate digoxin levels.

10. How does an anaphylactoid reaction reaction differ from anaphylaxis?

Anaphylaxis and anaphylactoid reactions produce identical clinical signs and symptoms but differ in the mechanism and predictability of the reaction. Anaphylaxis is an immunoglobulin E (IgE)-mediated event that occurs afer exposure in a previously sensitized individual. The anaphylactoid reaction is not IgE-mediated and does not require previous exposure to the inciting substance. Both reactions may cause various symptoms, including flushing, urticaria, angioedema, tachycardia, hypotension, syncope, shock, laryngeal edema, wheezing, diaphoresis, abdominal pain, diarrhea, and vomiting. The symptoms are due to intact cell-derived and basophil-derived mediators. A classic example of an anaphylactoid reaction is the response to radiocontrast.

A person who has had one anaphylactoid reaction has a 60% chance of a second reaction when exposed to the same agent. No specific characteristics identify a patient who may be at risk for an anaphylactoid reaction initially or on repeat exposure. Measures to decrease the repeat reactions include pharmacologic prophylaxis with diphenhydramine and corticosteroids.

11. Can orally administered drugs cause anaphylaxis?

Yes. Penicillin given orally or parenterally is the most common cause of anaphylaxis. The anaphylactic death rate is approximately 1–2/10,000 patients treated with penicillin. A personal or family history of allergies does not predict who will react to penicillin. A person with a history of any penicillin allergy is presumed to be allergic to all penicillins, unless a skin test to both major and minor determinants is negative. Cephalosporins cannot be considered a safe alternative because of cross-reactivity.

12. Which patients should not be given charcoal after an overdose? Which patients should not be induced to vomit?

Activated charcoal must not be given if ingestion of a corrosive substance is suspected (e.g., ammonia, bleach). In such patients it has no proved efficacy and obscures an endoscopic examination. The use of activated charcoal after acetaminophen overdose is generally not recommended because it binds to the antidote, N-acetyl-L-cysteine (NAC), in vitro. If ingestion of Tylenol and other agents is suspected, administration of activated charcoal within the first 4 hours may be useful.

Syrup of ipecac should not be used to induce emesis in patients who are comatose, experience seizures, or have an inadequate gag reflex. Suspected ingestion of corrosive substances is a contraindication to emesis, because exposure to the vomitus causes reinjury. Ingestion of poorly absorbed hydrocarbons (e.g., gasoline, kerosene) is not treated by emesis because the risk of aspiration outweighs the potential for central nervous system depression. Suspicion of coingestion of sharp, solid objects negates emesis therapy.

13. Name five drug overdoses that may cause arrhythmogenic death and thus require electrocardiographic (EKG) monitoring.

Drug toxicity may alter the intrinsic firing rate of pacemaker cells or conduction in one pathway, thus allowing the formation of a reentry circuit that triggers tachydysrhythmia. Dysrhythmias may result from both altered conduction and automaticity. Several drug overdoses may cause arrhythmogenic death, including (1) digoxin, (2) virtually all classes of antiarrhythmic drugs, (3) tricyclic antidepressants (overdoses prolong PR and QRS intervals and cause various other EKG abnormalities), (4) phenothiazine (overdoses cause dysrhythmia and hypotension), and (5) cocaine. Thus, cardiac monitoring is essential in cases of overdose or toxicity.

14. When should patients be treated for acetaminophen toxicity?

Patients should be treated for acetaminophin toxicity whenever it is suspected. Treatment is life-saving and nontoxic. If a patient presents within 4 hours of ingestion, gut decontamination may be used. NAC should be given within 8–10 hours of ingestion but may be effective up to 24 hours after ingestion. Therapy should be guided by levels corresponding to the Rumack-Matthew homogram but initiated promptly if toxicity is suspected. **Do not delay** therapy with NAC past 8–12 hours to await drug levels.

15. What is a toxicology screen? When is it cost-effective?

No single, inexpensive method detects all toxins. A toxicology screen does not provide blood levels of specific substances or drugs. Blood toxic screens generally detect the presence of benzodiazepines, barbiturates, cocaine, methadone, nicotine, caffeine, salicylates, and tricyclics. Qualitative evidence of metabolites of therapeutic agents and drugs of abuse is found in the urine rather than the serum.

A specific request for a blood level aids in management of toxicity due to acetaminophen, salicylates, carboxyhemoglobin, methemoglobin, methanol, ethylene glycol, lithium, iron, digoxin, theophylline, organophosphates, ethanol, phenytoin, lead, and arsenic.

Patients with an altered sensorium for whom the physical examination and available history fail to provide a cause should be suspected of having a toxic-metabolic disorder. Unexplained hypo- or hyperthermia, distinctive odors, miotic or mydriatic pupils, abdominal pain, nausea, vomiting, tremors, seizures, and coma are clues to poisoning syndromes. Various laboratory abnormalities may be due to drug toxicity, including unusual coloration of urine, hemolysis, coagulopathy, elevated levels of creatine phosphokinase (CPK), rhabdomyolysis, electrolyte abnormalities, and anion and/or osmolar gap.

16. What are the principles of treating drug overdoses?

1. Support the patient. Airway protection, oxygenation, and treatment of circulatory collapse should be initiated immediately.

2. Reduce further drug absorption. When appropriate, induced emesis, gastric lavage, oral activated charcoal, and/or cathartics should be used.

3. Enhance drug elimination. Alkalinization, diuresis, hemodialysis, and hemoperfusion are possibilities.

4. Give an antagonist or antidote, if available. Only 5% of poisons have specific antidotes.

5. Prevent recurrences. Education, psychiatric evaluation, and rehabilitation should be initiated to decrease recurrent ingestions.

17. What principles should be followed in prescribing drugs for elderly patients?

Factors that predispose older patients to adverse drug reactions include multisystem disease, greater severity of disease, female sex, small body size, hepatic or renal insufficiency, and previous drug reactions. The following principles are useful when prescribing medications to people over 65 years of age:

1. Ask about use of over-the-counter medications.

2. Simplify a patient's drug regimen whenever possible (avoid polypharmacy).

3. Remember that creatinine clearance, gastrointestinal motility, total body water, lean body mass, cardiac output, hepatic mass, and hepatic blood flow are decreased in the elderly.

4. In general, use smaller doses of medications (50% or less).

18. Which common drugs are likely to cause side effects in elderly patients and thus should be avoided?

Several medications place elderly patients at risk for adverse side effects. Any medication that may cause sedation, syncope, or confusion places the patient at risk for a fall. Other side effects to be avoided include urinary retention, anorexia, urinary incontinence, constipation, and dry mouth. Drugs to be avoided in the elderly patient include amitriptyline, propoxyphene, dipyridamole, chlorpropamide, chlordiazepoxide, diazepam, dipyridamole, indomethacin, methyldopa, propranolol, and muscle relaxants.

19. Which disease states lead to alterations in drug pharmacokinetics?

1. **Renal insufficiency** is associated with toxic levels of drugs that are cleared by urinary excretion. Commonly used antibiotics that require dosage adjustments in patients with renal insufficiency include aminoglycosides, penicillins and cephalosporins, and vancomycin. Reduced doses may be administered at normal intervals, or the usual dose may be administered less frequently.

2. **Liver disease** leads to altered pharmacokinetics in an unpredictable manner. Biotransformation of drugs metabolized primarily by the liver may be accelerated or impaired. Overall, hepatic drug clearance is often only mildly to moderately altered by liver dysfunction, and liver function tests do not predict the degree of alteration in drug clearance. However, patients with portocaval shunts do not have first-pass hepatic metabolism or high blood flow to the liver.

Concentrations of propranolol, lidocaine, meperidine, and phenytoin are notably increased in patients with liver failure.

3. **Hypotension and circulatory insufficiency** alter pharmacokinetics, because the body preserves blood flow to the heart and brain at the expense of other organs. The effective volume of distribution is smaller, and the central nervous system and heart are exposed to higher drug concentrations than found in the plasma. There are no useful methods to determine the exact alteration in drug dose in this setting. In patients with heart failure, lower doses of lidocaine, procainamide, and theophylline are used. Loading doses should be conservative, and the patient must be followed closely for indications of drug toxicity.

BIBLIOGRAPHY

1. Bochner BS, Lichtenstein LM: Anaphylaxis. N Engl J Med 324:1785–1790, 1991.
2. Ellenhan MJ, Barcelaux D: Medical Toxicology. Diagnosis and Treatment of Human Poisoning. New York, Elsevier, 1988.
3. Gentry CA, Paloucek EP, Rodvold KA: Prediction of acetaminophen concentrations in overdose patients using a Bayesian pharmacokinetic model. J Toxicol 32:17–30, 1994.
4. Hoffman RS, Smilkstein MJ, Howland MA, Goldfrank MR: Osmol groups revisited: Normal values and limitations. J Toxicol 31:81–93, 1994.
5. Jacobs DS, Kaston BL, et al: Laboratory Test Handbook, 2nd ed. Baltimore, Williams & Wilkins, 1990.
6. Montamat SC, Cuoack BJ, Vestal RE: Management of drug therapy in the elderly. N Engl J Med 321:303–309, 1991.
7. Talbert RL: Drug dosing in renal insufficiency. J Clin Pharmacol 34(2):99–110, 1994.
8. Willcox SM, Himmelstein DU, Woolhandler S: Inappropriate drug prescribing for the community-dwelling elderly. JAMA 272:292–296, 1994.

INDEX

Page numbers in **boldface** type indicate complete chapter.